Essentials of Exercise Physiology

ESSENTIALS OF EXERCISE PHYSIOLOGY

WILLIAM D. MCARDLE
Queens College — CUNY
Professor, Department of Health and Physical Education
Flushing, New York

FRANK I. KATCH
Professor, Department of Exercise Science
University of Massachusetts
Amherst, Massachusetts

VICTOR L. KATCH
Professor, Department of Movement Science
Division of Kinesiology
Associate Professor, Department of Pediatrics
School of Medicine
University of Michigan
Ann Arbor, Michigan

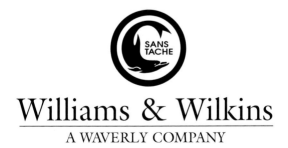

Williams & Wilkins

A WAVERLY COMPANY

BALTIMORE • PHILADELPHIA • LONDON • PARIS • BANGKOK
HONG KONG • MUNICH • SYDNEY • TOKYO • WROCLAW

Williams & Wilkins
Rose Tree Corporate Center, Building ll
1400 North Providence Road, Suite 5025
Media, PA 19063-2043 USA

EXECUTIVE EDITOR: *J. Matthew Harris*
DEVELOPMENT EDITOR: *Lisa Stead*
PROJECT EDITOR: *R. Lukens*
PRODUCTION MANAGER: *Michael DeNardo*

Library of Congress Cataloging-in-Publication Data

McArdle, William D.
    Essentials of exercise physiology / William D. McArdle, Victor L.
Katch, Frank I. Katch.
        p.   cm.
    Includes bibliographical references and index.
    1. Exercise—Physiological aspects.   I. Katch, Victor L.
II. Katch, Frank I.   III. Title.
QP301.M1149   1994
612'.044—dc20   93-47383
                                                 CIP

PRINTED IN THE UNITED STATES OF AMERICA

Print number: 5   4

DEDICATION

This book is dedicated to three very special people who have contributed in important ways over the years to our writing projects. John "Jack" Spahr, Sr. was a senior partner of the company when the first edition of *Exercise Physiology* was published in 1982, and he was there when we needed him most during publication of the third edition in 1991. Jack, you were a pillar of strength and reason at just the right times. His son, John Spahr, Jr. was a welcome addition to our team when Jack retired. His strong leadership at Lea & Febiger enabled us to work diligently during the preparation of the third edition of *Exercise Physiology* and the fourth edition of *Introduction to Nutrition, Exercise, and Health*. John really cared, and personally took us under his wing to be sure everything went off without a hitch. If John or Jack had promised that something was going to be done (even if it was left out of the contract), there was no need to worry because their word was as good as gold. A handshake and a look in the eye were as binding as words in a contract. That's just the way they were — honest to the letter — and we know they had our best interests at heart. We are thankful you gave the final OK to add color graphics to our last three books, and for providing us with the latest in computer technology to improve efficiency.

Tom Colaiezzi was production manager for the entire time we've been associated with Lea & Febiger. Tom pulled every string possible to make things happen when others said it just couldn't be done. Tom, we know you did lots of little extra things without our having to ask. You've been a true friend, and we know you were behind us every step of the way. Your dedication to technical excellence has been chiefly responsible for the artistic success of the seven book projects we worked on together. You always will be very special to us.

Besides being really terrific people to work with, all three of you made believers out of us by demonstrating that interrelationships between business goals, educational goals, and personal relationships need not be at odds, but can successfully work in harmony towards a common end. We were proud to be part of the Lea & Febiger family tradition. Your patience, encouragement, honesty, integrity, and always a sense of fair play made our close working relationship with you something special. We already miss you guys in so many ways, and we'll think of you often.

We also dedicate this book to three fine and loving gentlemen. During the past year, Professor Franklin M. Henry, Dr. Albert Behnke, and Professor Thomas K. Cureton, Jr. passed way. Each of these men was a pioneer and giant in our field, and has left a legacy that will endure. We were privileged to have known these men well since our graduate years, and we will miss their close association, guidance, friendship, and constant support as mentors and colleagues. "Doc," we'll always cherish our long walks and talks, and try to remember that "words have meaning — choose them carefully." Al, we promise to "carry the torch on to the next generation," and Tom, even though we were not your students, you were our teacher and trusted friend. All three of you played important roles in our lives.

PREFACE

Need for the text. With the success of the first three editions of *Exercise Physiology: Energy, Nutrition, and Human Performance* also came constructive criticism. Many of our colleagues who taught a one semester course believed that the existing text simply contained too much material that could not be covered in a one semester course. In addition to the need for a somewhat more compressed text, many felt there was also a need for a text that was more practical and applied in its approach to exercise physiology. Some instructors told us they wanted a text that clearly outlined the learning objectives and expectations so that it would be clear to the student what he or she should be able to do with the information once it was learned. It also was felt that a text emphasizing only the essentials did not have to follow a research-oriented format to document the material. Rather, a listing of relevant references at the end of each chapter would suffice. Within the context of practicality, there was a need to refocus text material and apply it more to teaching and exercise training situations. The suggestion was made to intersperse brief summaries, interpretations, and applications of the latest research in the interrelated areas of exercise, sports nutrition, weight control, and health. In addition, there was strong sentiment, with which we readily agreed, that a new textbook should be generously illustrated with graphics and photos to emphasize the sports, training, and physical performance focus of the book's contents. When we considered all of the suggestions, we felt strongly that we could design a new textbook that would continue to achieve high educational standards, yet meet the specific needs of certain students and faculty. This was the genesis of *Essentials of Exercise Physiology*.

Organization. The *Essentials* text is designed for a two-column format. This enables us to present current and relevant text with graphics, including the supplementary material close to the chapter's main text. We have added an introductory chapter to make it easier for students with limited background in the sciences to integrate the basics of the biology and chemistry of cellular organization and structure, energy transfer and biologic work, acid-base balance, and cellular transport within the study of exercise physiology.

The textbook contains eighteen chapters with six major sections. Although the flow of the sections and the chapters within each section seemed to the authors to progress logically for an essentials-oriented, one semester exercise physiology course, this structure is by no means "cast in stone." Chapters, as well as parts within certain chapters, can stand alone. In this way, students with prerequisite biology or physiology coursework would not be obliged to read the material for which they have been previously adequately prepared. This pertains to the introductory chapter on biology and chemistry basics, as well as portions of those chapters that deal with the physiology of the pulmonary, cardiovascular, and neuromuscular systems.

Section I contains four chapters that deal with energy transfer and physical activity. The presentation moves from a discussion of the basics of energy transfer at rest to the dynamics of energy release during various levels of physical activity up to the maximum. Where possible, comparisons are made between trained and untrained and the influence of age, gender, and specific training on these responses. Discussion also covers various methods for assessing energy expenditure during exercise, as well as the requirements and capacities for energy metabolism in diverse forms of physical activity.

Section II focuses on food energy and the concept of optimal nutrition and its role in exercise physiology, human performance, and good health. Practical recommendations and guidelines are presented for the active man and woman. The area of sports nutrition is explored with emphasis on the importance of fluid balance and dietary carbohydrate to sustain heavy training in both short and long term exercise performance.

In *Section III*, four chapters explore the physiologic support systems for physical activity. Major emphasis is placed on the structure, function, and exercise and training responses of the pulmonary, cardiovascular, neuromuscular, and endocrine systems.

Section IV considers training for muscular strength and conditioning for anaerobic and aerobic power. Also presented are practical ways to evaluate the functional capacities of these systems.

Section V discusses the impact of environmental factors of heat, cold, and altitude, as well as ergogenic aids such as caffeine, bicarbonate drinks, anabolic steroids, red blood cell reinfusion, and oxygen inhalation on physiology and exercise performance.

Three chapters in *Section VI* explore the underlying rationale for evaluating body composition among groups of highly trained men and women. Also discussed are the interrelated factors often associated with obesity, and the efficacy of diet and exercise as a treatment for the overfat condition. The final chapter is about exercise, aging, and health, with emphasis on how regular exercise relates to the risks for coronary heart disease.

Pedagogical Features. Overall, each chapter has been streamlined without sacrificing the appropriate detail required for an essentials text. Where possible, we have expanded our presentation to include applications that relate to both males and females, as well as children and older adults. Specific unique features of the text include:

- *Learning Objectives.* Each chapter is prefaced by a list of important student learning objectives specifically related to the material contained in the chapter. This provides the student with specific guideposts as to the important information within the chapter.
- *Marginal Notes, Data, and Illustrations.* There are over 500 marginal notes appearing throughout the chapters. These augment the thrust of the text material with the most up-to-date information, definitions, examples, data, and research findings on particular topics covered in the chapter.
- *Close-Ups.* A "close-up" feature within each chapter focuses on a timely and important exercise, sport, or clinical topic in exercise physiology related to the chapter's contents.
- *Visual Augmentation.* Illustrations and action photographs are liberally used to amplify the material presented within a particular figure or text section. We have tried very hard to integrate the graphic and photographic material to enhance overall readability and clarity of the presentation.
- *Chapter Summaries.* There is a list of summary statements in each chapter. These statements pull together the important concepts and information in the chapter.
- *Meaningful References.* An accessible group of up-to-date, as well as "classic" references, many of which are review articles on a specific topic, appear at the end of each chapter. These references can serve as a starting point for exploring a particular topic area in greater depth.
- *Relevant Appendices.* Appendices are located at the end of the text. These include:
  1. The metric system and constants in exercise physiology
  2. Metabolic computations in open-circuit spirometry
  3. Energy costs tables for physical activities
  4. Age- and gender-specific equations to predict percent body fat.
  5. Frequently cited journals in exercise physiology

Graphics. The graphics in the textbook were rendered by Bobby Starnes of Electragraphics, Inc., Blountville, Tennessee, simply the best electronic artist we know. To those who have ever tried to master the intricacies of modern computerized drawing tools, or are thinking of trying, we hope you are as fortunate in your search for artistic help as we were when we hooked up with Bobby Starnes. His creative energies gave zing and pep (and lots of color) to our initial renderings and ideas. It takes a special person to work long hours into the night to make sure our deadlines were met. We hope that the quality of the artwork has enhanced the educational relevance of the textbook.

The authors would like to acknowledge our executive editor Matt Harris, project editor Ray Lukens, production manager Mike DiNardo, development editor Lisa Stead, and the dedicated staff at Lea & Febiger for believing in this project and seeing that it all came to fruition on time. We would also like to acknowledge the staff at ALLSPORT for their help in securing first rate photos for the chapter openers, and to Mark Fox, (Box 113, Silverthorne, CO 80498) a superb phtographer whose many skills have enabled us to enhance our graphics with his excellent photographs.

STUDENT STUDY GUIDE AND WORKBOOK

The *Student Study Guide and Workbook* is a resource companion to the main textbook. Its purpose is to promote "active learning" by involving students in the learning process. There are four main sections to the study guide: Section I facilitates student understanding of text content by focusing on key terms and concepts (student-generated glossary), and on specific questions within each chapter. In order to answer the questions, students must read and understand the major points in the chapter. Also, a unique aspect of this section is the first crossword puzzles in exercise physiology. These puzzles facilitate learning in a fun and entertaining way. This section also includes 10 multiple choice and true/false questions to test the student's comprehension of the text. Section II includes the nutritive values of 2025 common foods, including fast-food items. It also includes a list showing the energy cost of over 240 physical activities. Section III contains practical assessment tests, including Health-Related Physical Fitness, Healthy Life-Style Assessment, Physical Readiness, Determining Desirable Body Weight, and different Flexiblity Tests. Section IV includes solutions to the crossword puzzles and answers to all chapter quizzes.

As an added feature, the *Food and Diet Analyzer*™ computer program, an interactive graphics diet analysis program designed for professional and educational use, can be purchased separately or in combination with the *Student Study Guide and Workbook*. The computer program analyzes foods or combinations of foods that may be classified as recipes, meals, menus, or complete diets. The analyses include the weight and percentage of the RDA according to age and gender for 28 nutrients, including the proportions of protein, carbohydrate, fat, and alcohol. Diabetic exchanges, based on food group and nutrient content, and nutrient densities and ratios, can be determined automatically. The *Food and Diet Analyzer*™ is an efficient, time-saving tool for analyzing and creating diets accurately. *Food and Diet Analyzer*™ also can indicate nutritive deficiencies and excesses, and identify the sources of these deficiencies and excesses. Analyses can be listed on the screen or printed in graphic or tabular form, and can be used to complete several of the self-assessment tests in the appendix of the workbook. The *Student Study Guide and Workbook* and *Food and Diet Analyzer*™ computer program can be ordered by filling out the single page, colored insert found with this book, or by mailing or faxing Fitness Technologies Press.

Fitness Technologies Press
1132 Lincoln Street
Ann Arbor, MI 48104
FAX (313)662-8153

Flushing, New York
Amherst, Massachusetts
Ann Arbor, Michigan

William D. McArdle
Frank I. Katch
Victor L. Katch

CONTENTS

ESSENTIALS OF EXERCISE PHYSIOLOGY

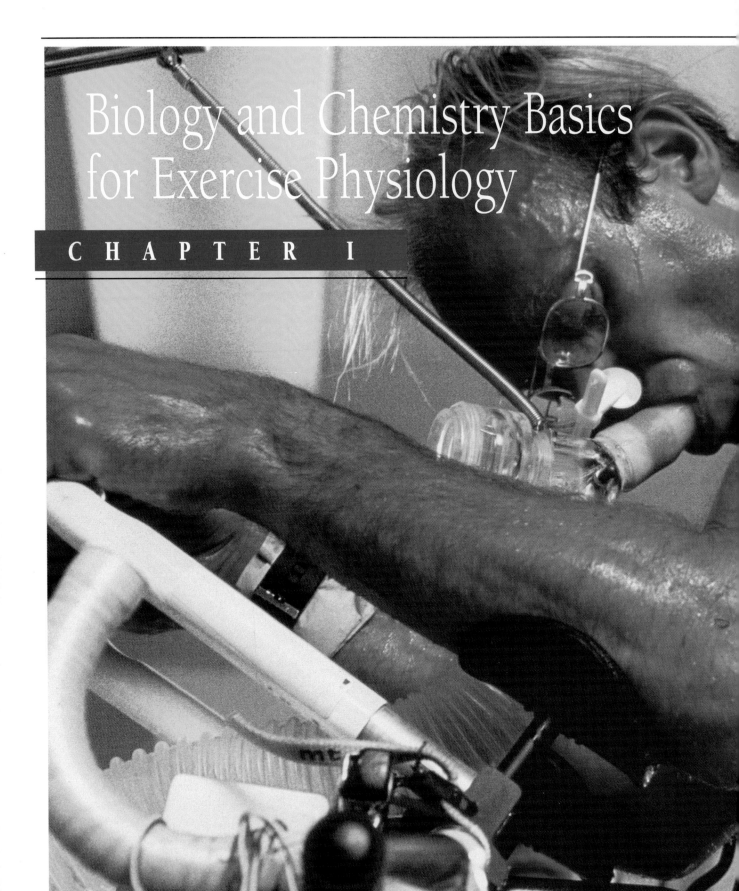

Biology and Chemistry Basics for Exercise Physiology

CHAPTER 1

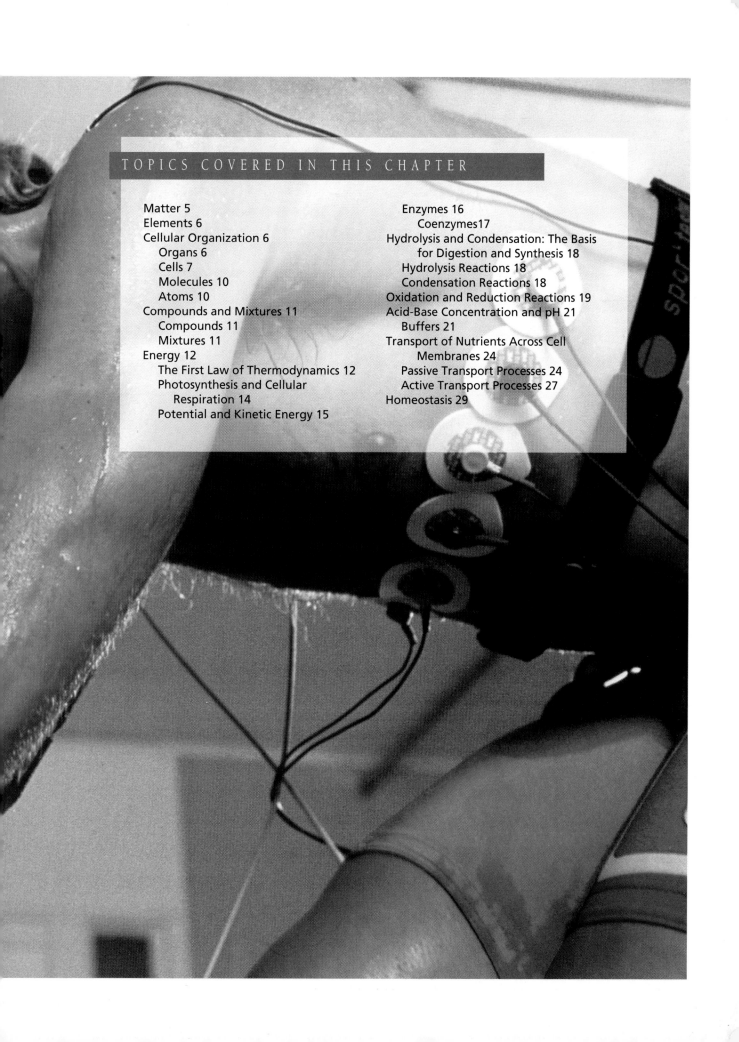

After reading this chapter you should be able to:

- Define the terms mass, weight, and density.

- Outline the general biologic organization of the human body.

- Discuss the role of the plasma membrane, nucleus, and mitochondria in cellular function.

- Explain the concept of energy and its role in various forms of biologic work.

- Compare and contrast the processes of photosynthesis and respiration.

- Explain the role of enzymes and coenzymes in the body's chemical reactions.

- Discuss the processes of oxidation and reduction and provide examples related to exercise energy metabolism.

- Define the terms acid, base, and pH, and describe how the body regulates acid-base balance.

- Outline the different ways chemicals are exchanged between the cell and its surroundings.

- Define homeostasis and give examples of this regulatory process during exercise.

Biology and chemistry form the foundation for understanding almost every aspect of exercise physiology. Sometimes the picture is fairly clear as in the role of the pulmonary and cardiovascular systems in supplying oxygen to the active muscles. Often, however, interactions are more complex, as during the digestion and absorption of carbohydrates, lipids, and proteins, or in the processes of energy transfer from these nutrients during diverse forms of physical activity.

In this introductory chapter, we review some basic definitions and concepts in biology and chemistry as they relate to energy expenditure and human exercise performance. Knowledge of these fundamentals will help you to appreciate what goes on "behind the scenes" as the various nutrients undergo chemical transformations during tissue synthesis or their conversion to useful energy while at rest or during physical activity.

MATTER

Chemistry is the science that studies the structure and composition of matter: the solids, liquids, and gases that are the basic building blocks of our universe. *Matter is defined as a substance (composed of atoms or molecules, or a mixture of the two) that occupies space and has mass.* All the biologic substances in the body are matter, and thus all of these substances have mass. A fundamental property of all matter is inertia, the resistance to change in speed or position when a force is applied. We clearly observe this resistance to movement when we try to move something heavy.

Mass

The mass of an object is the quantitative measure of its inertia or resistance to acceleration. Under ordinary circumstances, the mass of any object remains constant whether it is sub-merged under water or is nearly weightless beyond the earth's atmosphere. The greater the mass, the larger its inertia and the smaller the change produced when a force is applied.

Weight

The term weight is often used interchangeably (but imprecisely) to mean the same as mass; weight is related to mass but is not identical to it. *The weight of an object is equal to its mass and the gravitational attraction by the earth or other celestial body.* On earth, where gravitational force is fairly constant, differences between individuals in body weight are due to differences in body mass. On the surface of the moon, in contrast, with a smaller gravitational force, a person would weigh only one-sixth as much, yet the person's mass would remain unchanged. Even on earth, the weight of an object is slightly more at the South Pole (more gravitational pull) than at the Equator (less gravitational pull). Although the weight of an object changes according to where it is located, its mass remains the same. So, if you want to be precise, the next time you weigh yourself, remember that what you have measured is your mass and the attractive or gravitational force the earth exerts on this mass.

Density

Matter takes up space and occupies a volume. *The mass of a unit volume of a material substance is referred to as its density.* This is computed by the equation: density = mass ÷ volume, and is usually expressed as grams per cubic centimeter (g/cc). In nutrition studies, the physical density of a food is determined by its mass in relation to the volume it occupies. For example, the density of a fatty food is less than that of a food composed mostly of protein or carbohydrate (yet as we will see in Chapter 7, the caloric or "energy density" of the fat-laden food is nearly twice as high!).

The metric system. Scientific measurement is generally presented in terms of the metric system. This system uses units that are related to each other by the power of ten. The prefix centi- means one-hundredth, milli- means one thousandth, and the prefix kilo- is also derived from a word that means one thousand. Consequently, 1 kilogram (kg) is 1000 grams (g) or 2.2 pounds (lb). In general, we will use metric units throughout the text, although the English system will also appear where applicable.

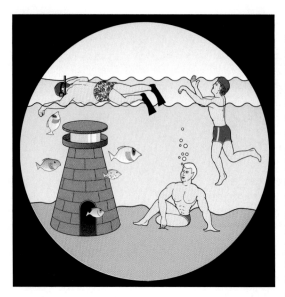

Why does one person sink and the other float?

High turnover rate of some elements. The mineral content of the body does not remain fixed. Some elements are continually replaced. During the growth cycle, for example, the mineral calcium is in a continual state of flux; more calcium is used than is excreted. Thus, there is a large turnover in bone during the first year of life. During adolescence, up to 32% of the skeletal mass per year can be rebuilt.

How elements are named. Each of the elements is abbreviatd by a one- or two-letter atomic symbol, a practice first used by the Swedish chemist Jons Berzelius in the early 1800s. Twelve elements are identified by the first letter of their name; most of the others are identified by the first two letters. In several cases the atomic symbol is derived from the Latin name for the element: Fe stands for iron (Latin *ferrum*), Pb for lead (Latin *plumbum*), Ag for silver (Latin *argentum*), and Na, the shorthand term for sodium, is from the Latin *natrium*.

The concept of density is also relevant when considering human body composition. For example, although two people may have the same body mass, their proportion of fat to muscle could differ radically. One person's fat content, for example, could be 38% of total mass, whereas the second person could possess one-tenth the fat, or only 3.8% of body mass. Because fat and muscle occupy different volumes per unit mass (i.e., they possess different densities), the volume occupied by each person varies considerably, depending on individual differences in body composition, even though body mass may be identical. Chapter 16 focuses on the concept of body density in relation to body fat content.

ELEMENTS

Matter in the universe is composed of fundamental materials called elements. Of the 105 elements which have been identified, 90 occur in nature, either free or in combination with other elements; the remaining 15 are produced artificially. *An important characteristic of an element is that it cannot be decomposed into a simpler substance by ordinary chemical processes.* Water, for example, is not an element because it can be chemically separated into the elements hydrogen and oxygen. As you will see in Chapter 6, minerals are the fundamental elements required by the body for optimal functioning.

Distribution of Elements in the Body. In humans, the most abundant elements are oxygen (O; 65%), carbon (C; 18%), hydrogen (H; 10%), and nitrogen (N; 3%). Combined, their composition by weight, shown in Figure 1-1, constitutes approximately 96% of body mass. These elements serve as the chief constituents of five of the six nutrients — carbo-

hydrates, lipids, proteins, vitamins, and water — and comprise the structural units for most biologically active substances in the body. The remaining group of mineral nutrients includes major minerals such as the elements calcium (1.5%), phosphorus (1.0%), potassium (0.4%), sulfur (0.3%), sodium and chlorine (0.2%), and magnesium as well as such exotic elements as vanadium, gold, silver, silicon, molybdenum, manganese, copper, cobalt, selenium, chromium, tin, and even arsenic. These elements are present in the body only in trace amounts, usually as integral parts of protein catalysts or enzymes (see "Enzymes" in this chapter). For example, copper (Cu) forms part of the enzymes associated with absorption and metabolism of the mineral iron. Copper is also intimately involved in the release of cholesterol from the liver; it helps to clot blood and, when bound to certain enzymes, aids in the synthesis of important neurotransmitters.

CELLULAR ORGANIZATION

Many types of cells make up biologic systems. The basic processes that sustain life among all cells are fairly similar, even though different cells carry out unique functions that necessitate special structures. Cells with different functions also contain essentially the same chemicals; they differ only in the proportion and arrangement of these chemicals. Figure 1-2 shows the complexity of the body's biologic organization. Humans are composed of a collection of diverse systems, each with highly specialized organs and tissues. The tissues are composed of many cells, and the cells are made up of molecules. Molecules, in turn, are constructed from individual atoms.

Organs

The body is a collection of eleven organ systems: the digestive, urinary, nervous, integumentary, skeletal,

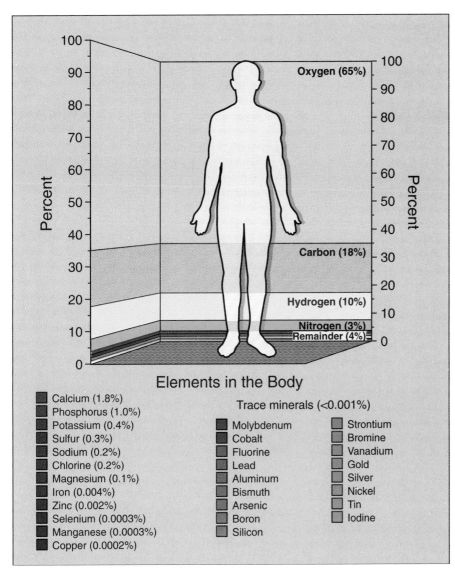

Figure 1-1. Elemental composition of the human body. The percentages represent the approximate contribution of the elements to the body mass of a typical 60 kg person.

Oxygen (65%)

Carbon (18%)

Hydrogen (10%)

Nitrogen (3%)
Remainder (4%)

Percent

Elements in the Body

Calcium (1.8%)
Phosphorus (1.0%)
Potassium (0.4%)
Sulfur (0.3%)
Sodium (0.2%)
Chlorine (0.2%)
Magnesium (0.1%)
Iron (0.004%)
Zinc (0.002%)
Selenium (0.0003%)
Manganese (0.0003%)
Copper (0.0002%)

Trace minerals (<0.001%)

Molybdenum
Cobalt
Fluorine
Lead
Aluminum
Bismuth
Arsenic
Boron
Silicon

Strontium
Bromine
Vanadium
Gold
Silver
Nickel
Tin
Iodine

muscular, endocrine, pulmonary, lymphatic, reproductive, and cardio-vascular. In turn, each organ system is made up of combinations of specialized tissues joined together to perform a common function. For example, specific cells make up the three main components of the integumentary system: the skin, hair, and nails. This system forms the body's outer protective layer to shield the deeper tissues from injury or invasion by outside organisms, as well as to respond to stimuli evoked by pressure, temperature, and pain. The skin also is the formation site of vitamin D. All the organ systems have their own particular and unique functions, yet each usually works in harmony with the others to maintain an optimal state of bodily function.

Cells

Below the level of the organ systems are the cells. *Cells represent the basic units of life;* they vary in size and shape depending on their specific function. Most have a diameter of approximately 10 micrometers (a micrometer, or µm, is 1/1000 of an inch), but an egg or ovum cell can be as large as 140 µm in diameter. Cell length can also vary tremendously, from approximately 8 µm for red blood cells, to a muscle cell 30 cm long, or a nerve cell that stretches up to 1 meter (100 cm) in length!

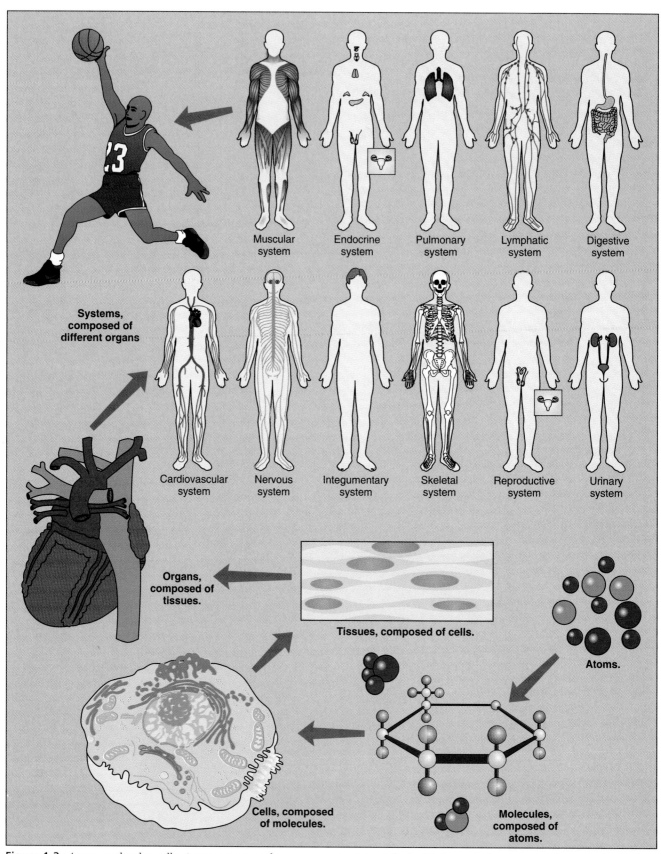

Figure 1-2. Atoms, molecules, cells, tissues, organs, and organ systems represent the body's increasingly more complex level of biologic organization.

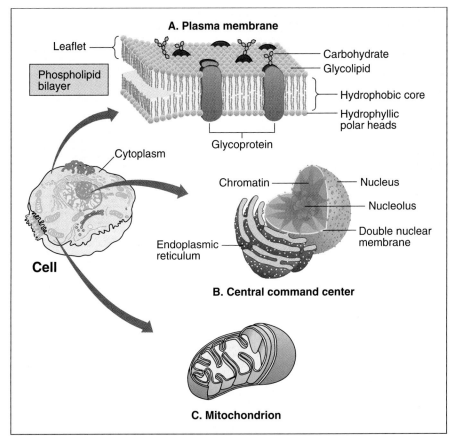

A. Plasma membrane

Leaflet

Phospholipid bilayer

Carbohydrate
Glycolipid
Hydrophobic core
Hydrophyllic polar heads

Glycoprotein

Cytoplasm

Cell

Chromatin
Endoplasmic reticulum

Nucleus
Nucleolus
Double nuclear membrane

B. Central command center

C. Mitochondrion

Figure 1-3. Three characteristic structures of living cells. *A.* The *plasma membrane*, a double "sandwich-type" structure composed of lipids (mostly phospholipids) and interspersed with proteins. Note that the bilayer can be split into two halves or leaflets. Each leaflet is responsible for binding specific protein structures. An elaborate network of tubules and microchannels serves as "inner scaffolding" to provide structure for the gel-like contents of the cell. *B.* The central command system, the *nucleus*, is the largest structure in the cell and regulates its many functions. Note that the endoplasmic reticulum joins the double nuclear membrane and is continuous with it. *C. Mitochondria*, the cell's "powerhouses", convert food nutrients into useful energy during aerobic metabolism. The size and number of mitochondria, as well as the enzymes that regulate energy metabolism, increase significantly with endurance training.

The Shape of Cells also Differs. The red blood cell is both oval (and thus adapted for carrying oxygen and carbon dioxide) and flat (for rapid uptake or release of these gases in appropriate tissues). Some digestive cells have many convolutions and depressions to increase their surface area-to-volume ratio and permit greater absorption of nutrients through their membranes. The epithelial cells on the inside of the mouth are flat and tightly packed to protect the underlying tissues from penetration by bacteria.

Although unique and often highly specific in function, cells share many structures in common. Figure 1-3 illustrates three common characteristics of living cells:

- *A plasma membrane,* a "sandwich-type" double structure made of lipids and proteins, separates the cell's contents from the surrounding extracellular fluid. The cell membrane is semipermeable, so only materials of certain sizes can be exchanged between the cell and its environment. The

bilayer serves as the basic constituent of the membrane; the core of the bilayer contains the fatty acid "tails" of the phospholipid, and the inner portion of the membrane prevents water-containing molecules from simply passing through the membrane. This part of the membrane is said to be *hydrophobic* (water-fearing). The outside of the bilayer membrane contains the polar "heads" of the phospholipid molecule. This part of the membrane is *hydrophilic* (water-loving); it is in continual contact with water on both the inside and outside of the cell.

- A central command center, the *nucleus,* is the largest structure in the cell and regulates its many functions. The nucleus contains chromatin, a precursor of the chromosomes that carry the hereditary material. The deoxyribonucleic acid (DNA) of the chromosomes directs cellular protein synthesis; ribonucleic

DNA. DNA is a highly specialized series of molecules called nucleic acids that exist in all cell nuclei. Nucleic acids code, store, and transmit the character of inherited traits of the organism through generations.

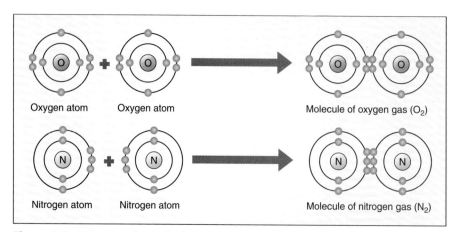

Figure 1-4. Molecules of specific elements are composed of identical atoms.

RNA. RNA is formed in the cell under the direction of DNA. This compound is the messenger by which the coded information in DNA is transmitted for the process of protein synthesis.

acid (RNA) is the messenger molecule responsible for translating the genetic instructions of DNA into proteins that carry out the cell's vital functions. The nucleus is surrounded by a plasma membrane that separates its cytoplasmic fluid from the rest of the cell. The endoplasmic reticulum joins the double nuclear membrane and is continuous with it. Communication takes place between the nucleus and the cellular fluid through pores or channels in the nuclear membrane and by way of microtubular channels in the endoplasmic reticulum.

• *Mitochondria,* the cell's "power plants," convert food nutrients into energy. In these structures, the potential energy in food is extracted and harvested within the energy-rich bonds of adenosine triphosphate (ATP), the unique energy currency of each cell. The mitochondria and other cellular organelles are bathed in cytoplasm, the intracellular watery medium containing minerals, enzymes, and other specialized solutions, compounds, and mixtures. The cytoplasm permits volleys of ionic charges to travel within the cell and also between cells and their surroundings.

Molecules

A molecule is defined as a minimum of two atoms bonded together strongly enough to create a stable identity. The molecule represents the smallest unit of a substance that still retains the compositional and chemical identity of that substance. Further fragmentation of the molecule involves breaking the chemical bonds that hold it together. The chemical properties of a molecule are changed by altering the configuration of its chemical bonds.

Figure 1-4 shows that a molecule made up of a single specific element always has identical atoms. Examples are the gases nitrogen ($N + N = N_2$) and oxygen ($O + O = O_2$), shown in the figure, as well as hydrogen ($H + H = H_2$) and chlorine gases ($Cl + Cl = Cl_2$).

Atoms

Molecules are composed of atoms which are particles up to 4 billionths of an inch in diameter that serve as the basic building blocks of matter. *The atom is the unit into which elements (matter) can be divided without the release of charged particles.* An atom consists of four main subatomic particles: nucleus, neutrons, protons, and electrons. The composition of atoms differs according to the number of subatomic particles they contain.

The dense core, or atomic nucleus, is the central portion of the atom. It can contain positively charged particles, called protons, and particles with a neutral electric charge, called neutrons. The protons and neutrons within the nucleus are bound tightly together and account for nearly 100% of the mass of the atom. Surrounding the nucleus is a cloud of electrons, negatively charged particles with almost no mass. Because opposite electric charges attract, the electrons are bound to the positively charged nucleus. An atom is usually electrically neutral; consequently, every atom has an equal number of positively charged protons and negatively charged electrons. For example, an atom of hydrogen has 1 proton and 1 electron; oxygen has 8 protons and 8 electrons; calcium has 20 protons and 20 electrons.

Ions. *An ion is any atom or group of atoms with a positive or negative electric charge.* If an atom holds fewer electrons than protons, it is positively charged and is referred to as a positive ion or *cation;* an example is the hydrogen ion, labeled H^+. An atom that has more electrons than protons (*anion*) is negatively charged, for example, the chloride ion (Cl^-). The strong acid, hydrochloric acid, (HCl), can separate or dissociate into the simple ionic form of H^+ and Cl^-. The reaction is written $HCl \rightarrow H^+ + Cl^-$. Similarly, a sodium cation (Na^+) and chloride anion (Cl^-) are present in solution when sodium chloride ($NaCl$), or table salt, dissolves and dissociates in water in the reaction $NaCl \rightarrow Na^+ + Cl^-$. Ions such as Na^+, Cl^-, and potassium (K^+) in solution are called *electrolytes* because these solutes dissociate into either positive or negative ions. More is said about the importance of electrolytes later in this chapter (see Oxidation-Reduction Reactions).

COMPOUNDS AND MIXTURES

Compounds

A compound is a substance formed from two or more different elements. The simple water molecule (H_2O), for example, is a compound formed from the union of one atom of oxygen (O) and two hydrogen atoms (H + H).

Mixtures

Most common materials are mixtures of various chemical compounds. *A mixture is created when two or more different substances are physically combined.* Mixtures differ from compounds in the following ways: (1) mixtures are not linked by chemical bonds; (2) mixtures can be separated into their individual components by physical processes such as filtering, straining, centrifugation, or distillation (evaporation); compounds can only be separated into their con-

stituent elements by chemical reactions in which bonds between atoms are broken; and (3) unlike a compound, a mixture is not a chemically pure substance. A mixture can be a heterogeneous substance such as a particular enzyme, hormone, or vitamin; it can also be a combination of food nutrients such as strawberries and whipped cream or chocolate chip cookies.

There are three types of mixtures:

Solutions. *A solution is a homogeneous mixture of either a gas, liquid, or solid composed of at least two substances.* Oxygen and carbon dioxide are in solution in the fluids of the body, as are the products of digestion as they are transported to and from different tissues. The air we breathe is a solution because it is a mixture of gases (approximately 79.04% nitrogen, 20.93% oxygen, and 0.03% carbon dioxide with trace amounts of several inert gases). The largest quantity of a substance in a solution is customarily called the solvent, while the smaller amount — usually a solid or gas — is the solute. In the body, water is the chief solvent. (Chapter 6 discusses this important substance.)

Suspensions. *A suspension is a mixture of substances that may have visible solutes, but with little chemical attraction for the solvent.* If a photograph is taken of blood flowing through the vascular system, the fluid looks like a well-mixed, heterogeneous solution. But if a sample is collected in a small tube and spun at high speed, there are three distinct parts. The top part, the plasma, is a relatively clear liquid representing about 55% of the sample. There is a minute middle layer of white blood cells (leukocytes) and platelets; and the third layer, consisting of red blood cells, settles to the bottom and occupies about 45% of the sample. The different layers of substances are the suspensions.

Colloids. *A colloid is similar to a suspension, but the substances in the mixture are often translucent and do not*

Atomic weight. The atomic weight of an atom is equal to the number of neutrons plus the number of protons.

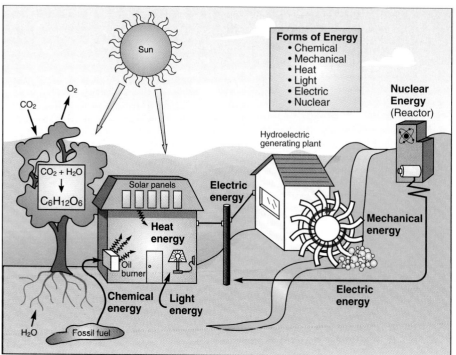

Figure 1-5. Interconversions of the six forms of energy.

precipitate like the solutes in blood. The cell cytoplasm and its lattice-like microstructures, for example, have a gel-like consistency which keeps the various molecules dispersed throughout this mixture. Many important metabolic reactions take place within the gel-like colloidal fluids of the cytoplasmic structures.

· · · · · · · · · · · · ·

ENERGY

All forms of biologic work are powered by the direct transfer of chemical energy. Performance in swimming, jogging, aerobic dancing, or competitive tennis is greatly influenced by our capacity to extract energy from food nutrients and ultimately transfer it to the contractile proteins of skeletal muscle. But unlike the physical properties of matter, it is difficult to define energy in concrete terms of size, shape, or mass. Rather, all forms of energy are associated with motion; this suggests a dynamic state related to change because the presence of

energy is revealed only when a change has taken place. Within this context, energy is related to the performance of work. As work increases, the transfer of energy increases so that a change occurs.

The First Law of Thermodynamics

One of the most important principles in chemistry, as related to work within biologic systems, is the first law of thermodynamics. The basic tenet of this principle states that energy is neither created nor destroyed, but instead, is transformed from one form to another without being used up. In essence, this is the immutable principle of the conservation of energy that applies to both living and nonliving systems. The large amount of chemical energy in fuel oil, for example, is readily converted to heat energy in the home oil burner. In the body, however, all the chemical energy trapped within the bonds of the food nutrients is not immediately lost as heat; rather, a large portion is conserved as chemical energy before it is changed into mechanical energy (and then ultimately heat energy) by the action of the musculoskeletal system. Figure 1-5 illustrates the interconversions for six different forms of energy.

The key point about the first law of thermodynamics is that energy is not produced, consumed, or used up in the body; it is merely transformed from one form into another as the various bodily systems undergo change in their many functions. For example, an increase in heart rate during exercise requires that a greater oxygen supply be delivered not only to the heart but also to the active muscles. The source of this energy is "waiting" to be put into play by certain chemical reactions; to sustain the effort, the energy supply must be maintained to keep pace with the new level of exertion. Thus, the total energy of the system has not been changed but "rearranged".

Biologic work. Biologic work encompasses all of the energy-requiring, life-sustaining processes of the cell.

· · · · · · · · · · · · ·

A decrease in useful energy. A physical or chemical process that releases energy to its surroundings is termed exergonic. Such reactions can be viewed as "downhill" processes; they result in a decline in free energy, that is "useful" energy for biologic work.

ATP — NATURE'S POWERFUL INGREDIENT

Animals and plants are as different as night and day, yet they share one important common biological trait; they each trap, store, and transfer energy through a complex series of chemical reactions that involve the compound adenosine triphosphate or ATP.

The history of the discovery of ATP reads like a mystery. It dates back to the 1860s in France, and the work of Louis Pasteur, a leading scientist of the day. During one of his experiments with yeast, Pasteur proposed that this micro-organism's ability to degrade sugar to carbon dioxide and alcohol (ethanol) was strictly a living (Pasteur termed it "vitalistic") function of the yeast cell. He hypothesized that if the yeast cell died, the fermentation process would cease.

In 1897, however, two German scientists, Eduard and Buchner, made a chance observation that showed Pasteur was wrong. Their discovery revolutionized the study of physiologic systems and represented the beginning of the modern science of biochemistry. Searching for therapeutic uses for protein, they concocted a thick paste of freshly grown yeast and sand in a large mortar and pressed out the yeast cell juice. The gummy liquid proved unstable and could not be preserved by techniques available at that time. One of the laboratory assistants suggested the addition of large amounts of yeast to the mixture — his wife used this technique to preserve fruit.

To everyone's surprise, what seemed a silly solution worked; the nonliving juice from the yeast cells converted the sugar to carbon dioxide and alcohol (that directly contradicted Pasteur's theorem). The epoch making finding later won Eduard the Nobel prize.

In 1905, the British biochemists Harden and Young observed, as had their German predecessors, that the fermenting ability of yeast juice decreased gradually with time and could be restored only by adding fresh boiled yeast juice or blood serum. What revitalized the mixture?

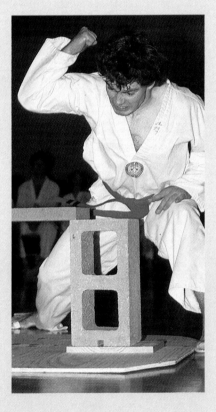

After prolonged research, inorganic phosphate, present in both liquids, was identified as the activating agent.

Other British scientists working with Harden and Young also played important roles in the final discovery of ATP. For example, when crude yeast juice was pressed through a gelatin film, a filtrate free of protein was obtained. This filtrate was completely inert as was the protein. But when the filtrate and protein were recombined, vigorous fermentation began. They called this combination "zymase": it was composed of the filtrate "cozmaze" and the protein residue "apozmase". Many years passed before the two components were accurately analyzed and identified as containing "coenzyme" compounds. In addition, the apomase actually consisted of many proteins, each a specific catalyst in the many reactions in the breakdown of sugar.

In 1929, the young German scientist, K. Lohmann, working in Otto Meyerhoff's laboratory, conducted a series of experiments into the "energy" source responsible for cellular reactions involving yeast and sugar. Working with yeast juice, Lohmann found that an unstable substance in the cozymase filtrate was necessary to break down the sugar. This energizing substance was made up of the nitrogen containing compound adenine linked to the sugar ribose and three phosphate groups. This is the compound we now call ATP. The potential energy is stored in the bonds, "high-energy bonds", which link the all-important phosphate groups in the ATP molecule — and it is the splitting of these phosphate bonds that releases the energy for all biologic work.

The function of ATP is amazing in terms of the variety of processes it powers in living cells. It is a ubiquitous compound found in micro-organisms, plants, and in animals ranging from nematodes to cockroaches and humans. Surprisingly, wherever ATP is found it is always in the same structure, regardless of the complexity of the organism. ATP truly is the fuel that powers all living organisms.

Photosynthesis and Cellular Respiration

The most fundamental examples of energy conversion in living cells are the processes of photosynthesis and respiration.

Photosynthesis. In the sun, with a temperature of several million degrees Fahrenheit, part of the potential energy stored in the nucleus of the hydrogen atom is released by the process of nuclear fusion. This energy, in the form of gamma radiation, is then converted to radiant energy.

Figure 1-6 illustrates that during photosynthesis, the plant pigment chlorophyll, contained in chloroplasts (the large organelles located in leaf cells), absorbs radiant (solar) energy to facilitate the synthesis of glucose from carbon dioxide and water. In addition, oxygen is released to the environment. Glucose and oxygen are subsequently used by animals in the process of respiration. In plants, carbohydrates also can be converted to fats and proteins. Animals then ingest the plant nutrients to serve their own energy needs. In essence, solar energy coupled with photosynthesis powers the animal world with food and oxygen.

Cellular Respiration. The process of respiration is the reverse of photosynthesis. During respiration, the chemical energy stored in glucose, lipid, or protein molecules is extracted in the presence of oxygen. A portion of the energy released can be conserved in other chemical compounds and then used by the body for its energy-requiring processes; the remaining energy flows to the environment as heat.

The energy released during cellular respiration is used to sustain biologic work. This can take one of three familiar forms as shown in Figure 1-7: mechanical work of muscle contraction, chemical work that involves the synthesis of cellular molecules, or transport work that concentrates various substances in the intracellular and extracellular fluids.

Mechanical work. The most obvious example of energy transformation in the body is the mechanical work generated by muscle contraction. The protein filaments of the muscle fibers directly convert chemical energy into mechanical energy. This is not the body's only form of mechanical work, however. In the cell nucleus, for example, contractile elements similar to those found in muscle literally tug at the chromosomes to facilitate the

An increase in useful energy. A physical or chemical process that stores or absorbs energy is termed endergonic. Such reactions can be viewed as "uphill" processes and they result in an increase in free energy for biologic work.

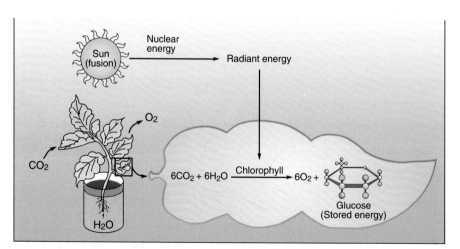

Figure 1-6. Photosynthesis is the plant's mechanism for synthesizing carbohydrates, lipids, and proteins. In this example, a glucose molecule is created from the union of carbon dioxide and water.

process of cell division. Mechanical work is also performed by specialized structures such as cilia that are part of many cells.

Chemical work. Chemical work is performed by all cells for growth and maintenance. Cellular components are continually synthesized as other components are destroyed.

Transport work. Much less conspicuous than mechanical or chemical work is transport work, or the biologic work of concentrating substances in the body. A continual expenditure of stored chemical energy is required to accomplish this "quiet" form of biologic work.

Potential and Kinetic Energy

Potential energy and kinetic energy are the two types that comprise the total energy of any system. Figure 1-8 illustrates that potential energy can be energy of position such as that possessed by water at the top of a hill before it flows downstream.

In this example, the energy change is proportional to the vertical drop of the water — the greater the vertical drop, the greater the potential energy at the top. Other examples of potential energy are light energy, electric energy, or bound energy within the internal structure of a nutrient. *When potential energy is released, it is transformed into kinetic energy, or energy of motion.* In some cases, the bound energy in one substance can be directly transferred to other substances to increase their potential energy. Energy transfers of this type are necessary for the body's chemical work of biosynthesis. In this process, specific building-block atoms such as carbon, hydrogen, oxygen, and nitrogen are activated and join other atoms and molecules to synthesize important biologic compounds such as cholesterol, enzymes, and hormones. Some of the newly created compounds serve structural needs, such as the protein-rich contractile elements of muscle or the fat-containing membranous covering of cells. Other energy-rich compounds can serve the cell's energy

Coupled reactions. Coupled reactions link exergonic with endergonic processes so that some of the energy is transferred to the endergonic process. In the body, such reactions conserve a large portion of the chemical energy in food nutrients in a usable form.

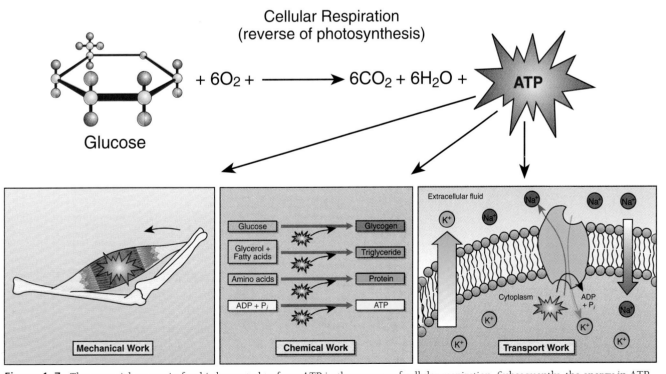

Figure 1–7. The potential energy in food is harvested to form ATP in the process of cellular respiration. Subsequently, the energy in ATP is used to power all forms of biologic work.

needs; this occurs, for example, when ATP is "split" apart during its own chemical breakdown.

. . . .

ENZYMES

An enzyme is a catalyst that accelerates the forward and reverse rates of chemical reactions within cells without being consumed or changed in the reaction. Within the fluids of a single cell there can be as many as four thousand different enzymes, each performing a specific function. Almost every chemical reaction within a cell is catalyzed by a specific enzyme. Enzymes make contact at precise locations on the surfaces of cell structures, and they can also work within the structure itself. Many enzymes also are operative outside the cell, such as in the bloodstream, in the digestive mixture, and in the fluids of the small intestine.

Enzymes are usually named for the function they perform. The suffix *-ase* is often appended to the specific molecule on which the enzyme operates. For example, hydro*lase* adds water during hydrolysis reactions, protease interacts with protein, oxi*dase* adds oxygen to a substance, and ribonucle*ase* splits apart RNA. What is truly remarkable is that enzymes do not all operate at the same rate; some operate slowly, while others act quite rapidly. Enzymes often work cooperatively among their binding sites. While one enzyme is "turned on" at a particular site, its neighbor is "turned off" until the job is completed; the operation can then be reversed, with one enzyme becoming inactive and the other active. Enzymes also can act along small regions of the *substrate* (any substance acted upon by an enzyme) and begin their task over again, each time working at a different rate than previously! Some enzymes delay when they begin to work. A good example is the precursor enzyme trypsinogen that is manufactured by the pancreas. After a delay, trypsinogen is secreted into the small intestine where it functions as the active enzyme trypsin to digest complex proteins to simple amino acids (referred to as proteolytic action). Without a delay in its activity, trypsinogen would literally digest the pancreatic tissue that produced it.

. . . .

Enzymes work extremely fast. In a typical mitochondrion, there may be as many as 10 billion enzyme molecules, each carrying out millions of operations within a short time period. During exercise, the rate of increase in enzyme activity within the cell speeds up tremendously. The increased rate of a catalyzed reaction can be 10^6 to 10^{12} times faster than an uncatalyzed reaction under similar conditions.

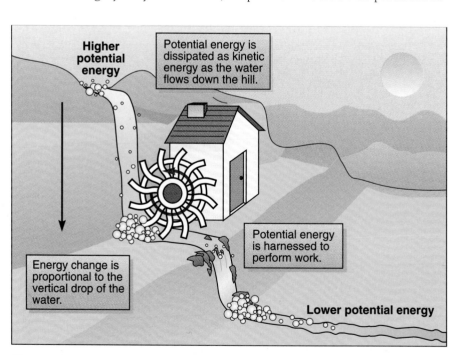

Figure 1-8. Potential energy to perform work is transformed into kinetic energy.

Other enzymes are inactivated once they perform their specific function. For example, once the blood-clotting enzymes have carried out their coagulation functions, they cease activity; if they did not, the blood vessels would become clogged with continually clotting blood.

A unique characteristic of an enzyme, as illustrated in Figure 1-9, is its interaction with one specific substrate to perform a specific function. The enzyme becomes turned on when its active site is joined in a "perfect fit" with the active site on the substrate. The example shows the sequence of steps for interaction of the enzyme maltase with its substrate maltose in the intestinal wall.

Step 1 is to achieve a fit between the active sites of the enzyme and substrate to form an enzyme-substrate complex.

Step 2 causes the enzyme to catalyze (speed up) the chemical reaction with the substrate. Note that a water molecule is liberated during this hydrolysis process.

Step 3 produces an end product. In the example, the major end product is glucose.

Because the enzyme-substrate interaction resembles a key fitting into a lock, it is known as the *lock and key mechanism*. This interactive process assures that the correct enzyme "mates" with its specific substrate to carry out a particular function. Once the enzyme and substrate are joined, a conformational change in shape of the enzyme takes place as it molds to its substrate.

The lock and key mechanism is essentially protective in that only the correct substrate becomes activated by the correct enzyme. A typical example involves the enzyme hexokinase, which accelerates a chemical reaction when it links with a glucose molecule. When this occurs, a phosphate molecule is transferred from ATP to a specific binding site on one of glucose's carbon atoms. Once the two binding sites join to form a glu-

cose-hexokinase complex, the substrate is degraded in stepwise fashion to less complex molecules in the process of energy metabolism. This process by which energy is extracted from carbohydrate, lipid, and protein molecules for use by the body is discussed in Chapter 2.

Coenzymes

Some enzymes are totally inactive in the absence of additional substances termed coenzymes. These are complex, nonprotein, organic substances that facilitate enzyme action by helping to bind the substrate with it specific enzyme.

The action of a coenzyme is less specific than an enzyme because the coenzyme can act in a number of different reactions. It can act as a "cobinder," or it can serve as a temporary carrier of intermediary products of the reaction. For example, the

Conformational change. Even if an enzyme happens to link with a substrate, unless the specific conformational change in the shape of the enzyme takes place, the enzyme will not interact chemically with the substrate.

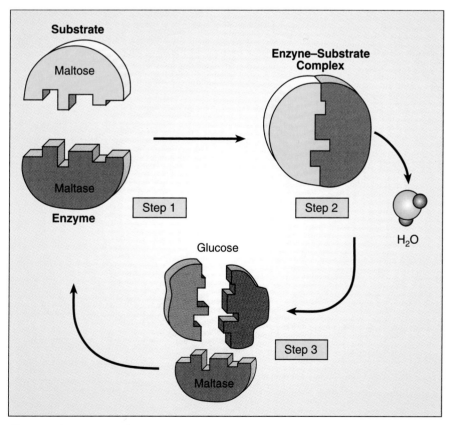

Figure 1-9. Sequence of steps in the "lock and key" mechanism of an enzyme with its substrate. The example shows how glucose is formed through the interaction of the enzyme maltase with its substrate maltose.

hydrogen atoms and electrons that are split from food fragments during energy metabolism are temporarily carried by the coenzyme *nicotinamine adeninedinucleotide* (or NAD$^+$) to form NADH. The electrons are then passed to special transporter molecules in another series of chemical reactions that ultimately deliver them to molecular oxygen.

HYDROLYSIS AND CONDENSATION: THE BASIS FOR DIGESTION AND SYNTHESIS

Hydrolysis Reactions

Hydrolysis is a basic process wherein complex organic molecules such as carbohydrates, lipids, and proteins are degraded, or catabolized into simpler forms that the body can easily assimilate. During the decomposition process of hydrolysis, energy is released when chemical bonds are broken by addition of the constituents of water (H$^+$ and OH$^-$) to the by-products of the reaction. Examples of hydrolysis are the digestion of the food nutrients: starches and disaccharides to monosaccharides, proteins to amino acids, and lipids to fatty acids. The hydrolysis of each nutrient is catalyzed by a specific enzyme. For the disaccharides lactose, sucrose, and maltose, for example, the specific enzymes are lactase, sucrase, and maltase, respectively. The lipid enzymes are called lipases; they degrade the lipid molecule when water is added, causing the fatty acids to be cleaved from their glycerol backbone. During the digestion of proteins, the protease enzymes require water to degrade the peptide linkages to their simple amino acids.

The general form for all hydrolysis reactions is as follows:

$$AB + HOH \longrightarrow A\text{-}H + B\text{-}OH$$

When water is added to the substance AB, the chemical bond that joins AB is decomposed to produce the breakdown products A-H (H is a hydrogen atom from water) and B-OH (OH is the remaining hydroxyl group from water). Figure 1-10A shows the hydrolysis reaction for the disaccharide sucrose to its end-product molecules glucose and fructose; also illustrated is the hydrolysis of a dipeptide (protein) into its two constituent amino acid units. Intestinal absorption occurs quickly following hydrolysis of the carbohydrate, lipid, and protein nutrients.

Condensation Reactions

Because the reactions illustrated for hydrolysis can also occur in the opposite direction, that is, they are reversible, the compound AB can be synthesized from A-H and B-OH in the process of condensation. In this building, or *anabolic,* process a molecule of water is formed. The structural components of the nutrients are bound together in condensation reactions to form more complex molecules. Figure 1-10B shows the condensation reaction for the synthesis of maltose from two glucose units and the creation of a more complex protein from two amino acid units. In the synthesis of proteins, note that a hydroxyl is removed from one amino acid, and a hydrogen from the other, to create a water molecule. For the protein, the new bond is called a *peptide bond.* A similar production of water occurs in the synthesis of complex carbohydrates from simple sugars, and for fats from the union of their glycerol and fatty acid components.

. . . .

OXIDATION AND REDUCTION REACTIONS

Literally thousands of simultaneous chemical reactions occur in the body that involve the transfer of electrons from one substance to another. *Oxidation reactions are those that involve the transfer of either oxygen atoms, hydrogen atoms, or electrons.* In oxidation reactions there is a loss of electrons with a corresponding gain in valence. When hydrogen is removed from a substance, for example, there is a net gain of valence electrons. In contrast, in reduction reactions, electrons are gained from a substance and there is a net loss of valence electrons from another substance.

Oxidation and reduction reactions are characteristically *coupled:* whenever oxidation occurs, the reverse reaction of reduction also takes place and the electrons lost from one substance are gained by the other. An oxidation-reduction reaction is also called a *redox* reaction. *Reduction involves any process in which the atoms in an element gain electrons with a corresponding decrease in valence.*

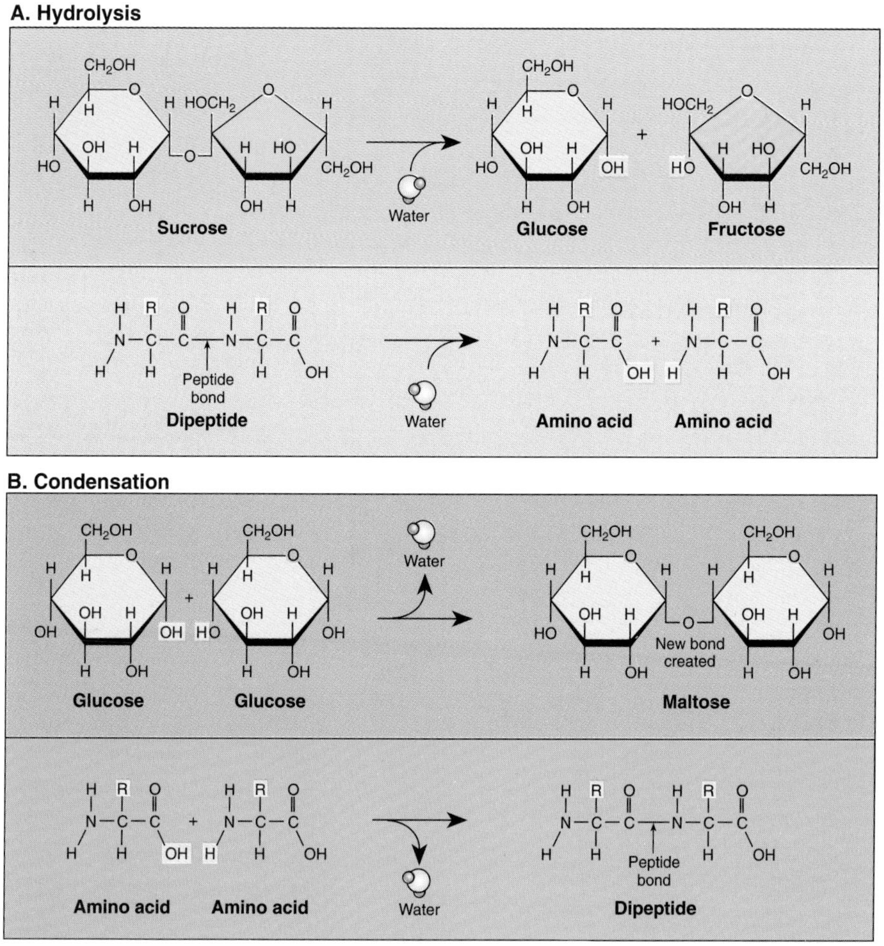

A. Hydrolysis

B. Condensation

Figure 1-10. *A. Hydrolysis* chemical reaction for the disaccharide sucrose to the end-product molecules glucose and fructose, and a hydrolysis reaction for a dipeptide (protein) into two amino acid end-product units. *B. Condensation* chemical reaction for the synthesis of maltose from two glucose units, and the creation of a protein dipeptide from two amino acid units. The latter reaction is the reverse of the hydrolysis reaction for the dipeptide. The symbol R represents the remainder of the amino acid molecule.

An excellent example of an oxidation reaction is the transfer of electrons in the mitochondria. Here, hydrogen atoms are oxidized and the removed electrons are passed by special carriers to be delivered ultimately to oxygen, which becomes reduced. The source of hydrogen is the carbohydrate, lipid, and protein nutrient substrates. The enzymes that speed up the redox reactions are called dehydrogenases or oxidases. Two of the hydrogen-accepting coenzymes are the vitamin-B containing nicotinamide-adenine dinucleotide (NAD$^+$) and *flavin adenine dinucleotide* (FAD). Energy in the form of ATP is harnessed during the transfer of electrons from NADH and FADH$_2$.

The transport of electrons by specific carrier molecules constitutes the respiratory chain. This is the final common pathway in aerobic (oxidative) metabolism and is referred to as *electron transport.* For each pair of hydrogen atoms, two electrons flow down the chain and reduce one atom of oxygen. To complete the process, oxygen also accepts hydrogen to form water. This coupled redox process constitutes the oxidation of hydrogen and subsequent reduction of oxygen. Much of the energy generated in cellular oxidation-reduction reactions is trapped or conserved as chemical energy to power the cell's various forms of biologic work.

Figure 1-11 illustrates a redox reaction during vigorous physical activity. As exercise intensifies, more hydrogen atoms are stripped from the carbohydrate substrate than can be oxidized in reactions in the respiratory chain that utilize oxygen. For energy metabolism to continue, these nonoxidized excess hydrogens must be "accepted" by a chemical other than oxygen. This is exactly the case, as a molecule of pyruvic acid, an intermediate compound formed in the initial phase of carbohydrate metabolism, temporarily accepts a pair of hydrogens (electrons). This reduction of pyruvic acid by accepting hydrogens forms a new compound called *lactic acid.* The more intense the exercise, the greater the flow of excess hydrogens to pyruvic acid, and lactic acid increases rapidly. During recovery, the excess hydrogens used to form lactic acid can now be oxidized (electrons removed and passed to NAD$^+$) and the pyruvic acid molecule is reformed. The enzyme that mediates this reaction is lactate dehydrogenase, or LDH.

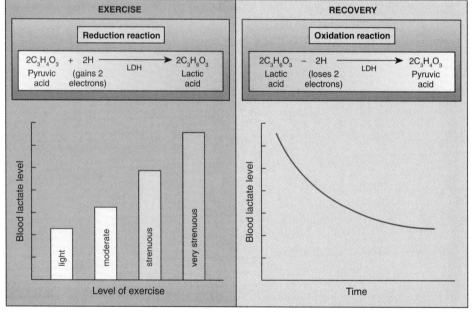

Figure 1-11. Example of a redox (oxidation-reduction) reaction. During progressively strenuous exercise when oxygen supply becomes inadequate, some pyruvic acid formed in energy metabolism gains two hydrogens (gains 2 electrons) and becomes *reduced* to a new compound lactic acid. In recovery when oxygen supply is adequate, lactic acid gives up two hydrogens (loses 2 electrons) and is *oxidized* back to pyruvic acid. This is an example of how a redox reaction enables energy metabolism to progress even though there is limited availability of oxygen in relation to exercise energy demands.

ACID-BASE CONCENTRATION AND pH

Acid. Any substance which ionizes in solution to give off hydrogen ions (H^+) is an acid. Acids taste sour, turn litmus indicators red, react with bases to form salts, and cause some metals to liberate hydrogen. Examples of acids in the body include hydrochloric, phosphoric, carbonic, citric, and carboxylic acids.

Base. A base is any substance that forms hydroxide ions (OH^-) in water solutions. Basic or alkaline solutions taste bitter, are slippery to the touch, turn litmus indicators blue, and react with acids to form salts. Examples of bases in the body include sodium and calcium hydroxides, and water solutions of ammonia that form ammonium hydroxide.

pH. The pH is a quantitative measure of the acidity or alkalinity (basicity) of a liquid solution. Specifically, pH refers to the concentration of protons, or H^+. Solutions with relatively more OH^- than H^+ have a pH above 7.0 and are called basic or alkaline. Conversely, solutions with more H^+ than OH^- have a pH below 7.0 and are termed acidic. Chemically pure or distilled water is considered neutral with equal amounts of H^+ and OH^- and thus a pH of 7.0. The pH scale shown in Figure 1-12 was devised in 1909 by the Danish chemist Sören Sörensen. It ranges from +1.0 to +14.0. The pH of body fluids ranges from a very low pH of 1.0 for the digestive acid hydrochloric acid to a slightly basic pH of between 7.35 and 7.45 for arterial and venous blood and most other body fluids.

Enzymes and pH. Many chemical processes in the body occur only at a specific pH. An enzyme that works at one pH becomes inactivated when the pH of its surroundings change. The fat-digesting enzyme gastric lipase, for example, is effective in the highly acidic stomach environment but ceases to function within the slightly alkaline small intestine. The same is true for salivary amylase, the enzyme that begins starch breakdown in the mouth. The pH of the salivary fluids ranges between 6.4 and 7.0. When passed to the stomach (pH 1.0 to 2.0), this enzyme ceases its digestive function and is itself digested like any other protein by the stomach acids. As a general rule, extreme changes in pH produce irreversible damage to enzymes. For this reason, the body's pH (acid-base) balance is maintained within narrow limits.

Buffers

The term buffering is used to designate reactions that minimize changes in H^+ concentration; the chemical or physiologic mechanisms that prevent this change are termed *buffers*. In the body, any decrease in pH is the result of an increase in H^+ concentration and is referred to as *acidosis*. Conversely, a decrease in H^+ concentration (increase in pH) is termed *alkalosis*. If the buffer system is unable to neutralize deviations in H^+, effective bodily function becomes disrupted with the end result of coma or death. Three mechanisms control the acid-base quality of our internal environment: chemical buffers, pulmonary ventilation, and kidney function.

Chemical Buffers. The chemical buffering system consists of a weak acid and a base or salt of that acid. The body's bicarbonate buffer, for example, consists of the weak carbonic acid and its salt, sodium bicarbonate. Carbonic acid is formed when the bicarbonate binds H^+. As long as H^+ concentration remains elevated, the reaction continually converts stronger acids to the weaker carbonic acid because the excess H^+ are bound in accordance with the general reaction:

pH and H^+. There is an inverse relation between pH and the concentration of H^+. Because the pH scale is logarithmic, a one-unit change in pH is associated with a tenfold change in H^+ concentration. For example, lemon juice and gastric juice (pH = 2.0) have 1000 times greater H^+ concentration than black coffee (pH = 5.0), while hydrochloric acid (pH = 1.0) is about one million times greater in H^+ concentration compared to blood (pH = 7.4)!

$$H^+ + Buffer \longrightarrow H\text{--}Buffer$$

The strong stomach acid, hydrochloric acid (HCl), is changed into the much weaker carbonic acid (H_2CO_3) by combining with sodium bicarbonate. As a result, only a slight reduction is noted in pH. If the body's buffer response is inadequate and stomach acidity remains elevated, many individuals seek "outside help" in the form of ingested neutralizing agents or antacids to provide buffering relief.

If, however, the concentration of H^+ decreases and the body fluids become more alkaline, the buffering reaction moves in the opposite direction. In the process, H^+ are released and acidity increases:

$$H^+ + Buffer \longleftarrow H\text{--}Buffer$$

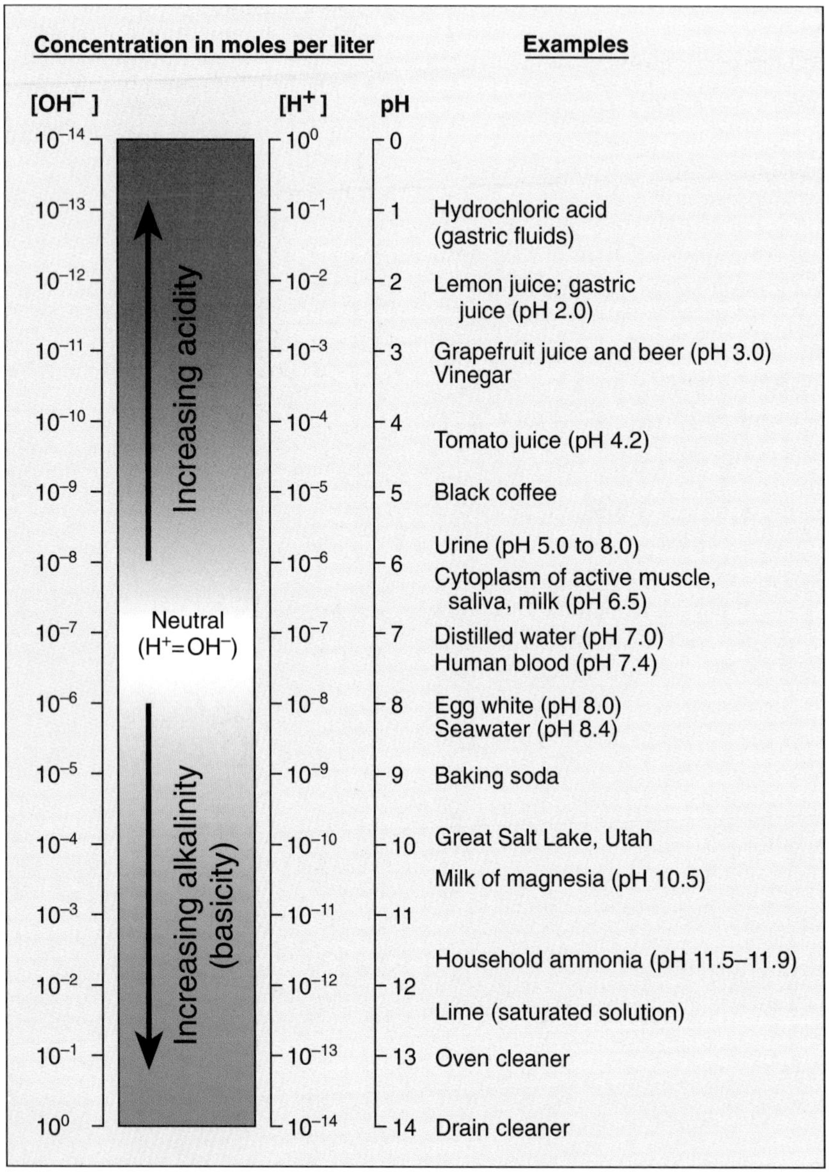

In addition to digestive juices, other acids are continually being produced in the body. Much of the carbon dioxide generated in energy metabolism reacts with water to form carbonic acid ($CO_2 + H_2O \rightarrow H_2CO_3$). This then dissociates into H^+ and HCO_3^-. Likewise, lactic acid, a strong metabolic acid, is buffered by sodium bicarbonate to form sodium lactate and the relatively weak carbonic acid; in turn, carbonic acid separates and increases the H^+ concentration of bodily fluids. Other organic acids such as fatty acids dissociate and liberate H^+, as do the sulfuric and phosphoric acids produced during protein breakdown.

Other chemical buffers available to the body include the phosphate buffers, consisting of phosphoric acid and sodium phosphate. These chemicals act in a manner similar to that of the bicarbonate system. The phosphate buffers regulate the acid-base quality of the kidney tubules and intracellular fluids, in which there is a relatively high concentration of phosphates. Carbonic acid is buffered by the protein-containing hemoglobin compound as well as by other plasma proteins.

Ventilatory Buffer. Any increase in H^+ concentration in body fluids stimulates the respiratory center to increase breathing. This adjustment causes a greater than normal amount of carbon dioxide to leave the blood. Carbon dioxide is transported dissolved in the blood and combined with water

Figure 1-12. The pH scale is a quantitative measure of the acidity or alkalinity (basicity) of a liquid solution. Blood pH is normally maintained at the slightly alkaline pH of 7.4. Even during the most vigorous exercise, values for blood pH rarely fall below a pH of 6.9.

as carbonic acid. Thus, reducing the carbon dioxide content of the body acts directly as a ventilatory buffer to reduce the quantity of carbonic acid. As a result, the body fluids become more alkaline. Conversely, reducing normal ventilation causes carbon dioxide to build up, and the fluids become more acidic.

Renal Buffer. The excretion of H^+ by the kidneys, although more time-consuming than the action of the chemical and ventilatory buffers, is required if the long-term acid-base quality of body fluids is to be maintained. Acidity is controlled by the renal buffer through alterations in the amount of bicarbonate ions, ammonia, and H^+ secreted into the urine and the alkali, chloride, and bicarbonate that is reabsorbed.

Diabetes and Acidosis. When insulin production is normal, energy is provided primarily from a mixture of carbohydrate and lipid. In diabetes, however, the lack of insulin limits carbohydrate utilization, and lipid becomes the major energy source. Such reliance on lipid for energy produces acid by-products, called keto-acids, that can lead to an acidotic condition. Additional water and sodium are lost as these acids are excreted by the kidneys. This limits the availability of sodium to form the strong chemical buffer sodium bicarbonate. If this imbalance continues, the person will eventually lapse into a coma from the resulting metabolic acidosis. Immediate countermeasures include ingestion of carbohydrate and injection of synthetic insulin to facilitate glucose transport into the cell.

Buffering and Strenuous Exercise. In strenuous exercise, large amounts of the metabolic by-product lactic acid leave active muscle and enter the bloodstream. Figure 1-13 shows the relationship between blood pH and blood lactic acid as a function of increasing intensities of exercise.

Notice that lactic acid begins to increase in the blood as exercise approaches 25% of maximum. Thereafter, there is a steady increase in blood lactate (and corresponding decrease in blood pH and bicarbonate). The blood pH can approach a low of 6.8 at the point of physical exhaustion. At this point, the individual can become disoriented and nauseated. Even though the body's buffering systems are attempting to maintain an acid-base balance throughout exercise (the bicarbonate buffers attempt to neu-

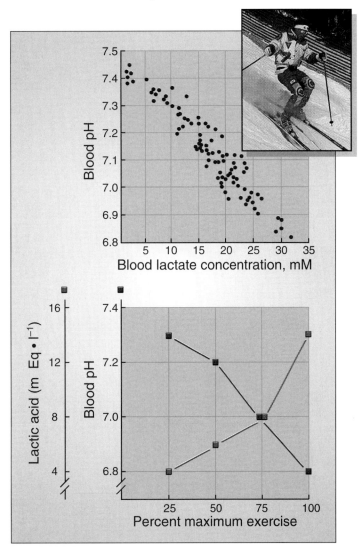

Figure 1-13. Top. The relationship between blood pH and blood lactic acid concentration at rest and during increasing intensities of short-duration exercise up to the maximum. Bottom. Blood pH and lactic acid concentration in relation to exercise intensity expressed as a percent of maximum. As blood lactic acid increases, there is an accompanying decrease in blood pH.

tralize the lactic acid), it is only when exercise ceases that the blood pH quickly stabilizes and returns to normal. In addition to the bicarbonate buffer, the protein-containing compound hemoglobin along with phosphate buffers serve as important neutralizing agents in the blood during vigorous physical activity.

• • • • • • • • • • • • • • • •

TRANSPORT OF NUTRIENTS ACROSS CELL MEMBRANES

At any moment, literally thousands of chemicals such as ions, vitamins, minerals, acids, salts, water, gases, hormones, and carbohydrate, protein, and lipid components traverse the bilayer plasma membrane as exchange takes place between the cell and its surroundings. The plasma membrane, however, is highly permeable to some substances but not to others. Such selective permeability allows the cell to maintain reasonable consistency in its chemical composition. When this equilibrium is disrupted, immediate adjustments occur to restore constancy in the cell's internal "milieu." This is accomplished by two processes: *passive transport* of substances through the cellular membrane, where no energy is required; and *active transport* through the membrane, where metabolic energy in the form of ATP is used to "power" the exchange of materials.

Passive Transport Processes

There are four types of passive transport: simple diffusion, facilitated diffusion, osmosis, and filtration. Figure 1-14 shows an example of each.

Simple Diffusion. In the cellular environment, simple diffusion involves the free and continuous net move-

A. Simple diffusion

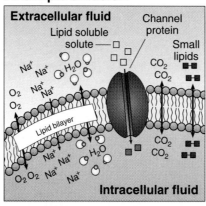

B. Facilitated diffusion

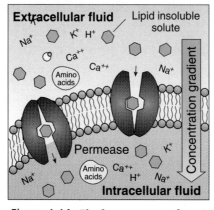

C. Osmosis

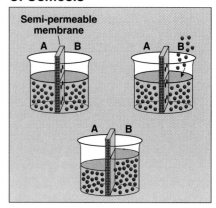

D. Filtration

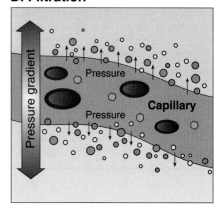

Figure 1-14. The four processes of passive transport. *A.* Simple diffusion. *B.* Facilitated diffusion. *C.* Osmosis. *D.* Filtration.

ment of molecules in aqueous solution across the plasma membrane. In the example, note that water molecules, small lipids, and gases move unimpeded from outside the cell through the lipid bilayer to the intracellular fluid. In *simple diffusion, a substance will move from an area of initial higher concentration to one of lower concentration until it becomes evenly dispersed.* This is an entirely passive process, powered only by the kinetic energy of the molecules themselves, with no expenditure of cellular energy. When sugar is added to water, for example, the sugar molecules dissolve and become evenly dispersed through their continuous, random movement. If the water is hot, diffusion speeds up because a higher temperature increases molecular movement and thus the rate of diffusion. If the particles stay within a closed system, they will eventually become evenly distributed throughout the solution and the net movement of particles will cease.

Simple diffusion across the plasma membrane occurs for water molecules, the dissolved gases such as oxygen, carbon dioxide, and nitrogen, small uncharged polar molecules such as urea and alcohol, and various lipid-soluble molecules. These substances diffuse so quickly because the plasma membrane consists of sheet-like, fluid structures composed mainly of lipids. This allows relatively small, uncomplicated molecules to traverse the membrane with ease. When a molecule of oxygen, for example, diffuses from a higher concentration outside the cell toward a lower concentration on the inside, it is said to move down or along its concentration gradient. It is this concentration gradient which determines the direction and magnitude of molecular movement. This is why the oxygen molecules continuously diffuse into cells. In contrast, the concentration of carbon dioxide, an end product of energy metabolism, is high within the cell; thus, carbon dioxide moves down its concentration gradient and continually diffuses from the cell into the blood.

Facilitated Diffusion. Unlike simple diffusion, in which molecules pass unaided through the semipermeable cell membrane, facilitated diffusion involves the passive, yet highly selective binding of lipid-insoluble molecules and other large molecules to a lipid-soluble carrier molecule. The carrier molecule is a protein called a transporter or *permease* that spans the plasma membrane; its function is to help transfer membrane-insoluble chemicals such as hydrogen, sodium, calcium, and potassium ions, as well as glucose and amino acids, down their concentration gradients across the plasma membrane.

The transport of glucose into the cell is an excellent example of facilitated diffusion. Glucose is a large, lipid-insoluble, uncharged molecule. Without its specific permease, it would have difficulty passing into the cell. With facilitated diffusion, however, the glucose molecule first attaches to a binding site on its specific permease in the plasma membrane. A structural change then occurs in the permease that creates a "passageway" enabling the glucose molecule to cross through the permease into the cytoplasm.

It is indeed fortunate that facilitated diffusion occurs, because glucose is an important energy fuel that should always be in ready supply. It is also fortunate that energy from ATP is not required to "power" glucose transport; if it were, this would only increase the demands on limited reserves of this high-energy compound. Consequently, facilitated diffusion should be considered an energy-conserving mechanism that spares cellular energy for other vital functions.

Osmosis. Osmosis is a special case of diffusion. It involves the *movement of water* through a selectively permeable membrane because of a difference in the concentration of water molecules on both sides of the membrane. Through this passive process, water is distributed throughout the fluid-con-

Faciliated diffusion moves chemicals rapidly. If simple diffusion were the only means for glucose to enter a cell, its maximum rate of uptake would be nearly 500 times slower compared to glucose transport by facilitated diffusion.

taining compartments (intracellular, extracellular, plasma) of the body.

In the example in Figure 1-14C, a semipermeable membrane separates compartments A and B. When there are an equal number of solute particles on sides A and B, the same water volume is present in both compartments. If a solute is added to an aqueous solution, the concentration of the solution increases by the amount of solute added; as more solute is added, its concentration of particles increases and the concentration of water molecules correspondingly decreases. In the example, adding the solute to side B forces water from side A to move through the semipermeable membrane to side B. When this happens, the volume of water now becomes greater on side B than side A. More water flows into an area where there are more particles, leaving less water on the side with fewer solute particles. Eventually, the concentration of solute particles on sides A and B becomes equal.

The total concentration of particles from all solutes in a solution is known as its osmolarity. In living tissue, there is always a difference in the osmolarity of the body's various fluid compartments. This is because the semipermeable membrane that separates different solutions retards the passage of many solute substances, particularly certain ions and intracellular proteins. This maintains a difference in solute concentration on both sides of the membrane. Because water diffuses freely through the plasma membrane, a net movement of water occurs as the system attempts to equalize osmolarity on both sides of the membrane. This often results in dramatic volume changes in the two fluid compartments. At some point, water is unable to gain further entry to the cell because the hydrostatic pressure of water on one side of the cell balances the pressure tending to draw water through the membrane. The pressure on one side of a membrane required to prevent the osmotic movement of

water from the other side is known as the *osmotic pressure* of the solution.

Altering the internal water volume of a cell changes its shape or "tone," a characteristic referred to as tonicity. When a cell neither loses nor gains water when placed in a solution, the solution is said to be *isotonic.* In isotonic solutions, the concentration of a nonpenetrating solute such as sodium chloride is equal on the inside and outside of the cell, and there is no net movement of water. An example of an isotonic solution is the body's extracellular fluid under normal conditions.

A solution is *hypertonic* if it contains a higher concentration of nonpenetrating solutes outside the cell membrane than inside. When this occurs, water migrates out of the cell by the process of osmosis and the cell shrinks in size. Hypertonic solutions are infused into the bloodstream when the objective is to decrease excessive accumulation of water in the tissues, a condition referred to as *edema.*

When the concentration of nondiffusible solutes outside the cell becomes diluted compared to that within the cell, the extracellular solution is considered *hypotonic.* In such cases, the cell takes on water by osmosis and appears bloated. If the condition goes uncorrected, cells can actually burst apart. Hypotonic solutions are administered during dehydration to return the tissues to isotonic conditions.

If the membrane is permeable to both the solute and water (sugar in water is a good example), then both solute and solvent molecules will diffuse until the sugar molecules are equally distributed. On the other hand, if the membrane is impermeable to the solute, then osmotic pressure will draw water in the direction that equalizes the solute concentration on both sides of the membrane. This movement of water will occur until solute concentration is equalized or until the hydrostatic pressure on one side of the membrane counteracts the force exerted by osmotic pressure. Examples of isotonic, hypertonic, and hypotonic solutions are illustrated in Figure 1-15.

Filtration. Filtration is a passive process whereby water and its solutes flow from a region of higher pressure to one of lower pressure. Filtration is the mechanism that allows plasma fluid and its solutes to move across the capillary membrane to literally bathe the tissues. The movement of plasma filtrate (the fluid portion of the blood with no significant amount of proteins) through the kidney tubules also occurs by filtration.

Active Transport Processes

If a substance is unable to move across the cell membrane by one of the four passive transport processes, then energy-requiring active transport processes come into play.

Sodium-Potassium Pump. Figure 1-16 illustrates the operation of the sodium-potassium pump, one of the active transport mechanisms for moving substances through semipermeable membranes. In this process, energy from ATP serves to "pump" ions "uphill" against their electrochemical gradients through the membrane. This is accomplished by a specialized carrier protein enzyme, sodium-potassium ATPase, which serves as the basic pumping mechanism. Recall that substances usually diffuse along their concentration gradients, from an area of higher to lower concentration. In the living cell, however, diffusion alone cannot provide for the optimal distribution of cellular chemicals. Charged particles such as sodium and potassium ions, and large amino acid molecules that are insoluble in the lipid bilayer, must often move against their concentration gradients to carry out their normal functions. Sodium ions, for example, exist in relatively low concentration inside the cell, so there is a tendency for Na^+ to remain there and not pass through the membrane barrier to the outside. In contrast, potassium ions normally exist in higher concentration inside the cell and the tendency is for extracellular K^+ to remain there. During

A. Isotonic solution

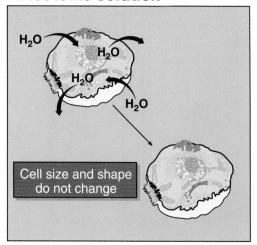

Cell size and shape do not change

B. Hypertonic solution

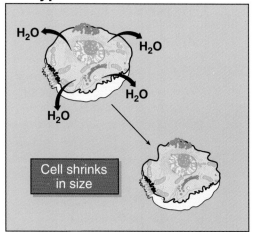

Cell shrinks in size

C. Hypotonic solution

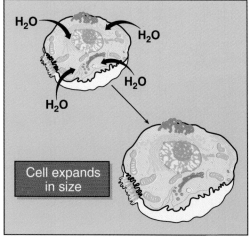

Cell expands in size

Figure 1-15. *A. Isotonic solution.* The cell retains its shape because the concentration of the solute is equal inside and outside the cell. *B. Hypertonic solutions* . The cell shrinks because there is a higher concentration of nonpenetrating solutes outside the cell membrane than inside. *C. Hypotonic solution.* The concentration of nondiffusible solutes in the solution is diluted compared to the concentration within the cell. The cell will actually take on water by osmosis, and can actually burst (lyse).

Figure 1-16. Operation of the sodium-potassium pump. This is a form of active transport that allows chemicals to move in a direction against their normal tendency for diffusion. In this example, sodium ions are pumped from the cytoplasm into the extracellular fluid, while potassium ions are pumped from the extracellular fluid into the cell.

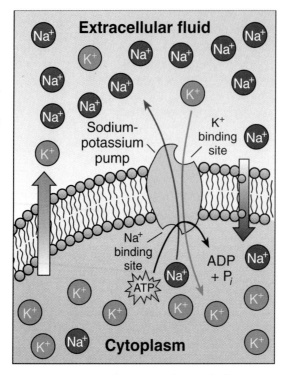

normal nerve and muscle function, however, both of these ions are continually moved against their concentration gradients so that Na^+ becomes concentrated extracellularly, whereas K^+ builds up within the cell. This ability of the sodium-potassium pump to counter the normal tendency of solutes to diffuse is indeed fortunate,

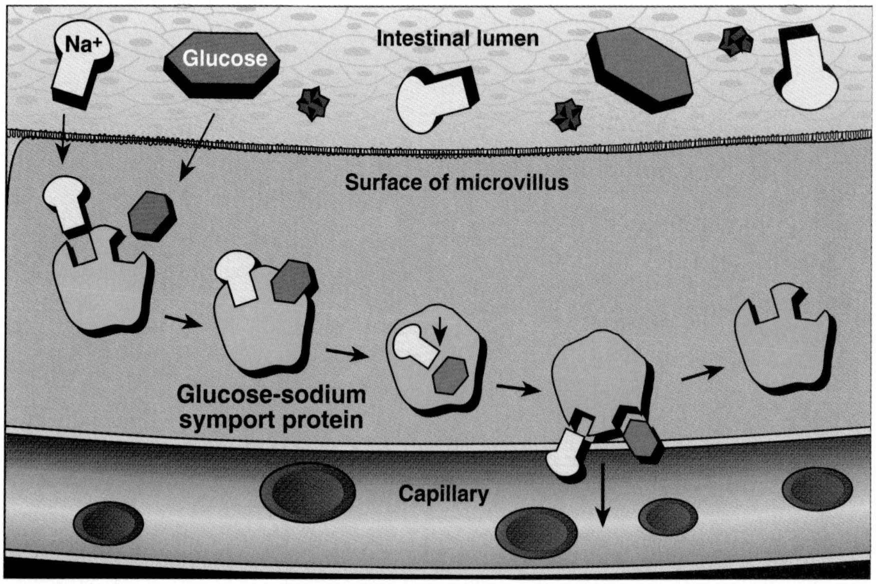

for it is this mechanism that establishes the normal electrochemical gradients so that nerve and muscle can be stimulated.

Coupled Transport In addition to its role in transporting sodium, potassium, and protein across cellular membranes, active transport is crucial in absorbing nutrients from the digestive tract and for reabsorbing important chemicals filtered by the kidneys. Absorption of glucose, for example, takes place by a form of active transport called coupled transport. In this process illustrated in Figure 1-17, a molecule of glucose and a Na^+ join together before they enter an intestinal villus; they then move in the same direction as they are "pumped" through the plasma membrane to the inside of the cell and finally into the bloodstream. Amino acids also join with Na^+ and pass through the intestinal villi. The simultaneous transport of two chemicals in the same direction is called *symport*, and each symport has its own specialized permease with a specific binding site for each substance. Coupled transport is unidirectional, so when the glucose-sodium and amino acid-sodium symports leave the intestine to enter the blood, they cannot move backward to re-enter the intestine.

Bulk Transport. Bulk transport is an energy-requiring process for moving large particles and macromolecules through cell membranes. There are two ways in which this is accomplished: exocytosis and endocytosis.

Exocytosis. This transfer process moves substances such as hormones, neurotransmitters, and mucous secretions from the intracellular to extracellular fluids. There are three distinct phases to exocytosis. First, the substance to be transferred is enclosed within a membranous, sac-like pouch. The pouch then migrates to the plasma membrane; once it fuses to the membrane, its contents are ejected into the extracellular fluids.

Figure 1-17. Example of coupled transport. A molecule of glucose and a sodium ion are carried together in a symport protein through the capillary's plasma membrane where they are then released into the bloodstream.

Endocytosis. In this transfer process of endocytosis substances are surrounded by the cell's plasma membrane which then pinches away and moves into the cytoplasm.

• • • • • • • • • • • • • •

HOMEOSTASIS

Homeostasis refers to the integration of self-regulating biologic processes that tend to maintain a stability or relative constancy in the internal environment. In essence, this stability is not static but rather a dynamic equilibrium or steady state as the body responds to continually changing internal and external conditions. When disruption of stability occurs within a biologic system, mechanisms of regulation respond to the change to establish a new balance. The unique aspect of biologic regulation, as contrasted to mechanical feedback regulation such as through gyroscopes or mechanical governors, is the greater flexibility and potential for adaptation in biologic systems. Homeostasis of blood temperature relates to the maintenance of a relative constancy of core temperature at about 37°C at rest. During exercise, the core temperature is regulated at a somewhat higher temperature. In addition, regular exercise training brings about adaptations in physiology (circulation, blood volume, sweating capacity) that facilitate the maintenance of an internal constancy. In general terms:

• Homeostatic regulatory mechanisms are activated by a stimulus caused by a change in the internal environment (e.g., blood gases, core temperature, circulating nutrients).

• Deviations from equilibrium are detected by means of sensor or receptor cells that then initiate responses to reverse the initial change and return the biologic system to homeostasis.

• Mechanisms for homeostasis operate by means of a general feedback. In essence, a change in one direction brings about a response to cause a change in the opposite direction to remove the stimulus. Thus, an increase in carbon dioxide in the blood during exercise stimulates the medulla to increase pulmonary ventilation. This adaptive response facilitates carbon dioxide elimination in the lungs. Consequently, this feedback mechanism provides for a relatively stable level of carbon dioxide in arterial blood delivered to tissues despite rather dramatic increases in this gas in the blood leaving the tissues.

ENERGY TRANSFER AND PHYSICAL ACTIVITY

SECTION I

There is a useful analogy for how a car and the human body obtain the energy to make them "go." In an automobile engine, the proper mixture of gasoline fuel with oxygen ignites to provide the energy necessary to drive the pistons. Various gears and linkages harness this energy to turn the wheels, and increasing or decreasing the energy supply either speeds up or slows down the engine. Similarly, the human body must continuously be able to extract the energy from its fuel and harness this energy to perform its many complex functions. Besides the considerable energy expended for muscular contraction during rest and various intensities of physical activity, the body expends substantial energy for other "quieter" forms of biologic work. This includes the energy required for the:

- Digestion, absorption, and assimilation of food nutrients
- Function of glands that secrete hormones at rest and during exercise
- Establishment of the proper electrochemical gradients along cell membranes for the transmission of signals from the brain through the nerves to the muscles
- Synthesis of new chemical compounds such as the thick and thin protein structures in skeletal muscle tissue that enlarges with resistance training.

During exercise, the ability to swim, jog or run, and roller skate and ski long distances is framed largely by the body's capacity to extract energy from food nutrients and transfer it to the contractile elements of skeletal muscle. This transfer occurs through thousands of complex chemical reactions that require a continual supply and utilization of oxygen. Such oxygen-requiring reactions are termed aerobic. In contrast, anaerobic chemical reactions generate energy rapidly for short periods and do not require oxygen. This rapid method of energy transfer is crucial for maintaining a high standard of performance in activities requiring all-out bursts of exercise such as sprinting in track and swimming, or stop-and-go activities like soccer, basketball, volleyball, and football. The crucial point to remember is that the direct transfer of chemical energy generated in aerobic and anaerobic reactions is required to power all forms of biologic work.

This Section, consisting of Chapters 2 to 5, presents an overview of areas related to energy transfer in general, and more specifically to energy transfer in exercise with a focus on:

- How cells extract the chemical energy bound within the food nutrients
- How this energy is transferred to sustain physiologic function during light, moderate, and strenuous exercise.

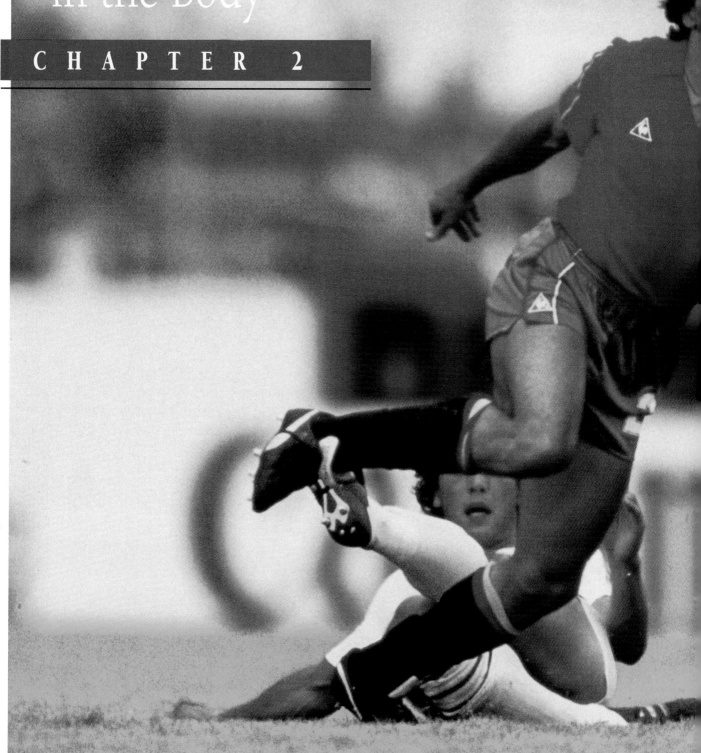

Energy Transfer
in the Body

CHAPTER 2

After reading this chapter you should be able to:

- Identify the high energy phosphates and discuss their roles in the various forms of biologic work.
- Outline the process of electron transport-oxidative phosphorylation and indicate the role of oxygen in energy metabolism.
- Describe the process by which anaerobic energy is provided to the cell in the breakdown of food, and discuss how lactic acid is formed.
- Discuss the role of the Krebs cycle in the breakdown of the food nutrients, and indicate the general pathways through which the macronutrients enter this cycle.
- Contrast the ATP yield from the breakdown of carbohydrates, lipids, and proteins.
- Discuss the statement, "Fats burn in a carbohydrate flame."

The human body must be continually supplied with chemical energy to perform its many complex functions. Energy derived from the oxidation of food is not released suddenly at some kindling temperature because the body, unlike a mechanical engine, cannot use heat energy. If this were the case, the body fluids would actually boil and our tissues would burst into flames. Rather, the chemical energy trapped within the bonds of carbohydrates, lipids, and proteins is extracted in relatively small quantities during complex, enzymatically-controlled reactions that occur in the relatively cool, watery medium of the cell. This process reduces the loss of energy as heat and provides for much greater efficiency in energy transformations. This enables the body to make direct use of chemical energy. In a sense, energy can be supplied to the cells as needed. The story of how the body maintains its continuous energy supply begins with adenosine triphosphate, the body's special carrier for free energy.

ATP IS THE ENERGY CURRENCY

The energy in food is not transferred directly to the cells for biologic work. Rather, this "nutrient energy" is harvested and funneled through the energy-rich compound *adenosine triphosphate* or ATP. The potential energy within the ATP molecule is then used for all of the cell's energy-requiring processes. In essence, this energy receiver-energy donor cycle represents the two major energy-transforming activities in the cell:

- To form and conserve ATP from the potential energy in food.
- To extract the chemical energy in ATP for biologic work.

Figure 2-1 shows the ATP molecule formed from a molecule of adenine and ribose, called adenosine, linked to three phosphate molecules. The bonds that link the two outermost phosphates are termed high-energy bonds because they represent a considerable quantity of potential energy within the ATP molecule.

When ATP joins with water in hydrolysis, it is catalyzed by the enzyme *adenosine triphosphatase*. During hydrolysis, the outermost phosphate bond is broken and a new compound called adenosine diphosphate or ADP is formed. In this reaction, approximately 7.3 kilocalories (kcal) of free energy (i.e., energy available for work) are liberated per mole of ATP degraded to ADP.

$$ATP + H_2O \xrightarrow{\text{ATPase}} ADP + P - 7.3 \text{ kcal per mole}$$

The free energy liberated in the hydrolysis of ATP is a measure of the energy difference between the reactants and the end products. Because considerable energy is generated in this reaction, ATP is referred to as a *high-energy phosphate* compound. Infrequently, additional energy is released when another phosphate is split from ADP. In some reactions of biosynthesis, the two terminal phos-

> **Energy.** From a broad perspective, energy can be viewed as the capacity or ability to do work.

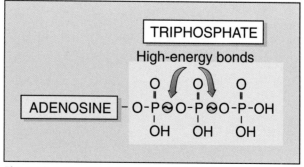

Figure 2-1. Simplified illustration of ATP, the energy currency of the cell. The symbol ⊖ represents the high-energy bonds.

phates from ATP are simultaneously donated in the construction of new cellular material. The remaining molecule with a single phosphate group is adenosine monophosphate or AMP.

The energy liberated during ATP breakdown is directly transferred to other energy-requiring molecules. In muscle, for example, this energy activates specific sites on the contractile elements causing the muscle fiber to shorten. *Because energy from ATP is harnessed to power all forms of biologic work, ATP is considered the cell's "energy currency."* Figure 2-2 illustrates the general role of ATP as energy currency.

The splitting of an ATP molecule takes place whether oxygen is available or not. This reaction is immediate, anaerobic, and energy-liberating. The cell's capacity for ATP breakdown enables it to generate energy for immediate use; this would not occur, however, if oxygen were required at all times for energy metabolism. For this reason, all types of exercise can be performed immediately without consuming oxygen, such as sprinting for a bus, driving a golf ball, or lifting a heavy barbell. The well known prac-

tice of holding one's breath during a sprint swim provides a clear example of ATP splitting without reliance on atmospheric oxygen. This same air-withholding maneuver, although not advisable, can be done during a 100-yard sprint on the track, lifting a barbell, or a dash up several flights of stairs. In each case, energy metabolism proceeds uninterrupted as the energy for muscular contraction is supplied predominantly from anaerobic sources.

••••••••••••••

CP IS THE ENERGY RESERVOIR

Only a small quantity of ATP is actually stored within the cell. Thus, it must be continually resynthesized at the rate it is used. This situation provides a sensitive mechanism for regulating energy metabolism in the cell. By maintaining only a small amount of ATP, its relative concentration (and corresponding concentration of ADP) is altered rapidly with any increase in a cell's energy demands. Any change in energy requirement (that is, a disturbance in the cell's current state of activity)

Rapid energy release. Anaerobic energy release can be viewed as an emergency or back-up power source that is called upon when the body requires energy in excess of what can be generated aerobically.

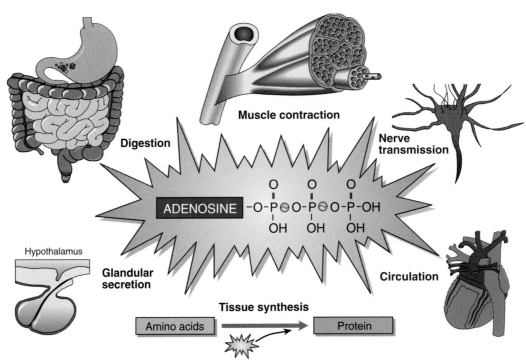

Figure 2-2. ATP is the energy currency that powers all forms of biologic work.

immediately stimulates the breakdown of stored energy-containing compounds to provide energy for ATP resynthesis. This is why energy transfer increases rapidly at the start of exercise. And as one might expect, the increase in energy transfer depends on the intensity of the exercise. In going from sitting in a chair to walking, for example, the energy transfer increases about four-fold. However, when changing from a walk to an all-out anaerobic sprint, the energy transfer can rapidly increase 120 times!

ATP: A Limited Currency. Although ATP serves as the energy currency for *all* cells, its quantity is limited. In fact, only about 85 g (3 oz) of ATP is stored in the body at any one time. This would provide only enough energy for performing all-out exercise for several seconds. Thus, ATP must be constantly resynthesized to continuously supply energy for biologic work. Some energy for ATP resynthesis is supplied directly and rapidly by the anaerobic splitting of a phosphate molecule from another energy-rich compound called *creatine phosphate* or CP. This molecule is similar to ATP because a large amount of energy is released when the bond is split between its creatine and phosphate molecules. Figure 2-3 presents a schematic illustration of the release and use of the phosphate-bond energy in ATP and CP.

In both reactions, the arrows point in opposite directions to indicate that the reactions are reversible. In other words, creatine (C) and phosphate (P) can be joined again to reform CP. This is also true of ATP where the union of ADP and P reforms ATP. Resynthesis of ATP occurs if sufficient energy is available to rejoin an ADP molecule with one P molecule. The breakdown of CP can supply this energy. Cells store CP in considerably larger quantities than ATP. The mobilization of CP for energy is almost instantaneous and does not require oxygen. For this reason, CP is considered a "reservoir" of high-energy phosphate bonds.

THE HIGH-ENERGY PHOSPHATES

The energy released from the breakdown of the energy-rich phosphates ATP and CP can sustain all-out exercise, such as running, cycling, or swimming, for approximately 5 to 8 seconds. In the 100-meter sprint, the body cannot maintain maximum speed for longer than this duration. During the last few seconds of the race, the runners are actually slowing down, and the winner is often the one who slows down least! From an energy standpoint, the winner is the one who is better able to supply and use this short-term supply of phosphate-bond energy. Mobilization of energy from the combined phosphate pool of ATP + CP is important in determining one's ability to generate and sustain maximum power for a relatively short duration.

In almost all sports, the capacity of the ATP-CP energy system plays an important role in the success or failure of some phase of performance. If an all-out effort must continue beyond 8 seconds, or if moderate exercise continues for much longer periods, an additional energy source is required to resynthesize ATP. If this does not happen, the "fuel" supply will become depleted and movement will cease. As will be discussed shortly, the foods we eat and store for ready access in the body provide the energy for continually recharging the cellular supply of ATP and CP.

The Source of Energy is Important. Identification of the predominant source(s) of energy required for a particular sport or physical activity provides the basis for an effective physiologic training program. For example, sports such as football and baseball require a high energy output

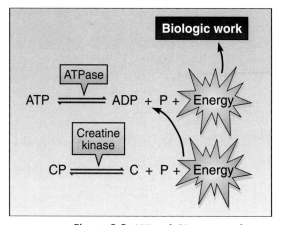

Figure 2-3. ATP and CP are anaerobic sources of phosphate-bond energy. The energy liberated from the hydrolysis (splitting) of CP is used to rebond ADP and P to form ATP.

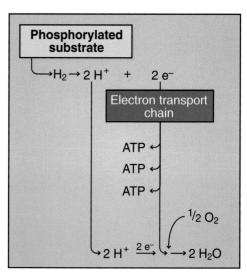

Figure 2-4. A general scheme for the oxidation (removal of electrons) of hydrogen and accompanying electron transport. In this process, oxygen is reduced (gain of electrons) and water is formed.

for brief periods of time. These performances rely almost exclusively on energy transfer from the high energy phosphate system. Paying close attention to developing this system is important in training for optimal performance in these sports.

Transfer of Energy by Chemical Bonds. An important point about human energy dynamics involves the transfer of energy by means of chemical bonds. Potential energy is released by the splitting of bonds and conserved by the formation of new bonds. Some energy lost by one molecule can be transferred to the chemical structure of another molecule and not appear as heat. Compounds relatively low in potential energy can be "juiced-up" by energy transfer from the high-energy phosphates to accomplish biologic work.

Adenosine triphosphate serves as the ideal energy-transfer agent. In one respect, ATP "traps" in its phosphate bonds a large portion of potential energy in the original food molecule. It also readily transfers this energy to other compounds to raise them to a higher level of activation. This transfer of energy in the form of phosphate bonds is termed *phosphorylation.* The energy for phosphorylation is ultimately generated by the oxidation ("biologic burning") of carbohydrates, lipids, and proteins consumed in the diet.

CELLULAR OXIDATION

Recall from Chapter 1 that when a molecule accepts electrons from an electron donor it is said to be reduced. The molecule that gives up the electron is said to be oxidized. Oxidation (giving up an electron) and reduction (accepting an electron) reactions are coupled in that for every oxidation there is a reduction reaction. In essence, *cellular oxidation-reduction is the crucial mechanism for energy metabolism in the body.* In this process, hydrogen atoms are

continually stripped from the carbohydrate, lipid, and protein nutrients. Carrier molecules within the cell's "energy factories," the mitochondria, remove electrons from hydrogen (oxidation) and eventually pass them to oxygen (reduction). In this oxidation-reduction process high energy phosphates are produced in the form of ATP.

Electron Transport

Figure 2-4 illustrates the general scheme for the oxidation of hydrogen and the accompanying electron transport to oxygen. During cellular oxidation, hydrogen atoms are not merely turned loose in the cell fluid. Rather, the release of hydrogen from the nutrient substrate is catalyzed by highly specific *dehydrogenase* enzymes. The electrons (energy) from hydrogen are picked up in pairs by the coenzyme part of the dehydrogenase that is usually the vitamin B (niacin)-containing coenzyme, *nicotinamide adeninedinucleotide* or NAD^+. While the substrate is being oxidized and losing hydrogen (electrons), NAD^+ is gaining a hydrogen and two electrons and being reduced to NADH; the other hydrogen appears in ionized form in the cell fluid as H^+.

The other important electron acceptor in the oxidation of the food fragments is *flavin adenine dinucleotide,* or FAD. Flavin adenine dinucleotide is derived from the B-vitamin riboflavin. This coenzyme also catalyzes dehydrogenations and accepts pairs of electrons. Unlike NAD^+, however, FAD accepts both hydrogens to become $FADH_2$.

The NADH and $FADH_2$ formed in the breakdown of the food nutrients are energy-rich molecules because they carry electrons that have a high-energy-transfer potential. On the inner membranes of the mitochondria, pairs of electrons carried by NADH and $FADH_2$ are then passed in "bucket brigade" fashion by the *cytochromes,* a series of iron-protein electron carriers. The iron por-

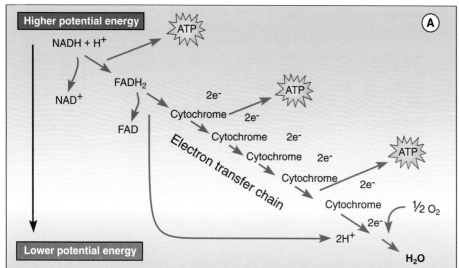

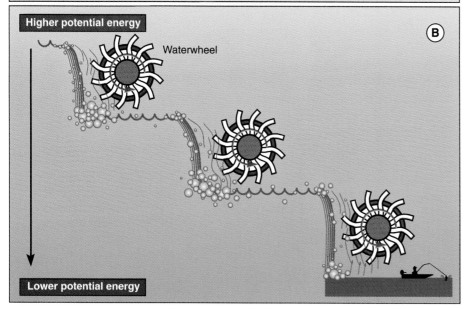

Figure 2-5. Examples of harnessing potential energy. *A. In the body.* The electron transfer chain involves the removal of electrons from hydrogens and their ultimate delivery to oxygen. In this oxidation-reduction process, much of the chemical energy stored within the hydrogen atom is not dissipated to kinetic energy, but rather is conserved in forming ATP. *B. In industry.* Energy from falling water is harnessed to turn the waterwheel which in turn is used to perform mechanical work.

tion of each cytochrome can exist in either its oxidized (ferric or Fe^{+++}) or reduced (ferrous or Fe^{++}) ionic state. By accepting an electron, the ferric portion of a specific cytochrome becomes reduced to its ferrous form. In turn, this donates its electron to the next *cytochrome,* and so on down the line. The cytochromes transfer electrons by shuttling between these iron forms.

The transport of electrons by specific carrier molecules constitutes what is known as the respiratory chain. This is the final common pathway where the electrons extracted from hydrogen are passed to oxygen. For each pair of hydrogen atoms, two electrons flow down the chain and reduce one atom of oxygen to form water. Of the five specific cytochromes, only the last one, cytochrome oxidase (cytochrome A3), can discharge its electron directly to oxygen. Figure 2-5A shows the route for the oxidation of hydrogen and the accompanying electron transport and energy transfer in the respiratory chain. Free energy is released in the respiratory chain in relatively small amounts. In several of the electron transfers, energy is conserved by the formation of high-energy phosphate bonds.

Oxidative Phosphorylation

Oxidative phosphorylation refers to how ATP becomes synthesized during the transfer of electrons from NADH and $FADH_2$ to molecular oxygen. This important process represents the cell's primary means for extracting and trapping chemical energy in the form of high-energy phosphates. *Over 90% of ATP synthesis is accomplished in the respiratory chain by oxidative reactions coupled with phosphorylation.*

In a way, the process of oxidative phosphorylation can be likened to a waterfall divided into several separate cascades by the intervention of waterwheels at different heights. As depicted in Figure 2-5B, the waterwheels harness the energy of the falling water; similarly, the electrochemical energy generated in electron transport from one respiratory chain component to the next is harnessed and transferred (or coupled) to ADP. The energy in NADH is transferred to ADP to reform ATP at three distinct coupling sites during electron transport (Fig. 2-5A). This oxidation of hydrogen and subsequent phosphorylation can be formulated as follows:

$$NADH + H^+ + 3\ ADP + 3\ P + 1/2\ O_2 \rightarrow NAD^+ + H_2O + 3\ ATP$$

Note in the above reaction that for each $NADH + H^+$, there are three ATP formed. However, if hydrogen is originally donated by $FADH_2$ only two molecules of ATP are formed for each hydrogen pair oxidized. This occurs because $FADH_2$ enters the respiratory chain at a lower energy level at a point beyond the site of the first ATP synthesis.

Efficiency of Electron Transport and Oxidative Phosphorylation

Approximately 7 kcal of energy are stored for each mole of ATP formed. Because 3 moles of ATP are generated in the oxidation of 1 mole of NADH, about 21 kcal (7 kcal / mole x 3) are conserved as chemical energy. Since a total of 52 kcal are liberated during the oxidation of a mole of NADH, the relative efficiency of electron transport-oxidative phosphorylation for harnessing chemical energy is approximately 40% (21 kcal ÷ 52 kcal x 100). The remaining 60% of the energy is lost to the body as heat. Considering that a steam engine transforms its fuel into useful energy with an efficiency of only about 30%, the value of 40% for the human body represents a relatively high efficiency rate.

Role of Oxygen in Energy Metabolism

Three prerequisites must be met for the continual resynthesis of ATP during coupled oxidative phosphorylation. These conditions are:

(1) A reducing agent in the form of NADH (or $FADH_2$) must be available.

(2) An oxidizing agent, oxygen, must be present in the tissues.

(3) Enzymes must be present in sufficient concentration to make the energy transfer reactions "go."

In strenuous exercise, when the rate of oxygen delivery (condition #2) or its rate of utilization (condition #3) may be inadequate, a relative imbalance is created between the release of hydrogen and its final acceptance by oxygen. In this condition, electron flow down the respiratory chain begins to "back up" with an accumulation of hydrogens bound to NAD^+ and FAD. As is discussed in a subsequent section, the compound pyruvic acid temporarily binds these excess hydrogens (electrons) to form lactic acid; this permits continuation of coupled oxidative phosphorylation by electron transport.

The role of oxygen in energy metabolism is clearly to serve as the final electron acceptor in the respiratory chain and combine with hydrogen to form water. This process of coupled oxidative phosphorylation with oxygen serving as the final electron and H$^+$ acceptor is referred to as aerobic metabolism. In one sense, this term is misleading because oxygen does not participate directly in the synthesis of ATP. The presence of oxygen at the "end of the line," however, largely determines one's capability for ATP production and hence the ability to sustain exercise. Chapter 5 describes the method to measure an individual's maximum capacity for aerobic energy transfer during exercise.

Part 1 PHOSPHATE BOND ENERGY

SUMMARY

1. The energy contained within the chemical structure of carbohydrates, lipids, and proteins is not released in the body suddenly at some kindling temperature; rather, it is released slowly in small quantities during complex, enzymatically–controlled reactions. This allows for greater efficiency during the energy transfer processes.

2. About 40% of the potential energy in the food nutrients is transferred to the high energy compound ATP. When the terminal phosphate bond of ATP is broken, the free energy liberated is harnessed to power all forms of biologic work. Although the supply of ATP in the muscles is limited to about 85 g, ATP is still considered the body's energy currency,

3. Creatine phosphate interacts with ADP to form ATP. Thus, CP serves as an energy reservoir to replenish ATP rapidly. Collectively, ATP and CP are referred to as the high energy phosphates.

4. Phosphorylation is the process by which energy is transferred in the form of phosphate bonds. During phosphorylation, ADP and creatine are continually recycled into ATP and CP.

5. Cellular oxidation occurs in the mitochondria and involves the transfer of electrons from hydrogen to oxygen. This results in the release and transfer of chemical energy to form the high–energy phosphates.

6. In the aerobic resynthesis of ATP, oxygen's primary role is to serve as the final electron acceptor in the respiratory chain and to combine with hydrogen to form water. In terms of energy transfer, this is the cell's "main event."

EXPRESSING METABOLIC DATA: THE PROBLEM OF SCALING

All living species differ in body size and shape. For example, an elephant weighs 100,000 times more than a mouse, and the smallest shrew when fully grown, is only one-tenth the weight of the mouse and one-millionth the weight of the elephant! These differences in structure play an important role in determining the differences in the biologic function of species. The exact relationship between structure and function depends on the variables under consideration. For example, should the heart and circulation, or metabolic processes be fundamentally different in an elephant compared to a mouse simply because of differences in body size? Stated another way, will the resting metabolic rate of the elephant be proportionally larger (100,000 times larger) than the mouse? And what consequences do changes in size have in terms of function? That is, what effect do changes in the size of the pulmonary, cardiovascular, and muscular systems have on the functional capacity of these systems? Such questions are called questions of scaling, and have direct application to exercise physiology. In the above example, if the resting metabolic rate of the mouse is 0.003 kcal · min^{-1}, is it reasonable to predict that the metabolic rate of the elephant at rest would be scaled proportionally by 100,000 times, or 300 kcal · min^{-1}?

The question of scaling takes on added importance when trying to compare different functions of persons of different sizes. For example, how should we compare, equate, or evaluate the metabolic rate of an obese person compared to a leaner counterpart? Do we assume that the metabolic rate of an overfat person is proportionally higher simply because of an increased body size? Or is the metabolic rate also altered because of differences in function caused by their obesity, independent of their absolute size?

One approach to this problem is to identify the specific relationship between body size and function by plotting these variables on a bivariate scale. When biological variables are plotted on regular graph paper they often plot as a non-linear or curved line, but as a straight line

plotted on logarithmic coordinates. Many observations relating biological variables to body size conform to the general equation: $y = a x^b$, where $\log y = \log a + b \log x$

This equation is often called an allometric scaling equation. The exponent b is the slope (rate of change in one variable per unit change in the other variable) of the line that can be either positive or negative. When we buy vegetables, for example, the amount we pay increases in direct proportion to the amount we buy. This is a simple proportionality, and a plot would show a straight line relationship with a slope of 1.00. A biological example of this linear relationship is blood volume in mammals. The blood makes up a constant and proportional fraction of the total body mass, and the larger the animal the more blood it will have (and this volume will increase in direct proportion to changes in body mass). This is shown in the insert figure along with other examples of allometric relationships. If one of the variables increases at a slower rate than would be indicated by simple proportionality, the line will have a slope less than 1.00. A well-known example is metabolic rate that increases with body size, but at a rate less than would be predicted by simple proportionality. In this case, the slope of the plotted line is 0.75. This means we should not expect the metabolic rate of the elephant to be 100,000 lager than the mouse, but rather larger by a function equal to the body weight raised to the 0.75 power. This suggests that we should compare people's metabolic rate relative to body weight$^{0.75}$.

It has become convention in exercise physiology, however, to express metabolic rate or oxygen uptake relative to body weight not raised to *any* power. In essence, the expression of oxygen uptake in $mlO_2 \cdot$ kg-body mass$^{-1} \cdot$ min^{-1} makes the assumption that the oxygen uptake is proportional to the body mass (which we know is not correct). Nevertheless, use of this proportional expression is almost universal and is used as a way to "equate" the energy metabolism of people who may differ vastly in body size. While the error in using this proportional expression can be great when applied to individuals at the extremes of the body weight continuum (jockeys vs sumo wrestlers, or ballet dancers vs heavyweight lifters), the error is probably acceptable for most normal weight individuals.

The energy released in the breakdown of the food nutrients serves one crucial purpose — to phosphorylate ADP to reform the energy-rich compound ATP (Fig. 2-6). Although the breakdown of various food nutrients during energy metabolism is geared toward generating phosphate-bond energy, the specific pathways of degradation differ depending on the nutrients metabolized. In the sections that follow, we show how the potential energy in the food nutrients is extracted and utilized to synthesize ATP.

ENERGY RELEASE FROM CARBOHYDRATE

The primary function of carbohydrate is to supply energy for cellular work. Our discussion of nutrient energy metabolism begins with carbohydrates for three reasons:

- Carbohydrate is the only nutrient whose stored energy can be used to generate ATP anaerobically. This is important in vigorous exercise that requires rapid energy release above levels supplied by aerobic metabolic reactions. In this case, stored glycogen and blood glucose must supply the main portion of energy for ATP resynthesis.
- During light and moderate aerobic exercise, carbohydrate supplies about one-half of the body's energy requirements.
- A continual breakdown of some carbohydrate is required so that lipid nutrients can be processed through the metabolic mill and used for energy. It is not uncommon in high intensity, prolonged aerobic exercise such as marathon running for a participant to experience fatigue — a state associated with a depletion of glycogen in the muscles and liver.

The complete breakdown of one mole of glucose to carbon dioxide and water yields a maximum of 686 kcal of chemical free energy, or energy available for work.

$$C_6H_{12}O_6 + 6O_2 \rightarrow 6CO_2 + 6H_2O + 686 \text{ kcal per mole}$$

In the body, however, the complete breakdown of glucose is accompanied by the conservation of energy in the form of ATP. Because 7.3 kcal are required to synthesize each mole of ATP from ADP and inorganic phosphate, it would be theoretically possible to form 94 moles of ATP per mole of glucose by coupling all of the energy in glucose to phosphorylation (686 kcal ÷ 7.3 kcal/mole = 94 moles). In the muscles, however, only about 40% or 277 kcal of the total 686 kcal is actually conserved in phosphate bonds with the remainder dissipated as heat. Consequently, about 38 moles of ATP (not 94 moles) are regenerated in glucose breakdown (277 kcal ÷ 7.3 kcal/mole = 38 mole) with an accompanying gain in free energy of 277 kcal. In the following sections we will show exactly how and where the ATP is formed in the energy transfer process. You should also note that

The anaerobic macronutrient. During high-intensity, fatiguing exercise in which anaerobic reactions predominate, carbohydrates are the main source of energy supply.

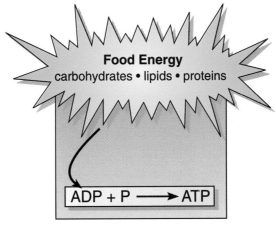

Figure 2-6. The potential energy in food is used to resynthesize ATP.

there is a difference in the total ATP yield between glucose and glycogen. There is an additional ATP generated when glycogen is metabolized. Furthermore, as will be discussed shortly, it requires the energy from 2 ATP to initiate the breakdown of the glucose molecule. Consequently, the net ATP yield from glucose breakdown is 36 ATP.

Anaerobic vs. Aerobic. There are two stages for glucose degradation in the body. The first involves the rapid breakdown of a glucose molecule to two molecules of pyruvic acid. These reactions involve energy transfers that do not require oxygen and are termed anaerobic. In the second phase of glucose catabolism, the pyruvic acid molecules are further degraded to carbon dioxide and water. Energy transfers from these reactions involve electron transport and the accompanying oxidative phosphorylation. Thus, these chemical reactions are referred to as aerobic.

Anaerobic Energy from Glucose: Glycolysis

When a glucose molecule enters a cell to be used for energy, it undergoes a series of chemical reactions collectively termed *glycolysis.* When this series of reactions starts with stored glycogen the process is called *glycogenolysis.* These reactions, summarized in Figure 2-7, occur in the watery medium of the cell outside of the mitochondrion. In a sense, this process represents a more primitive form of energy transfer that is well developed in amphibians, reptiles, fish, and marine mammals. In skeletal muscle the breakdown of stored glycogen for energy is regulated and limited by the enzyme *phosphorylase.* The activity of this enzyme is greatly influenced by the action of *epinephrine,* a hormone of the sympathetic nervous system.

In the first reaction, ATP acts as a phosphate donor to phosphorylate glucose to glucose 6-phosphate. In most tissues of the body, the glucose molecule is "trapped" in the cell. The glucose molecule can now be linked together, or *polymerized,* with other glucose molecules to form glycogen, the storage form of glucose. This process is dependent on the enzyme *glycogen synthetase.* In energy metabolism, however, glucose 6-phosphate is changed to fructose 6-phosphate. At this stage, no energy has been extracted, yet energy has been incorporated into the original glucose molecule at the expense of one molecule of ATP. In a sense, phosphorylation has "primed the pump" so that energy metabolism can proceed. Then, controlled by the enzyme *phosphofructokinase* (PFK), the fructose 6-phosphate molecule gains an additional phosphate and is changed to fructose 1, 6-diphosphate. It is the activity level of PFK that probably places a limit on the rate of glycolysis during all-out exercise. Fructose 1, 6-diphosphate then splits into two phosphorylated molecules with three carbon chains; these are further degraded in five successive reactions to pyruvic acid.

Substrate-Level Phosphorylation. Most of the energy generated in the reactions of glycolysis is insufficient to resynthesize ATP and is lost to the body as heat. In reactions 7 and 10, the energy released from the glucose intermediates is sufficient to stimulate the direct transfer of a phosphate group to ADP. This generates a total of four molecules of ATP. Because two molecules of ATP were lost in the initial phosphorylation of the glucose molecule, the *net* energy transfer from glycolysis results in a gain of two molecules of ATP. These specific energy transfers from substrate to ADP by phosphorylation do not require oxygen. Rather, energy is directly transferred to phosphate bonds in the anaerobic process called substrate-level phosphorylation. This process of energy conservation during glycolysis operates at an efficiency of about 30%.

Only about 5% of the total ATP generated in the complete breakdown of the glucose molecule is formed during glycolysis. Due to the high concentration of glycolytic enzymes and the speed of these reactions, however, significant energy for muscle contraction can be provided rapidly from glycolysis. The athlete sprinting at the end of the mile run relies heavily on this form of anaerobic energy transfer. It is important to remember that this rapid form of energy transfer is possible *only* from the breakdown of the body's carbohydrate stores by glycolytic reactions.

Hydrogen Release. During glycolysis, two pairs of hydrogen atoms are stripped from the substrate and their electrons passed to NAD^+ to form NADH (Fig. 2-7). Normally, if these electrons were processed directly through the respiratory chain, three molecules of ATP would be generated for each molecule of NADH oxidized. The mitochondrion, however, is impermeable to NADH formed in the cytoplasm during glycolysis. Consequently, the electrons from extramitochondrial NADH must be shuttled indirectly into the mitochondria. In skeletal muscle, this route ends with electrons being passed to FAD to form $FADH_2$ at a point below the first formation of ATP (see Fig. 2-5A). Thus, in skeletal muscle, two, rather than three, ATP molecules are formed when cytoplasmic NADH is oxidized by the respiratory chain. Because two molecules of NADH are formed in glycolysis, four molecules of ATP are generated aerobically by subsequent electron transport-oxidative phosphorylation.

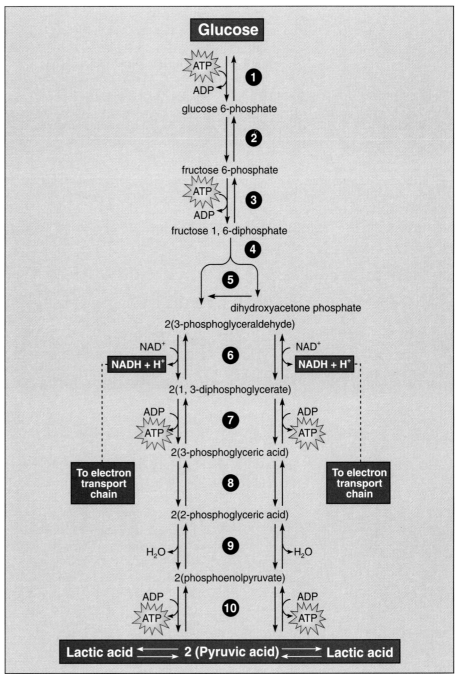

Figure 2-7. Glycolysis: a series of 10, enzymatically–controlled chemical reactions involving the anaerobic breakdown of glucose to two molecules of pyruvic acid. Lactic acid is formed when the oxidation of NADH does not keep pace with its formation in glycolysis.

Formation of Lactic Acid. Sufficient oxygen is available to the cells during moderate levels of energy metabolism. Consequently, the hydrogens (electrons) stripped from the substrate and carried by NADH are oxidized within the mitochondria and passed to oxy-

Always some lactic acid. Even at rest some lactic acid is continually formed by the energy metabolism of red blood cells. This is because these cells contain no mitochondria and thus drive their energy from the glycolytic process.

Lactic acid formation permits glycolysis to continue. The temporary storage of hydrogen with pyruvic acid to form lactic acid is a unique aspects of energy metabolism because it allows glycolysis to continue to generate ATP anaerobically.

A muscle fiber for sprinters. Fast-twitch muscle fibers are rich in the glycolytic enzyme PFK making them ideally suited for generating anaerobic energy via glycolysis.

Named for a Nobel laureate. The Krebs cycle was named after the chemist Hans Krebs, who was awarded the Nobel Prize in 1953 for his pioneering studies of these vital metabolic processes.

gen to form water. In a biochemical sense a "steady state," or more precisely a "steady rate," exists because hydrogen is oxidized at about the same rate as it is made available. Biochemists frequently refer to this condition as *aerobic glycolysis* with pyruvic acid being the end product.

In strenuous exercise, when the energy demands exceed either the oxygen supply or its rate of utilization, all of the hydrogen joined to NADH cannot be processed through the respiratory chain. Continued release of anaerobic energy in glycolysis depends on the availability of NAD$^+$ for the oxidation of 3-phosphoglyceraldehyde (see reaction 6 in Fig. 2-7); otherwise, the rapid rate of glycolysis would "grind to a halt." Under conditions of *anaerobic glycolysis*, NAD$^+$ is "freed-up" as pairs of "excess" hydrogens combine temporarily with pyruvic acid in an additional step, catalyzed by the enzyme *lactic dehydrogenase,* to form lactic acid in the reversible reaction shown in Figure 2-8.

The temporary storage of hydrogen with pyruvic acid is a unique aspect of energy metabolism because it provides a ready "sump" or storage bin for the disappearance of the end products of anaerobic glycolysis. Also, once lactic acid is formed in the muscle, it diffuses rapidly to the blood where it is buffered to lactate and carried away from the site of energy metabolism. In this way, glycolysis can proceed to supply additional anaerobic energy for the resynthesis of ATP. This avenue for extra energy is only temporary, however, because as the level of lactic acid in the blood and muscles increases, the regeneration of ATP cannot keep pace with its utilization. When this occurs, fatigue sets in and exercise performance is diminished. Fatigue is probably mediated by increased acidity, which inactivates various enzymes involved in energy transfer, as well as diminishes some aspect of the muscle's contractile properties.

Lactic acid should not be viewed as a metabolic "waste product." To the contrary, it is a valuable source of chemical energy that accumulates and is retained in the body during heavy physical exercise. When sufficient oxygen is once again available, as in recovery or when the pace of exercise is slowed, hydrogens attached to lactic acid are scavenged by NAD$^+$ and subsequently oxidized with the formation of ATP. Consequently, lactic acid is readily reconverted to pyruvic acid and used as an energy source. In addition, the potential energy in the lactate and pyruvate molecules formed in muscle during exercise can be conserved, with the carbon skeletons of these molecules used for glucose synthesis in the Cori cycle illustrated in Figure 2-9. This cycle not only provides a means for lactic acid removal, but it also uses this compound to resynthesize blood glucose and muscle glycogen (*gluconeogenesis*).

Aerobic Energy From Glucose: The Krebs Cycle

Because the anaerobic reactions of

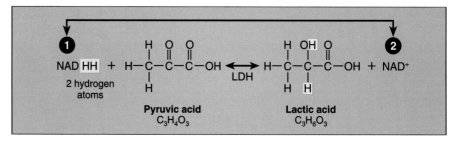

Figure 2-8. The formation of lactic acid occurs when excess hydrogens from NADH combine temporarily with pyruvic acid (1). This frees up NAD$^+$ to accept additional hydrogens generated in glycolysis (2). LDH = lactate dehydrogenase.

glycolysis release only about 10% of the energy within the glucose molecule, an additional means is available for extracting the remaining energy. This occurs when the pyruvic acid molecules are irreversibly converted to acetyl-CoA which is a form of acetic acid. This intermediate compound acetyl-CoA enters the second stage of carbohydrate breakdown known as the *Krebs cycle* (or more descriptively, the citric acid or tricarboxylic acid cycle). As shown schematically in Figure 2-10, the main function of the Krebs cycle is to degrade the acetyl-CoA substrate to carbon dioxide and hydrogen atoms within the mitochondria. The hydrogen atoms are then oxidized in processes involving electron transport-oxidative phosphorylation with the subsequent regeneration of ATP. Figure 2-11 shows that pyruvic acid is prepared for entrance into the Krebs cycle by joining with the vitamin B-derivative coenzyme A (A stands for acetic acid) to form the 2-carbon compound acetyl-CoA. In the process, two hydrogens are released and their electrons transferred to NAD^+; one molecule of carbon dioxide is formed as follows:

$$Pyruvic\ acid + NAD^+ + CoA \rightarrow Acetyl–CoA + CO_2 + NADH + H^+$$

When the acetyl portion of acetyl-CoA joins with oxaloacetic acid, it forms citric acid, the same 6-carbon compound found in citrus fruits, that then proceeds through the Krebs cycle. The Krebs cycle is continued because the original oxaloacetic molecule is retained and joins with a new acetyl fragment.

For each molecule of acetyl-CoA that enters the Krebs cycle, two carbon dioxide molecules and four pairs of hydrogen atoms are cleaved from the substrate. One molecule of ATP is also regenerated directly by substrate level phosphorylation from Krebs cycle reactions (see reaction 7 in Fig. 2-11). As summarized at the bottom of Figure 2-11, four hydrogens are released when acetyl-CoA is formed from the two pyruvic acid molecules created in glycolysis, and 16 hydrogens are released in the Krebs cycle. *The most important function of the Krebs cycle is to generate electrons (hydrogens)*

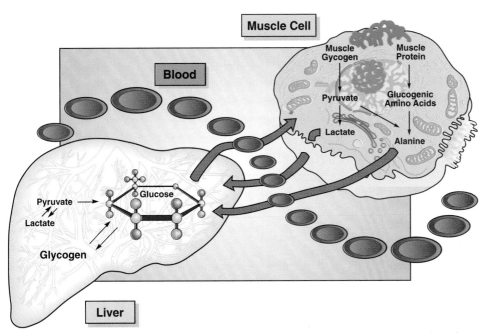

Figure 2-9. The Cori cycle is a biochemical process in the liver by which the lactic acid released from the active muscles is synthesized to glucose. This gluconeogenic process enables the body to maintain carbohydrate reserves.

for their passage to the respiratory chain by means of NAD+ and FAD.

Oxygen does *not* participate directly in the reactions of the Krebs cycle. The major portion of the chemical energy in pyruvic acid is transferred to ADP through the aerobic process of electron transport-oxidative phosphorylation. As long as there is an adequate oxygen supply with enzymes and substrate available, NAD+ and FAD are regenerated and Krebs cycle aerobic metabolism proceeds unimpeded.

Net Energy Transfer From Glucose Breakdown

Figure 2-12 summarizes the pathways for energy transfer during the breakdown of a glucose molecule in skeletal muscle. A net gain of 2 ATP is formed from substrate phosphorylation in glycolysis and, similarly, 2 ATP are generated during acetyl-CoA degradation in the Krebs cycle. The 24 released hydrogen atoms can be accounted for as follows:

- Four hydrogens (2 NADH) gen-

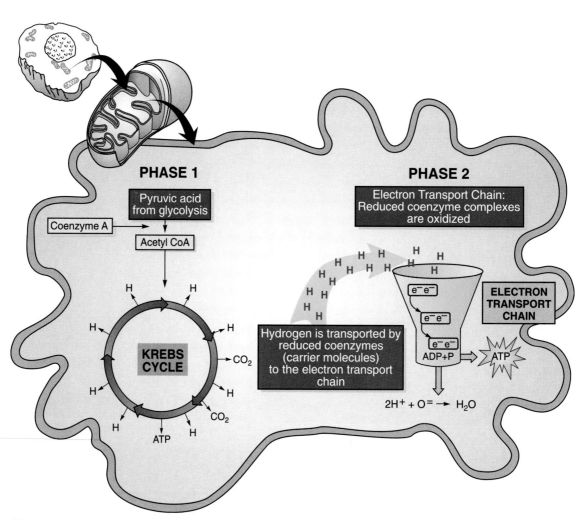

Figure 2-10. *Phase 1*. In the mitochondria, the Krebs cycle generates hydrogen atoms in the breakdown of acetyl CoA. *Phase 2*. Significant quantities of ATP are regenerated when these hydrogens are oxidized via the aerobic process of electron transport-oxidative phosphorylation (electron transport chain).

erated outside the mitochondria during glycolysis yield 4 ATP (6 ATP in heart muscle) during oxidative phosphorylation

- Four hydrogens (2 NADH)released in the mitochondria as pyruvic acid is changed to acetyl-CoA yield 6 ATP

- Twelve of the 16 hydrogens (6 NADH) released in the Krebs cycle yield 18 ATP
- Four remaining hydrogens join to FAD (2 $FADH_2$) in the Krebs cycle and yield 4 ATP.

The total ATP yield from the complete breakdown of glucose is 38.

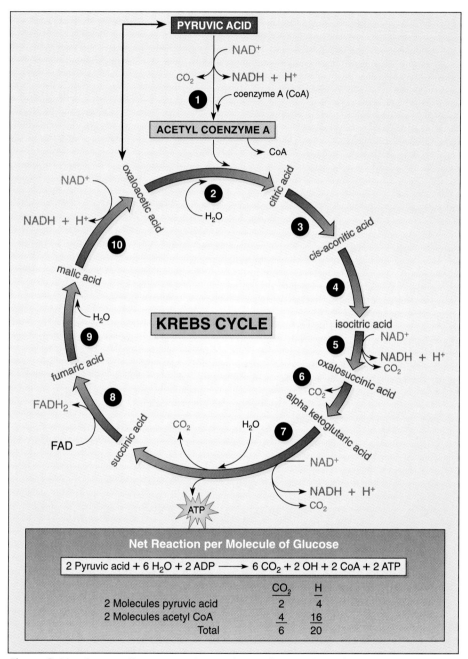

Figure 2-11. Schematic illustration and quantification for the release of H and CO_2 in the mitochondrion during the breakdown of one molecule of pyruvic acid. All values have doubled when computing the net gain of H and CO_2 from pyruvic acid breakdown because two molecules of pyruvic acid are formed from one glucose molecule in glycolysis.

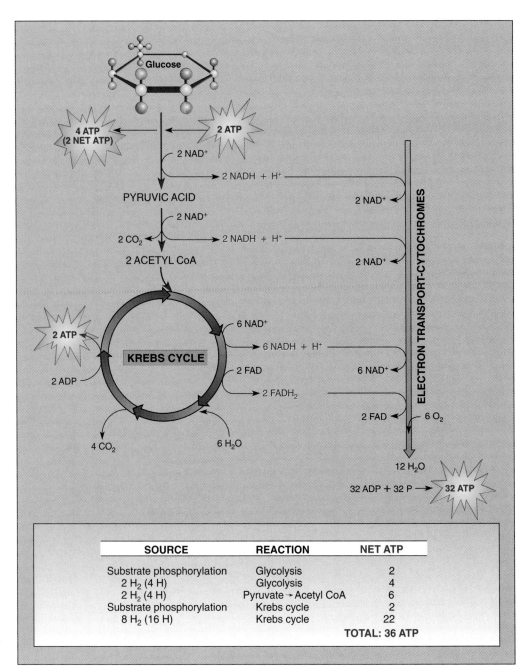

Figure 2-12. There is a net yield of 36 ATP from energy transfer during the complete oxidation of one glucose molecule through glycolysis, the Krebs cycle, and electron transport.

In the figure:

Glucose

4 ATP (2 NET ATP) ← ← 2 ATP

2 NAD⁺

→ 2 NADH + H⁺ —— 2 NAD⁺

PYRUVIC ACID

2 NAD⁺

2 CO₂ ← → 2 NADH + H⁺ —— 2 NAD⁺

2 ACETYL CoA

ELECTRON TRANSPORT-CYTOCHROMES

KREBS CYCLE

2 ATP ←

2 ADP

6 NAD⁺

→ 6 NADH + H⁺ —— 6 NAD⁺

2 FAD

→ 2 FADH₂ —— 2 FAD ← 6 O₂

4 CO₂   6 H₂O

12 H₂O

32 ADP + 32 P → 32 ATP

SOURCE	REACTION	NET ATP
Substrate phosphorylation	Glycolysis	2
2 H₂ (4 H)	Glycolysis	4
2 H₂ (4 H)	Pyruvate → Acetyl CoA	6
Substrate phosphorylation	Krebs cycle	2
8 H₂ (16 H)	Krebs cycle	22
	TOTAL: 36 ATP	

However, because 2 ATP are required to initially phosphorylate glucose, the net ATP yield from the complete breakdown of the glucose molecule in skeletal muscle is 36 molecules of ATP. Of these, 4 ATP molecules are formed directly from substrate phosphorylation via glycolysis and the Krebs cycle, and 32 ATPs are generated during oxidative phosphorylation.

ENERGY RELEASE FROM LIPID

Stored fat represents the body's most plentiful source of potential energy. Relative to other nutrients, the quantity of fat available for energy is almost unlimited. The actual fuel reserves from stored fat in an average young adult male represent about 90,000 to 110,000 kcal of energy. In contrast, the carbohydrate energy reserve is less than 2000 kcal.

Prior to energy release from fat, the triglyceride molecule is cleaved in the process of hydrolysis into glycerol and three fatty acid molecules. This fat breakdown or *lipolysis* is catalyzed by the enzyme lipase as follows:

FFA. Because plasma concentrations of these hormones are increased during exercise due to the activation of the sympathetic nervous system, this mechanism for lipase activation provides the muscle with an energy-rich substrate. It appears that lipase activation (and thus the regulation of

Lipoprotein lipase. This fat-degrading enzyme is attached to capillary walls and facilitates the hydrolysis of triglyceride into its glycerol and fatty acid components.

$$\text{Triglyceride} + 3H_2O \xrightarrow{\text{lipase}} \text{Glycerol} + 3 \text{ Fatty acids}$$

Adipocytes: The Site of Fat Storage and Mobilization

Although some fat is stored in all cells, the most active supplier of fatty acid molecules is adipose tissue. *Adipocytes,* or fat cells, are specialized for the synthesis and storage of triglycerides. Triglyceride fat droplets occupy as much as 95% of the cell's volume. Once the fatty acids diffuse from the adipocyte into the circulation and become bound to plasma albumin, these free fatty acid (FFA) are then delivered to active tissues where they are metabolized for energy. The utilization of fat as an energy substrate varies closely with blood flow in the active tissue. As blood flow increases with exercise, more FFA are removed from adipose tissue and delivered to active muscle. Hence, greater quantities of this nutrient are utilized for energy.

Depending on a person's state of nutrition and fitness, including the intensity and duration of physical activity, 30 to 80% of the energy for biologic work is usually derived from intra- and extracellular fat (Chapter 3 includes a more complete discussion of this topic).

The activation of lipase and subsequent lipolysis and mobilization of FFA from adipose tissue is augmented by the hormones epinephrine, norepinephrine, glucagon, and growth hormone. The injection of epinephrine into the blood, for example, results in a rapid increase in plasma

fat breakdown) is catalyzed by an intracellular mediator called adenosine 3',5'-cyclic monophosphate or *cyclic AMP.* Cyclic AMP is activated by the various fat mobilizing hormones which themselves do not enter the cell. Alterations in lipase activity may partly explain the enhanced utilization of fat observed with aerobic exercise training. A more detailed evaluation of hormone regulation in exercise is presented in Chapter 11.

Breakdown of Glycerol and Fatty Acids

Figure 2-13 summarizes the pathways for the degradation of the glycerol and fatty acid fragments of the triglyceride molecule. Glycerol can be accepted into the anaerobic reactions of glycolysis as 3-phosphoglyceraldehyde and degraded to pyruvic acid. In this process, ATP is formed by substrate-level phosphorylation, hydrogen atoms are released to NAD^+, and pyruvic acid is oxidized in the Krebs cycle. In total, 19 ATP molecules are synthesized in the complete breakdown of the glycerol molecule. Glycerol also serves an important function in providing carbon skeletons for glucose synthesis. This gluconeogenic role of glycerol is important when carbohydrate is restricted in the diet, or in long-term exercise that places a significant drain on glycogen reserves.

The fatty acid molecule undergoes transformation to acetyl-CoA in the mitochondrion by a process called *beta oxidation*. This process involves the successive release of 2-carbon acetyl fragments split from the long chain of the fatty acid. ATP is used to phosphorylate the reactions, water is added, hydrogens are passed to NAD^+ and FAD, and the acetyl fragment joins with coenzyme A to form acetyl-CoA. This is the same acetyl unit generated from glucose breakdown. Beta oxidation is repeated over and over until the entire fatty acid molecule is degraded to acetyl-CoA so it can enter the Krebs cycle directly to be metabolized. The hydrogens released during fatty acid catabolism are oxidized through the respiratory chain.

It is important to note that the breakdown of fatty acids is directly associated with oxygen uptake. Oxygen must be available to accept hydrogen so beta oxidation can proceed. Fat catabolism is halted under anaerobic conditions because hydrogen remains with NAD^+ and FAD.

Total Energy Transfer From Fat Breakdown

For each 18-carbon fatty acid molecule, 147 molecules of ADP are phosphorylated to ATP during beta oxidation and Krebs cycle metabolism. Because there are three fatty acid molecules in each triglyceride molecule,

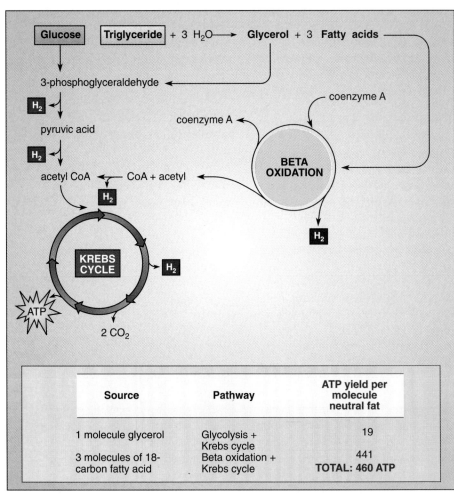

Source	Pathway	ATP yield per molecule neutral fat
1 molecule glycerol	Glycolysis + Krebs cycle	19
3 molecules of 18-carbon fatty acid	Beta oxidation + Krebs cycle	441
		TOTAL: 460 ATP

Figure 2-13. General scheme for the breakdown of the glycerol and fatty acid fragments of a triglyceride molecule. Glycerol enters the energy pathways in the reactions of glycolysis. The fatty acid fragments are prepared for entrance into the Krebs cycle through the process of beta oxidation. The released hydrogens from glycolysis, beta oxidation, and Krebs cycle metabolism go to the electron transport chain.

441 ATP molecules are formed from the fatty acid component of fat (3 x 147 ATP). Also, because 19 molecules of ATP are formed during glycerol catabolism, a total of 460 molecules of ATP are generated for each fat molecule catabolized for energy. This is a considerable energy yield because only 36 ATP are formed during the catabolism of a glucose molecule in skeletal muscle. The efficiency of energy conservation for fatty acid oxidation is about 40%, a value similar to that of glucose.

ENERGY RELEASE FROM PROTEIN

Protein can play an important role as an energy substrate during endurance-type exercise, as well as during intense physical training. To provide energy, the amino acids (primarily leucine, isoleucine, valine, glutamine, and aspartate) must first be converted to a form that can readily enter the pathways for energy release. Whereas the liver is the main site for nitrogen removal (a process known as *deamination*), the skeletal muscles also contain the enzymes for removing nitrogen in amino acids and passing it to other compounds in the process of *transamination*. This is how amino acids can be used directly in muscle for energy. In fact, the levels of these enzymes for transamination adapt to physical training which may further facilitate the use of protein as an energy substrate. Once the amino or nitrogen-containing group is removed from the amino acid, the remaining "carbon skeleton" is usually one of the reactive compounds that can contribute to the formation of high-energy phosphate bonds. Alanine, for example, loses its amino group and gains a double-bond oxygen to form pyruvic acid; glutamine forms alpha ketoglutaric acid; and aspartate forms oxaloacetic acid — all of these end products are Krebs cycle intermediates.

THE METABOLIC MILL

The Krebs cycle plays a much more important role than simply the degradation of pyruvic acid produced during glucose catabolism. The Krebs cycle allows fragments of other organic compounds formed from the breakdown of lipids and proteins to be effectively metabolized for energy. As illustrated in Figure 2-14, the deaminated residues of amino acids can enter the Krebs cycle at various intermediate stages, whereas the glycerol fragment of fat catabolism gains entrance via the glycolytic pathway. Fatty acids are oxidized by beta oxidation to acetyl-CoA which then directly enters the Krebs cycle.

This sketch of the "metabolic mill" also shows the interconversions among fragments of the various nutrients and the possible routes for substrate synthesis. Excess carbohydrates, for example, provide the glycerol and acetyl fragments for the synthesis of fat. Acetyl-CoA also can function as the starting point for the synthesis of cholesterol and many hormones. Because the conversion of pyruvic acid to acetyl-CoA is *not* reversible (notice the one-way arrow in Fig. 2-14), fatty acids cannot be used to synthesize glucose. Amino acids with carbon skeletons resembling Krebs cycle intermediates are deaminated and synthesized to glucose in the process termed gluconeogenesis. This role in glucose synthesis is especially true for the amino acid alanine (see Chapter 6).

FATS BURN IN A CARBOHYDRATE FLAME

One interesting aspect of the metabolic mill is that the breakdown of fatty acids somewhat depends on a continual background level of carbohydrate breakdown. Acetyl-CoA enters the Krebs cycle by combining with oxaloacetic acid (generated

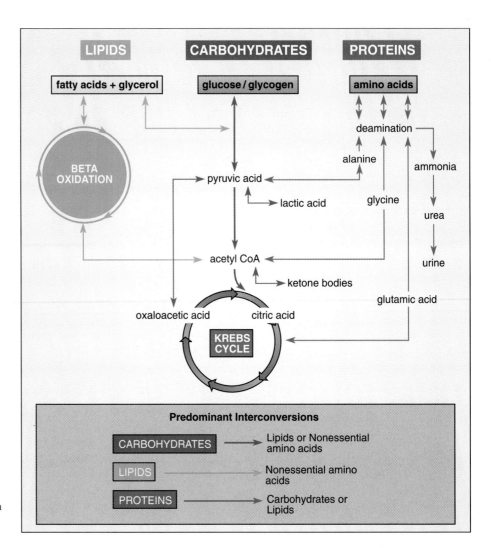

Figure 2-14. The "metabolic mill": important interconversions between carbohydrates, lipids, and proteins.

Within the figure:

LIPIDS   CARBOHYDRATES   PROTEINS

fatty acids + glycerol   glucose / glycogen   amino acids

BETA OXIDATION

pyruvic acid

lactic acid

deamination

alanine

glycine

ammonia

urea

urine

acetyl CoA

ketone bodies

glutamic acid

oxaloacetic acid   citric acid

KREBS CYCLE

Predominant Interconversions

CARBOHYDRATES	→	Lipids or Nonessential amino acids
LIPIDS	→	Nonessential amino acids
PROTEINS	→	Carbohydrates or Lipids

Carbohydrate intake is crucial. Although gluconeogenesis provides a metabolic option for making glucose from non-carbohydrate sources, this process cannot maintain glycogen stores unless carbohydrates are regularly consumed in the diet.

mainly by carbohydrate catabolism) to form citric acid. The degradation of fatty acids by the Krebs cycle continues only if sufficient oxaloacetic acid is available to combine with acetyl-CoA formed during beta oxidation. The pyruvic acid formed during glucose breakdown may play an important role in furnishing this oxaloacetic intermediate (refer to Fig. 2-14). When carbohydrate levels fall, oxaloacetic acid levels may become inadequate to sustain a high level of fat breakdown. In this sense, "fats burn in a carbohydrate flame."

It also is likely that there may be a rate limit to fatty-acid utilization by the exercising muscle. Although this limit can be greatly enhanced by aerobic-type exercise training, the aerobic muscle power generated only by fat breakdown never appears to equal that generated by combined fat and

carbohydrate breakdown. Thus, the maximum power output of muscle declines when muscle glycogen becomes depleted.

An appreciable reduction in carbohydrate availability, which could occur in prolonged exercise such as marathon running, consecutive days of heavy training, inadequate caloric intake, dietary elimination of carbohydrates (as advocated with high-fat, low-carbohydrate "ketogenic diets"), or diabetes, seriously limits the capacity for energy transfer. This occurs although large amounts of fatty acid substrate are available in the circulation. In instances of extreme carbohydrate restriction or depletion, the acetate fragments produced in beta oxidation begin to build up in the extracellular fluids because they cannot be accommodated in the Krebs cycle. These fragments are readily converted to ketone bodies, some of which are excreted in the urine. If this condition of ketosis persists, the acid quality of the body fluids can increase to potentially toxic levels.

REGULATION OF ENERGY METABOLISM

Each of the biochemical pathways involved in energy metabolism is precisely controlled by specific enzymes. The control of these enzymes thus controls ATP formation. Each pathway has at least one enzyme that is considered "rate-limiting" because it controls the speed of the reactions in that pathway. By far, the concentration of cellular ADP is the most important factor that modulates the rate-limiting enzymes that control the breakdown of carbohydrates, lipids, and proteins for energy release in the cell. *Under normal conditions, the transfer of electrons and subsequent release of energy are tightly coupled to ADP phosphorylation.* In general, unless ADP is available and phosphorylated to ATP, electrons do not shuttle down the respiratory chain to oxygen. This particular mechanism for respiratory control makes sense because any increase in ADP signals a need for energy to restore the ATP levels. Conversely, a low level of cellular ADP indicates a relatively low energy requirement. From a broader perspective, the level of ADP serves as a cellular feedback mechanism to maintain a relative constancy or homeostasis in the level of energy currency available for biologic work. Other rate-limiting modulators include cellular levels of phosphate, pH, cyclic AMP, calcium, and citrate.

SUMMARY

1. The carbohydrate, lipid, and protein food nutrients provide a ready source of potential energy so ADP and free phosphate can rejoin to form ATP.

2. The complete breakdown of 1 mole of carbohydrate liberates 686 kcal of energy. Of this, about 277 kcal or 40% is conserved in the bonds of ATP; the remainder is dissipated as heat.

3. In the reactions of glycolysis in the cell cytoplasm, 2 ATP are formed (net gain) in the anaerobic process of substrate–level phosphorylation.

4. In the second stage of carbohydrate breakdown that occurs within the mitochondria, pyruvic acid is converted to acetyl–CoA, which is then processed through the Krebs cycle. The hydrogens released during glucose breakdown are oxidized by the respiratory chain and the energy generated is coupled to phosphorylation.

5. A total of 36 ATP molecules are formed (net gain) in the complete breakdown of one carbohydrate molecule in skeletal muscle.

6. A biochemical "steady rate" is said to exist when hydrogen atoms are oxidized at the rate they are formed. In heavy exercise when the oxidation of hydrogen does not keep pace with its rate of production, lactic acid is formed when pyruvic acid temporarily combines with hydrogen.

7. The complete breakdown of a lipid molecule yields about 460 ATP molecules. These reactions are primarily aerobic because fatty acid metabolism is directly associated with oxygen uptake.

8. Protein can serve as an important energy substrate. After nitrogen is removed from the amino acid molecule in the process of deamination, the remaining carbon skeleton can enter the Krebs cycle for the aerobic production of ATP.

9. Numerous interconversions are possible among the various food nutrients. The exception is fatty acids that cannot be used for the synthesis of glucose.

10. A certain level of carbohydrate breakdown is required so fats can be continually metabolized for energy in the metabolic mill. To this extent, "fats burn in a carbohydrate flame."

11. ADP is the most important factor that controls the rate of breakdown of carbohydrate, lipid, and protein for energy release in the cell.

Åstrand, P. O., and Rodahl, K.: *Textbook of Work Physiology*. 3rd ed. McGraw-Hill. 1986.

Björntorp, P. Importance of fat as a support nutrient for energy: Metabolism of athletes. In *Foods, Nutrition and Sports Performance*. Edited by C. Williams, and J. T. Devlin. London, E. & F. N. Spon, 1992.

Brooks, G.A.: Physical activity and carbohydrate metabolism. In *Physical Activity, Fitness, and Health*. Edited by C. Bouchard, et al., Champaign, IL, Human Kinetics, 1994.

Brooks, G. A., and Fahey, T. D.: *Exercise Physiology: Human Bioenergetics and its Applications*. New York, Wiley, 1984.

Cerretelli, P.: Energy sources for muscular exercise. *Int. J. Sports Med.*, 13 (Suppl. 1): S106, 1992.

Chasiotis, D.: Role of cyclic AMP and inorganic phosphate in the regulation of muscle glycogenolysis during exercise. *Med. Sci. Sports Exerc.*, 20: 545, 1988.

Coggan, A.R., et al. Plasma glucose kinetics during exercise in subjects with high and low lactate thresholds. *J. Appl. Physiol.*, 73: 1873, 1992.

Hargreaves, M., et al.: Influence of sodium on glucose bioavailalbility during exercise. *Med. Sci. Sports Exerc.*, 26: 365, 1994.

Horton, E. S., and Terjung, R. L. (Eds.):*Exercise, Nutrition, and Energy Metabolism*. New York, Macmillan, 1988.

Hultman, E., et al.: Biochemistry of fatigue. *Biomed. Biochim. Acta,* 45: 597, 1986.

Lehninger, A. L.: *Principles of Biochemistry*. New York, Worth Publishers, 1982.

Mainwood, G. W., and Renaud, J. M.: The effect of acid-base on fatigue of skeletal muscle. *Can. J. Physiol. Pharmacol.*, 63: 403, 1985.

MacRae, H.S-H., et al.: Effects of training on lactate production and removal during progressive exercise. *J. Appl. Physiol.*, 72: 1649, 1992.

Marieb, E. N.: *Human Anatomy and Physiology*. Redwood City, Benjamin Cummings, 1989.

McArdle, W. D., et al.: *Exercise Physiology: Energy, Nutrition, and Human Performance,* 3rd ed. Philadelphia, Lea & Febiger, 1991.

McCann, D.J., et al.: Phosphocreatine kinetics in humans during exercise and recovery. *Med. Sci. Sports Exerc.*, 27(3): 378, 1995.

McCully, K.K., et al.: Simultaneous invivo measurements of HbO_2 saturation and PCr kinetics after exercise in normal humans. *J. Appl. Physiol.*, 77: 5, 1994.

Mudio, D.M., et al.: Effects of dietary fat on metabolic adjustments to maximal $\dot{V}O_2$ and endurance in runners. *Med. Sci. Sports Exerc.*, 26: 81, 1994.

Romijn, J.A., et al.: Regulations of endogenous fat and carbohydrate metabolism in relation to exercise intensity and duration. *Am. J. Physiol.*, 265: E380, 1993.

Stefanick, M.L., and Wood, P.D.: Physical activity, lipid and lipoprotein metabolism, and lipid transport. In *Physical Activity, Fitness, and Health*. Edited by C. Bouchard, et al. Champaign, IL, Human Kinetics, 1994.

Stryer, L.: *Biochemistry,* 2nd ed. San Francisco, Freeman, 1988.

Vander, A. J., et al.: *Human Physiology,* 2nd ed. New York, McGraw-Hill, 1985.

Weltman, A.: *The Blood Lactate Response to Exercise*. Human Kinetics Publishers, Champaign, IL, 1995.

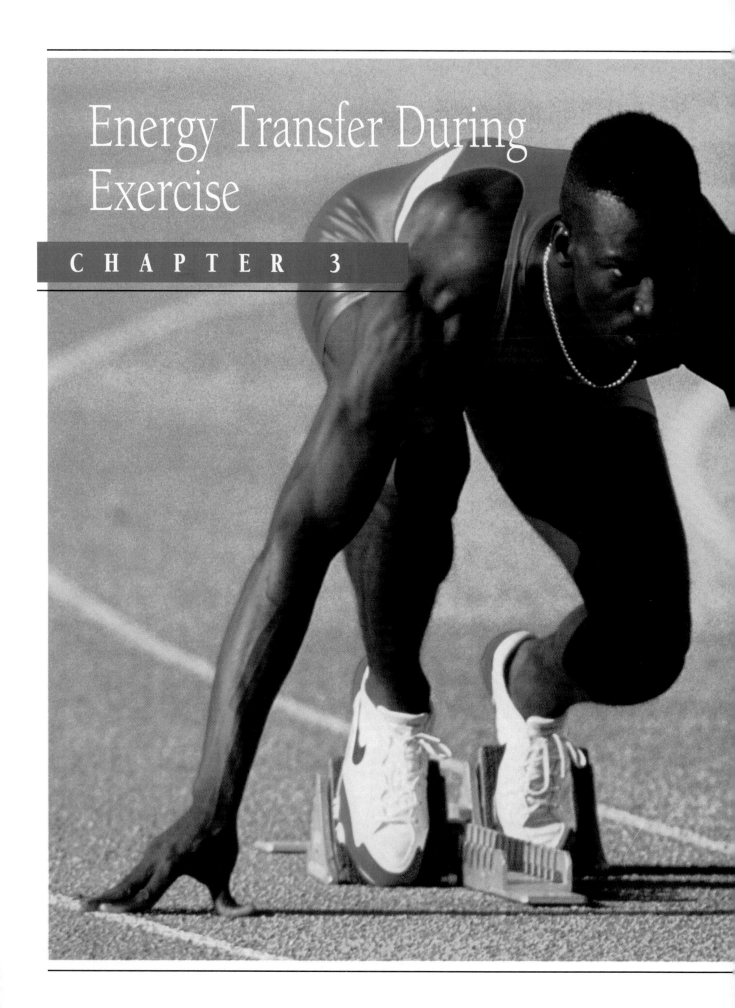

Energy Transfer During Exercise

CHAPTER 3

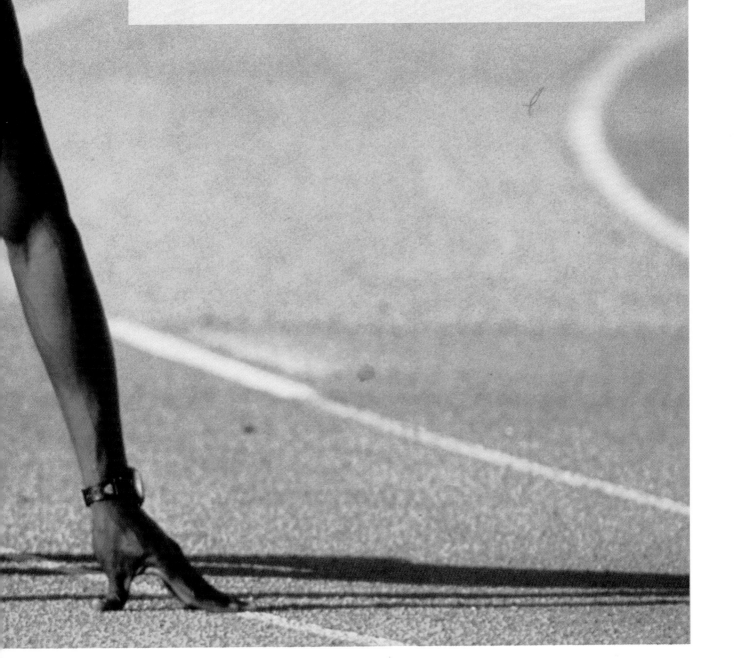

After reading this chapter you should be able to:

- Identify the body's three energy systems and outline the relative contribution of each in terms of exercise intensity and duration. Relate your discussion to specific sport activities.

- Discuss the blood lactate threshold indicating differences between sedentary and aerobically trained individuals.

- Outline the time course for oxygen uptake during 10-minutes of moderate exercise.

- Draw a figure that indicates the relationship between oxygen uptake and exercise intensity during progressively increasing increments of exercise up to the maximum.

- Differentiate between the two types of muscle fibers in the body.

- Discuss differences in recovery oxygen uptake from moderate and exhaustive exercise. Indicate the major factors that account for the EPOC in each form of exercise.

- Outline the optimal recovery procedures from steady-rate and non-steady-rate exercise.

Physical activity clearly provides the greatest demand for energy. In sprint running, cycling, and swimming, for example, the energy output may be as much as 120 times greater in the working muscles than when at rest. In contrast, during less intense but sustained exercise such as marathon running, the energy requirement still increases about 20 to 30 times above rest. The relative contributions of the body's various means for energy transfer thus differ markedly depending on exercise duration and intensity, and the fitness of the participant. In the following sections, the discussion centers on how the body's various energy systems interact during different intensities of exercise.

IMMEDIATE ENERGY: THE ATP-CP SYSTEM

Performances of short duration and high intensity such as the 100-meter sprint, 25-meter swim, smashing a tennis ball during the serve, or lifting a heavy weight require an immediate and rapid supply of energy. This energy is provided almost exclusively from the high-energy phosphates ATP and CP stored within the specific muscles activated during exercise. Approximately 5 millimoles (mmol) of ATP and 15 mmol of CP are stored within each kilogram of muscle. For a 70-kg person with a muscle mass of 30 kg, this amounts to between 570 and 690 mmol of high-energy phosphates. If we assume that 20 kg of muscle are activated during exercise, there is sufficient stored phosphate energy to power a brisk walk for 1 minute, a slow run for 20 to 30 seconds, or an all-out exercise such as sprint running and swimming for about 6 seconds. In the 100-meter dash, for example, the body cannot maintain maximum speed for longer than about 6 seconds and the runner may actually be slowing down in the last portion of the race. In such activities that are performed "all-out," the quantity of intramuscular phosphate may significantly influence one's ability to generate intense energy for short durations.

All sports require utilization of the high-energy phosphates, but many activities rely almost exclusively on generating energy rapidly from the stored phosphagens. For example, success in wrestling, apparatus routines in gymnastics, weight lifting, most field events like discus, shot put, pole vault, hammer, and javelin, baseball, and volleyball all require a brief but maximal effort during the performance. It is difficult to imagine what an end run in football or a pole vault would look like without the capacity to generate energy rapidly from the stored phosphagens. For more sustained activities like ice hockey, soccer, field hockey, lacrosse, and basketball, additional energy must be generated to replenish the muscles' stores of ATP. For this purpose, the stored carbohydrates, lipids, and proteins stand ready to continually recharge the phosphate pool.

SHORT-TERM ENERGY: THE LACTIC ACID SYSTEM

The high-energy phosphates must continually be resynthesized at a rapid rate for strenuous exercise to continue beyond a brief period. In such intense exercise, the energy to phosphorylate ADP comes mainly from glucose and stored glycogen during the anaerobic process of glycolysis with the resulting formation of lactic acid. In a way, this mechanism of lactic acid formation "buys time" to allow for the rapid formation of ATP by substrate-level phosphorylation. This occurs when the oxygen supply is inadequate or the energy demands outstrip cellular capacity for the aerobic resynthesis of ATP. The anaerobic energy from glycolysis for ATP resynthesis can be thought of as reserve fuel that is brought into use by the athlete "kicking" the last phase of a mile run.

Phosphagens. This term is used to identify the high energy phosphates ATP and CP.

It is also of critical importance during a 440-yard run or 100-yard swim or in multiple sprint sports such as ice hockey, field hockey, and soccer that energy be provided rapidly in excess of that supplied by the stored phosphagens. If the intensity of "all-out" exercise is decreased (thereby extending the period of exercise), there is a corresponding decrease in the rate of buildup of lactic acid and its final concentration in both the blood and muscle.

Lactate Accumulation. Lactic acid does not build up at all levels of exercise. Figure 3-1 illustrates the general relationship between oxygen uptake expressed as a percentage of maximum, and blood lactate during light, moderate, and heavy exercise in endurance athletes and untrained subjects. During light and moderate exer-

ATP required for muscular contraction is made available predominantly through energy generated by the oxidation of hydrogen. Any lactic acid formed in light exercise is rapidly oxidized. Consequently, blood lactate remains fairly stable even though oxygen uptake increases.

Lactate begins to rise in an exponential fashion at about 55% of the healthy, untrained person's maximal capacity for aerobic metabolism. The usual explanation for the increase in lactic acid is based on the assumption of a relative tissue hypoxia in heavy exercise. Under conditions of oxygen deficiency, the energy requirement is partially met by a predominance of anaerobic glycolysis as the release of hydrogen begins to exceed its oxidation down the respiratory chain. Consequently, excess hydrogens are passed to pyruvic acid and lactic acid is formed. The increase in lactic acid formation becomes greater as exercise becomes more intense and the muscle cells cannot meet the additional energy demands aerobically. This pattern is essentially similar for trained individuals except for the threshold for lactate buildup, termed the *blood lactate threshold*, which occurs at a higher percentage of the athlete's aerobic capacity. This favorable response could be due to the endurance athlete's genetic endowment (e.g., type of muscle fiber, page 66.) or specific local adaptations with training that favor production of less lactic acid, as well as a more rapid removal rate at any particular exercise level.

Research has shown that capillary density, as well as the size and number of mitochondria, increase with endurance training. The concentration of various enzymes and transfer agents involved in aerobic metabolism also increases, and this training response remains unaffected by the aging process. Such favorable alterations certainly enhance the cell's capacity to generate ATP aerobically, especially through the breakdown of fatty acids. This may extend the per-

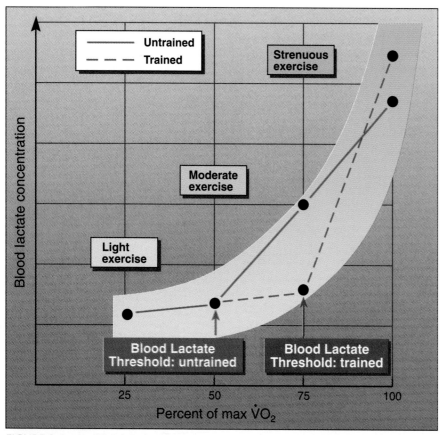

FIGURE 3-1. Blood lactate concentration at different levels of exercise expressed as a percentage of maximal oxygen uptake for trained and untrained subjects.

cise in both groups, the energy demands are adequately met by biochemical reactions that rely primarily on oxygen. Stated in another way, the centage of one's maximum that can be sustained before the blood lactate threshold. World-class endurance athletes, for example, perform at sustained exercise intensities that represent 85 to 90% of their maximum capability for aerobic metabolism!

There are alternative explanations for the accumulation of lactate in the blood during exercise. It is possible that under the conditions of rapid glycolysis, NADH production may exceed the transport capacity for shuttling hydrogens (and electrons) down the respiratory chain. This imbalance in hydrogen release and subsequent oxidation would cause pyruvate to accept the excess hydrogens to form lactic acid. This would occur regardless of the availability of oxygen. Another explanation for lactate accumulation is the tendency for the enzyme *lactate dehydrogenase* (LDH) in fast-twitch muscle fibers to favor conversion of pyruvic acid to lactic acid. The LDH in slow-twitch fibers, on the other hand, favors the conversion of lactic acid to pyruvic acid. Therefore, recruitment of the fast-twitch fibers (as occurs in more intense exercise), would favor lactate formation independent of tissue oxygenation.

The lactic acid formed in one part of an active muscle can be oxidized by other fibers in the same muscle or by less active neighboring muscle tissue. This adjustment would certainly help to keep lactate levels low during exercise, and also would provide an important means for glucose conservation in prolonged work. The concept of the blood lactate threshold and its relation to endurance performance is developed more fully in Chapter 8.

Lactate-Producing Capacity. The ability to generate a high lactic acid level in all-out exercise is increased with specific "anaerobic training" and subsequently reduced with detraining. Well-trained "anaerobic" athletes performing maximal short-term exercise can generate blood lactate levels that are 20 to 30% higher than in untrained subjects under similar circumstances. The mechanism for this response is unknown, but it may be caused by large differences in motivation levels accompanying the trained state as well as about a 20% increase in enzymes involved in glycolysis, specifically phosphofructokinase, observed as a result of anaerobic-type training. It is also likely that the increased intramuscular glycogen stores that accompany the trained state allow for a greater contribution of energy via anaerobic glycolysis. Although increases in enzymes of the anaerobic pathway take place with sprint-type training, these changes are not as impressive as the 2 to 3-fold increase in aerobic enzymes with endurance training.

LONG-TERM ENERGY: THE AEROBIC SYSTEM

Although the energy released in glycolysis is rapid and does not require oxygen, relatively little ATP is resynthesized in this manner. It is, instead, the aerobic metabolic reactions that provide the important final stage for energy transfer, especially if vigorous exercise is longer than 2 to 3 minutes.

Oxygen Uptake During Exercise

The curve in Figure 3-2 illustrates oxygen uptake during each minute of a relatively slow jog continued at a steady pace for 10 minutes. The usage of oxygen by the cells, referred to as *oxygen uptake*, is indicated on the vertical axis (Y-axis) on the graph; the horizontal or X-axis shows exercise time. Oxygen uptake during any minute can easily be determined by locating the time on the X-axis and its corresponding point for oxygen uptake on the Y-axis. For example, after 4 minutes of running, the oxygen uptake is about $1.6 L \cdot min^{-1}$.

Oxygen uptake rises rapidly during the first minutes of exercise. Between the third and fourth minute a plateau is reached, and the oxygen uptake

Oxygen uptake and body size. To adjust for the effects of variations in body size on oxygen uptake (that is, bigger people consume more oxygen), oxygen uptake is often expressed in terms of body mass, as milliliters of oxygen per kilogram of body mass per minute, or $ml \cdot kg^{-1} \cdot min^{-1}$, or about $250 ml \cdot min^{-1}$ (one-fourth of a liter).

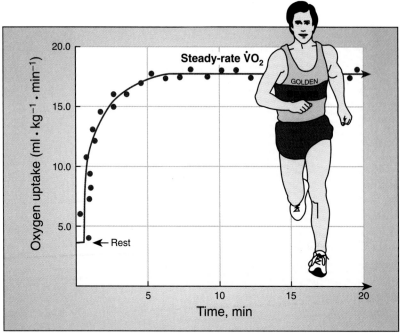

FIGURE 3-2. Time course of oxygen uptake during continuous jogging at a relatively slow pace. The dots along the curve represent measured values of oxygen uptake determined by open-circuit spirometry described in Chapter 4.

mile pace is a magnificent accomplishment in terms of the many physiologic functions involved. One of these important functions is delivering adequate oxygen to the exercising muscles. Another is the cells' ability to use this oxygen in the aerobic process of energy metabolism.

Oxygen Deficit. The upward trending curve of oxygen uptake shown in Figure 3-2 does not increase instantaneously to a steady rate at the start of exercise. The oxygen uptake is considerably below the steady-rate level in the beginning stages of work, even though the energy required to perform the exercise remains essentially unchanged throughout the exercise period. This temporary lag in oxygen uptake occurs because the muscle's immediate energy source is *always* provided directly from ATP, which does not require oxygen for its breakdown. Only in the subsequent reactions of energy transfer does oxygen become important as it serves as an electron acceptor to combine with the hydrogens generated during glycolysis, beta oxidation of fatty acids, and the reactions of the Krebs cycle. Whenever there is an increase in exercise intensity, there is always an oxygen deficit, regardless of the level or mode of exercise.

The oxygen deficit quantitatively is the difference between the total oxygen actually consumed during exercise and the amount that would have been consumed had a steady rate of aerobic metabolism been reached immediately at the start of exercise. The energy provided during the deficit phase of exercise most likely represents non-aerobic energy. Stated in energy terms, the deficit represents the immediate energy from the stored high-energy phosphates plus anaerobic energy from glycolysis that is utilized until a steady rate is reached between oxygen uptake and the energy demands of exercise.

Figure 3-3 depicts the relationship between the size of the oxygen deficit and the contribution of energy from

remains relatively stable throughout the exercise period. The flat portion or plateau of the oxygen uptake curve is generally considered the *steady rate*. This steady rate reflects a balance between the energy required by the working muscles and the rate of ATP production through aerobic metabolism. In this region, oxygen-consuming reactions supply the energy for exercise, and any lactic acid produced is either oxidized or reconverted to glucose in the liver and possibly the kidneys. Under steady-rate metabolic conditions, lactic acid accumulation is minimal.

There Are Many Levels of Steady Rate. Steady-rate exercise for the athlete could be exhausting for an untrained person. For some of us, lying in bed, working around the house, and playing an occasional round of golf represent the spectrum of activity for which adequate oxygen can be utilized to maintain a steady rate. A champion marathon runner, on the other hand, can run 26 miles in slightly more than 2 hours and still be in steady rate! This 5-minute-per-

Limited duration of steady rate. Theoretically, once a steady rate is attained, exercise could continue indefinitely if the individual so desired. However, factors other than motivation place a limit on the duration of steady-rate work. These include the loss of important body fluids in sweat and depletion of essential nutrients, especially blood glucose and glycogen stored in the liver and active muscles.

both the ATP-CP and lactic acid energy systems. The high-energy phosphates become substantially depleted by exercise that generates about a three- to four-liter oxygen deficit. Consequently, this intensity of exercise can continue only on a "pay-as-you-go" basis and ATP must continually be replenished through the breakdown of the food nutrients by oxidative phosphorylation or glycolysis. Interestingly, lactic acid begins to increase in exercising muscle well before the phosphates reach their lowest levels. This means that glycolysis contributes anaerobic energy in the early stages of vigorous exercise even before the full utilization of the high-energy phosphates. Thus, energy for exercise is not merely the result of a series of energy systems that "switch on" and "switch off" like a water faucet. Rather, a muscle's energy supply represents a smooth blend between nonaerobic and aerobic sources with considerable overlap from one source of energy transfer to another.

Oxygen Deficit in the Trained and Untrained. It is generally observed that the steady-rate oxygen uptake during light and moderate exercise is similar in trained and untrained individuals. The trained person, however, reaches a steady rate more rapidly and hence has a smaller oxygen deficit for the same exercise compared to the untrained person. Consequently, the total oxygen consumed during exercise is greater for the trained person and the anaerobic component of energy transfer proportionately smaller.

Maximal Oxygen Uptake (max $\dot{V}O_2$)

Figure 3-4 depicts the curve of oxygen uptake during a series of constant-speed runs up six hills, each progressively steeper than the next. In the laboratory, these "hills" can be simulated by increasing the elevation of a treadmill, increasing the height of a step bench, or increasing the resistance to pedaling a bicycle ergometer. Each successive hill (equivalent to an

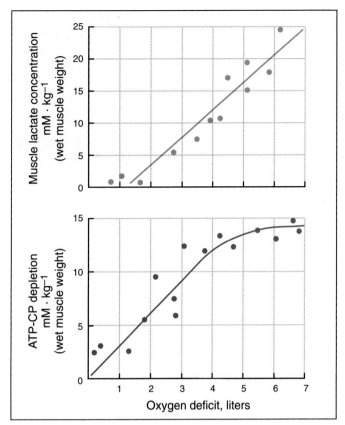

FIGURE 3-3. Muscle ATP and CP depletion and muscle lactate concentration in relation to the oxygen deficit. (Adapted from Pernow, B. and Karlsson, J.: Muscle ATP, CP and lactate in submaximal and maximal exercise. In *Muscle Metabolism During Exercise.* Edited by B. Pernow, and B. Saltin. New York, Plenum Press, 1971.)

increase in exercise load) requires a greater energy output, and thus, an additional demand on the person's capacity for aerobic metabolism. Climbing the first several hills, the increases in oxygen uptake are linear and in direct proportion to the severity of exercise. Although the runner is able to maintain speed running up the last two hills, the oxygen uptake does not increase to the same extent observed previously. As noted, there is no increase in oxygen uptake for the run up the last hill. *The point when the oxygen uptake plateaus and shows no further increase (or increases only slightly) with an additional workload is called the maximal oxygen uptake or simply max* $\dot{V}O_2$.

The max $\dot{V}O_2$ represents a good approximation of an individual's

The rapid attainment of steady rate. An individual who is trained by predominantly aerobic exercise reaches a steady rate more rapidly compared to someone who is untrained. This facilitated level of aerobic metabolism early in exercise may be the result of training-induced cellular adaptations that are known to increase the capacity of muscle to generate ATP aerobically.

Criterion for max $\dot{V}O_2$. Max $\dot{V}O_2$ is measured as the region where work continues to increase but oxygen uptake levels off or even declines slightly.

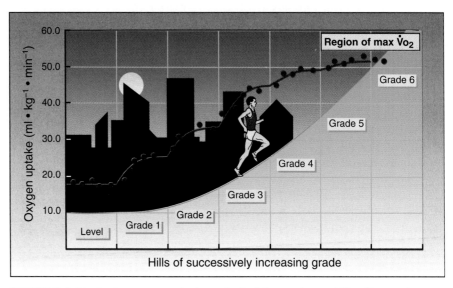

FIGURE 3-4. Maximal oxygen uptake is reached while running up hills of increasing slope. This occurs in the region where a further increase in exercise intensity is unaccompanied by an additional increase in oxygen uptake. The dots represent measured values of oxygen uptake during running up each of the hills.

An important endurance component. The max $\dot{V}O_2$ is important in determining a person's capacity to sustain high-intensity exercise for longer than 4 to 5 minutes.

capacity for the aerobic resynthesis of ATP. Additional exercise above the max $\dot{V}O_2$ can be accomplished only by the energy transfer reactions of glycolysis with the resulting formation of lactic acid. Under such conditions, performance deteriorates and the individual eventually will be unable to continue at that exercise level. A good example of performance decrement is the runner or swimmer who starts out too fast in a race, or who begins the "kick" to the finish too soon. The large build up of lactic acid, due to the additional anaerobic muscular effort, disrupts the already high energy transfer rate for the aerobic resynthesis of ATP. To borrow an analogy from business economics, supply (aerobic resynthesis of ATP) is unable to meet the demand (energy required for muscular effort); consequently, there is an imbalance between requirements and production (lactic acid accumulates), and performance is compromised.

In subsequent chapters, we discuss various aspects of max $\dot{V}O_2$, including its measurement and role in exercise performance.

FAST- AND SLOW-TWITCH MUSCLE FIBERS

Exercise physiologists have studied the functional and structural characteristics of human skeletal muscle with surgical biopsy. This invasive procedure uses a special needle to puncture the muscle and obtain approximately 20 to 40 mg (the size of a grain of rice) of tissue for chemical and microscopic analysis. Two distinct *types* of fiber have been identified in human skeletal muscle. The proportion of each fiber type within a particular muscle probably remains fairly constant throughout life.

Fast-twitch Fiber. This muscle fiber, also called a *type II* fiber, possesses a high capacity for anaerobic production of ATP during glycolysis. The contraction speed is rapid for these fibers. Fast-twitch muscle fibers are

To quantify the amount of exercise performed, it is necessary to view physical activity much like a physicist views work. The physicist defines work as the application of force through a given distance in the formula:

$$Work\ (W) = Force\ (F) \times Distance\ (D)$$

where F is a constant force, and D is the distance through which the force is applied.

For example, if your body mass is 70 kg, and you jump vertically 0.5 meters, you have accomplished 35 kilogram-meters (kg-m) of work (70 kg x 0.5 m = 35 kg-m). Work can be expressed in many different units of measurements, the most common of which are kilogram-meters (kg-m), foot-pounds (ft-lbs), joules (J), Newton-meters (Nm), and kilocalories (kcal).

Work performed per unit time (T) is power (P) and is expressed as:

$$P = F \times D/T$$

Calculation of Work on a Treadmill

The treadmill is a moving conveyor belt with variable angle of incline and speed. Work performed on the treadmill equals the weight (mass) of the person (F) times the vertical distance (D) the person would have been raised in walking up the incline. The vertical distance (D) equals the sine of the treadmill angle (theta or Ø) multiplied by A, the distance traveled along the incline.

Work = Body Mass (Force) x Vertical distance

where, Vertical distance = Sine of angle Ø x Distance (A)
A = Treadmill speed x Time

For example, if the angle Ø is 8° (this angle can be measured with an inclinometer, or it can be determined by knowing the percent grade of the treadmill), the sine of

angle Ø is equal to 0.1392 (see insert). The value of A is calculated as the speed of the treadmill multiplied by the time spent exercising. For example, the distance traveled (A) on the incline while walking at 5000 m per hr for 1 hour is 5000 m (5000 m · hr⁻¹ x 1 hr = 5000 m).

If a person with a body mass of 50 kg walked on a treadmill at an incline of 8° (percent grade = approximately 14%) for 60 min at 5000 m per hr, the work accomplished would be calculated as follows:

$$W = F \times D\ (Sine\ Ø \times A)$$

$$W = 50\ kg \times (0.1392 \times 5000\ m)$$
$$W = 34,800\ kg\text{-}m$$

The expression for power would be 34,800 kg-m/60 min or 580 kg-m · min⁻¹.

Calculation of Work on a Bicycle Ergometer

The mechanically braked ergometer has

Ø (deg)	Sine Ø	Tangent Ø	Percent grade
1	0.0175	0.0175	1.75
2	0.0349	0.0349	3.49
3	0.0523	0.0523	5.23
4	0.0698	0.0698	6.98
5	0.0872	0.0872	8.72
6	0.1045	0.1051	10.51
7	0.1219	0.1228	12.28
8	0.1392	0.1405	14.05
9	0.1564	0.1584	15.84
10	0.1736	0.1763	17.63
15	0.2588	0.2680	26.80
20	0.3420	0.3640	36.40

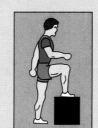

a flywheel with a belt around it connected with a small spring at one end to an adjustable tension lever at the other end. A pendulum balance indicates the resistance on the flywheel while it is turning. By increasing the tension on the belt, more

friction is applied to the flywheel, and there is an increase in resistance. The force (friction on the flywheel) is determined as the braking power and is given in kg or kilopounds (kp; force acting on the 1 kg mass at the normal acceleration of gravity). The distance traveled is the number of pedal revolutions times the flywheel circumference.

For example, if a person pedals a bicycle ergometer (flywheel circumference of 6 meters) at 60 revolutions per min for 1 min, the distance (D) covered is 360 m each minute. If the frictional resistance on the flywheel is 2.5 kg, the total work performed is computed as follows:

$$W = F \times D$$

W = Frictional resistance x Distance traveled
W = 2.5 kg x 360 m
W = 900 kg-m

The power generated by the effort would be 900 kg-m in 1 min or 900 kg-m · min⁻¹.

Calculation of Work During Bench Stepping

In bench stepping, only the vertical (positive) work can be calculated. Distance is computed as bench height times the number of times the person steps; the force is the body mass.

For example, if a 70 kg person steps on a bench 0.375 meters high (1.23 ft) at 30 steps per min for 10 min, the total work is calculated as follows:

$$W = F \times D$$

W = Body Mass x (Vertical distance per min x 10 min)
W = 7875 kg-m

Power is computed as 7875 kg-m/ 10 min = 787 kg–m · min⁻¹

activated in short-term, sprint activities that depend almost entirely on anaerobic metabolism for energy. The metabolic capabilities of fast-twitch fibers are also important in the stop-and-go or change-off-pace sports such as basketball, soccer, lacrosse, and field hockey, which at times require rapid energy that only can be supplied through anaerobic metabolism.

Slow-twitch Fiber. The slow-twitch or *type II* fiber has a contraction speed about half as fast as its fast-twitch counterpart. Slow-twitch fibers possess numerous mitochondria and a high concentration of the enzymes required to sustain aerobic metabolism. Their capacity to generate ATP aerobically is much greater than that of fast-twitch fibers. So, slow-twitch fibers are active in endurance activities that depend almost exclusively on aerobic metabolism. Middle-distance running or swimming, or sports such as basketball, field hockey, and soccer, require a blend of both aerobic and anaerobic capacities, and they activate both types of muscle fibers.

From the preceding discussion, do you think that the predominant fiber type in specific muscles is an important factor that determines success in a particular sport or activity? This idea is discussed more fully in Chapter 10, as well as other considerations concerning each type of muscle fiber and various subdivisions.

THE ENERGY SPECTRUM OF EXERCISE

Figure 3-5 illustrates the relative contribution of anaerobic and aerobic energy sources during various durations of maximal exercise. Although these data were originally obtained from laboratory experiments that involved running and bicycling, they easily can be related to other activities by drawing the appropriate relationships in terms of time. For example, a 2- to 7-second period of all-out exercise represents most offensive and defensive maneuvers in football, a "solo dash" in soccer and ice hockey, or a fast-break layup in basketball. All-out exercise for about 1 minute incorporates the 400-meter dash in track, the 100-meter swim, and possibly a long rally in tennis.

It is useful to consider energy transfer as a continuum. At one extreme, the total energy for exercise is supplied almost entirely by the intramuscular phosphagens. In intense exercise that lasts 2 minutes, about half of the energy is supplied by the ATP-CP and lactic acid systems, and aerobic reactions supply the remainder. In activities of this length, the athlete ought have a high capacity for both aerobic and anaerobic metabolism. Intense exercise of an intermediate duration performed for 4 to 10 minutes requires an increasingly greater demand for aerobic energy. Examples include certain middle distance running and swimming events, basketball, rugby, soccer, field hockey, and lacrosse. Performances of 2 hours or longer, such as distance running, swimming, and cycling, or recreational jogging or hiking, rely predominantly on a constant supply of aerobic energy with little need to provide energy from glycolysis and subsequent lactic acid formation.

From a practical standpoint, the correct approach to exercise training is to analyze an activity in terms of its specific energy components and then gear training to improve those systems to assure optimal physiologic and metabolic adaptations. It is safe to conclude that an improved capacity for energy transfer translates into improved exercise performance.

OXYGEN UPTAKE DURING RECOVERY: THE "OXYGEN DEBT"

After exercise, bodily processes do not immediately return to resting levels. In "light" exercise (e.g., golf, archery, slow dancing), recovery to resting conditions is rapid and often

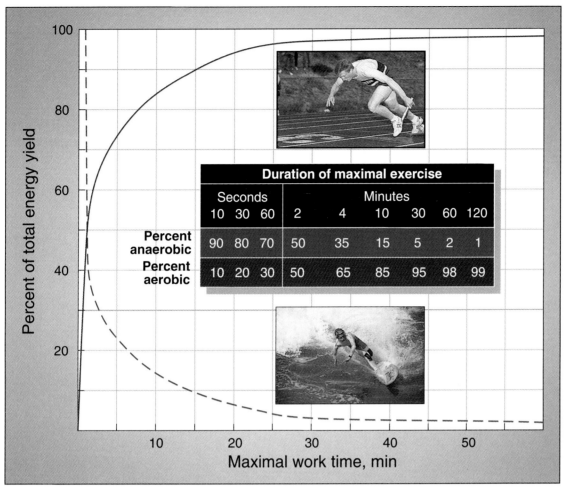

Duration of maximal exercise								
Seconds			Minutes					
10	30	60	2	4	10	30	60	120
Percent anaerobic 90	80	70	50	35	15	5	2	1
Percent aerobic 10	20	30	50	65	85	95	98	99

FIGURE 3-5. Relative contribution of aerobic and anaerobic energy metabolism during maximal physical effort of various durations. Note that about 2.0 minutes of maximal effort requires about 50% of the energy from both aerobic and anaerobic processes. At a world-class 4 minute mile pace, approximately 65 percent of the energy is derived from aerobic metabolism, with the remainder generated from anaerobic processes. (Adapted from Åstrand, P. O., and Rodahl, K.: *Textbook of Work Physiology*. New York, McGraw-Hill Book Company, 1977.)

proceeds unnoticed. If the activity is particularly stressful, however, such as running full speed for 800 meters or trying to swim 200 meters as fast as possible, it takes considerable time for the body to return to rest. The difference in recovery from both light and strenuous exercise is associated largely with the specific metabolic and physiologic processes that result from each form of exercise.

The oxygen uptake during recovery was originally termed the oxygen debt by Archibald Vivian Hill, the British Nobel physiologist. Contem-

porary theory no longer employs this term. Instead, the post-exercise oxygen uptake is referred to as recovery oxygen uptake or excess post-exercise oxygen consumption (EPOC). Regardless of the term used, the reference is to the total oxygen consumed following exercise in excess of a baseline level.

In light exercise (Figure 3-6, Panel A), where the oxygen deficit is small and the steady-rate oxygen uptake achieved rapidly, the recovery oxygen uptake is also small as recovery is rapid. In moderate to heavy aerobic exercise (Panel B) it takes longer to reach a steady rate and the oxygen deficit is considerably greater than in

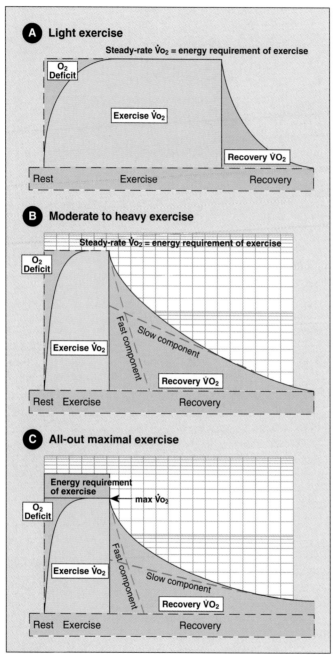

FIGURE 3-6. Oxygen uptake during exercise and in recovery from (**A**) light steady-rate exercise, (**B**) moderate to heavy steady-rate exercise, and (**C**) exhaustive exercise where one cannot attain a steady-rate of aerobic metabolism. The first phase of recovery occurs rapidly; the second phase is much slower and may take considerable time to return to resting conditions. Note that in exhaustive exercise, the oxygen requirement of the exercise is greater than the actual exercise oxygen uptake.

light exercise. Consequently, it takes longer to return to the resting level in recovery. For this more strenuous exercise, there is an initial rapid decline in the oxygen uptake in recovery (as in recovery from light exercise) that is followed by a more gradual decline to the baseline. In both Panel A and B, the oxygen deficit and recovery oxygen uptake are computed the same way, with the steady-rate oxygen uptake representing the oxygen (energy) requirement of the exercise. During the exhausting exercise illustrated in Panel C, a steady rate of aerobic metabolism cannot be attained. In this situation, anaerobic energy transfer is large, lactic acid accumulates, and considerable time is required for complete recovery. In this type of exercise no steady-rate is achieved as the energy requirement exceeds the maximal or peak oxygen uptake. In this case, the true oxygen deficit is difficult to determine. No matter how intense the exercise (golf, tennis, sailing, wrestling, cross-country skiing, sprint running, sailboarding, or surfing), there is always oxygen consumed in recovery in excess of the resting value. This quantity of oxygen is indicated by the shaded area under the recovery curve and is calculated as the total oxygen consumed in recovery minus the total oxygen that would normally be consumed at rest during the recovery period.

If a total of 5.5 liters of oxygen are consumed in recovery until the resting value of 0.31 liters per minute is reached, and the recovery required 10 minutes, the recovery oxygen uptake would be 5.5 liters minus (0.31 L x 10 min), or 2.4 liters. This result means that the preceding exercise plus the metabolic activities that occurred during recovery caused the uptake of an additional 2.4 liters of oxygen before reaching the pre-exercise state. An important assumption that underlies the calculation of the recovery oxygen uptake is that resting oxygen uptake remains essentially unchanged during exercise and recovery. This assumption is not entirely correct, especially in recovery from strenuous exercise.

The recovery curves in Figure 3-6 illustrate two fundamentals of oxygen uptake during recovery:

- If the exercise was primarily aerobic (with little disruption in body temperature), about half the total recovery oxygen uptake is repaid in 30 seconds; after several minutes, recovery is complete (fast component).
- Recovery from strenuous exercise (lactic acid and body temperature increased considerably) is quite different. In addition to the fast component of the recovery oxygen uptake, a second phase, the slow component, occurs. This phase of recovery, depending on the intensity and duration of exercise, may take up to 24 hours before the preexercise oxygen uptake level is re-established.

Metabolic Dynamics of the Recovery Oxygen Uptake

A precise biochemical explanation of the recovery oxygen uptake, especially the role of lactic acid, is not possible because the specific chemical dynamics of oxygen debt are still unclear.

Traditional Concepts. The term "oxygen debt" (used to explain the recovery oxygen uptake) was first coined by A.V. Hill in 1922. Hill, as well as others, discussed energy metabolism during exercise and recovery in financial-accounting terms. They suggested that the body's carbohydrate stores were likened to energy "credits." If these stored credits were expended during exercise, then a "debt" was incurred. The greater the energy "deficit," or use of available stored energy credits, the larger the energy debt incurred. The recovery oxygen uptake, therefore, was thought to represent the metabolic cost of repaying this debt — hence "oxygen debt".

Hill argued that the accumulation of lactic acid during the anaerobic component of exercise represented the utilization of the stored energy credit, glycogen. The ensuing oxygen debt was believed to serve two purposes: (1) to re-establish the original carbohydrate stores (credits) by resynthesizing approximately 80% of the lactic acid back to glycogen (gluconeogenesis) in the liver (Cori cycle), and (2) to catabolize the remaining lactic acid through the pyruvic acid-Krebs cycle pathway. The ATP generated in this process presumably was used to power the resynthesis of glycogen from lactic acid. This early explanation of the dynamics of recovery oxygen uptake has often been termed the "lactic acid theory of oxygen debt."

In 1933, following Hill's work, researchers at Harvard's famous Fatigue Laboratory attempted to explain their observations that the initial portion of the recovery oxygen uptake was consumed before blood lactic acid began to decrease. In fact, they showed that it was possible to incur an oxygen debt of almost 3 liters without any appreciable elevation in lactic acid. To resolve these findings, two phases of oxygen debt were proposed: (1) alactic or *alactacid* oxygen debt (without lactic acid buildup), and (2) lactic acid or *lactacid* oxygen debt (lactic acid buildup). It is noteworthy that these two explanations were based on speculation; the researchers were unable to measure ATP and CP replenishment or the relationship between lactic acid and glucose and glycogen levels. Essentially, the following model has served to explain the energetics of oxygen debt for nearly 60 years:

- **Alactacid debt.** The alactacid portion of the oxygen debt depicted for steady-rate exercise in panels A and B of Figure 3-6 or for the rapid phase of recovery from strenuous exercise (bottom graph), was attributed to the

Recovery oxygen uptake. The oxygen consumed in excess of the resting value during recovery from exercise has been called the "oxygen debt." This term was used because the excess oxygen was thought to represent the metabolic cost of repaying the stored energy (glycogen) used during the deficit, or anaerobic, phase of exercise. We now know that a large portion of the oxygen used in recovery is required for a variety of physiologic processes (circulation, ventilation, hormonal and temperature effects) that are actually elevated during recovery. Hence, the term recovery oxygen uptake more accurately describes the dynamics of the recovery process.

restoration of the high-energy phosphates ATP and CP depleted during exercise. The energy for this restoration supposedly comes from the aerobic breakdown of the food nutrients during recovery. A small portion of the recovery oxygen is also used to reload the muscle myoglobin as well as the hemoglobin in the blood returning from previously active tissues.

- **Lactacid debt**. In keeping with A.V. Hill's explanation, the major portion of the lactic acid oxygen debt was thought to represent the reconversion of lactic acid to glycogen in the liver.

Controversy About the Traditional Explanation. Several relationships must be established to verify that an aerobic energy deficit in exercise is temporarily compensated for by anaerobic energy sources which are then resynthesized in recovery as theorized by Hill. We now know that only a moderate relationship exists between the degree of anaerobiosis in exercise (oxygen deficit) and the excess oxygen uptake in recovery (oxygen debt).

Acceptance of the traditional explanation for the lactacid phase of the oxygen debt as Hill and others speculated requires proof that the major portion of lactic acid produced in exercise is actually resynthesized to glycogen in recovery. This fact, however, has never been proved. To the contrary, when radioactive-labeled lactic acid is infused into rat muscle, more than 75% of this substrate appears as radioactive carbon dioxide, whereas only 25% is synthesized to glycogen. In confirming experiments in humans, no substantial replenishment of glycogen was observed 10 minutes after strenuous exercise, even though blood lactate levels were significantly reduced. Apparently, a major portion of lactic acid is oxidized for energy. It is well established that heart, liver, kidney, and skeletal muscle tissues use lactate as an energy substrate during both exercise and recovery.

Contemporary Concepts. There is no doubt that the elevated aerobic metabolism in recovery is required to restore the body's processes to their pre-exercise condition. Following light to moderately intense exercise, the recovery oxygen uptake serves to replenish the high-energy phosphates depleted by the preceding exercise, whereas in strenuous exercise, some oxygen is used to resynthesize a portion of lactic acid to glycogen. *However, a significant portion of the recovery oxygen uptake following strenuous exercise is attributed to physiologic processes that actually take place during recovery.* The considerably larger recovery oxygen uptake in relation to oxygen deficit in exhaustive exercise is probably the result of factors such as an elevated body temperature. It is common for core temperature to increase by about 3° C (5.4° F) during vigorous, longer duration exercise, and can remain high for several hours in recovery. This thermogenic "boost" directly stimulates metabolism to cause an appreciable increase in recovery oxygen uptake.

Other factors affect recovery oxygen uptake. Perhaps as much as 10% of the recovery oxygen goes to reload the blood as it returns from the exercised muscles. An additional 2 to 5% restores the oxygen dissolved in body fluids, as well as the oxygen bound to myoglobin in the muscle itself. During intense exercise, the volume of air breathed per minute increases 8 to 15 times above resting levels, and when exercise ceases, breathing still remains elevated during recovery. Thus, the respiratory muscles require more oxygen for the work of breathing during recovery than they normally require at rest. The heart also works harder and requires a greater oxygen supply in recovery. Tissue repair and the redistribution of the ions of calcium, potassium, and sodium within the muscle and other body compartments require energy (active transport), whereas the residual effects of the hormones epinephrine, norepinephrine, and thyroxine released in exercise may continue to augment metabolism for a considerable time in recovery.

In essence, all of the physiologic systems that are activated to meet the demands of an increase in muscular activity also increase their own particular need for oxygen during recovery. The recovery oxygen uptake reflects both the anaerobic metabolism of exercise, as well as the respiratory, circulatory, hormonal, ionic, and thermal adjustments that occur in recovery as a consequence of the prior exercise.

Implications of EPOC for Exercise and Recovery

Understanding the dynamics of the recovery oxygen uptake provides a basis for structuring exercise intervals during training and optimizing recovery from strenuous exercise. No appreciable lactate accumulates with either steady-rate aerobic exercise or brief 5- to 10-second bouts of all-out work powered by the high energy phosphates. Consequently, recovery is rapid (fast component), and work can begin again with little recovery. In contrast, longer periods of anaerobic exercise powered by glycolysis are performed at the expense of lactate buildup in the blood and exercising muscles, as well as a significant disruption in other physiologic processes. In this situation, recovery oxygen uptake consists of both fast and slow components, and considerably more time is required for complete recovery. This can pose a problem in sports such as basketball, hockey, soccer, tennis, and badminton, because a performer pushed to a high level of anaerobic metabolism may not fully recover during brief rest periods such as times out, between points, or even half-time breaks.

Procedures for speeding recovery from exercise can generally be categorized as either *active* or *passive*. In active recovery (often called "cooling-down" or "tapering-off"), submaximal aerobic exercise is performed immediately after the exercise in the belief that this continued movement in some way prevents muscle cramps, stiffness, and facilitates the recovery process. In contrast, a person usually lies down in passive recovery with the hope that complete inactivity may reduce the resting energy requirements and thus "free" oxygen for the recovery process. Modifications of active and passive recovery have included the use of cold showers, massages, specific body positions, ice application, and ingesting cold fluids.

Optimal Recovery from Steady-Rate Exercise. For most people, exercise at an oxygen uptake below 55 to 60% of max $\dot{V}O_2$ can generally be performed in a steady rate with little lactate buildup. Recovery from this intensity of exercise entails the resynthesis of high-energy phosphates, replenishment of oxygen in the blood, body fluids, and muscle myoglobin, and a small energy cost to sustain circulation and ventilation. Recovery is most rapid with passive procedures under these conditions because exercise would only serve to elevate total metabolism and delay the recovery.

Optimal Recovery from Non Steady-Rate Exercise. When exercise intensity exceeds about 55 to 60% of max $\dot{V}O_2$, a steady rate of aerobic metabolism is no longer maintained, lactic acid formation exceeds its rate of removal, and blood lactate accumulates. As work intensity increases, the level of lactate rises sharply and the exerciser soon becomes exhausted. Although the precise mechanisms of fatigue during intense anaerobic exercise are not fully understood, the level of blood lactate does provide a fairly objective indication of the relative

Blood lactate is not a waste product. Lactic acid has often been called a metabolic "waste product." To the contrary, lactic acid is not treated as an unwanted chemical and then excreted from the body. Instead, it is a valuable potential source of energy that is retained at relatively high concentrations during intense exercise. When there is sufficient oxygen during recovery, lactic acid is readily converted back to pyruvic acid and then used for energy. This is the way the body preserves about 90% of energy from the original glucose molecule for later use as an aerobic energy source.

Causes of Excess Postexercise Oxygen Consumption (EPOC) with Heavy Exercise.

- Resynthesize ATP and CP
- Resynthesize lactate to glycogen (Cori cycle)
- Oxidize lactate in energy metabolism
- Restore oxygen to blood
- Effects of elevated core temperature
- Effects of hormones
- Effects of elevated heart rate, ventilation, and other levels of physiologic function

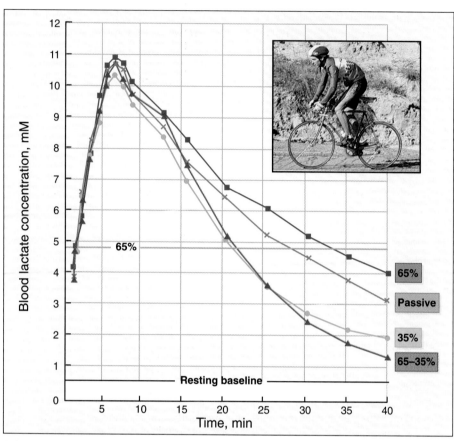

FIGURE 3-7. Blood lactate concentration following maximal exercise during passive and active exercise recoveries at 35% and 65%, and a combination of 35% and 65% of max $\dot{V}O_2$. The horizontal dashed line indicates the level of blood lactate produced by exercise at 65% of max $\dot{V}O_2$ without previous exercise. (Adapted from Dodd, S., et al.: Blood lactate disappearance at various intensities of recovery exercise. *J. Appl. Physiol.: Respirat. Environ. Exercise Physiol.*, 57:1462, 1984.)

strenuousness of exercise and may also reflect the adequacy of the recovery process.

Lactic acid removal is accelerated by performing active aerobic exercise in recovery. Apparently, the optimal level of exercise in recovery is between 30 and 45% of the max $\dot{V}O_2$ for bicycle exercise, and 55 to 60% of max $\dot{V}O_2$ when the recovery involves treadmill running. The variation between these two forms of exercise is probably caused by the more localized nature of bicycling which is generally reflected by a lower lactate threshold in this activity.

Figure 3-7 illustrates blood lactate recovery patterns for trained men who performed 6 minutes of supermaximal work on a bicycle ergometer.

Active recovery involved 40 minutes of continuous exercise at either 35 or 65% of max $\dot{V}O_2$. A combination of 65% of max $\dot{V}O_2$ performed for 7 minutes followed by 35% of max $\dot{V}O_2$ for 33 minutes also was used to evaluate whether a higher-intensity exercise interval early in recovery would expedite the removal of lactic acid from the tissues to the blood. Clearly, moderate aerobic exercise performed in recovery facilitated lactate removal compared to passive recovery. The combination of higher intensity exercise followed by lower intensity exercise was of no more benefit than a single exercise bout of moderate intensity. It is noteworthy that if exercise in recovery is too intense and above the lactate threshold, it is of no added benefit and may even prolong recovery by increasing lactic acid formation. In a practical sense, if left to their own choice, people voluntarily select their own optimal intensity of recovery exercise.

It is not entirely clear why active recovery is a better choice than passive recovery. Most likely, the facilitated removal of lactate occurs because of an increased perfusion of blood through "lactate-using" organs like the liver and heart. In addition, increased blood flow through the muscles in active recovery certainly enhances lactate removal because muscle tissue can use this substrate and oxidize it during the Krebs cycle.

Intermittent Exercise

Several approaches can enable a person to perform significant amounts of normally exhaustive exercise, while at the same time, reduce the deleterious effects of anaerobic energy transfer through glycolysis and subsequent lactic acid buildup. One is to train the aerobic systems to increase their capacity to sustain exercise at a high rate of aerobic energy transfer. A dramatic example of this high steady-rate capability is the performance of elite marathon runners, distance swimmers, and cross-country skiers who compete at close to 90% of their max $\dot{V}O_2$. Another approach to performing exercise that would normally cause exhaustion within 3 to 5 minutes if performed continuously is to exercise in an *intermittent* manner using a pre-established spacing of exercise and rest intervals.

This technique of exercise and rest intervals is popular in physical fitness and conditioning programs and is known as *interval training*. Here, various exercise-to-rest intervals using "supermaximal" exercise are applied to overload the various systems of energy transfer. For example, with all-out exercise bouts of up to 8 seconds, the intramuscular phosphates provide

the major portion of energy, with little demand on the glycolytic pathway. Therefore, recovery is rapid (fast component), and another bout of heavy exercise can begin after only a brief recovery period.

Table 3-1 summarizes the results of one series of laboratory experiments using various combinations of exercise and rest intervals during intermittent exercise. On one day, the subject ran at a speed that would normally exhaust him within 5 minutes. About 0.8 mile was covered during this continuous run, and the runner attained a maximal oxygen uptake of 5.6 liters per minute. A relative state of exhaustion plus a high level of anaerobic metabolism were verified by the high blood lactate level shown in the last column of the table.

On another day, the same fast speed was maintained, but the exercise was performed intermittently with periods of 10 seconds of exercise and 5 seconds of recovery. With a 30-minute protocol of intermittent exercise, the actual duration of running amounted to 20 minutes and the distance covered was 4 miles compared to less than 5 minutes and 0.8 miles when the run was performed continuously! This exercise capability is even more impressive if one

TABLE 3-1. Results of an experiment dealing with intermittent exercise*

Exercise: Rest Periods	Total Distance Run (yards)	Average Oxygen Uptake ($l \cdot min^{-1}$)	Blood Lactate Level (mg · 100 ml blood^{-1})
4 min continuous	1422	5.6	150
10 s exercise 5 s rest	7294	5.1	44
10 s exercise 10 s rest	5468	4.4	20
15 s exercise 30 s rest	3642	3.6	16

* From data of Christenson, E.H., et al.: Intermittent and continuous running. *Acta Physiol. Scand.*, 50:269, 1960, as reported in Åstrand, P.O., and Rodahl, K.: *Textbook of Work Physiology*. New York, McGraw-Hill, 1970, p. 384.

considers that the blood lactate level remained low although the oxygen uptake was quite high, averaging 5.1 liters per minute (91% of max $\dot{V}O_2$) throughout the 30-minute period. Thus, a relative balance was achieved between the energy requirements of exercise and the level of aerobic energy transfer within the muscle during the exercise and rest intervals.

Clearly, by manipulating the duration of exercise and rest intervals, a specific energy transfer system can be emphasized and overloaded. When the rest interval was extended from 5 to 10 seconds, the oxygen uptake averaged 4.4 liters per minute; with 15-second exercise and 30-second recovery intervals, only a 3.6 liter oxygen uptake was noted. In each case of 30 minutes of intermittent exercise, however, the runner achieved a longer distance and a much lower lactate level compared to the same exercise performed continuously. It is clear that coaches and athletes need to consider both exercise *and* rest intervals in optimizing workouts.

A practical example of applying the exercise-to-rest interval (called the *E to R method*) involves the conventional sit-up. There are two basic ways to train to improve sit-up capacity. In one method, the person does as many sit-ups as possible in a specified time period. For purposes of illustration, suppose a person completed 41 consecutive sit-ups in 2 minutes. If the person now switched methods of performing sit-ups and applied the E to R method, this is what would occur. If 6 sit-ups were done in 10 seconds, and the person repeated the sequence of sit-ups and a 20 to 30 seconds rest 10 times, total sit-ups would equal 60 (6 sit-ups x 10 repeat bouts). If the person were ambitious and performed 20 bouts of sit-ups, the total would obviously double. While the added rest intervals do add to the duration of the sit-up training, the total number of completed sit-ups becomes significantly greater than a single bout of doing as many as possible. The E to R method is a sure "winner" in terms of producing significant gains in exercise performance. The same E to R method can be applied to other types of performances such as push-ups, various flexibility exercises, and workouts with resistance equipment.

The specific application of the principles of intermittent exercise to both aerobic and anaerobic training and sports performance is discussed more fully in Chapter 14.

SUMMARY

1. The major energy pathway for ATP production differs depending on the intensity and duration of exercise. In intense exercise of short duration (100-meter dash, weight lifting), energy is derived primarily from the already present stores of intramuscular ATP and CP (immediate energy system). For intense exercise of longer duration (1 to 2 min), energy is generated mainly from the anaerobic reactions of glycolysis (short-term energy system). As exercise progresses beyond several minutes, the aerobic system predominates and oxygen uptake becomes an important factor (long-term energy system).

2. A steady rate of oxygen uptake represents a balance between the energy requirements of the exercising muscles and the aerobic resynthesis of ATP. The oxygen deficit is the difference between the oxygen requirement and the actual oxygen consumed.

3. The maximum capacity for the aerobic resynthesis of ATP is quantitatively measured as the maximum oxygen uptake or max $\dot{V}O_2$. This is one of the important indicators of one's ability to sustain high intensity exercise with undue fatigue.

4. Humans possess different types of muscle fibers, each with unique metabolic and contractile properties. The two major fiber types are: (1) low glycolytic-high oxidative, slow-twitch fibers, and (2) low oxidative-high glycolytic, fast-twitch fibers.

5. By understanding the energy spectrum of exercise, it is possible to optimally train for specific improvement of the appropriate energy system.

6. Following exercise, the oxygen uptake remains elevated above the resting level. This is called recovery oxygen uptake or oxygen debt and it reflects the metabolic characteristics of the preceding exercise, as well as the physiologic alterations caused by that exercise.

7. Moderate exercise performed during recovery (active recovery) from strenuous exercise facilitates the recovery process compared to passive procedures. In most situations, this recovery is reflected in a faster removal of lactic acid.

8. Adding rest intervals to shorter bouts of high intensity exercise can significantly enhance a variety of exercise performances (E to R method).

SELECTED REFERENCES

Bahr, R.: Effects of supramaximal exercise on excess postexercise oxygen consumption. *Med. Sci. Sports Exerc.*, 24: 66, 1992.

Bahr, R.: Excess postexercise oxygen consumption — magnitude, mechanisms and practical implications. *Acta Physiol. Scand (Suppl.)*, 605: 1, 1992.

Barstow, T.J.: Characterization of $\dot{V}O_2$ kinetics during heavy exercise. *Med. Sci. Sports Exerc.*, 26: 1327, 1994.

Brooks, G.A.: Physical activity and carbohydrate metabolism. In *Physical Activity, Fitness, and Health.* Edited by C. Bouchard, et al., Champaign, IL, Human Kinetics, 1994.

Bouchard, C., et al.: Genetics of aerobic and anaerobic performances. In *Exercise and Sport Sciences Reviews.* Vol. 20. Edited by J. O. Holloszy. Baltimore, Williams & Wilkins, 1992.

Coggan, A. R., et al.: Endurance training decreases plasma glucose turnover and oxidation during moderate-intensity exercise, *J. Appl. Physiol.,* 68: 990, 1990.

Dodd, S., et al.: Blood lactate disappearance at various intensities of recovery exercise. *J. Appl. Physiol,* 57: 1462, 1984.

Falk, B., et al.: Blood lactate concentration following exercise: effects of heat exposure and of active recovery in heat-acclimatized subjects. *Int. J. Sports Med.* 16: 7, 1995.

Gaesser, G. A., and Brooks, G. A.: Metabolic basis of excess post-exercise oxygen consumption: a review. *Med. Sci. Sports Exerc.,* 16: 29, 1984.

Gladden, L. B.: Lactate uptake by skeletal muscle. In *Exercise and Sport Sciences Reviews.* Vol. 17. Edited by K. B. Pandolf. Baltimore, Williams & Wilkins, 1989.

Hochachka, P.W. *Muscles as molecular and metabolic machines.* CRC Press. Boca Raton, FL. 1994.

Holloszy, J. O., and Coyle, E. F.: Adaptations of skeletal muscle to endurance training and their metabolic consequences. *J. Appl. Physiol.,* 56: 831, 1984.

Jacobs, I.: Blood lactate: Implications for training and sports performance. *Sports Med.,* 3: 10, 1986.

Jacobs, I., et al.: Sprint training effects on muscle myoglobin, enzymes, fiber types, and blood lactate. *Med. Sci. Sports Exerc.,* 19: 368, 1987.

Katz, A., and Sahlin, K.: Role of regulation of glycolysis and lactate production in human skeletal muscle. In *Exercise and Sport Sciences Reviews.* Vol. 18. Edited by K. B. Pandolf and J. O. Holloszy. Baltimore, Williams and Wilkins, 1990.

MacRae, H. S-H., et al.: Effects of training on lactate production and removal during progressive exercise. *J. Appl. Physiol.,* 72: 1649, 1992.

McArdle, W. D., et al.: *Exercise Physiology: Energy, Nutrition, and Human Performance.* 3rd ed. Philadelphia, Lea & Febiger, 1991.

Minotti, J. R., et al.: Training-induced skeletal muscle adaptations are independent of systemic adaptations. *J. Appl. Physiol.,* 68: 289, 1990.

Oscai, L. B., and Palmer, W. K.: Adipose tissue adaptation to exercise. In *Exercise, Fitness and Health. A Consensus of Current Knowledge.* Edited by C. Bouchard, et al., Illinois, Human Kinetics, 1990.

Poole, D.C.: VO_2 slow component: physiological and functional significance. *Med. Sci. Sports Exerc.,* 26: 1354, 1994.

Quinn, T.J., et al.: Postexercise oxygen consumption in trained females: effort of exercise duration. *Med. Sci. Sports Exerc.* 26: 908, 1994.

Stainsby, W. N., and Brooks, G. A.: Control of lactic acid metabolism in contracting muscles and during exercise. In *Exercise and Sport Sciences Reviews.* Vol 18. Edited by K. B. Pandolf. Baltimore, Williams & Wilkins, 1990.

Weltman, A., et al.: Reliability and validity of a continuous incremental treadmill protocol for the determination of lactate threshold, fixed blood lactate concentrations and $\dot{V}O_2$ max. *Int. J. Sports Med.,* 11:26, 1990.

Whipp, B.J.: The slow component of O_2 uptake kinetics during heavy exercise. *Med. Sci. Sports Exerc.,* 26: 1319, 1994.

Wolfe, R.R., and Grorge, S.: Stable isotopic tracers as metabolic probes in exercise. In *Exercise and Sport Sciences Reviews.* Vol. 21. Edited by J. O. Holloszy. Baltimore, MD, Williams & Wilkins, 1993.

Energy Expenditure at Rest and During Physical Activity

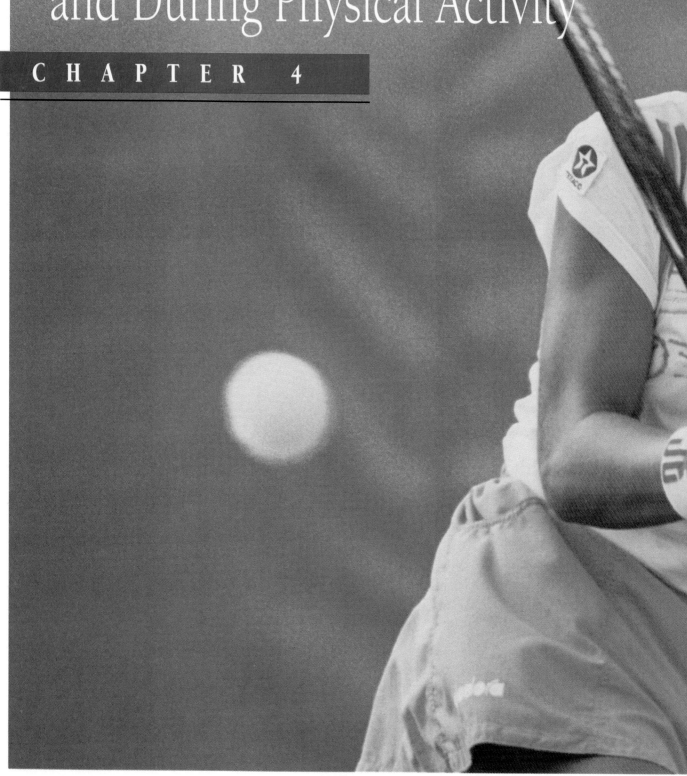

After reading this chapter you should be able to:

- Define the terms direct calorimetry, indirect calorimetry, closed-circuit spirometry, and open-circuit spirometry.
- Define RQ and discuss how it is used to quantify calorie release in energy metabolism, and the nature of the food mixture metabolized.
- Discuss the difference between RQ and R, and factors that affect the R.
- Define BMR and discuss factors that affect it.
- Indicate the role of body weight in the energy cost of different forms of physical activity.
- Discuss the factors that contribute to an individual's total daily energy expenditure.
- Outline the different classification systems for rating the strenuousness of physical activities.
- Discuss the concept of exercise economy, and highlight differences in running economy between trained and untrained individuals and children and adults.
- Graphically display the relationship between walking velocity and energy expenditure, and list important factors that affect the energy cost of walking.
- Graphically display the relationship between running velocity and energy expenditure, and discuss how air density, runner's body surface, and head wind affect energy cost.
- Discuss the reasons why the economy for swimming is significantly lower than the economy for running.

I n this chapter we discuss the direct and indirect measurement of human energy expenditure. In addition, important factors are presented that influence energy expenditure at rest and during the stress of various forms of physical activity. Specific emphasis is placed on the common exercise activities of walking, running, and swimming, and the factors that influence the economy of such activities.

CHAPTER 4

Part 1 — MEASUREMENT OF HUMAN ENERGY EXPENDITURE

HEAT PRODUCED BY THE BODY

Two techniques, direct and indirect calorimetry, are used to determine the energy generated by the body both at rest and during physical activity.

Direct Calorimetry

The heat produced by the body can be measured in a calorimeter similar to the one used to determine the energy content of food (refer to Figure 7-1). The human calorimeter illustrated in Figure 4-1 consists of an airtight chamber with an oxygen supply in which a person can live and work for an extended period. A known volume of water at a specified temperature is circulated through a series of coils at the top of the chamber. Because the entire chamber is well insulated, the heat produced and radiated by the individual is absorbed by the circulating water. The change in water temperature over a particular time period is directly proportional to the individual's energy metabolism. To provide adequate ventilation, the person's exhaled air is continually drawn from the room and passed through chemicals that remove moisture and absorb carbon dioxide. Oxygen is then added to the air and recirculated through the chamber.

Indirect Calorimetry

All energy-releasing reactions in the body ultimately depend on the utilization of oxygen. By measuring a person's oxygen uptake, it is possible to obtain an indirect estimate of energy expenditure. Indirect calorimetry is highly accurate, and compared to direct calorimetry, it is relatively simple and much less expensive in terms of maintenance, supplies, and personnel required.

There are two common methods of indirect calorimetry; these are *closed-circuit spirometry* and *open-circuit spirometry*. With the closed-circuit method, the subject breathes and rebreathes from a prefilled container of oxygen. The open-circuit method is the most widely used technique to measure oxygen uptake, especially during exercise. In open-circuit spirometry, the subject inhales ambient air that has a constant composition of oxygen (20.9%), carbon dioxide (0.03%), and nitrogen (79.0%), with the remainder inert gases. The changes in oxygen and carbon dioxide percentages in expired air compared

Human calorimeter. The direct measurement of heat production in humans is of considerable theoretical importance, yet its use and application are rather limited. The calorimeter is relatively small and quite expensive, accurate measurements of heat production are time-consuming, and its use is generally not applicable for energy determinations during common sports, occupational, or recreational activities.

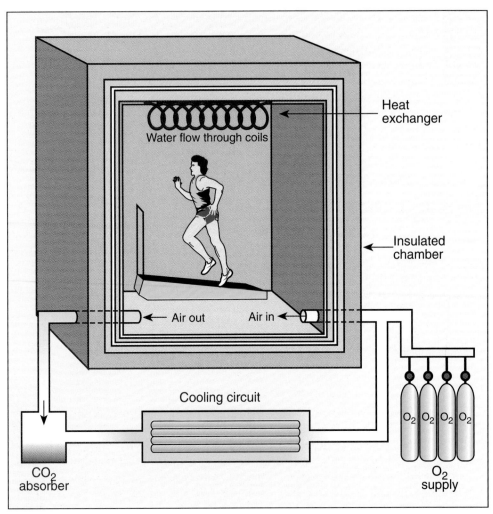

FIGURE 4-1. The body's heat production is measured directly in the human calorimeter.

to inspired ambient air indirectly reflect the ongoing process of energy metabolism. Thus, analysis of two factors — the volume of air breathed during a specified time period, and the composition of exhaled air — provides a useful way to measure oxygen uptake and infer energy expenditure. In Appendix 2 we present the step-by-step procedure for computing oxygen uptake.

Three common indirect calorimetry procedures are used to measure oxygen uptake during various physical activities:

- Portable spirometry
- Bag technique
- Computerized instrumentation.

Portable Spirometry. Two German scientists in the early 1940's developed a lightweight, portable system to deter-

mine indirectly the energy expended during a variety of physical activities, including many war-related operations such as traveling over different terrain with full battle gear, operating transportation vehicles including tanks and aircraft, and activities that soldiers would encounter during actual combat operations. The box-shaped apparatus shown in Figure 4-2 weighs approximately 3 kg and is usually carried on the back during the measurement period. The subject breathes through a two-way valve that allows inspiration of ambient air, while exhaled air passes through a meter to measure air volume. Samples of exhaled air are simultaneously collected in small rubber bags attached to the meter. Oxygen uptake is computed by measuring how much air was breathed through the meter, and analyzing the sample of expired air for oxygen and carbon dioxide content. Energy expenditure expressed in kcal is then computed from the oxygen uptake. An advantage of the portable spirometer is that it gives a person considerable freedom to move while being measured. The portable spirometer was used to estimate the energy expenditure for many of the recreational and household activities listed in Appendix 3 and in the *Student Study Guide and Workbook* (Section II).

Bag Technique. The subject shown in Figure 4-3A is riding a stationary bicycle ergometer. During the period of measurement, the subject inhales and exhales through a two-way breathing valve. Ambient air is breathed in through one side of the valve and air is exhaled through the other side into a collection bag. The volume of exhaled air is then analyzed for its composition of oxygen and carbon dioxide. Energy expenditure can be computed from oxygen uptake just as it is when using the portable spirometer. Figure 4-3B illustrates oxygen uptake being measured by the bag technique during an activity requiring the lifting of boxes of different weight and size.

Computerized Instrumentation. Recent advances in computer and microprocessor technology enable the exercise scientist to efficiently measure metabolic and cardiovascular response to exercise. A computer is interfaced with at least three instruments: a system to continuously sample the airflow from the subject, a meter to record the volume of air breathed, and oxygen and carbon dioxide analyzers to measure the composition of the expired gas mixture. The computer is pre-programmed to perform the metabolic calculations based on electronic signals it receives from the instruments. A printed or graphic display of the data is provided throughout the measurement period. More advanced systems include automated blood pressure, heart rate, and temperature monitors, as well as preset instructions to regulate the speed, duration, and workload of treadmills, bicycle ergometers, steppers, rowers, and other exercise devices. Figure 4-4 shows examples of the automated and computerized measurement of metabolic and physiologic responses.

The system illustrated in Figure 4-5 shows that all of the components for

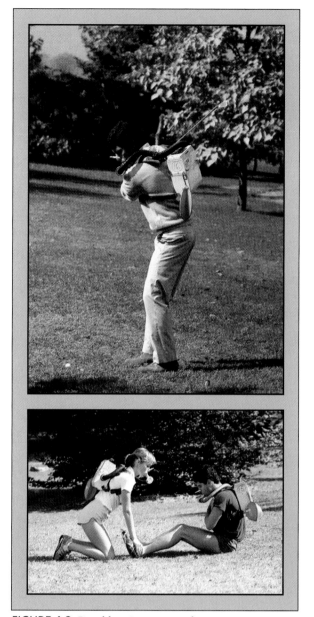

FIGURE 4-2. Portable spirometer used to measure oxygen uptake by the open-circuit method during golf and calisthenics exercise.

Good results require good data. Regardless of the sophistication of a particular automated system, the output data are only as good as the accuracy of the measuring devices. In large part, this depends on careful and frequent calibration of the electronic equipment using previously established reference standards.

metabolic measurement — ventilation meter and O_2 and CO_2 analyzers — are miniaturized to fit into the headpiece that the subject wears. The device even contains a voice-sensitive chip that provides feedback on duration of exercise, energy expenditure, heart rate, and ventilation. The microprocessor in the headpiece can store up to several hours of exercise data.

Caloric Transformation for Oxygen. Oxygen uptake can be readily converted to a corresponding value for energy expenditure. *Approximately 4.82 kcal of heat energy is liberated when 1 liter of oxygen is consumed by burning a mixture of carbohydrates, lipids, and proteins.* This value, 4.82 kcal per liter of oxygen, varies only slightly depending on the food mixture being oxidized. For convenience in calculations, therefore, a value of *5 kcal per liter of oxygen consumed* can be used as an appropriate conversion factor. This amount, 5 kcal, is important because it enables us to determine the body's energy release at rest or during steady-rate exercise simply by measuring oxygen uptake.

Weir Calculation of Energy Expenditure. In 1949, J. Weir presented a simple and accurate method for determining caloric expenditure from ventilation and expired oxygen percent. Weir

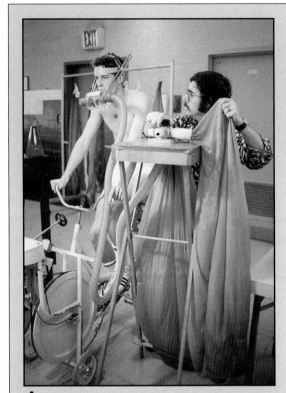

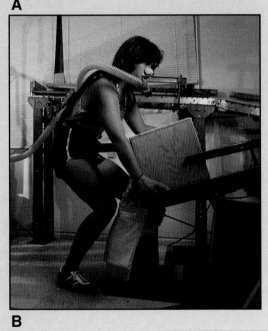

FIGURE 4-3. Measurement of oxygen uptake by open-circuit spirometry (bag technique) during (*A*) stationary cycle ergometer exercise and (*B*) during box loading and unloading.

showed that if the total caloric production due to protein breakdown is assumed to be 12.5%, a reasonable percentage, caloric expenditure can be calculated from the following formula:

$$\text{Kcal} \cdot \text{min}^{-1} = \dot{V}_{E\ STPD} \times (1.044 - 0.0499 \times \%\ O_{2\ Expired}),$$
where $\%\ O_{2\ Expired}$ is the expired oxygen percentage and $\dot{V}_{E\ STPD}$ is the expired ventilation in STPD units (see Appendix C)

Table 4-1 presents the "Weir factors" for different percentages of oxygen in expired air. Suppose, for example, the expired air contained 16.0% oxygen; reading from Table 4-1, the Weir Factor would be 0.2456. This factor is then multiplied by the ventilation volume to obtain the caloric expenditure. If the $\dot{V}_{E\ STPD} = 50\ L \cdot \text{min}^{-1}$, then the kcal $\cdot \text{min}^{-1}$ would be 12.28 (50 L $\cdot$ min^{-1} x 0.2456).

THE RESPIRATORY QUOTIENT

Because of inherent chemical differences in the composition of carbohydrates, lipids, and proteins, different amounts of oxygen are required to oxidize completely the carbon and hydrogen atoms in the molecule to the end products carbon dioxide and water. Thus, the quantity of carbon dioxide produced in relation to the oxygen uptake varies depending on the substrate metabolized. This ratio of metabolic gas exchange is termed the respiratory quotient or RQ.

$$RQ = CO_2 \text{ produced} \div O_2 \text{ uptake}$$

The RQ is useful to know during rest and steady-rate aerobic exercise because it is a convenient guide to the nutrient mixture being catabolized for energy. It also is necessary to know the value for RQ to estimate precisely the body's heat production. This is because the caloric equivalent for oxygen varies somewhat depending on the nutrient that is oxidized.

RQ for Carbohydrate

Because the ratio of hydrogen to oxygen atoms in carbohydrates is always the same as in water, that is 2:1, all the oxygen consumed by the cells is used to oxidize the carbon in the carbohydrate molecule to carbon dioxide. Consequently, during the complete oxidation of a glucose molecule, six molecules of car-

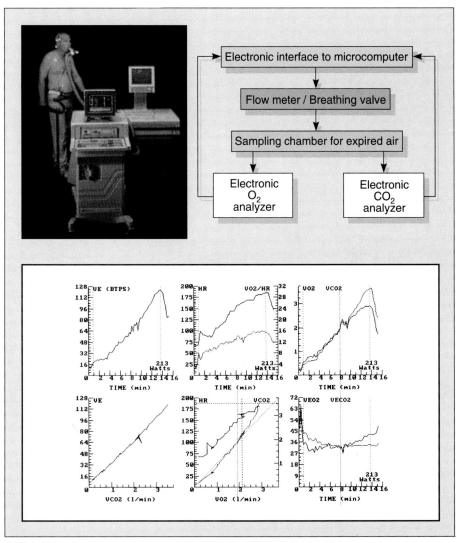

FIGURE 4-4. Computerized systems approach for the collection, analysis, and output of physiologic and metabolic data. Photos courtesy of SensorMedics Corporation, Anaheim, CA.

bon dioxide are produced and six molecules of oxygen are consumed. The overall equation for this reaction is:

$$C_6H_{12}O_6 + 6\,O_2 \rightarrow 6\,CO_2 + 6\,H_2O$$

Because the gas exchange in this reaction is equal (that is, there are an equal number of CO_2 molecules produced to O_2 molecules consumed), the RQ for carbohydrate is unity or 1.00:

$$RQ = 6\,CO_2 \div 6\,O_2 = 1.00$$

RQ for Lipid

The chemical composition of lipids differs from carbohydrates because lipids contain considerably fewer oxygen atoms in proportion to atoms of carbon and hydrogen. Consequently, when fat is degraded, relatively more oxygen is required to oxidize fat to carbon dioxide and water. When palmitic acid, a typical fatty acid, is oxidized to carbon dioxide and water, 16 carbon dioxide molecules are produced for every 23 oxygen molecules con-

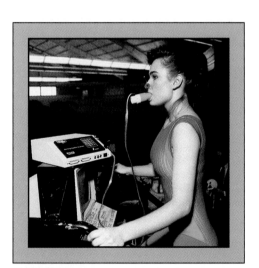

FIGURE 4-5. Miniaturized metabolic system. In future models, a headpiece will contain all of the electronic instrumentation, including the microcomputer, so it is easily transportable during physical activity. Photo courtesy of P. Howard, AeroSport Inc., Ann Arbor, MI.

TABLE 4-1. Calculation of energy expenditure by use of the Weir factors*

% O₂ Exp	Weir Factor	% O₂ Exp	Weir Factor
14.50	.3205	17.00	.1957
.60	.3155	.10	.1907
.70	.3105	.20	.1857
.80	.3055	.30	.1807
.90	.3005	.40	.1757
15.00	.2955	.50	.1707
.10	.2905	.60	.1658
.20	.2855	.70	.1608
.30	.2805	.80	.1558
.40	.2755	.90	.1508
.50	.2705	18.00	.1468
.60	.2556	.30	.1308
.70	.2606	.20	.1368
.80	.2556	.30	.1308
.90	.2506	.40	.1268
16.00	.2456	.50	.1208
.10	.2406	.60	.1168
.20	.2366	.70	.1109
.30	.2306	.80	.1068
.40	.2256	.90	.1009
.50	.2206	19.00	.0969
.60	.2157	.10	.0909
.70	.2107	.20	.0868
.80	.2057	.30	.0809
.90	.2007	.40	.0769
		.50	.0710

* The Weir factor is computed as 1.044 − 0.0499 x % O_2 EXPIRED. Use this calculation for accurate determination of the Weir factor if the O_2 EXPIRED is not shown in the table. The accuracy of the computation of kcal is within ± 1 percent of actual values when the subject has a steady-rate $\dot{V}O_2$ and their diet averages about 12.5% protein.

sumed. This exchange is summarized by the equation:

$$C_{16}H_{32}O_2 + 23O_2 \longrightarrow 16CO_2 \div 16H_2O$$
$$RQ = 16CO_2 \div 23O_2 = 0.696$$

Generally, the RQ value for lipid is considered to be 0.70.

RQ FOR PROTEIN

In the body, proteins are not simply oxidized to carbon dioxide and water during energy metabolism. Rather, the protein is first deaminated in the liver and the nitrogen and sulfur fragments are excreted in the urine and feces. The resulting "keto acid" fragments are then oxidized to carbon dioxide and water to provide energy to sustain metabolism. As in the case of fat metabolism, these short-chain keto acids require more oxygen for complete combustion in relation to carbon dioxide produced. The protein albumin oxidizes as follows:

$$C_{72}H_{112}N_2O_{22}S + 77O_2 \longrightarrow 63CO_2 + 38H_2O + SO_3 + 9CO(NH_2)_2$$
$$RQ = 63CO_2 \div 77O_2 = 0.818$$

The general value for the RQ of protein is 0.82.

RQ FOR A MIXED DIET

During activities that range from complete bed rest to light, aerobic exercise such as golf, billiards, archery, or slow-pace walking, the RQ seldom reflects the oxidation of pure carbohydrate or pure fat. Instead, a mixture of these nutrients is usually used, and the RQ is intermediate in value between 0.70 and 1.00. For most purposes, an RQ of 0.82 from the metabolism of a mixture of 40% carbohydrate and 60% fat can be assumed, and the caloric equivalent of 4.825 kcal per liter of oxygen can be applied in energy transformations. By use of this midpoint value, the maximum error possible in estimating energy metabolism from steady-rate oxygen uptake would only be about 4%.

Table 4-2 presents the energy expenditure per liter of oxygen uptake for different nonprotein RQ values. (The nonprotein value assumes that the metabolic mixture is comprised only of carbohydrate and fat.) Also included are the corresponding percentages and grams of carbohydrate and lipid utilized for energy. The table is used as follows:

Suppose the oxygen uptake during 30 minutes of steady-rate exercise averaged 3.22 L $\cdot$ min^{-1} with CO$_2$ production of 2.78 L $\cdot$ min^{-1}. The RQ would be computed as $\dot{V}CO_2 \div \dot{V}O_2$ (2.78 ÷ 3.22) or 0.86. From Table 4-2 this RQ value (left column) corresponds to an energy equivalent of 4.875 kcal per liter of oxygen uptake or an exercise energy output of 13.55 kcal $\cdot$ min^{-1} (2.78 L O$_2$ $\cdot$ min^{-1} x 4.875 kcal). Based on a nonprotein RQ, 54.1% of the calories were derived from the combustion of carbohydrate and 45.9% from fat. The total calories expended during the 30-minute exercise period was 406 kcal (13.55 kcal $\cdot$ min^{-1} x 30).

. . . .

RESPIRATORY EXCHANGE RATIO (R)

The calculation of RQ is based on the assumption that the exchange of O$_2$ and CO$_2$ measured at the lungs reflects the actual gas exchange from nutrient metabolism in the cell. This assumption is reasonably valid at rest and under steady-rate, mild to moderate exercise conditions. Factors that disturb the normal metabolic relationship between these gases, however, may spuriously alter this exchange ratio. For example, an

TABLE 4-2. Thermal equivalents of oxygen for the non-protein respiratory quotient, including percent kcal and grams derived from carbohydrate and fat*

Nonprotein RQ	Kcal per Liter O₂ Uptake	Percentage Kcal Derived from		Grams per Liter O₂ Uptake	
		Carbohydrate	Fat	Carbohydrate	Fat
0.707	4.686	0.0	100.0	0.000	.496
.71	4.690	1.1	98.9	.012	.491
.72	4.702	4.8	95.2	.051	.476
.73	4.714	8.4	91.6	.900	.460
.74	4.727	12.0	88.0	.130	.444
.75	4.739	15.6	84.4	.170	.428
.76	4.750	19.2	80.8	.211	.412
.77	4.764	22.8	77.2	.250	.396
.78	4.776	26.3	73.7	.290	.380
.79	4.788	29.9	70.1	.330	.363
.80	4.801	33.4	66.6	.371	.347
.81	4.813	36.9	63.1	.413	.330
.82	4.825	40.3	59.7	.454	.313
.83	4.838	43.8	56.2	.496	.297
.84	4.850	47.2	52.8	.537	.280
.85	4.862	50.7	49.3	.579	.263
.86	4.875	54.1	45.9	.621	.247
.87	4.887	57.5	42.5	.663	.230
.88	4.887	60.8	39.2	.705	.213
.89	4.911	64.2	35.8	.749	.195
.90	4.924	67.5	32.5	.791	.178
.91	4.936	70.8	29.2	.834	.160
.92	4.948	74.1	25.9	.877	.143
.93	4.961	77.4	22.6	.921	.125
.94	4.973	80.7	19.3	.964	.108
.95	4.985	84.0	16.0	1.008	.090
.96	4.998	87.2	12.8	1.052	.072
.97	5.010	90.4	9.6	1.097	.054
.98	5.022	93.6	6.4	1.142	.036
.99	5.035	96.8	3.2	1.186	.018
1.00	5.047	100.0	0	1.231	.000

*From Zuntz, H.: *Pflugers Acrh. Physiol.,* 83:557, 1901.

increase in carbon dioxide elimination occurs during hyperventilation (see Chapter 8) because the response of breathing is disproportionately high in relation to the metabolic demands of a particular exercise intensity. With over-breathing, the normal level of CO_2 in the blood is reduced because the CO_2 is "blown off" in the expired air. This increase in carbon dioxide elimination is not accompanied by a corresponding increase in oxygen uptake; thus, there is a disproportionate increase in the gaseous exchange ratio that cannot be attributed to the oxidation of foodstuffs. In such cases, the ratio of carbon dioxide produced to oxygen consumed usually increases above 1.00. Respiratory physiologists have termed the ratio of carbon dioxide produced to oxygen consumed under conditions when the exchange of oxygen and carbon dioxide at the lungs no longer reflects the oxidation of specific foods in the cells, the *Respiratory Exchange Ratio* or R. The value for R (ratio of CO_2 produced to O_2 consumed) is calculated in exactly the same manner as the RQ.

Exhaustive exercise presents another situation in which R can rise significantly above 1.00. The lactic acid generated during anaerobic exercise is buffered or "neutralized" by sodium bicarbonate in the blood to maintain the proper acid-base balance in the reaction:

It is also possible to obtain relatively low R values. For example, carbon dioxide tends to be retained in the cells

$$HLa + NaHCO_3 \longrightarrow NaLa + H_2CO_3 \longrightarrow H_2O + CO_2 \longrightarrow Lungs$$

Carbonic acid, a weaker acid, is formed during this process. In the pulmonary capillaries, carbonic acid breaks down to its components, carbon dioxide and water, and the carbon dioxide exits through the lungs. This buffering process adds "extra" carbon dioxide to that quantity normally released during energy metabolism, and the R moves toward and above 1.00.

and body fluids following very strenuous anaerobic exercise to replenish the bicarbonate used to buffer lactic acid. This action reduces the quantity of expired carbon dioxide (less CO_2 expired in relation to O_2 consumed) and may cause the respiratory exchange ratio to dip temporarily below 0.70.

SUMMARY

PART 1

1. Direct and indirect calorimetry are the two methods for determining the body's rate of energy expenditure. With direct calorimetry, the actual heat production is measured in an insulated calorimeter. Indirect calorimetry infers energy expenditure from measurements of oxygen uptake and carbon dioxide production, using either closed-circuit or open-circuit spirometry.

2. Because of their chemical composition, carbohydrates, lipids, and proteins require different amounts of oxygen in relation to carbon dioxide produced during oxidation. The ratio of CO_2 produced to O_2 consumed is called the respiratory quotient or RQ. This ratio provides an important clue to the nutrient mixture catabolized for energy. The RQ for carbohydrate is 1.00, for lipid it is 0.70, and for protein it is 0.82.

3. For each RQ value, there is a corresponding calorific value for each liter of oxygen consumed. This value provides for a high degree of accuracy in determining energy expenditure during steady-rate exercise. A value of 5 kcal per liter of O_2 consumed can serves as a rough estimation of the calorific value for oxygen when estimating energy expenditure.

4. In strenuous exercise, the RQ may not be representative of specific substrate utilization because of nonmetabolic production of carbon dioxide, as occurs during the buffering of lactic acid. When this occurs, there is a disproportionate increase in the amount of CO_2 produced to O_2 consumed. Under such situations, the R is used to denote the ratio of gaseous exchange.

Many obese individuals complain that they do not necessarily consume more food than their lean counterparts, but the food they consume results in greater fat deposition. If correct, this would suggest a defective thermogenic or energy generating response in obesity that contributes to a greater storage of calories (kcal) per kcal ingested. This could result in long-term weight gain for an obese person compared to a lean person, even if the food (energy) intake of the two were identical.

The possibility that the obese might have a defective thermogenic response has been the focus of considerable research over the last few years. One proposed mechanism for a blunted thermogenesis (that leads to greater energy storage per quantity of energy ingested) is based on the possibility that obese individuals have increased insulin resistance and a reduced rate of nonoxidative glucose disposal, which has a greater energy cost than does glucose oxidation. This means that obese individuals who are insulin resistant may have a reduced rate of glucose storage per amount of food ingested. This would lead to a greater energy conservation over time and an increase in body weight.

The typical procedure to measure energy conservation is to administer the same amount of food to a group of obese and nonobese people and then measure the energy expenditure for several hours. Only a relatively small increase in total energy expenditure in response to the meal would indicate the potential for greater energy storage per kcal of food ingested.

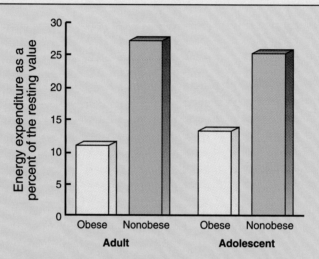

Thermic effect of a meal for adult and adolescent obese and nonobese subjects. The lower values for the obese show that for a given energy intake they expend less energy (i.e., store more kcal) than the nonobese subjects.

The insert bar graph presents the results of two experiments, one performed on obese adults and the other on obese adolescents. Each experiment had a non obese control group of the same age and gender. Each of the groups was administered the same food load, and the energy expenditure was monitored for up to 3 hours after eating. As illustrated in the graph, both the obese adults and adolescents had a significantly blunted thermogenic response. This smaller increase in metabolic rate in response to a food challenge in obesity may help to explain the relative ease of weight gain (and difficulty for weight loss) on a given kcal intake among the obese.

Consider the following example to illustrate the effects of a reduced thermogenesis in response to food. Suppose an obese and nonobese person each consumed 2500 kcal daily, but the obese person had a blunted thermogenic response to the meal similar to that observed in the adolescent study illustrated in the insert graph. Over a year, the obese person would store an extra 18,750 kcal compared to the normal-weight individual. This corresponds to a potential weight gain of nearly 5.5 lbs or about a 25 lb difference between the obese and nonobese person over a 5-year period!

References

Katch, V.L., et al. Reduced short-term thermic effects of a meal in obese adolescent girls. *Eur. J. Appl. Physiol.* 65:535, 1992.

Segal, K. R., et al. Comparison of thermic effects of constant and relative caloric loads in lean and obese men. *Am. J. Clin Nutr.* 51:14, 1990.

Figure 4-6 illustrates that daily energy expenditure is determined by three factors:

- Resting metabolic rate, which includes basal and sleeping conditions plus the added cost of arousal
- Thermogenic influence of food consumed
- Energy expended during physical activity and in recovery

basal metabolic rate (BMR) and is usually determined by measuring oxygen uptake under three standardized laboratory conditions. First, no food is eaten for at least 12 hours prior to measurement to eliminate the energy required for digestion and absorption of food. Abstaining from food in this manner is referred to as the *postabsorptive state*. Second, no undue muscular exertion should have occurred

Components of Daily Energy Expenditure

Resting Metabolic Rate (~60-75%)
- sleeping metabolism
- basal metabolism
- arousal metabolism

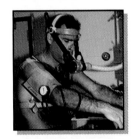

Thermic Effect of Feeding (~ 10%)

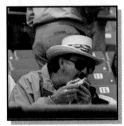

Thermic Effect of Physical Activity (~15-30%)

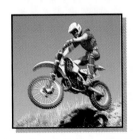

FIGURE 4-6. Components of the daily energy expenditure.

ENERGY EXPENDITURE AT REST: BASAL METABOLIC RATE

For each individual, there is a minimum energy requirement to sustain the body's functions in the waking state. This requirement is called the

for at least 12 hours prior to determining the BMR. Third, the subject lies quietly in a dimly lit, temperature-controlled room during the test. Oxygen uptake is measured after the person has been lying quietly for 30 to 60 minutes.

Basal oxygen uptake. Values for oxygen uptake during the BMR test usually range between 160 and 290 ml per minute (0.80 to 1.45 kcal · min⁻¹); depending upon a variety of factors, especially a person's size.

The measurement of BMR under controlled laboratory conditions provides a convenient method to study the relationship between energy expenditure and body size, gender, and age. The BMR also establishes an important energy baseline for implementing a sound program of weight control by food restraint, exercise, or the effective combination of both.

Influence of Body Size on Resting Metabolism

When individuals who differ in body size are compared for basal energy metabolism, this value is usually expressed in terms of surface area and not of body mass. The results of numerous experiments have provided data on average values of BMR per unit surface area in men and women of different ages.

Figure 4-7 reveals that BMR is not equal between genders, but averages 5 to 10% lower in women at all ages. This lower BMR can be attributed to a woman's larger percentage of body fat and smaller muscle mass. However, the BMR differences are essentially eliminated when the BMR is expressed per unit of "fat-free" or lean body mass. Whereas this observation may be of some theoretical importance, the curves shown in Figure 4-7 still describe the BMR in men and women adequately. From ages 20 to 40, average values for BMR are 38 kcal per square meter (m^2) of surface per hour for men, and 36 kcal for women. If one desires a more precise estimate of BMR, the actual average value for a specific age can be read directly from the curves. By using the values for heat production in Figure 4-7 in conjunction with the appropriate value for sur-

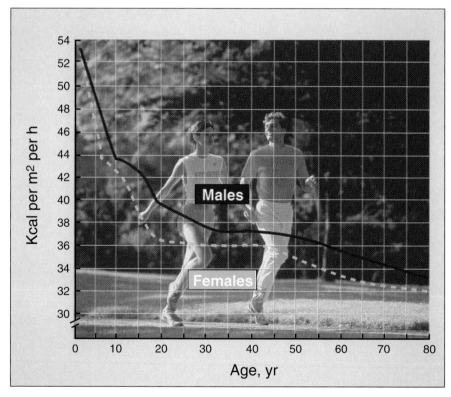

FIGURE 4-7. Basal metabolic rate as a function of age and gender. (Data from Altman, P. L., and Dittmer, D.: *Metabolism*. Bethesda, MD, Federation of American Societies for Experimental Biology, 1968.)

face area, it is easy to estimate resting metabolism in kcal per minute and convert this to a total daily requirement. The nomogram in Figure 4-8 provides a simplified method for computing surface area based on stature and mass.

To determine surface area with the nomogram, locate stature on Scale I and body mass on Scale II. Connect the two points with a straight edge. The intersection at Scale III gives the surface area in square meters. For example, if stature is 185 cm and mass is 75 kg, surface area according to Scale III on the nomogram is 1.98 m^2.

Estimate Daily Resting Energy Expenditure

To estimate one's approximate energy expenditure or kcal requirement during rest, multiply the appropriate average kcal per unit surface area per hour from Figure 4-7 by the surface area determined from the nomogram in Figure 4-8. Then multiply this value by 24 to estimate the energy requirement for 24 hours.

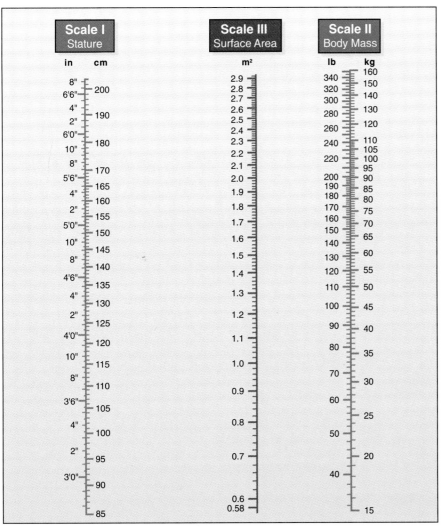

FIGURE 4-8. Nomogram to estimate body surface area from stature and mass. (Reproduced from "Clinical Spirometry," as prepared by Boothby and Sandiford of the Mayo Clinic, through the courtesy of Warren E. Collins, Inc., Braintree, MA.)

Dietary Induced Thermogenesis

For most people, food has a stimulating effect on energy metabolism attributable mainly to the energy-requiring processes of digesting, absorbing, and assimilating the various nutrients. This dietary induced thermogenesis reaches a maximum within 1 hour after a meal, and it can vary between 10 and 15% of the ingested food energy depending on the quantity and type of food eaten. While considerable variability exists among individuals, the magnitude of dietary induced thermogenesis can vary between 10 and 35% of the ingested food energy in normal individuals depending on both the quantity and type of food eaten. A meal of pure protein, for example, elicits the greatest thermic effect and is nearly 25% of the total calories of the meal itself.

The calorie-burning effect of protein ingestion has been used by some to argue for a high-protein diet for weight reduction. They maintain that fewer calories are ultimately available to the body with a meal high in protein compared to a lipid or carbohydrate meal of similar caloric value. Although this point may have some validity, other factors must be considered in formulating a prudent weight loss program — not to mention the potentially harmful strain on kidney and liver function brought on by excessive protein intake. For one thing, well-balanced nutrition requires a blend of macronutrients as well as appropriate quantities of vitamins and minerals. In addition, if exercise is combined with food restriction for weight loss, carbohydrate intake is important to provide energy for exercise and to conserve the lean tissue often lost through dieting.

Research indicates that individuals who have poor control over their body weight often have a blunted thermic response to eating. Undoubtedly, this could contribute to a considerable accumulation of body fat over a period of years. The important point, however, is that if a person's life-style includes regular periods of moderate physical activity, the thermogenic effect represents only a small portion of the total daily energy expenditure. It also appears that exercising after eating augments an individual's normal thermic response to food intake. This certainly would support the wisdom of "going for a brisk walk" after eating, especially for those interested in weight control.

Exercise augments thermogenesis. In one study, exercising 30 minutes after eating breakfast nearly doubled the thermogenic effect of the meal compared to the effect of eating without subsequent exercise.

Thermic effect of protein. Part of the elevated thermic response to dietary protein is thought to be due to the "extra" energy required to convert certain amino acids into glucose.

SUMMARY

PART 2

1. A person's total daily energy expenditure is the sum of the energy required in basal and resting metabolism, thermogenic influences (especially the thermic effect of food), and the energy generated in physical activity.
2. The BMR is the minimum energy required to maintain vital functions in the waking state. The BMR is only slightly lower than the resting metabolism and is proportionate to the surface area of the body. It is also related to age, and generally is higher for men than for women; these influences are largely due to variation in lean body mass and percent body fat.
3. Dietary induced thermogenesis refers to the increase in energy metabolism attributable to the digestion, absorption, and assimilation of food nutrients. A blunted thermogenic response to eating may contribute to weight gain.

An understanding of resting energy metabolism provides an important frame of reference for the potential to increase daily energy output. According to numerous surveys, about one-third of a person's waking hours is spent in resting activities such as watching television, lounging around the home, and engaging in activities that are little more intense than resting conditions. This means that the total daily energy expenditure has the potential to be considerably greater than the basal requirement, depending of course on the intensity, duration, and type of physical activity performed.

Researchers have measured the energy expended during such varied activities as brushing teeth, cleaning house, mowing the lawn, walking the dog, driving a car, playing ping-pong, bowling, dancing, swimming, sawing, and physical activity during space flight. Consider an activity such as rowing continuously at 30 strokes a minute for 30 minutes. How can we determine how many calories are "burned" during the 30 minutes?

If the amount of oxygen consumed averaged 2 liters per minute during each minute of rowing, then in 30 minutes the rower would consume 60 liters of oxygen. A reasonably accurate estimate of the energy expended in rowing can be made because the utilization of 1 liter of oxygen generates about 5 kcal of energy. In this example, the rower generated 300 kcal (60 liters x 5 kcal) during the exercise period. This value is considered the *gross energy expenditure*.

All this energy, however, cannot be attributed solely to the energy expended during rowing because the 300 kcal value also includes the resting requirement during the 30 minutes. By knowing the exerciser's size (body mass = 81.8 kg; stature = 183 cm), surface area can be determined from the nomogram in Figure 4-8. The value for surface area, 2.04 m^2, when multiplied by the average BMR for gender (38 kcal/m^2/h x 2.04 m^2), gives the resting metabolism per hour. This amounts to approximately 78 kcal per hour, or 39 kcal "burned" over a 30-minute period. Based on these computations, the *net energy expenditure* can be determined solely for rowing. It is equal to the total energy expenditure (300 kcal) minus the requirement for rest (39 kcal), resulting in a net energy expenditure for rowing of approximately 261 kcal (300 kcal gross − 39 kcal rest).The net kcal values would be computed in similar fashion for other physical activities.

Some investigators have measured the daily energy expenditure for men and women in a variety of occupations. This is done by determining the time spent in each activity and the energy expended for the activity. An accurate assessment of the time spent in activities is kept by diary, and energy expenditure is measured with the portable spirometer shown in Figure 4-2. Because it is impractical to carry the spirometer constantly day after day, frequent observations are made for a representative time period. For the miner listed in Table 4-3, who spent 12 hours during the week loading coal, the energy cost of the task ranged from 5.5 to 7.2 kcal per minute. For purposes of computation, an average value of 6.3 kcal per minute was used to represent the energy cost during this time. The total of 26,460 kcal expended during the 1-week period averaged 3780 kcal per day. This value includes the energy expended during the 8-hour work shift, the energy cost of an 8-hour sleeping period, as well as the remaining 8-hour period spent in nonoccupational activities.

Caloric cost of exercise. The portable spirometer shown in Figure 4-2 has been used extensively to determine the energy cost of most daily chores and occupational activities, while the balloon and computer techniques have measured oxygen uptake in activities such as cycling, swimming, skiing, walking, jogging, running, dancing, rowing, and resistance training.

A considerable energy output. The competitive efforts of elite athletes during a marathon generate a steady rate energy expenditure of about 25 kcal per minute for the duration of the run. Among elite rowers, a 5 to 7 min competition generates about 36 kcal per minute!

TABLE 4-3. Energy expended by a coal miner during one week*

Activity	Time Spent in 1 Week (h)	(min)	Rate of Energy Expended (kcal · min⁻¹)	Energy in 1 Week (kcal)
Sleep				
in bed	58	30	1.05	3690
Nonoccupational				
Sitting	38	37	1.59	3680
Standing	2	16	1.80	250
Walking	15	0	4.90	4410
Washing and dressing	5	3	3.30	1000
Gardening	2	0	5.00	600
Cycling	2	25	6.60	960
Work				
Sitting	15	9	1.68	1530
Standing	2	6	1.80	230
Walking	6	43	6.70	2700
Cutting	1	14	6.70	500
Timbering	6	51	5.70	2340
Loading	12	6	6.30	4570
Total	168	h		
26,460				
Average daily energy expenditure				3780

The rate of energy expended is in units of $kcal \cdot min^{-1}$.

* Data from Garry, R. C., et al.: Expenditure of energy and the consumption of food by miners and clerks. *Medical Research Council Report No. 289.* Fife, Scotland, H.M.S.O., 1955.

If you weigh more, it costs more. The effect of added weight on energy expenditure occurs whether a person gains weight "naturally" as body fat, or as an acute added load, such as sports equipment or a weighted vest worn on the torso.

Weight-bearing exercise. In weight-bearing exercise such as walking, running, and cross-country skiing, participants must transport their body mass during the activity. This makes the cost of the exercise closely linked to body mass.

ENERGY COST OF RECREATION AND SPORT ACTIVITIES

Table 4-4 lists several examples to illustrate the large variation in energy cost that occurs with participation in various types of physical activities.

Notice, for example, that volleyball requires about 3.6 kcal per minute, or 216 kcal hourly, for a person weighing 71.4 kg (157 lb). The same person will expend more than twice this amount of energy, or 546 kcal per hour, while swimming the front crawl. Viewed somewhat differently, 25 minutes of swimming requires about the same number of calories as participating in recreational volleyball for 1 hour. If the pace of the swim or volleyball game is increased, the energy expenditure will rise proportionally.

Effect of Body Mass

Body size often plays an important role with respect to exercise energy requirements, just as it does for BMR. Figure 4-9 illustrates that heavier people generally expend more energy to perform the same activity than people who weigh less. This is because the energy expended during *weight-bearing* exercise increases in proportion to body mass. The relationship is so high that energy expenditure during walking or running can be predicted from body mass with almost as much accuracy as if the actual oxygen uptake were measured. In *non-weight-bearing* exercise such as stationary cycling, on the other hand, there is little relationship between body mass and the energy cost of exercise.

A practical application of these findings is that walking and other forms of

TABLE 4-4. Gross energy cost for selected recreational and sports activities in relation to body mass*

Activity	kg lb	50 110	53 117	56 123	59 130	62 137	65 143	68 150	71 157	74 163	77 170	80 176	83 183
Volleyball		l2.5	2.7	2.8	3.0	3.1	3.3	3.4	3.6	3.7	3.9	4.0	4.2
Aerobic dancing		6.7	7.1	7.5	7.9	8.3	8.7	9.2	9.6	10.0	10.4	10.8	11.2
Cycling, leisure		5.0	5.3	5.6	5.9	6.2	6.5	6.8	7.1	7.4	7.7	8.0	8.3
Tennis		5.5	5.8	6.1	6.4	6.8	7.1	7.4	7.7	8.1	8.4	8.7	9.0
Swimming, slow crawl		6.4	6.8	7.2	7.6	7.9	8.3	8.7	9.1	9.5	9.9	10.2	10.6
Touch football		6.6	7.0	7.4	7.8	8.2	8.6	9.0	9.4	9.8	10.2	10.6	11.0
Running, 8-min. mile		10.8	11.3	11.9	12.5	13.1	13.6	14.2	14.8	15.4	16.0	16.5	17.1
Skiing, uphill racing		13.7	14.5	15.3	16.2	17.0	17.8	18.6	19.5	20.3	21.1	21.9	22.7

*Data from *Student Study Guide and Workbook*.
Note: Energy expenditure is computed as the number of minutes of participation multiplied by the kcal value in the appropriate body weight column. For example, the kcal cost of one hour of tennis for a person weighing 150 pounds is 444 kcal (7.4 kcal x 60 min).

weight-bearing exercise provide a substantial caloric expenditure for heavier people.

Notice in Table 4-4 that the energy expended in playing tennis or volleyball for a person weighing about 83 kg is considerably greater than for a person 20 kg lighter. When the caloric cost is expressed in terms of body mass, that is, as kcal per minute per kilogram of body mass ($kcal \cdot min^{-1} \cdot kg^{-1}$), the difference in caloric cost is reduced considerably between men and women of different sizes. Although the average energy expenditure during recreational tennis may be 0.109 $kcal \cdot min^{-1} \cdot kg^{-1}$ regardless of race, gender, or body mass, keep in mind that the total energy expended by the heavier player is greater, simply because the body mass itself must be transported, and this requires proportionately more energy. Appendix 3 and Section II of the *Student Study Guide and Workbook* presents a comprehensive list of the gross energy expended in relation to body mass during household, recreational and sport, and occupational and industrial activities. These figures represent average values that can vary consider-

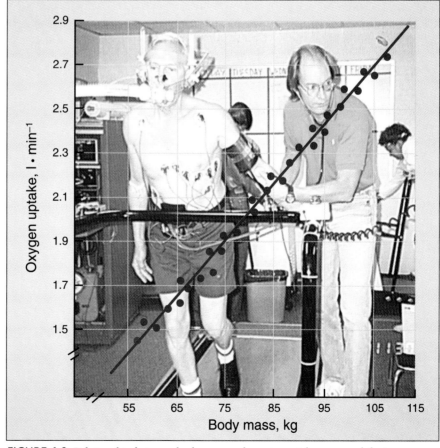

FIGURE 4-9. Relationship between body mass and oxygen uptake measured during submaximal, brisk treadmill walking. (From Applied Physiology Laboratory, Queens College, Flushing, N. Y.) Photo courtesy of Dr. Jay Graves.

ably depending on skill and pace of performance.

How to Use Appendix 3 and *Section II of the Student Study Guide and Workbook.* Refer to the column closest to the person's body mass. Multiply the number in this column by the number of minutes spent in an activity. Suppose an individual weighs 62.3 kg (137.4 lb) and spends 30 minutes playing a casual game of billiards. To determine the energy cost of participation, multiply the caloric value per minute (2.6 kcal) by 30 to obtain the 30-minute gross expenditure of 78 kcal. If the same individual does aerobic dance for 45 minutes, the gross energy expended would be calculated as 6.4 kcal x 45 minutes or 288 kcal.

AVERAGE DAILY RATES OF ENERGY EXPENDITURE

A committee of the United States Food and Nutrition Board proposed various norms to represent average rates of energy expenditure for men and women in the United States. These standards apply to people whose occupations could be considered between sedentary and active, and who participate in some recreational activities such as weekend swimming, golf, and tennis. As shown in Table 4-5, the *average daily energy expenditure is 2700 kcal for men and 2000 kcal for women between the ages of 23 and 50.* As seen in the lower part of the table, about 75% of the average person's day is spent in fairly sedentary activity. This predom-

TABLE 4-5. Average daily rates of energy expenditure for men and women living in the United States*

	Age (yr)	Mass (kg)	Mass (lb)	Stature (cm)	Stature (in)	Energy Expenditure (kcal)
Men	15–18	66	145	176	69	2800
	19–22	70	154	177	70	2900
	23–50	70	154	178	70	2700
	51+	70	154	178	70	2400
Women	15–18	55	120	163	64	2100
	19–22	55	120	163	64	2100
	23–50	55	120	163	64	2000
	51+	55	120	163	64	1800

Average daily rates of energy expenditure for men and women living in the United States*

Activity	Time (h)
Sleeping and lying down	8
Sitting	6
Standing	6
Walking	2
Recreational activity	2

* Data from Food and Nutrition Board, National Research Council, *Recommended Dietary Allowances,* 8th rev. ed., National Academy of Sciences, Washington, DC, 1980.

inance of physical inactivity has prompted some sociologists to refer to the modern-day American as *homo sedentarius.*

CLASSIFICATION OF WORK

All of us at one time or another have done some type of physical work that we would classify as exceedingly "difficult." This might be walking up a long flight of stairs, shoveling a snow-filled driveway, running to catch a bus, loading and unloading furniture on a truck, digging a deep trench, skiing through a snow storm, or running in soft beach sand. There are two factors to consider in rating the difficulty of a particular task. The first is the duration of the activity, and the second is the intensity of the effort. Both factors can vary considerably. For example, two people of the same body size could expend an equal amount of energy completing the same task. One might exert extreme effort over a short period, while the other could exert less effort over a longer period. This can be illustrated for running a 26-mile marathon at various speeds. One runner might run at maximum pace and complete the race in a little more than 2 hours. Another runner of about the same fitness might select a slower, more leisurely pace and complete the run in 3 hours. In these examples, the *intensity* of exercise is the factor distinguishing how the work is completed. In another situation, two people may run at the same speed, but one may run twice as long as the other. Here, exercise *duration* becomes the important consideration.

Several classification systems have been proposed for rating the intensity of work. The five-level classification system presented in Table 4-6 rates the difficulty of exercise based on energy expended by average men and women performing a physical activity throughout a workday. The energy intensity that corresponds to a particular rating is expressed in kcal per minute and *METs,* a MET being

defined as a multiple of the resting metabolism. *One MET represents an average person's resting metabolism or oxygen uptake.* It is not directly measured but is assumed to equal an oxygen uptake of $3.5 \text{ ml} \cdot \text{kg}^{-1} \cdot \text{min}^{-1}$. It is possible to use the MET concept to estimate the oxygen cost of exercise for a particular individual if body mass and the MET level of exercise are known. For example, if your body mass is 75 kg and you are exercising at a level of 10 METs, your oxygen uptake will equal $35 \text{ ml} \cdot \text{kg}^{-1} \cdot \text{min}^{-1}$ ($3.5 \text{ ml} \cdot \text{kg}^{-1} \cdot \text{min}^{-1}$ x 10) or a total of 2.625 L $\cdot \text{min}^{-1}$ ($35 \text{ ml} \cdot \text{kg}^{-1} \cdot \text{min}^{-1}$ x 75 kg). If we apply the calorific value for oxygen of 5 kcal per liter O_2, then you will be expending about $13.1 \text{ kcal} \cdot \text{min}^{-1}$ while exercising ($2.635 \text{ L} \cdot \text{min}^{-1}$ x 5 kcal). The use of METs is justified for quick screening purposes in estimating exercise intensity and energy demands. However, if more precision is required the various techniques of indirect calorimetry should be applied.

Most tasks require only a moderate energy expenditure. As a frame of reference for evaluating the intensity of effort, most industrial jobs and household tasks require an energy expenditure that is less than 3 times resting level, or the equivalent of 3 METs.

TABLE 4-6. Five-level classification of physical activity based on exercise intensity*

Level	Energy Expenditure			
Men				
	kcal · min⁻¹	l · min⁻¹	ml · kg⁻¹ · min⁻¹	METs
Light	2.0–4.9	0.40–0.99	6.1–15.2	1.6–3.9
Moderate	5.0–7.4	1.00–1.49	15.3–22.9	4.0–5.9
Heavy	7.5–9.9	1.50–1.99	23.0–30.6	6.0–7.9
Very heavy	10.0–12.4	2.00–2.49	30.7–38.3	8.0–9.9
Unduly heavy	12.5–	2.50–	38.4–	10.0–
Women				
	kcal · min⁻¹	l · min⁻¹	ml · kg⁻¹ · min⁻¹	METs
Light	1.5–3.4	0.30–0.69	5.4–12.5	1.2–2.7
Moderate	3.5–5.4	0.70–1.09	12.6–19.8	2.8–4.3
Heavy	5.5–7.4	1.10–1.49	19.9–27.1	4.4–5.9
Very heavy	7.5–9.4	1.50–1.89	27.2–34.4	6.0–7.5
Unduly heavy	9.5–	1.90–	34.5–	7.6–

* l · min⁻¹ based on 5 kcal per liter of oxygen; ml · kg⁻¹ · min⁻¹ based on 65-kg man and 55-kg woman; one MET is equivalent to the average resting oxygen uptake.

PART 3

1. Energy expenditure can be expressed in gross as well as net terms. Total or gross values include the resting energy requirement, whereas net energy expenditure is the energy cost of the activity per se excluding the value for resting metabolism.

2. It is possible to classify different occupations as well as athletic groups by daily rates of energy expenditure. Within any classification, however, there is large amount of variability due to energy expended in recreational pursuits. In addition, heavier individuals expend more energy in most physical activities than lighter counterparts.

3. The average daily energy expenditure is estimated to be 2700 to 2900 kcal for men and 2000 to 2100 for women between the ages of 15 and 50 years. Great variability in daily energy expenditure exists, however, and this difference is largely determined by one's physical activity level.

4. Different classification systems exist for rating the strenuousness of physical activities. These include the ratings based on (1) the energy cost expressed in kcal $\cdot$ min^{-1}, (2) the oxygen requirement in L $\cdot$ min^{-1}, or (3) multiples of the resting metabolic rate or METs.

ENERGY EXPENDITURE DURING WALKING, RUNNING, AND SWIMMING

The total energy expended each day depends largely on the type and duration of one's physical activity. The following sections detail the energy expenditure of the popular activities—walking, running, and swimming. Aside from being competitive sports, these exercises take on special significance because they are commonly prescribed in programs for weight control, physical conditioning, and cardiac rehabilitation.

ECONOMY OF MOVEMENT

The concept of economy can generally be viewed as the relationship between energy input and resulting energy output. In an economic sense, economy of operation relates to the cost required to produce goods in relation to the money generated from the sale of such goods. In another context, the auto industry is always striving to optimize the aerodynamic design of its vehicles to improve economy of operation which is reflected in the important miles-per-gallon rating. In terms of economy of human movement, the basic concern is the quantity of energy required to perform a particular task in relation to the quality of the performance. In a sense this is illustrated in assessing the ease of movement of highly trained athletes. It does not require a trained eye to qualitatively discriminate the ease of effort in comparisons of elite swimmers, skiers, cyclists, and dancers with less skilled counterparts who seem to expend considerable "wasted energy" to perform the same task. (Refer to Appendix 3 for a discussion of estimating the actual *mechanical efficiency* of human movement.)

A fairly simple and commonly used means to establish differences among individuals in the economy of physical effort is to evaluate the *oxygen uptake* while performing a particular exercise.

This approach is useful during steady rate exercise where the oxygen consumed during the activity closely mirrors the energy expended. For example, at a given submaximal speed of running, cycling, or swimming, an individual with greater economy for movement consumes less oxygen to perform the task. This is important in longer-duration exercise where success largely depends on the aerobic capability of the individual and the oxygen requirements of the task. *All else being equal, any adjustment in training that improves the economy of effort directly translates into improved endurance performance.*

No single biomechanical factor can account for individual variation in running economy. Even among trained runners, significant variation is observed in economy at a particular speed. At least for well-trained runners, it would seem that the best procedure is to let them run at the stride length they have selected through years of practice; this generally produces the most economical running performance blended to individual variations in body mass, inertia of limb segments, and anatomic development. Consequently, there is no "best" style characteristic of elite runners! Biomechanical analysis may help some athletes correct or "fine tune" minor irregularities in movement patterns while running. This would certainly be of considerable practical importance to the competitive runner. An ideal training program enhances both the economy of movement and the aerobic capacity to perform the exercise task.

Running Economy: Children and Adults, Trained and Untrained

In general, boys and girls are less economical in running compared to adults because they require between 20 to 30% more oxygen per unit of body mass to run at a given speed. These differences have been attributed to greater stride frequency among children, as well as to differences in mechanics that could contribute to their inferior movement economy. As shown in Figure 4-10B, the decreasing steady-rate $\dot{V}O_2$ values at a given speed indicate that running economy improves steadily from ages 10 to 18 years. This in part helps to explain the relatively poor performance of young children in distance running, as well as the progressive improvement in the endurance performance of children throughout adolescence. This occurs even though the aerobic capacity in relation to body mass (ml $O_2 \cdot kg^{-1} \cdot min^{-1}$; Fig. 4-10A) remains relatively constant during this time.

At a particular speed, elite endurance runners generally run at an oxygen uptake that is lower than less trained or less successful counterparts of the same age. This has been shown for 8 to 11-year-old cross-country runners as well as adult marathoners. Distance athletes as a group tend to run

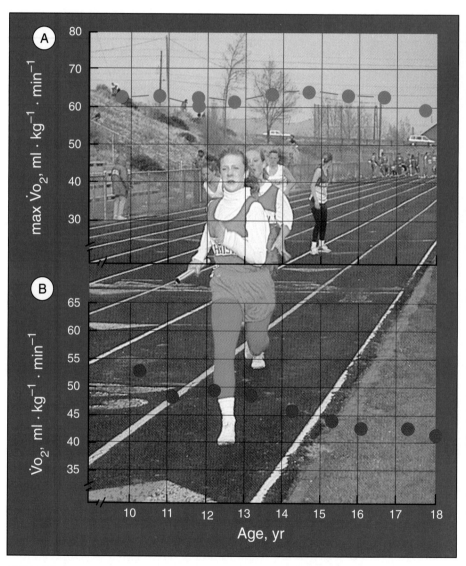

FIGURE 4-10. Effects of growth on (*A*) aerobic capacity and (*B*) submaximal oxygen uptake during running at 202 m · min⁻¹. (Adapted from Daniels, J., et al.: Differences and changes in $\dot{V}O_2$ among runners 10 to 18 years of age. *Med. Sci. Sports,* 10:200, 1978.)

with between 5 to 10% more economy than well-trained middle-distance runners.

ENERGY EXPENDITURE DURING WALKING

Walking is the most common form of exercise. For most individuals, it represents the major type of physical activity that falls outside the realm of sedentary living. Figure 4-11 displays the energy expenditure during walking at slow and fast speeds and running. The relationship between walking speed and oxygen uptake is approximately linear between speeds of 3.0 and 5.0 kilometers per hour (1.86 to 3.10 mph); at faster speeds, walking becomes less economical and the relationship curves in an upward direction that indicates a greater energy cost per unit of distance traveled. This finding accounts for the observation that, per unit distance traveled,

the total calories expended are greater at the faster but less efficient walking speeds.

Competition Walking

The energy expenditure of Olympic-caliber walkers has been studied at various speeds while walking and running on a treadmill. In actual competition, the walking speed of these athletes averaged 13.0 kilometers per hour (11.5 to 14.8 km · h^{-1} or 7.1 to 9.2 mph) over distances ranging from 1.6 to 50 km. This was a relatively fast speed, because the winner of the 20-km walk at the 1992 Barcelona Olympics averaged a record 14.4 km per hour (8.9 mph) during this 12.4-mile walk. As illustrated in Figure 4-12, the break point in economy of locomotion between walking and running for these competitive racewalkers is about 8.0 km · hr^{-1}. These data, plus biomechanical evidence, support the contention that the crossover speed at which running

Specificity of max$\dot{V}O_2$. The attainment of similar values for max$\dot{V}O_2$ in both racewalking and running in elite competitive walkers further supports the model for aerobic training specificity because in nontrained subjects, aerobic capacity measured during a graded walking test is generally 5 to 15% lower compared to that achieved with running.

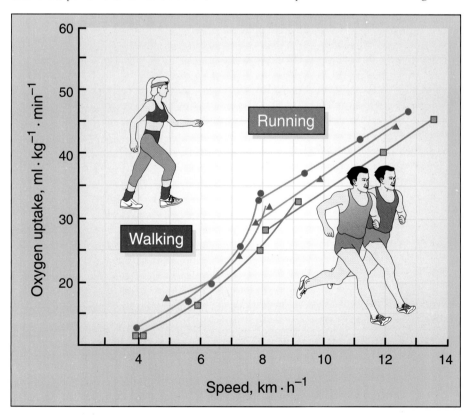

FIGURE 4-11. Relationship between oxygen uptake and speed of horizontal walking and running. Different symbols represent values from various studies reported in the literature. (Adapted from Falls, H. B., and Humphrey, L. D.: Energy cost of running and walking in young adult women. *Med. Sci. Sports,* 8:9, 1976.)

becomes more economical than walking remains about the same for both conventional walking and competitive styles of walking (Figure 4-12). For racewalkers the oxygen uptake during treadmill walking at competition speeds was only slightly lower than the highest oxygen uptake measured for these athletes during treadmill running. Also, the relationship between oxygen uptake and walking at speeds above 8 km per hour (4.97 mph) was approximately linear, but the slope of the line was twice as steep compared to running at the same speeds. Although these athletes were able to walk at velocities up to 16 km per hour (9.94 mph) and attain oxygen uptakes as high as those achieved while running, *the economy of walking faster than 8 km per hour was one-half of that for running at similar speeds.*

Competition walkers are able to achieve such high yet uneconomical rates of movement compared with conventional walking by use of a special gait that involves a "rolling" of the hips. Among elite race walkers, variations in economy for walking contribute more to performance in this sport than previously observed among competitive runners.

Effects of Body Mass

At horizontal walking speeds ranging from 3.2 to 6.4 km per hour (2.0 to 4.0 mph), energy expenditure can be predicted with reasonable accuracy for people who differ considerably in body mass. The predicted values for energy expenditure are listed in Table 4-7; these are accurate to within 15% of the actual energy expenditure for both men and women of different sizes.

On a daily basis, therefore, estimates of the energy expended in walking could be in error by only about 50 to 100 kcal, assuming that the person walks 2 hours each day. The table is

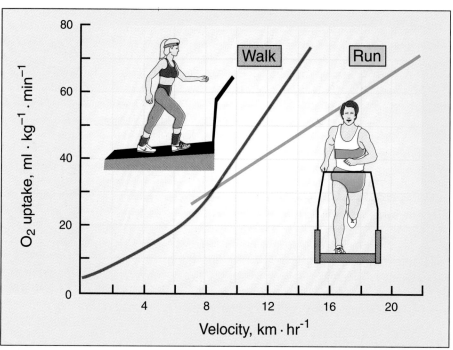

FIGURE 4-12. Relationship between oxygen uptake and horizontal velocity for walking and running in competition walkers. (Adapted from Menier, D. R., and Pugh, L. G. C. E.: The relation of oxygen intake and velocity of walking and running in competition walkers. *J. Physiol.*, 197:717, 1968.)

easy to use, is formulated on sound research, and is relatively accurate for assessing the caloric cost of walking within the speed range indicated and for body masses up to 91 kg (200 lb). For heavier individuals, extrapolations can be made but with some loss in accuracy.

Effects of Terrain and Walking Surface

The influence of terrain and surface on the energy cost of walking is summarized in Table 4-8. Economy is similar for level walking on a grass track or on a paved surface. Walking in the sand, however, is almost twice as costly as walking on a hard surface, while walking in soft snow elevates the metabolic cost 3-fold compared to similar walking on a treadmill. Certainly, a brisk walk along a beach or in freshly fallen snow provides an excellent exercise stress in programs designed to "burn up" calories or improve physiologic fitness.

Effects of Footwear

It is considerably more costly to carry weight on the feet or ankles than to carry similar weight attached to the torso. For example, for an increment in weight equal to 1.4% of body mass placed on the ankles, the energy cost of walking increases an average of 8% or nearly 6 times more than if the same weight is carried on the torso. In a practical sense, the energy cost of locomotion during walking and running is significantly increased by wearing boots compared to running shoes. Simply adding an additional 100 g to each shoe causes a 1% increase in oxygen uptake during moderate running. The implications of these findings for the design of running shoes, hiking and climbing boots, and work boots traditionally required in professions such as mining, forestry, fire fighting, and the military seems clear — small changes in shoe weight produce large changes in the economy of locomotion.

TABLE 4-7. Prediction of energy expenditure (kcal · min^{-1}) based on speed of level walking and body mass*

Speed			Body Mass						
		kg	36	45	54	64	73	82	91
mph	km · hr^{-1}	lbs	80	100	120	140	160	180	200
2.0	3.22		1.9	2.2	2.6	2.9	3.2	3.5	3.8
2.5	4.02		2.3	2.7	3.1	3.5	3.8	4.2	4.5
3.0	4.83		2.7	3.1	3.6	4.0	4.4	4.8	5.3
3.5	5.63		3.1	3.6	4.2	4.6	5.0	5.4	6.1
4.0	6.44		3.5	4.1	4.7	5.2	5.8	6.4	7.0

* Data from Passmore, R., and Durnin, J.V.G.A., Human energy expenditure. *Physiol. Rev.,* 35: 801, 1955.
How to use the chart: A 54 kg (120 lb) person who walks at 3.0 mph (4.83 km · hr^{-1}) expends 3.6 kcal · min^{-1}. A total of 216 kcal would be expended if the person walked for 60 min.

Use of Hand-Held and Ankle Weights

The impact force on the legs while running is equal to about 3 times body mass whereas the level of leg shock with walking is only about 30 percent of this value.

Walking. For many men and women the use of ankle weights increases the energy cost of walking to values usually observed for running. This is beneficial to people who desire to use only walking as a relatively low-impact training modality, yet require intensities of effort higher than can be provided at normal walking speeds. Hand-held weights also increase the metabolic (caloric) and physiologic (cardiovascular) cost of walking. There is some indication, however, that this procedure disproportionately elevates systolic blood pressure, perhaps due to the elevated intramuscular tension with gripping the weight. For individuals with existing hypertension or coronary heart disease, this could restrict the use of hand-held weights.

Cushioning makes a difference. Shoes with differing cushioning properties affect the economy with a softer-soled running shoe reducing the oxygen cost of running by about 2.4% compared to a similar shoe with a firmer cushioning system— even though the softer-soled shoe averaged 31 g heavier per pair.

TABLE 4-8. Effect of Different Terrain on the Energy Expenditure of Walking Between 5.2 and 5.6 km · h^{-1}

Terrain[a]	Correction Factor[b]
Paved road (similar to grass track)	0.0
Plowed field	1.5
Hard snow	1.6
Sand dune	1.8

a First entry from Passmore, R., and Dumin, J.V.G.A.: Human energy expenditure. *Physiol. Rev.* 35:801, 1955. Last three entries from Givoni, B., and Goldman, R.F.: Predicting metabolic energy cost. *J. Appl. Physiol.* 30:429, 1971.
b The correction factor is a multiple of the energy expenditure for walking on a paved road or grass track. For example, the energy cost of walking in a plowed field is 1.5 times that of walking on the paved road.

Running. Simply increasing the unweighted running speed or distance is probably a more desirable alternative than using hand or ankle weights if running is the preferred mode of exercise. This will certainly reduce the injury potential from increased impact force in the weighted condition and eliminate the added discomfort of carrying weights.

. . . .

ENERGY EXPENDITURE DURING RUNNING

Running can be performed at various intensities depending on terrain, weather, training goals, and the performer's fitness level. The energy expenditure for running has been quantified in one of two ways:
- During performance of the actual activity
- On a treadmill in the laboratory where running speed and grade can be precisely controlled.

Jogging and running are essentially qualitative terms that relate to the speed at which movement is performed. This difference is determined largely by the relative aerobic energy demands required in raising and lowering the body's center of gravity and accelerating and decelerating the limbs during the run. At identical running speeds, a highly conditioned distance runner runs at a lower percentage of maximal aerobic capacity than an untrained runner, even though the oxygen uptake during the run may be similar for both people. Thus, the demarcation between what is considered jogging and running depends on the fitness level of the participant; a jog for one person could be a run for another.

Independent of fitness, however, it is more economical from an energy standpoint to discontinue walking and to begin to jog or run at speeds greater than about 8 km per hour (5 mph). This was illustrated in Figure 4-11 which shows the relationship between oxygen uptake and horizontal walking and running for men and women at speeds ranging from 4 to 14 km per hour (2.5 to 8.7 mph). The lines relating oxygen uptake and speed of walking and running indicate that the "break point" between the economy of walking and running occurs at about 8 km per hour (5.0 mph).

The Economy of Running

The data for running shown in Figure 4-11 illustrate an important principle in relation to running speed and energy expenditure. Because the relationship between oxygen uptake and speed of running is linear (it is only about 3% more costly to run at a fast compared to slow pace), the total caloric cost of running a given distance at a steady-rate oxygen uptake is about the same whether the pace is fast or slow. In simple terms, if one runs a mile at a speed of 10 miles per hour, it requires about twice as much energy per minute as running at 5 miles per hour; however, the runner finishes the mile in 6 minutes whereas running at the slower speed requires twice the time or 12 minutes. Consequently, the net energy cost of the mile is about the *same,* regardless of whether it is run at a fast or slow pace.

For horizontal running, the net energy cost (that is, excluding the resting requirement) per kilogram of body mass per kilometer traveled is approximately 1 kcal or $1 \ kcal \cdot kg^{-1} \cdot km^{-1}$. Thus, for an individual who weighs 78 kg, the net energy requirement for running 1 km would be about 78 kcal, regardless of the running speed. Expressed in terms of oxygen uptake, this would amount to 15.6 liters of oxygen consumed per kilometer (1 liter O_2 = 5 kcal). In comparing the energy cost of locomotion per unit distance traveled, it is well documented that for both men and women it is more costly to run than to walk a given distance.

Energy Cost Values

Table 4-9 presents values for the *net* energy expended during running for 1 hour at various speeds.

Running speeds are expressed as kilometers per hour, miles per hour, as well as the number of minutes required to complete one mile at a particular running speed. The boldface values are the net calories expended to run one mile for a given body mass; this energy requirement is fairly constant and *independent* of running speed. Thus, for a person who weighs 62 kg, running a 26-mile marathon requires about 2600 kcal whether the run is completed in just over 2 hours or 4 hours!

For a heavier person, the energy cost per mile increases proportionately. This certainly supports the role of weight-bearing exercise as a caloric stress for the overfat individual who may want to increase energy expenditure for purposes of weight control. For example, if a 102-kg person jogs 5 miles each day at any comfortable pace, 163 kcal are expended for each mile completed, or a total of 815 kcal for the 5-mile run. Increasing or decreasing the speed (within the broad range of steady-rate paces) simply alters the length of the exercise period; it has little effect on the total energy expended.

Effects of Air Resistance

Anyone who has run into a head wind intuitively knows that more energy is expended trying to maintain a

TABLE 4-9. Net energy expenditure per hour for horizontal running in relation to velocity and body mass[a]

[a] The table is interpreted as follows: For a 50-kg person, the *net* energy expenditure for running for 1 hour at 8

Body kg	Mass lb	km·hr⁻¹[b] mph min per mile Kcal per mile	8 4.97 12:00	9 5.60 10:43	10 6.20 9:41	11 6.84 8:46	12 7.46 8:02	13 8.08 7:26	14 8.70 6:54	15 9.32 6:26	16 9.94 6:02
50	110	**80**	400	450	500	550	600	650	700	750	800
54	119	**86**	432	486	540	594	648	702	756	810	864
58	128	**93**	464	522	580	638	696	754	812	870	928
62	137	**99**	496	558	620	682	744	806	868	930	992
66	146	**106**	528	594	660	726	792	858	924	990	1056
70	154	**112**	560	630	700	770	840	910	980	1050	1120
74	163	**118**	592	666	740	814	888	962	1036	1110	1184
78	172	**125**	624	702	780	858	936	1014	1092	1170	1248
82	181	**131**	656	738	820	902	984	1066	1148	1230	1312
86	190	**138**	688	774	860	946	1032	1118	1204	1290	1376
90	199	**144**	720	810	900	990	1080	1170	1260	1350	1440
94	207	**150**	752	846	940	1034	1128	1222	1316	1410	1504
98	216	**157**	784	882	980	1078	1176	1274	1372	1470	1568
102	225	**163**	816	918	1020	1122	1224	1326	1428	1530	1632
106	234	**170**	848	954	1060	1166	1272	1378	1484	1590	1696

km·hr⁻¹ or 4.97 mph is 400 kcal; this speed represents a 12-minute per mile pace. Thus, 5 miles would be run in 1 hour and 400 kcal would be expended. If the pace was increased to 12 km·hr⁻¹, 600 kcal would be expended during the hour of running.

[b] Running speeds are expressed as kilometers per hour (km.hr⁻¹), miles per hour (mph), and minutes required to complete each mile (min per mile). The values in **boldface type** are the *net* calories expended to run 1 mile for a given body mass, independent of running speed.

given pace compared with running in calm weather or with the wind at one's back. The magnitude of the effect of air resistance on the energy cost of running varies with three factors:

- Air density
- The runner's projected surface area
- The square of the wind velocity

Depending on running speed, overcoming air resistance accounts for 3 to 9% of the total energy requirement of running in calm weather. Running into a head wind creates an additional energy expense. For example, the average oxygen uptake while running at 15.9 km per hour in calm conditions was 2.92 liters per minute. This increased by 5.5% to 3.09 liters per minute against a 16-km per hour (9.9 mph) "head wind" and 4.1 liters per minute while running against the strongest wind (41 mph); this represented a 41% additional expenditure of energy to maintain running velocity! This influence of headwind on the oxygen cost of running verifies the wisdom of some athletes who select to run in a more aerodynamically desirable position (drafting) directly behind a competitor.

Some may argue that the negative effects of running into a headwind are counterbalanced on one's return with the tailwind. This is not the case, however, as the energy cost of cutting through a headwind is significantly greater than the reduction in exercise oxygen uptake observed with an equivalent wind velocity at one's back. Wind tunnel tests have shown that modification of clothing or even trimming one's hair can improve aerodynamics and reduce wind resistance effects by up to 6%, significantly increasing running performance. In competitive bicycling, clothing and helmets as well as the rider's body position on the bicycle are continually being modified in an attempt to reduce the effects of air resistance on energy cost.

At higher altitudes, wind velocity has less effect on energy expenditure than it does at sea level due to the reduced air density at higher elevations. For speed skaters, for example, the oxygen cost of skating at a particular speed is always lower at altitude compared to sea level. Overcoming air resistance at altitude only becomes important at the faster skating speeds. In all likelihood, this altitude-effect would also be the case for running, cross-country skiing, and cycling.

Treadmill Versus Track Running

Although the treadmill is used almost exclusively to evaluate the physiology of running, a question exists concerning the validity of this procedure for determining the energetics of running and for relating this to performance on a track. For example, is the energy required to run a given speed or distance on a treadmill the same as that required to run on a track in calm weather? To answer this question, eight distance runners were studied on both a treadmill and track at three submaximal speeds of 180, 210, and 260 meters per minute (6.7, 7.8, and 9.7 mph), and during a graded exercise test to determine possible differences between treadmill and track running on both submaximal and maximal oxygen uptake.

From a practical as well as a statistical standpoint, there were no measurable differences in the aerobic requirements of submaximal running (up to 286 m per min) on the treadmill or track (either on level or up a grade), or between the maximal oxygen uptake measured in both forms of exercise under similar environmental conditions. It is still possible, however, that at the faster running speeds achieved during endurance competition, the influence of air resistance becomes considerable and the oxygen cost of track running may become greater compared to "stationary" running on a treadmill at the same speed.

Marathon Running

The first place finisher in the men's division of the 1992 New York City Marathon set a course record of

2:08:1.The average speed of 4:53 minutes per mile over the 26.2 mile course is an outstanding achievement in terms of human performance. Not only does this pace require a steady-rate aerobic metabolism that exceeds the aerobic capacity of the average male college student, but it also represents about 85 to 90% of the marathoners aerobic power that must be maintained for just over 2 hours! These athletes have an average aerobic capacity of approximately 4.4 liters per minute or 70 to 84 ml · kg^{-1} · min^{-1}.

Two long-distance runners were measured during a marathon to determine the energy expenditure per minute and the total caloric cost of the run. For these racers, oxygen uptake was determined every 3 miles by use of the balloon technique of open-circuit spirometry. Their marathon times were 2 h: 36 min: 34 s and 2 h: 39 min: 28 s; their maximal oxygen uptakes measured during treadmill running were 4.43 liters per minute (70.5 ml · kg^{-1} · min^{-1}) and 4.66 liters per minute (73.9 ml · kg^{-1} · min^{-1}), respectively. During the marathon, the first runner maintained an average speed of 270.5 m per minute (10.0 mph), which required an oxygen uptake equal to 80% of his maximal aerobic power. For the second runner, whose average speed was slower at 266.1 m per minute (9.92 mph), the aerobic energy requirement per minute averaged 78.3% of maximum. For both men, the energy requirement for running the marathon was between 2300 to 2400 kcal.

For distance runners who train up to 100 miles a week, or slightly less than the distance of four marathons at close to competitive speeds, the weekly caloric expenditure from exercise is about 10,000 kcal. For the serious marathon runner who trains year-round, the total energy expended in training for 4 years prior to an Olympic competition would be close to two million calories! It is not surprising then that these superior athletes have such a low quantity of body fat (3 to 5% of body mass for men). As illustrated in

Table 4-9, the total expenditure of energy for a marathon run remains fairly constant for individuals of similar body size, regardless of running speed. Obviously, persons with low aerobic capacities must maintain a slower running speed; thus, they will need more time to finish the marathon.

. . . .

ENERGY EXPENDITURE DURING SWIMMING

Swimming exercise differs in several important respects from walking or running. One obvious difference in swimming is that energy must be expended to maintain buoyancy and at the same time to generate horizontal movement by the use of the arms and legs, either in combination or separately. Other differences include the requirements for overcoming the *drag forces* that impede the movement of an object through a fluid. *The amount of drag depends on the fluid medium and on the size, shape, and velocity of the object.* All of these differences contribute to a significantly lower economy in swimming compared to running. *Within this framework, the energy cost of swimming a given distance is about four times greater than running the same distance.*

Methods of Measurement

Energy expenditure has been computed from oxygen uptake measured by open-circuit spirometry during portions of the swimming performance. In studies conducted in the pool, the researcher walks alongside the swimmer and carries the portable gas collection equipment. In another form of swimming exercise illustrated in Figure 4-13A, the subject remains stationary and attached or "tethered" to a cable and pulley system by means of a belt worn around the waist. The amount of weight attached to the cable can be increased periodically, thereby forcing the swimmer to exert more effort to keep from being pulled back.

Figure 4-13B shows a subject swimming in a flume or "swim-mill." Water is circulated and its velocity can vary from a slow swimming speed to a near-record pace for a free-style sprint. Also, water temperature in the 38,000-liter swim-mill can be varied from 10 to 40°C, and photographic analysis of stroke mechanics is possible through windows on the side of the flume beneath the water's surface. Values for aerobic capacity measured by either tethered, free, or flume swimming are essentially identical. This means that either of these modes can be used to evaluate the functional capacity of the aerobic system during swimming.

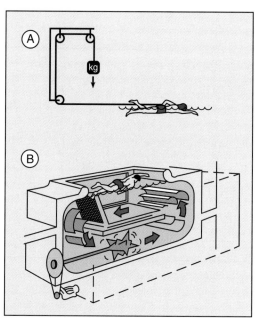

FIGURE 4-13. *(A)* Measurement of energy expenditure during tethered swimming. *(B)* The swimming flume (Adapted from Àstrand, P. O., and Englesson, S.: A swimming flume. *J. Appl. Physiol.,* 33:514, 1972.)

Energy Cost and Drag

The total drag force encountered by the swimmer consists of three components:

- **Wave drag** is caused by waves that build up in front of and form hollows behind the swimmer as he or she moves through the water. This component of drag is not a significant factor when swimming at slow velocities, but its influence becomes greater at faster swimming speeds.

- **Skin friction drag** is produced as the water slides over the surface of the skin. Even at relatively fast swimming velocities, the quantitative contribution of skin friction drag to the total drag is probably small. However, recent research supports the common practice of swimmers "shaving down" to reduce skin friction drag. Removal of body hair reduced drag, thus decreasing the energy cost and physiologic demands during swimming at a particular speed.

- **Viscous pressure drag** contributes substantially to counter the propulsive efforts of the swimmer at slow velocities. It is caused by the separation of the thin sheet of water, or boundary layer, adjacent to the swimmer. The pressure differential created in front of and behind the swimmer represents the viscous pressure drag. Its effect is probably reduced in highly skilled swimmers who have learned to "streamline" their stroke. Such streamlining with improved stroke mechanics reduces the separation region by moving the separation point closer to the trailing edge of the water. This is similar to what occurs when an oar slices through the water with the blade parallel rather than perpendicular to the flow of water.

Energy Cost, Swimming Velocity, and Skill

Elite swimmers are able to swim a particular stroke at a given velocity at a lower oxygen uptake than are relatively untrained or recreational swimmers. This is illustrated in Figure 4-14A for the breaststroke, front crawl, and back crawl with subjects representing three levels of ability. One subject was a recreational swimmer who did not participate in swimming training; the trained subject swam on a daily basis and was a top Swedish swimmer; the elite swimmer was a European champion. Except for the breaststroke, the elite swimmer was able to swim at a given speed with a lower oxygen uptake than his trained and untrained counterparts. Figure 4-14B shows that for the two trained athletes swimming at any particular speed, the breaststroke was the most costly; this was followed by the backstroke, with the front crawl being the least "expensive" of the three strokes.

Effects of Buoyancy: Men Versus Women

Women of all ages possess on the average significantly more total body fat than men. Because fat floats and muscle and bone sink, the average woman therefore gains a hydrodynamic lift and floats more easily than her male counterpart. It is likely that this difference in body fat and thus in buoyancy is partly responsible for the greater economy for swimming observed in women. For example, women can swim a given distance at a lower energy cost than men; expressed another way, women can achieve a higher swimming velocity than men for the same level of energy expenditure.

It is also possible that the distribution of body fat in women is such that their legs float high in the water, making them more horizontal or

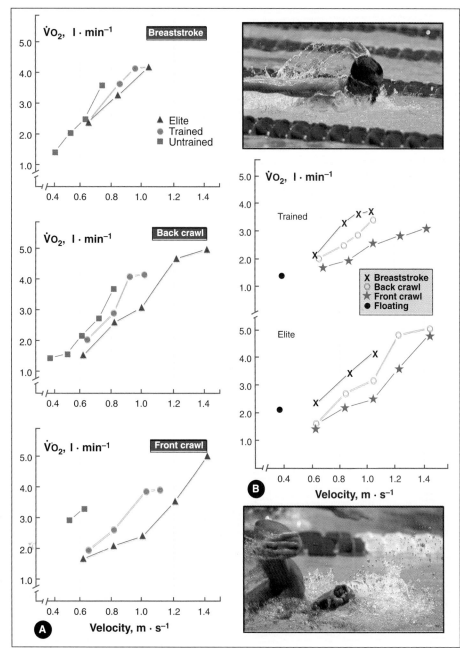

FIGURE 4-14. *A.* Oxygen uptake as a function of speed for the breaststroke, front crawl, and back crawl in subjects who represented three levels of skill ability. *B.* Oxygen uptake for two trained swimmers during three competitive strokes. (From Holmér, I.: Oxygen uptake during swimming in man. *J. Appl. Physiol.*, 33: 502, 1972.). Photos courtesy of John Urbanchek, Varsity men's swim coach, University of Michigan.

"streamlined," whereas the leaner men's legs tend to swing down and float lower in the water. This lowering of the legs to a deeper position would increase body drag and thus reduce swimming economy.

Such differences in flotation may also help explain the "gender difference" in swimming economy and that present swimming performances of women are more closely approaching those of men. The potential hydrodynamic benefits enjoyed by women become especially noteworthy in longer distances where swimming economy and body insulation are important. In fact, the record for swimming the English Channel of 7 hours: 40 minutes is presently held by a female compared to the men's record of 8 hours: 12 minutes!

SUMMARY

PART 4

1. The relationship between walking speed and oxygen uptake is essentially linear. Walking surface also has an influence because walking on sand requires about twice the energy expenditure as walking on hard surfaces. The energy cost is proportionally larger for heavier people.

2. It is more economical from an energy standpoint to jog-run rather than to walk at speeds that exceed 8 km · h^{-1} (5 mph). The difference between jogging and running depends on the fitness level of the participant; a jog for one person may be a run for another.

3. For many people, hand-held and ankle weights can increase the energy cost of walking to values usually observed for running. This would benefit those desiring to use only walking as a low-impact form of exercise training.

4. The total caloric cost for running a given distance is about the same whether the pace is fast or slow. For horizontal running, the net energy expenditure is about 1 kcal · kg^{-1} · km^{-1}.

5. Overcoming air resistance accounts for 3 to 9% of the total energy cost of running in calm weather. This percentage increases considerably if a runner attempts to maintain pace while running into a head wind.

6. Children generally require significantly more oxygen to transport their body mass while running compared to adults. This relatively lower running economy accounts for the poor endurance performance of children compared to adults with similar aerobic capacity.

7. The energy required to run a given distance or speed on a treadmill is about the same as that required to run on a track under identical weather conditions.

8. The energy expended to swim a given distance is about four times greater than to run the same distance. This is because the swimmer must expend considerable energy to maintain buoyancy and overcome the various drag forces that impede movement.

9. Elite swimmers expend fewer calories to swim a given stroke at any velocity.

10. There are significant gender differences for body drag, economy, and net oxygen uptake during swimming. Women swim a given distance at about 30% lower energy cost than men.

Ainsworth, B. E., et al.: Compendium of Physical Activities: classification of energy costs of human physical activities. *Med. Sci. Sports Exerc.*, 25: 71, 1993.

Armstrong, N., and Welsman, J.R.: Assessment and interpretation of aerobic fitness in children and adolescents. *Exerc. Sport Sci. Rev.*, 22: 435, 1994.

Bacharach, D. W. and von Duvillard, S. P.: Intermediate and long-term anaerobic performance of elite alpine skiers. *Med. Sci. Sports Exerc.*, 27(3): 305, 1995.

Belko, A., et al.: Effect of energy and protein intake and exercise intensity on the thermic effect of food. *Am. J. Clin. Nutr.*, 43: 863, 1986.

Bilodeau, B., et al.: Effect of drafting on heart rate in cross-country skiing. *Med. Sci. Sports Exerc.*, 26: 637, 1994.

Carpenter, W.H., et al.: Total energy expenditure in 4 to 6 year old children. *Am. J. Physiol.*, 27: E706, 1993.

Coyle, E. F., et al.: Cycling efficiency is related to the percentage of type I muscle fibers. *Med. Sci. Sports Exerc.*, 24: 782, 1992.

Crandall, C.G., et al.: Evaluation of the Cosmed K2 portable telemetric oxygen uptake analyzer. *Med. Sci. Sports Exerc.*, 26: 108, 1994.

Cureton, K. J., and Sparling, P. B.: Distance running performance and metabolic response to running in men and women with excess weight experimentally equated. *Med. Sci. Sports*, 12: 288, 1980.

Durnin, J. V. G. A., and Passmore, R.: *Energy, Work and Leisure*. London, Heinemann, 1967.

Evans, B.W., et al.: Metabolic and hemodynamic responses to walking with hand weights in older

individuals. *Med. Sci. Sports Exerc.*, 26: 1047, 1994.

Ferraro, R. et al.: Energy cost of physical activity on a metabolic ward in relationship to obesity. *Am J. Clin. Nutr.* 53: 1368, 1991.

Franklin, B. A.: Exercise testing, training and arm ergometry. *Sports Med*, 2:109, 1985.

Jansson, E.: On the significance of the respiratory exchange ratio after different diets during exercise in man. *Acta Physiol. Scand.*, 114: 103, 1982.

Kannagi, T., et al.: An evaluation of the Beckman Metabolic Cart for measuring ventilation and aerobic requirements during exercise. *J. Cardiac Rehab.*, 3: 38, 1983.

Kashiwazaki, H., et al.: Correlations of pedometer readings with energy expenditure in workers during free-living daily activities. *Eur. J. Appl. Physiol.*, 54: 585, 1986.

Katch, V., et al.: Basal metabolism of obese adolescents: age, gender and body composition effects. *Int. J. Obes.*, 9: 69, 1985.

Keys, A., et al.: Basal metabolism and age of adult men. *Metabolism*, 22: 579, 1973.

LeBlanc, J., et al.: Hormonal factors in reduced post prandial heat production of exercise trained subjects. *J. Appl. Physiol.*, 56: 772, 1984.

Livesey, B., and Elia, M.: Estimation of energy expenditure, net carbohydrate utilization and net fat oxidation and synthesis by indirect calorimetry: evaluation of errors with special reference to detailed composition of fuels. *Am. J. Clin. Nutr.*, 47: 608, 1988.

Meredith, C. N., et al.: Body composition and aerobic capacity in young and middle-aged endurance-

trained men. *Med. Sci. Sports Exerc.*, 19: 557, 1987.

Poehlman, E.T., et al.: Endurance exercise in aging humans: effects on energy metabolism. *Exerc. Sport Sci. Rev.*, 22: 75, 1994.

Poehlman, E. T., et al.: Resting metabolic rate and post prandial thermogenesis in highly trained and untrained males. *Am. J. Clin. Nutr.*, 47: 793, 1988.

Rumpler, W. et al.: Repeatability of 24-hour energy expenditure measurements in humans by indirect calorimetry. Am J. Clin. Nutr. 51: 147, 1990.

Schutz, Y., et al.: Diet-induced thermogenesis measured over a whole day in obese and non-obese women. *Am. J. Clin. Nutr.*, 40: 542, 1984.

Segal, K. R., et al.: Thermic effects of food and exercise on lean and obese men of similar lean body mass. *Am. J. Physiol.*, 252: E110, 1987.

Snellen, J. W.: Studies in human calorimetry. In *Assessment of Energy Metabolism in Health and Disease*. Columbus, OH, Ross Laboratories, 1980.

Thompson, J.L., et al.: Daily energy expenditure in male endurance athletes with differing energy intakes. *Med. Sci. Sports Exerc.*, 27(3): 347, 1995.

Trembly, A., et al.: Diminished dietary thermogenesis in exercise-trained human subjects. *Eur. J. Appl. Physiol.*, 52: 1, 1983.

Wilmore, J. A., et al.: An automated system for assessing metabolic and respiratory function during exercise. *J. Appl. Physiol.*, 40: 619, 1976.

After reading this chapter you should be able to:

- Discuss the terms specificity and generality as they apply to exercise performance and physiologic function.

- Describe the procedures to administer two practical "field tests" to evaluate the power output capacity of the high energy phosphates (immediate energy system).

- Describe a commonly used test to evaluate the power output capacity of glycolysis (short-term energy system).

- Define maximal oxygen uptake (max $\dot{V}O_2$) and describe the physiologic significance of this fitness measure.

- Define what is meant by a graded exercise test.

- List the criteria that indicate a person has reached a "true" max $\dot{V}O_2$ during a graded exercise test.

- Outline 3 commonly used treadmill protocols to assess aerobic capacity.

- Indicate how each of the following affect maximal oxygen uptake:
  (1) mode of exercise , (2) heredity, (3) state of training, (4) gender,
  (5) body composition, and (6) age.

- Describe the procedures to administer a submaximal walking "field test" to predict max $\dot{V}O_2$.

- List the assumptions when predicting maximal oxygen uptake from submaximal exercise heart rate.

We all possess the capability for anaerobic and aerobic energy metabolism, although the capacity for each form of energy transfer varies considerably among individuals. This between–individual variability underlies the concept of *individual differences* in metabolic capacity for exercise. It also appears that a person's capacity for energy transfer (and for many other physiologic functions) is not simply a general factor, but depends highly on the form of exercise used for training and evaluation. A high maximum oxygen uptake in running, for example, does not necessarily assure a similar metabolic power when different muscle groups are activated as in swimming and rowing. This is an example of *specificity* of metabolic capacity. Individuals with a high aerobic power in one activity may also possess an above average aerobic power in other activities in relation to other individuals. This is an illustration of the *generality* of physiologic function and performance. In this chapter, the capacity of the various energy transfer systems discussed in Chapters 2 and 3 are evaluated, with special reference to measurement, specificity, and individual differences.

Figure 5-1 illustrates the specificity–generality concept with respect to energy capacities. The non-overlapped areas represent specificity of physiologic function, and the overlapped areas represent generality of function. For each of the energy systems there is more specificity than generality; it is rare to find individuals who possess tremendous capabilities in markedly different types of activities (e.g., sprinting and long-distance running). Yet, there are many world-class triathletes who appear to possess "metabolically generalized" capacities for a variety of aerobic activities. This "generalized" aerobic fitness capacity, however, is the result of long hours of highly specific train-

ing in *each* of the triathlete's grueling physical training activities.

Because of specificity, training for high aerobic power probably contributes little to one's capacity to generate anaerobic energy, and vice versa. *The effects of systematic training are highly specific in terms of neurologic, physiologic, and metabolic demands.* Terms such as "speed," "power," and "endurance" must therefore be defined carefully within the context of the specific movement patterns and the specific metabolic and physiologic requirements of an activity.

● ● ● ● ● ● ● ● ● ● ● ● ● ●

OVERVIEW OF ENERGY TRANSFER CAPACITY DURING EXERCISE

All-out exercise for up to 2 minutes duration is powered mainly by the immediate and short-term energy systems. Both systems operate anaerobically because their transfer of chemical energy does not require oxygen. Generally, there is greater reliance on

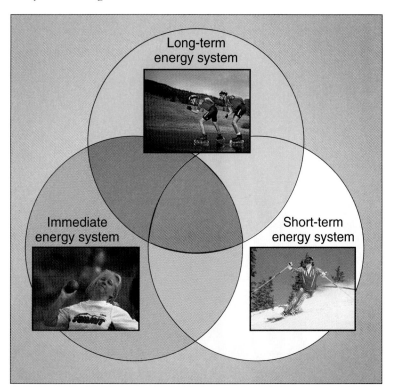

FIGURE 5-1. Illustration to represent the Specificity-Generality concept of the three energy systems. If only two systems are considered, their overlap represents generality and the remainder is specificity.

anaerobic energy for fast movements or when there is resistance to movement at a given speed. This principle is shown in Figure 5-2 which illustrates the relative involvement of the anaerobic and aerobic energy transfer systems for different durations of all-out exercise. At the initiation of movement performed at high or low speed, the stored phosphates, ATP and CP, provide immediate and nonaerobic energy for muscle contraction. After the first few seconds of movement, an increasingly greater proportion of energy is generated by the glycolytic energy system. For exercise to continue, although at a lower intensity, a greater demand is then placed on the aerobic metabolic pathways for purposes of ATP resynthesis.

Some activities require the capacity of more than one energy system, whereas others rely predominately on a single system of energy transfer. All activities use some percentage from each of the energy systems, however, depending on intensity and duration. Of course the higher the intensity and shorter the time, the greater the demand on anaerobic energy transfer.

ANAEROBIC ENERGY: THE IMMEDIATE AND SHORT-TERM ENERGY SYSTEMS

Evaluation of the Immediate Energy System

Performance tests that cause maximal activation of the ATP-CP energy system have been developed to provide practical "field tests" to evaluate this capacity for immediate energy transfer. These tests are generally referred to as *power tests;* power in this context is defined as the time-rate of doing work, or work accomplished per unit time. The formula for power output is:

$$P = F \times D \div T$$

In the equation, F is the force generated, D is the distance through which the force is moved, and T is the duration of the exercise period. Power is usually expressed in watts — one watt is equal to 0.73756 ft lb · sec^{-1} or 6.12 kg-m · min^{-1}. The following assumptions underlie the use of performance estimates of the ATP-CP system of energy delivery:

- Under conditions of maximal power output, all of the ATP is regenerated by the ATP-CP system and accordingly, all power generated during this time can be attributed to this system
- There is enough ATP and CP to support maximal performance for approximately 6 to 8 seconds

Stair-Sprinting Power Tests. Researchers have proposed that muscular short-term power can be measured by sprinting up a flight of stairs. As illustrated in Figure 5-3, the subject runs up a staircase as fast as possible taking three steps at a time. The external work done in this test is the total vertical distance the body is lifted up the stairs; this distance for six stairs is usually about 1.05 m.

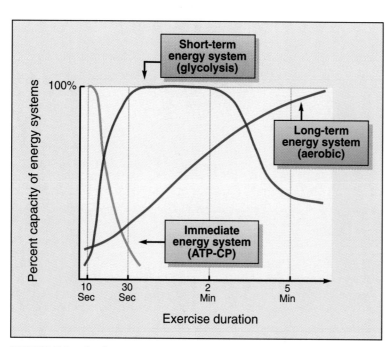

FIGURE 5-2. The three energy systems and their percentage contribution to total energy output during all-out exercise of different durations.

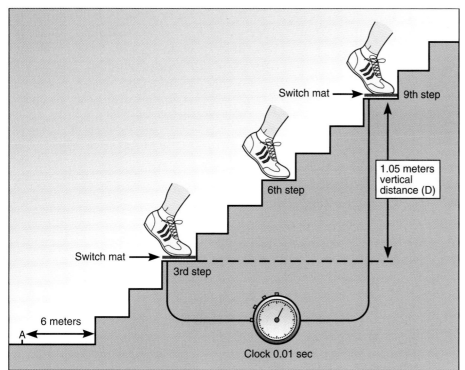

FIGURE 5-3. Stair-sprinting power test. The subject begins at point A and runs as rapidly as possible up a flight of stairs, taking three steps at a time. The time to cover the distance between stair 3 and stair 9 is recorded to the nearest 0.01 sec by the use of electric switch mats placed on the steps. Power output is the product of the subject's mass (F) and vertical distance covered (D), divided by the time (T). (Modified from Mathews, D. K., and Fox, E. L.: *The Physiological Basis of Physical Education and Athletics.* Philadelphia, W. B. Saunders, 2nd Edition, 1976.).

The power output of a 65-kg woman who traverses six steps in 0.52 seconds is computed as follows:

$$F = 65 \text{ kg}$$
$$D = 1.05 \text{ m}$$
$$T = 0.52 \text{ sec}$$
$$\text{Power} = [65 \text{ kg} \times 1.05 \text{ m}] \div 52 \text{ sec}$$
$$\text{Power} = 131.3 \text{ kg-m or}$$
$$1287 \text{ watts}$$

Because the power score in the stair-sprinting test is greatly influenced by the person's body mass, the heavier person will necessarily have a higher power score if several individuals achieve the same speed. This implies that the heavier person has a more highly developed immediate energy system than a lighter person who may cover the same vertical distance in the same time. Because there is no direct evidence to support this contention, caution is urged in interpreting differences in stair-sprinting power scores and making inferences about individual differences in ATP-CP energy capacity. The test may be better suited for evaluating individuals of similar body mass, or the same people before and after a specific training regimen designed to develop rapid anaerobic leg power.

Jumping-Power Tests. For years, *jumping tests* such as the *Sargent jump-and-reach test* or a *standing broad jump* have been common elements in many physical fitness test batteries. The Sargent jump is scored as the difference between a person's standing reach and the maximum jump-and-touch height. In the case of the broad jump, the score is the horizontal distance covered in a leap from a semicrouched position. Although both tests purport to measure leg power, they probably fail to achieve this goal. For one thing, with the jump tests, power generated in propelling the body from the crouched position occurs only in the time the feet are in contact with the surface. It is doubtful whether this brief period is sufficient to evaluate a person's ATP and CP power capacity. Also, a small or essentially no relationship has been established between jump-test scores and ATP-CP levels or depletion patterns.

TABLE 5-1. Correlations among tests that are supposed to measure immediate nonaerobic power output[a]

Variables	40-Yard Dash	Sargent Jump and Reach	Power Bicycle Test
Stair-sprinting power test	−0.88[b]	0.56	0.69
40-yard dash	–	−0.48[b]	−0.62[b]
Sargent jump and reach	–	–	.31

[a] From the Applied Physiology Laboratory, University of Michigan, (N = 31 males).
[b] A negative correlation coefficient means that for the group of individuals, a high score earned on one test is associated with a low score on the other test. For the correlations with the 40-yard dash, a negative correlation means a good performance on one test is associated with a low 40-yard run time, and a low score in running (time) is a good performance.

Interchangeable Expressions for Energy and Work.

1 Foot-pound (ft-lb) = 0.13825 kilogram-meters (kg-m)

1 Kg-m = 7.233 ft-lb = 9.8066 joules

1 Kilocalories (kcal) = 3.0874 ft-lb = 426.85 kg-m = 4.186 kilojoules (kJ)

1 Joule (J) = 1 Newton-meter (Nm)

1 Kilojoule (kJ) = 1000 J = 0.23889 kcal

Other Power Tests. As indicated in Figure 5-2, any performance involving all-out exercise of 6 to 8 seconds duration can probably be considered indicative of the person's capacity for immediate power from the high-energy phosphates in the specific muscles activated in the performance. Other examples of such tests are sprint running or cycling, shuttle runs, or even more localized movements such as arm cranking or simulated stair climbing, rowing, or skiing.

Relationships Among Power Tests. If the various power tests measure the same general metabolic capacity, then individuals ranking high on one test should rank correspondingly high on a second or third test. Although information on this topic is incomplete, the available data indicate that those who do well on one power performance test tend to do well on another performance test, but the correlation is generally not strong. Table 5-1 shows the interrelationship (expressed statistically as a correlation coefficient) among several tests that supposedly measure immediate power output.

The relationship ranges from poor to good, indicating some commonalty between tests and suggesting that each may be measuring a similar metabolic quality. Of practical significance is the fairly strong relationship between scores on the stair-sprinting power test and the 40-yard dash. Clearly, almost the same information can be obtained by sprint running on a track compared with the more elaborate set-up in the stair sprint.

Several factors may explain why the interrelationship among the other test scores is not high. For one thing, *human performance is highly task-specific.* From a metabolic and performance standpoint, this means the best sprint runner is not necessarily the best sprint swimmer, sprint cyclist, "stair sprinter," or "arm cranker." Even though the energy to power each performance is generated by the same metabolic reactions, these reactions are isolated within the specific muscles activated by the exercise. Furthermore, each specific test requires different neurologic or skill components that tend to cause the individual scores to be more variable.

We have suggested that power tests might be used to show changes in an athlete's performance resulting from specific training. Such tests also offer an excellent means for self-testing and motivation, and often provide the actual exercise for training the immediate energy system. With many football teams, for example, the 40-yard dash is routinely used as a criterion to evaluate a player's speed. Although there are many types of "speed" that need to be evaluated, these test scores may provide some information for the evaluation of a player. It should be emphasized that it has yet to be established that 40-yard speed in a straight line is related to overall football ability for players at similar positions! A run test of shorter duration (up to 20 yards), or one with frequent changes in direction, may turn out to be an equal or more suitable performance measure.

Evaluation of the Short-Term Energy System

As was shown in Figure 5-2, when all-out exercise continues longer than a few seconds, increasingly more energy for ATP resynthesis is generated from the short-term energy system through the anaerobic reactions of glycolysis. This is not to say that aerobic metabolism is unimportant at this stage of exercise or that the oxygen-consuming reactions have not been "switched-on." To the contrary, Figure 5-2 shows an increase in the contribution of aerobic energy very early in exercise. But it is in all-out exercise that the energy requirement significantly exceeds the energy generated by the oxidation of hydrogen in the respiratory chain. This means that the anaerobic reactions of glycolysis predominate and large quantities of lactic acid accumulate within the active muscle and ultimately in the blood.

Unlike tests for maximal oxygen uptake, no specific criteria exist to indicate that a person has reached a maximal anaerobic effort. In fact, it is highly likely that one's score on such a test is influenced by the level of self motivation as well as the test environment. The level of blood lactate is the most common indicator of the activation of the short-term energy system.

Performance Tests of Glycolytic Power. Performances requiring substantial activation of the short-term energy system are those demanding maximal work for up to 3 minutes duration. All-out runs and cycling exercise have usually been used to test this energy capacity, although weight lifting (repetitive lifting of a certain percentage of maximum) and shuttle and agility-runs have also been used. Because of the effects that factors such as age, skill, motivation, and body size have on physical performance, it is difficult to select a suitable criterion test and to develop appropriate norms to evaluate the glycolytic energy system. Also, within the framework of exercise specificity, short-term anaerobic capacity for an arm and upper body activity like rowing or swimming cannot be adequately assessed with a test that makes maximum use of only the leg muscles. The performance test *must* be similar to the activity for which the energy capacity is being evaluated. In most cases the actual activity can serve as the test.

An all-out cycling test of short duration to estimate the power and capacity of the anaerobic energy systems was first described in 1973 as the *Katch test*. This work was extended in subsequent years and resulted in a test where the frictional resistance against the bicycle's flywheel was preset at a high load (6 kp for men and 5 kp for women), and subjects attempted to turn as many revolutions as possible in 40 seconds. Pedal revolution rate was recorded continuously, with the peak power achieved representing *anaerobic power* and the total work done representing *anaerobic capacity.* A later modification of this procedure, the *Wingate test*, involves 30 seconds of all-out supermaximal exercise performed on either an arm-crank or leg-cycle ergometer. The frictional resistance during exercise is based on body mass (0.075 of resistance per kg body mass) and is applied only after initial inertia and unloaded frictional resistance to pedaling are overcome (about 3 sec). Timing of the test is then begun and pedal revolutions are counted. The assessment of *peak power output* represents the highest mechanical power generated during any 3- to 5-second period of the test; *average power output* is the arithmetic average of the total power generated during the 30-second test period. *Rate of fatigue,* or the rate of decline in power relative to the peak value, can also be computed. As in the Katch test, the underlying assumption for this testing is that the value for peak power output represents the energy-generating capacity of high-energy

> **Supermaximal exercise.** In this form of performance, the exercise level is set above the intensity that elicits the max $\dot{V}O_2$.

Percentile Norms for Average Power and Peak Power for Physically Active Young Adult Men and Women

	Average Power Watts (W)		Peak Power Watts (W)	
% Rank	Male	Female	Male	Female
90	662	470	822	560
80	618	419	777	527
70	600	410	757	505
60	577	391	721	480
50	565	381	689	449
40	548	367	671	432
30	530	353	656	399
20	496	336	618	376
10	471	306	570	353

	$W \cdot kg\ BW^{-1}$		$W \cdot kg\ BW^{-1}$	
	Male	Female	Male	Female
90	8.24	7.31	10.89	9.02
80	8.01	6.95	10.39	8.83
70	7.91	6.77	10.20	8.53
60	7.59	6.59	9.80	8.14
50	7.44	6.39	9.22	7.65
40	7.14	6.15	8.92	6.96
30	7.00	6.03	8.53	6.86
20	6.59	5.71	8.24	6.57
10	5.98	5.25	7.06	5.98

Maud, P.J., and Schultz, B.B.: Norms for the Wingate anaerobic test with comparisons in another similar test. *Res. Q. Exerc. Sport,* 60:144, 1989.

phosphates, whereas the average power score represents glycolytic capacity. Some of the highest reported all-out cycle ergometer power scores have been produced by elite volleyball and ice hockey players.

Figure 5-4 presents the relative contribution of each metabolic pathway during three different duration all-out cycle ergometer tests. The lower portion shows the results in estimated kilojoules of energy (1 kJ = 4.2 kcal), and the upper portion shows the results in percent of the total work output. Note the progressive change in the percentage contribution of each of the energy systems to the total work output as the duration of effort changes.

Performance scores on the Wingate or Katch test are reproducible, and validity is moderate using a variety of other measures of "anaerobic capacity." The mechanism is unknown to explain the relatively poorer performance of children on this test compared to adolescents and young adults. It is possible that both lower concentrations and rate of utilization of muscle glycogen in children provide part of the answer.

Blood Lactate Levels. As was shown previously in Figure 3-1, the blood lactate level remains relatively low during steady-rate exercise up to about 55% of the maximum oxygen uptake. As the max $\dot{V}O_2$ is approached, however, there is a precipitous increase in blood lactic acid.

The data in Figure 5-5 were obtained from 10 college men who performed nine all-out bicycle ergometer rides of different durations on the Katch test on different days. The subjects were highly motivated; many were involved in conditioning programs and some were varsity athletes. The men were unaware of the duration of each test but were instructed and urged to turn as many revolutions as possible. Venous blood lactate was measured before and immediately after each test and throughout recovery. The plotted points are the average of the values for blood lactate just at the end of exercise for each of the tests. Blood lactate levels increased in direct proportion with the duration (and total work output) of the all-out exercise. At the end of 3 minutes of cycling, the amount of lactate in the blood was highest and averaged about 140 mg in each 100 ml of blood.

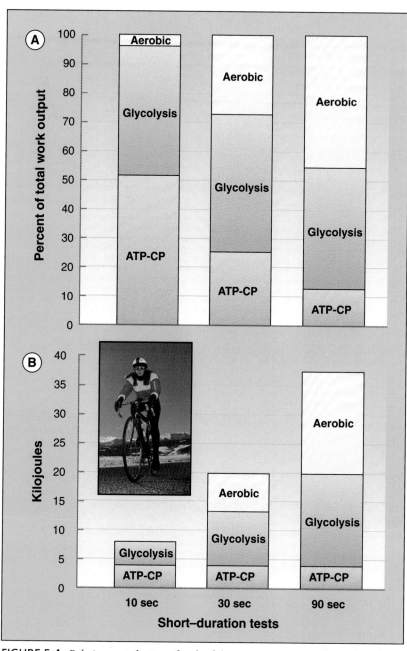

FIGURE 5-4. Relative contribution of each of the energy systems to the total work accomplished in three tests of short-duration. (*A*) Percent of total work output. (*B*) Kilojoules of energy. Test results based on the Katch Test protocol (see p. 121). (Data from the Applied Physiology Laboratory, University of Michigan.)

Glycogen Depletion. Because the short-term energy system largely depends on glycogen stored in the specific muscles activated by exercise, the pattern of glycogen depletion in these muscles also provides an indication of the contribution of glycolysis to exercise. Figure 5-6 illustrates that the rate of glycogen depletion in the quadriceps femoris muscle during bicycle exercise is closely related to exercise intensity.

With steady-rate exercise at about 30% of max $\dot{V}O_2$, a considerable reserve of muscle glycogen remains, even after 180 minutes of exercise. Because metabolism in this relatively light exercise is essentially aerobic, large quantities of fatty acids are used for energy and the drain is only moderate on stored glycogen. At the two heaviest workloads, however, the most rapid and pronounced glycogen depletion is observed. This makes sense from a metabolic standpoint because glycogen is the only stored nutrient that provides anaerobic energy for the resynthesis of ATP; clearly, this substrate has high priority in the "metabolic mill" during strenuous exercise.

Changes in total muscle glycogen such as those illustrated in Figure 5-6 may not give a precise indication of the degree of glycogen breakdown in specific fibers within the muscle. Depending on the intensity of exercise, glycogen depletion occurs selectively in fast- and slow-twitch fibers. For example, during all-out exercise such as 1-minute sprints on a bicycle ergometer at a very heavy load, the fast-twitch fibers are activated to provide the predominant power for the exercise. Glycogen content in these fibers is almost totally depleted because of the anaerobic nature of this work. In contrast, during moderate to heavy prolonged aerobic exercise, the slow-twitch fibers are always the first to become glycogen-depleted. This specificity in glycogen utilization (and depletion) makes it difficult to evaluate glycolyt-

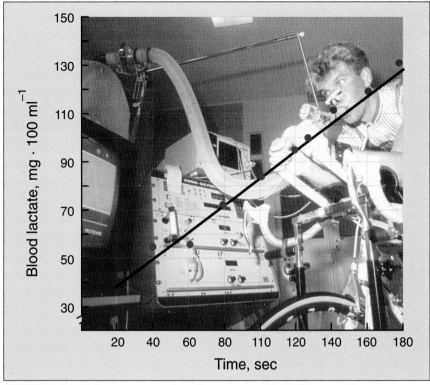

FIGURE 5-5. Pedaling a stationary bicycle ergometer at the highest possible power output causes blood lactate to increase in direct proportion to the duration of exercise for up to 3 minutes. Each value represents the average of 10 subjects. (Data from the Applied Physiology Laboratory, University of Michigan.).

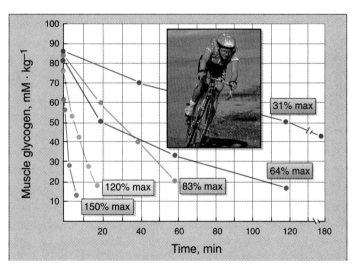

FIGURE 5-6. Glycogen depletion from the vastus lateralis portion of the quadriceps femoris muscle in bicycle exercise of different intensities and durations. Exercise at 31% of max$\dot{V}O_2$ (the lightest workload) caused some depletion of muscle glycogen, but the most rapid and largest depletion occurred with exercise that ranged from 83% to 150% of max $\dot{V}O_2$. (Adapted from Gollnick, P. D.: Selective glycogen depletion pattern in human muscle fibers after exercise of varying intensity and at varying pedaling rates. *J. Physiol.*, 241:45, 1974.)

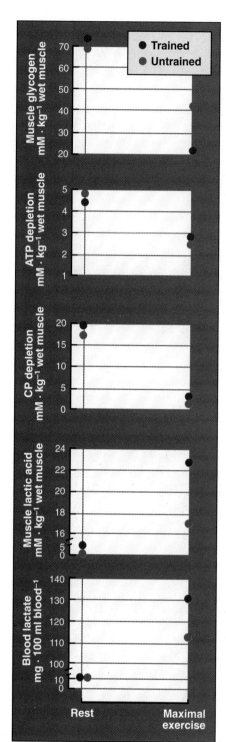

Figure 5-7. Depletion of anaerobic substrates (ATP, CP, and glycogen) and increases in muscle and blood lactic acid in short-term maximal exercise for trained and nontrained subjects. The trained subjects exhibited a greater increase in anaerobic metabolism (higher levels of lactic acid) and a depletion in glycogen, while the reduction of the high-energy phosphates ATP and CP was essentially the same as for the nontrained. (From Karlsson, J., et al.: Muscle metabolites during submaximal and maximal exercise in man. *Scand. J. Clin. Invest.*, 26:382, 1971.)

ic involvement from changes in a muscle's total glycogen content before and after exercise.

Individual Differences in Anaerobic Energy Transfer Capacity

Several factors contribute to differences among individuals in their capacity to generate short-term anaerobic energy. These include differences in previous training, motivation, and the capacity to buffer acid metabolites.

Effects of Training. A comparison of the anaerobic capabilities of trained and untrained subjects is presented in Figure 5-7. Following short-term supermaximal exercise on the bicycle ergometer, the trained subjects always exhibited higher levels of muscle and blood lactic acid, as well as greater depletion of muscle glycogen. In short-term, intense forms of exercise, better performances are usually associated with higher levels of blood lactate. These results support the belief that training for short-term, all-out exercise enhances one's capacity to generate energy from the glycolytic system. This is important because in sprint-and middle-distance activities, individual differences in anaerobic capacity can account for large performance differences.

Buffering of Acid Metabolites. Lactic acid accumulates when anaerobic energy transfer predominates; this causes an appreciable increase in the acidity of muscle and blood and has a dramatic negative influence on the intracellular environment. The immediate effect is on the contractile capa-

bility of exercising muscles. This had led to the speculation that anaerobic training may enhance short-term energy capacity by the mechanism of increasing the body's alkaline reserve. This would theoretically enable greater lactic acid production because it could be buffered more effectively. Although this reasoning seems appealing, only a small increase in alkaline reserve has been noted in athletes compared to sedentary counterparts. There also is no appreciable change in alkaline reserve following hard physical training. The general consensus is that trained people have a buffering capability within the range expected for healthy untrained individuals.

It is interesting that relatively short-term, high-intensity exercise performance can be enhanced significantly by temporarily altering acid-base balance in the direction of alkalosis. This was achieved by ingesting a buffering solution of sodium bicarbonate prior to an 800-meter race. The significantly faster run times were accompanied by higher levels of blood lactate and extracellular H^+ which suggested an increased anaerobic energy contribution. More is said of this procedure in Chapter 14 concerning the possible ergogenic effects.

Motivation. Individuals with greater "pain tolerance," "toughness," or ability to "push" beyond the discomforts of fatiguing exercise definitely accomplish more anaerobic work. These people usually generate greater levels of blood lactate and glycogen depletion; they also score higher on tests of short-term energy capacity. *Motivational factors, which are difficult to categorize or quantify, play a key role in superior performance at all levels of competition.*

• • • • • • • • • • • • • •

AEROBIC ENERGY: THE LONG-TERM ENERGY SYSTEM

The results in Figure 5-8 illustrate that persons who engage in sports that require sustained, high-intensity exercise generally have a large capacity for aerobic energy transfer.

The highest maximal oxygen uptakes are generally recorded for men and women who compete in distance running, swimming, bicycling, and cross-country skiing. These athletes have almost double the aerobic capacity of a sedentary group! This is not to say that the max $\dot{V}O_2$ is the only determinant of aerobic exercise capacity. Other factors, especially those at the muscular level such as the number of capillaries, enzymes, and fiber type, exert a strong influence on one's capacity to sustain a high percentage of aerobic exercise (i.e., achieve a high lactate threshold). The max $\dot{V}O_2$ however, does provide useful information about the capacity of the long-term energy system. In addition, the attainment of max $\dot{V}O_2$ requires integration of the ventilatory, cardiovascular, and neuromuscular systems; this gives significant physiologic as well as metabolic meaning to the max $\dot{V}O_2$. *For these reasons, max $\dot{V}O_2$ has become fundamental measures in exercise physiology.*

Measurement of Maximal Oxygen Uptake

The max $\dot{V}O_2$ can be determined by a variety of exercise tasks that activate large muscle groups as long as the exercise is of sufficient intensity and duration to engage maximal aerobic energy transfer. The usual forms of exercise include treadmill walking or running, bench stepping, or cycling. The max $\dot{V}O_2$, however, has also been measured during free, tethered, and flume swimming and swimbench ergometry, as well as during simulated rowing, skiing, stair climbing, as well as ice skating and arm-crank exercise. Considerable research effort has been directed toward the development and standardization of tests for maximal aerobic power and toward the establishment of norms for this measure in relation to age, gender, state of training, and body composition.

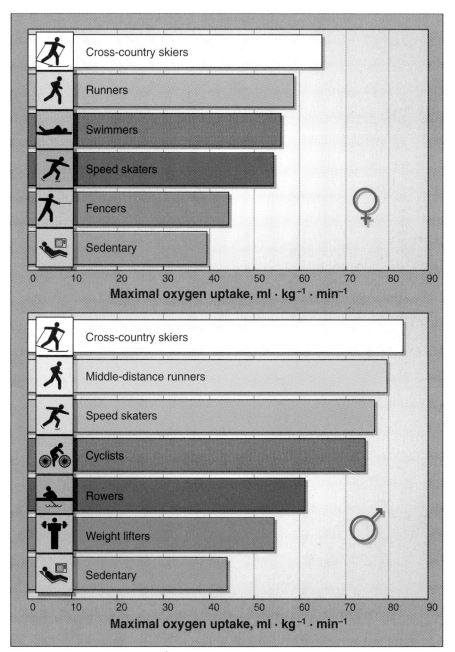

Figure 5-8. Maximal oxygen uptake of male and female Olympic-caliber athletes in different sport categories in comparison to healthy sedentary subjects. (Adapted from Saltin, B., and Åstrand, P. O.: Maximal oxygen uptake in athletes. *J. Appl. Physiol.*, 23:3523, 1967.)

Criteria for Max $\dot{V}O_2$. To be reasonably sure that a person has reached the maximum capacity for aerobic metabolism during specific exercise (i.e., achieved a "true" max $\dot{V}O_2$), a levelling-off or peaking-over in oxygen uptake should be achieved (Fig. 5-9).

When this generally accepted criterion for the attainment of max $\dot{V}O_2$ is not met, or the test performance

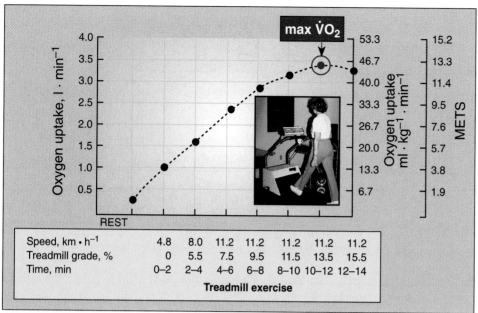

Speed, km · h⁻¹		4.8	8.0	11.2	11.2	11.2	11.2	11.2
Treadmill grade, %		0	5.5	7.5	9.5	11.5	13.5	15.5
Time, min		0–2	2–4	4–6	6–8	8–10	10–12	12–14

Treadmill exercise

FIGURE 5-9. Peaking over in oxygen uptake with increasing intensity during treadmill exercise. Each point represents the average oxygen uptake of 18 sedentary males. The region where oxygen uptake fails to increase the expected amount, or even decreases slightly with increasing exercise intensity, represents the max$\dot{V}O_2$. (Data from the Applied Physiology Laboratory, University of Michigan. Photo courtesy of J. Graves, Exercise Science Laboratory, Syracuse University).

> **Different terms but the same fitness component.** The terms stamina, endurance fitness, cardiovascular fitness, and aerobic fitness refer to the body's ability to generate ATP aerobically.

appears limited by local factors (muscle fatigue in the arms or legs) rather than central circulatory dynamics, the term peak $\dot{V}O_2$ is usually used. *Peak $\dot{V}O_2$ refers to the highest value of oxygen uptake measured during the test.*

The max $\dot{V}O_2$ test shown in Figure 5-9 involved progressive increases in treadmill exercise, and the test was terminated when the subject would not complete the full duration of a particular exercise block. For the average oxygen uptake values of 18 subjects plotted in Figure 5-9, the highest oxygen uptake was reached before the subjects attained their maximum exercise level. This peaking-over criterion substantiates that a max $\dot{V}O_2$ has been reached.

In many instances, however, a peaking-over or slight decrease in oxygen uptake with increasing levels of exercise is not observed at the highest exercise level. Often, the highest oxygen uptake or "peak $\dot{V}O_2$" is recorded in the last minute of exercise to

exhaustion without showing the plateau criterion required to objectify the attainment of max $\dot{V}O_2$. Consequently, additional criteria have been suggested based on both metabolic and physiologic responses.

- Max $\dot{V}O_2$ is considered to have been reached when oxygen uptake fails to increase by some value usually expected from previous observations with the particular test.
- It is also argued that to accept an oxygen uptake value as being maximum, blood lactic-acid levels should reach 70 or 80 mg per 100 ml of blood (about 8 to 10 mmol), or higher.
- Less precise but more easily measured criteria are usually applied that are reasonable indicators that the oxygen uptake is near-maximum. These include the attainment of near age-predicted maximum heart rate, or a respiratory exchange ratio (R) in excess of 1.00.

Tests of Aerobic Power

Numerous tests have been devised and standardized for the measurement of max $\dot{V}O_2$. Performance on these tests should be independent of muscle strength, speed, body size, and skill, with the exception of specialized tests such as swimming, rowing, and ice skating.

The max $\dot{V}O_2$ test may require a continuous 3- to 5-minute "super-maximal" effort, but it usually consists of increments in effort (referred to as *graded exercise*) to the point where the subject will no longer continue to exercise. Some researchers have perhaps imprecisely termed this end point "exhaustion". It should be

Max$\dot{V}O_2$ OF OLYMPIC WHEELCHAIR-DEPENDENT ATHLETES

Most able-bodied individuals have never considered the psychological trauma, physical limitations, and societal constraints that confront the physically challenged. When an able-bodied person suffers a physical disability and loses the use of his or her legs, the effort to merely survive and function at a level close to "normal" becomes heroic. To many, however, normal is neither sufficient nor acceptable. Many physically challenged individuals want to function as they did before being injured and this includes athletic competition. Indeed, for many, a wheelchair is not a hindrance but rather a support and even a training device.

Athletics notwithstanding, a sedentary lifestyle has been suggested as a major cause of cardiovascular disease for wheelchair-dependent people. For these individuals, upper body exercise training provides an important tool to combat the risk of cardiovascular disease. The upper body max $\dot{V}O_2$ of highly trained wheelchair-dependent athletes serves as an indication of the level of physiologic function that is attainable in the wheelchair-dependent population. Data on these athletes are also useful in setting aerobic training goals for individuals, and specific modes of testing may be available to evaluate sport-specific training for the diverse sports practiced by these men and women.

While studies of the physical work capacity and aerobic power of wheelchair-dependent men and women are limited, and testing procedures vary, recent data on 40 male French olympic wheelchair-dependent subjects are revealing. Athletes from 8 different sports were tested for max $\dot{V}O_2$ using their own general purpose wheelchair while on a treadmill. A continuous progressive exercise protocol was applied with 2-min exercise bouts. At the beginning of each bout, the workload was increased either by the speed $(2.0 \text{ km} \cdot \text{h}^{-1})$ at a constant treadmill grade, or by increasing treadmill grade by 1% with constant velocity. The max $\dot{V}O_2$ data $(\text{ml} \cdot \text{kg}^{-1} \cdot \text{min}^{-1})$ by sport are presented in the insert graph. The highest values were achieved by the track and field athletes followed by the swimmers. To compare these values with those of able-bodied athletes (measured during treadmill running or stationery bicycling) of approximately the same age, the reader is referred to Fig. 5–8. Remember, however, that values for aerobic capacity during upper body exercise are generally about 70% of those achieved during running and bicycling.

Reference

Veeger, H. E. J., et al. Peak oxygen uptake and maximal power output of Olympic wheelchair-dependent athletes. *Med. Sci. Sports Exerc.* 23:1201, 1991.

kept in mind that it is the performer who, for whatever reason, terminates the test. This decision is often influenced by a variety of psychologic or motivational factors that may not necessarily reflect true physiologic strain. We have found that it takes considerable urging and prodding to get subjects to the point at which acceptable criteria can be demonstrated for the attainment of max $\dot{V}O_2$. Practical experience has shown that high motivation and a relatively large anaerobic output are generally required to demonstrate a plateau in oxygen uptake during the max $\dot{V}O_2$ test. This applies to untrained people in particular who do not normally perform strenuous exercise with its associated discomforts.

Comparison of Tests. Maximal oxygen uptake tests are usually performed in one of the following ways:

- Continuously — with no rest between exercise increments
- Discontinuously — with the subject resting several minutes between exercise periods

The data in Table 5-2 show the results of a systematic comparison of max $\dot{V}O_2$ scores measured by six common continuous and discontinuous treadmill and bicycle procedures.

Although there was only a small 8-ml difference in max $\dot{V}O_2$ between the continuous and discontinuous bicycle tests, the max $\dot{V}O_2$ during bicycle exercise averaged 6.4 to 11.2% below values on the treadmill. The largest difference between any of the three treadmill running tests was only 1.2%. The walking test, on the other hand, elicited max $\dot{V}O_2$ scores about 7% above values on the bicycle but 5% below the average for the three running tests.

A common complaint of subjects on both the continuous and discontinuous bicycle tests was a feeling of intense local discomfort in the thigh muscles during heavy exercise. In the walking test, the common complaint was severe local discomfort in the lower back and calf muscles, especially walking at the higher treadmill elevations. Local discomfort was not common in the running tests, and subjects complained more of a general fatigue that was usually categorized as feeling "winded." From a standpoint of ease of administration, the continuous treadmill run appears to be the test of preference for testing the aerobic capacity of large numbers of healthy subjects. The total time to administer the test averaged a little over 12 minutes, whereas discontinuous running tests averaged about 65 minutes. Subjects seemed to "tolerate" the continuous test well and preferred the shorter time period for testing. In fact, research indicates that max $\dot{V}O_2$ can be reached with a continuous exercise protocol where exercise intensity is increased progressively in 15-second intervals. With this approach, the total test time for either bicycle or treadmill exercise averages about 5 minutes!

TABLE 5-2 Average maximal oxygen uptakes for 15 college students during continuous and discontinuous tests on the bicycle and treadmill*

Variable	Bike continuous	Bike, continuous	Treadmill, discontinuous walk-run	Treadmill, continuous walk	Treadmill, discontinuous run	Treadmill, continuous run
Max $\dot{V}O_2$, ml · min^{-1}	3691 ± 453	3683 ± 448	4145 ± 401	3944 ± 395	4157 ± 445	4109 ± 424
Max $\dot{V}O_2$, ml · kg^{-1} · min^{-1}	50.0 ± 6.9	49.9 ± 7.0	56.6 ± 7.3	566 ± 7.6	55.5 ± 7.6	55.5 ± 6.8

Values are means ± standard deviations

* Adapted from McArdle, W. D., et al.: Comparison of continuous and discontinuous treadmill and bicycle tests for max $\dot{V}O_2$. *Med. Sci Sports.*, 5:156, 1973.

Commonly Used Treadmill Protocols. Six commonly used treadmill protocols for the assessment of aerobic capacity in both normals and cardiac patients are summarized in Figure 5-10.

A feature common to these tests is the manipulation of exercise duration and treadmill speed and grade. The Harbor treadmill protocol (example F) is a unique application, and is referred to as a *ramp test*. With this procedure, the grade is increased each minute up to 10 minutes by a constant amount that ranges from a 1 to 4% grade depending on the exerciser's fitness. This relatively quick procedure produces a linear increase in oxygen uptake to the maximum level and is well tolerated by both normal persons and monitored cardiac patients.

Factors that Affect Maximal Oxygen Uptake

Many factors influence the maximal oxygen uptake score. Of these, the most important are the mode of exercise and the person's heredity, state of training, body composition, gender, and age.

Mode of Exercise. Variations in max $\dot{V}O_2$ during different forms of exercise reflect the quantity of muscle mass activated during the performance. In experiments in which the max $\dot{V}O_2$ was determined on the same subjects during different forms of exercise, the highest max $\dot{V}O_2$ was obtained with treadmill exercise. Bench-stepping, however, generated max $\dot{V}O_2$ scores identical to values obtained on the treadmill and significantly higher than those obtained on the bicycle ergometer. With arm-crank exercise, the aerobic capacity value reaches only about 70% of one's treadmill performance. For skilled but untrained swimmers, the maximal oxygen uptake during swimming was generally about 20% below treadmill

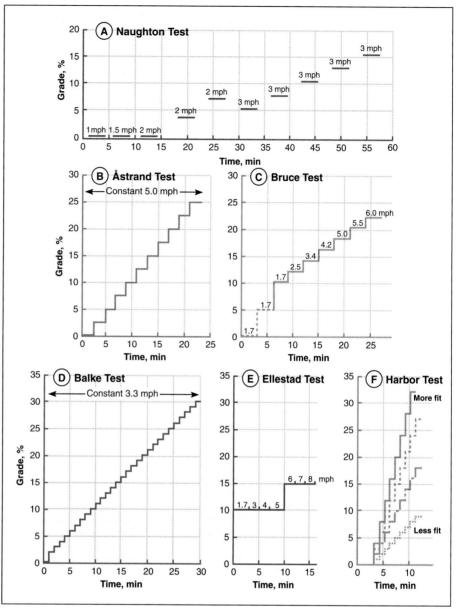

FIGURE 5-10. Six commonly used treadmill procedures. *(A) Naughton protocol.* Three minute exercise periods of increasing intensity alternate with 3 minutes of rest. The exercise periods vary in grade and speed. *(B) Åstrand protocol.* The speed is constant at 5 mph. After 3 minutes at 0% grade, the grade is increased 2 1/2% every 2 minutes. *(C) Bruce protocol.* Grade and/or speed are changed every 3 minutes. The 0% and 5% grades are omitted in healthier subjects. *(D) Balke protocol.* After one minute at 0% grade and one minute at 2% grade, the grade is increased 1% per minute, all at a speed of 3.3 mph. *(E) Ellestad protocol.* The initial grade is 10% and the later grade is 15% while the speed is increased every 2 or 3 minutes. *(F) Harbor protocol.* After 3 minutes of walking at a comfortable speed, the grade is increased at a constant preselected amount each minute: 1%, 2%, 3%, or 4%, so that the subject reaches max$\dot{V}O_2$ in approximately 10 minutes. (From Wasserman, K., et al.: *Principles of Exercise Testing and Interpretation.* 2nd Edition. Philadelphia, Lea & Febiger, 1994.)

values. There is a definite *test specificity* in this form of exercise because trained collegiate swimmers achieved max $\dot{V}O_2$'s swimming that were only

11% below their treadmill values, and some elite competitive swimmers can equal or even exceed their treadmill max $\dot{V}O_2$ scores during a swimming test. Similarly, a distinct exercise and training specificity is noted among competitive racewalkers who are capable of achieving an oxygen uptake during walking that is similar to their max $\dot{V}O_2$ values during treadmill running. Furthermore, if competitive cyclists are permitted to cycle at the fast pedal frequencies at which they compete, they also are able to achieve max $\dot{V}O_2$ values equivalent to their treadmill scores.

In the laboratory, the treadmill is the apparatus of choice for determining max $\dot{V}O_2$ in healthy subjects. Exercise intensity is easily determined and regulated. Compared to other forms of exercise, the treadmill makes it easier for subjects to achieve one or more of the criteria for establishing that the max $\dot{V}O_2$ has in fact been attained. Under field conditions outside of the laboratory, bench stepping or bicycle exercise are suitable alternatives.

Heredity. The question is frequently raised concerning the relative contribution of natural endowment to physiologic function and exercise performance. For example, to what extent does heredity determine the extremely high aerobic capacities of the endurance athletes displayed in Figure 5-8? Certainly these exceptionally high levels of functional capacity do not *only* reflect the effects of training. Although the answer is far from complete, some researchers have focused on the question of how genetic variability accounts for differences between individuals in physiologic and metabolic capacity.

Studies were made of 15 pairs of identical twins (who presumably had the same heredity since they came from the same fertilized egg) and 15 pairs of fraternal twins (who do not differ from ordinary siblings because they result from the separate fertilization of two eggs) raised in the same city and whose parents were of similar socioeconomic backgrounds. It was concluded that heredity alone accounted for up to 93% of the observed differences in aerobic capacity as measured by the max $\dot{V}O_2$! In addition, the capacity of the short-term energy system of glycolysis and the maximum heart rate were shown to be genetically determined by about 81 and 86%, respectively. Subsequent investigations of larger groups of brothers, fraternal twins, and identical twins have shown a significant but smaller effect of inherited factors on aerobic capacity and endurance performance.

The genetic effect is estimated at about 25–40% for max $\dot{V}O_2$, 50% for maximum heart rate, and 70% for physical working capacity. Muscle fiber composition of identical twins is similar, whereas wide variation exists in fiber type among fraternal twins and brothers. Future research might determine the upper limit of genetic determination, but available data currently indicate a significant contribution from inherited factors to both functional capacity and exercise performance. It now appears that a large portion of the sensitivity of maximal aerobic and anaerobic power, as well as the adaptations of most muscle enzymes to training, is genotype-dependent. In other words, members of the same twin-pair generally show the same response to training. Genetic makeup plays such a predominant role in determining the training response that it is almost impossible to predict a particular individual's response to a given training stimulus.

State of Training. The max $\dot{V}O_2$ score must be evaluated relative to the person's state of training at the time of measurement. Improvements in aerobic capacity with training generally range between 6 and 20%, although increases have been reported as large as 50% above pretraining levels. This subject is discussed further in Chapter 12.

Gender. Max $\dot{V}O_2$ values for women are typically 15 to 30% below scores for men. Even among trained athletes, this difference ranges between 15 and 20%. These differences, however, are considerably larger if the max $\dot{V}O_2$ is expressed as an absolute value ($L \cdot min^{-1}$) rather than relative to body mass ($ml \cdot kg^{-1} \cdot min^{-1}$). Among world class male and female cross-country skiers, for example, a 43% lower max $\dot{V}O_2$ value for women (6.54 vs. 3.75 $L \cdot min^{-1}$) is reduced to 15% (83.8 vs. 71.2 $ml \cdot kg^{-1} \cdot min^{-1}$) when the body mass of the athletes is used in the ratio expression of max $\dot{V}O_2$.

The apparent gender difference in max $\dot{V}O_2$ has generally been attributed to differences in body composition and hemoglobin content. Untrained young adult women, for example, generally possess about 25% body fat whereas the corresponding value for men averages 15%. Although trained athletes have a lower percentage of fat, trained women still possess significantly more body fat than their male counterparts. Thus, the male is generally able to generate more total aerobic energy simply because he possesses a relatively large muscle mass and less fat than the female.

Probably due to their higher level of testosterone, men also have a 10 to 14% greater concentration of hemoglobin than women. This difference in the oxygen-carrying capacity of the blood potentially enables the male to circulate more oxygen during exercise and thus gives him a slight edge in aerobic capacity.

Although lower body fat and higher hemoglobin provide the male with some advantage in aerobic power, we must look for other factors to explain fully the difference between the genders. One possible explanation is the difference in the normal physical activity level between the typical or "average" male and "average" female. It can be convincingly argued that due to social constraints, the opportunities for women to exercise have been considerably less than for men. In fact, even among prepubertal children, boys are significantly more active in daily life than female counterparts. Despite these possible limitations, however, the aerobic capacity of physically active females is generally higher than that of sedentary males. In fact, female cross-country skiers have max $\dot{V}O_2$ scores 40% higher than untrained males! Considerable variability exists even among the so-called "normal" population, and the max $\dot{V}O_2$ scores of many women exceed the values for the less-fit men.

Body Composition. It is estimated that 70% of the differences in max $\dot{V}O_2$ scores among individuals can be explained simply by differences in body mass, 4% by differences in stature, and 1% by variations in lean body mass. Thus, it is usually not meaningful to compare exercise performance or the absolute value for oxygen uptake among individuals who differ in body size (mass or stature) or body composition (body fat and lean body mass). This has led to the common practice of expressing oxygen uptake in terms of body size — either in relation to surface area, body mass, lean body mass, or limb volume.

Table 5-3 presents some typical values for an untrained man and woman who differ considerably in body mass. The percent difference is 43% in the max $\dot{V}O_2$ when the aerobic capacity is expressed in liters per minute. When the max $\dot{V}O_2$ is expressed in relation to body mass ($ml \cdot kg^{-1} \cdot min^{-1}$), women still have about a 20% lower max $\dot{V}O_2$. If aerobic

Heritability is a controlling factor. While a vigorous program of physical training will enhance a person's level of fitness regardless of genetic background, it is clear that the limits for developing fitness capacity are also linked to natural endowment.

TABLE 5-3 Different ways of expressing oxygen uptake

Variable	Female	Male	Female vs male % difference
Max $\dot{V}O_2$, $1 \cdot min^{-1}$	2.00	3.50	-43
Max $\dot{V}O_2$, $ml \cdot kg^{-1} \cdot min^{-1}$	40.0	50.0	-20
Max $\dot{V}O_2$, $ml \cdot kgLBM^{-1} \cdot min^{-1}$	53.3	58.8	-9.0
Body mass, kg	50	70	-29
Percent body fat	25	15	+67
Lean body mass, kg	37.5	59.5	-37

capacity is expressed in relation to lean body mass, however, the difference between the two subjects is reduced still more. This is especially true when men and women of equal training status are compared. Findings such as these have also been noted for men and women during arm-cranking exercise. When oxygen uptake values during maximal exercise were corrected for variations in arm and shoulder size, no difference in peak $\dot{V}O_2$ was observed between the genders. These findings suggest that the differences in aerobic capacity between men and women are largely a function of the size of the contracting muscle mass. On the other hand, one must not be misled into believing that simply expressing the aerobic or endurance performance capacity by some measure of body composition will automatically "adjust" such criterion measures for the observed gender differences. The crucial test is to ascertain whether the gender differences are real (i.e., biological in origin) or are due to factors other than true inherited characteristics.

Age. The maximal oxygen uptake is not spared the effects of aging. Although inferences from cross-sectional studies of people of different ages are somewhat limited, the available data provide insight into the possible effects of aging on physiologic function.

Absolute values. As shown in Figure 5-11, the maximal oxygen uptake expressed in liters per minute rapidly increases during the growth years. Longitudinal studies of children and aerobic power have been few. The available data indicate that the absolute max $\dot{V}O_2$ ranges from about $1.0 \text{ L} \cdot \text{min}^{-1}$ at age 6 years to about $3.2 \text{ L} \cdot \text{min}^{-1}$ at 16 years. Average max $\dot{V}O_2$ in girls peaks at about age 14 and begins to decline thereafter. At age 14, the differences in max $\dot{V}O_2$ ($\text{L} \cdot \text{min}^{-1}$) between males and females approximates 25%, and will reach 50% by age 16 years.

Relative values. When expressed relative to body mass, the max $\dot{V}O_2$ remains constant at about $53 \text{ ml} \cdot \text{kg}^{-1} \cdot \text{min}^{-1}$ between the ages of 6 and 16 years for boys. On the other hand, relative max $\dot{V}O_2$ gradually decreases with age in girls from $52.0 \text{ ml} \cdot \text{kg}^{-1} \cdot \text{min}^{-1}$ at age 6 to $40.5 \text{ ml} \cdot \text{kg}^{-1} \cdot \text{min}^{-1}$ at age 16 years. The most commonly offered explanation for the discrepancy in relative max $\dot{V}O_2$ between boys and girls as they advance in age is the relatively greater accumulation of body fat in females.

After age 25, the max $\dot{V}O_2$ declines steadily at about 1% per year, so that by age 55 it is about 27% below values reported for 20-year-olds. The data in the insert graph indicate that while active adults retain a relatively high max $\dot{V}O_2$ at all ages, a progressive decline in this physiologic capacity occurs with advancing years. In one study of 8 women who averaged about 80 years of age, max $\dot{V}O_2$ averaged $13.4 \text{ ml} \cdot \text{kg}^{-1} \cdot \text{min}^{-1}$ or about 3.7 METs! Research is accumulating, however, to indicate that one's habitual level of physical activity is more a determinant of aerobic capacity than chronological age per se. The age-related effects on physiologic function are discussed more fully in Chapter 18.

• • • • • • • • • • • • •

PREDICTION OF MAXIMAL OXYGEN UPTAKE

The direct measurement of max $\dot{V}O_2$ requires an extensive laboratory and specialized equipment, as well as considerable motivation on the part of the subject. Consequently, these tests are not suitable for measuring large groups of untrained subjects outside of the laboratory. In addition, such heavy exercise could pose a potential hazard to adults who have not received proper medical clearance, or who are exercised without appropriate safeguards or supervision. In view of these considerations, tests have been devised to predict the max $\dot{V}O_2$ from performance measures such as walking and

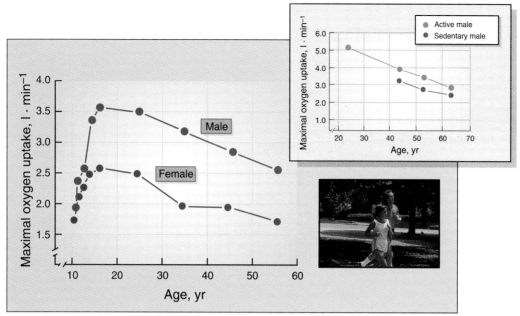

FIGURE 5-11. Maximal oxygen uptake as a function of age and level of activity in male and female subjects. (From Hermansen, L.: Individual differences. In *Fitness, Health, and Work Capacity*. International Standards for Assessment. Edited by L.A. Larson. New York, Macmillan Publishing Co., 1974. The inset graph was redrawn from tabled data of Åstrand, P.O., and Rodahl, K.R.: *Textbook of Work Physiology*. New York, McGraw-Hill Book Co., 1970.)

running endurance, or from easily obtained heart rates during or immediately following exercise. The tests are easy to administer, can be used with large groups of men or women, and they usually require only submaximal exercise.

female, 1 = male; T_1 is time for the 1-mile track walk expressed as minutes and hundredths of a minute; HR_{1-4} is the heart rate in beats $\cdot$ min^{-1} at the end of the last quarter mile.

The equation to predict max $\dot{V}O_2$, expressed in ml $\cdot$ kg^{-1} $\cdot$ min^{-1}, is:

$$Max\ \dot{V}O_2 = 132.853 - (0.0769\ x\ W) - (0.3877\ x\ A) + (6.315\ x\ G) - (3.2649\ x\ T_1) - (0.1565\ x\ HR_{1-4})$$

Walking Tests

In the 1980s, walking tests were developed on a large sample of males and females to predict max $\dot{V}O_2$. In one study, the following equation was developed to predict max $\dot{V}O_2$ from walking speed and other variables.

In terms of prediction error, most individuals' max $\dot{V}O_2$ will lie within 0.335 L $\cdot$ min^{-1} or 4.4 ml $\cdot$ kg^{-1} $\cdot$ min^{-1} of the predicted value. Because the study population ranged in age from 30 to 69 years, this prediction method is applicable to a large segment of the population.

$$Max\ \dot{V}O_2 = 6.9652 + (0.0091\ x\ W) - (0.0257\ x\ A) + (0.5955\ x\ G) - (0.224\ x\ T_1) - (0.0115\ x\ HR_{1-4})$$

In this equation, max $\dot{V}O_2$ is in L $\cdot$ min^{-1}; W is body weight in pounds; A is age in years; G is gender: 0 =

To illustrate this walking prediction test, suppose the following data were collected on a 30 year old female:

Body weight = 155.5 lb; T_1 = 13.56 min; HR_{1-4} = 145 beats $\cdot$ min^{-1}

Substituting in the equation to predict max $\dot{V}O_2$ in ml $\cdot$ kg^{-1} $\cdot$ min^{-1} results in a value of 42.3 as follows:

tion. These latter variables are in themselves related to the run-walk and max $\dot{V}O_2$ scores. To avoid spurious relationships, the proper statisti-

$$Max\ \dot{V}O_2 = 132.853 - (0.0769 \times 155.5) - (0.3877 \times 30.0) + (6.315 \times 0) - (3.2649 \times 13.56) - (0.1565 \times 145)$$
$$Max\ \dot{V}O_2 = 132.853 - (11.96) - (11.63) + (0) - (44.27) - (22.69)$$
$$Max\ \dot{V}O_2 = 42.3\ ml \cdot kg^{-1} \cdot min^{-1}$$

Endurance Runs

Like walking tests, runs of various durations or distances can be used to evaluate aerobic fitness. Such tests are based on the reasonable notion that the distance one is able to run in a specified time (in excess of 5 or 6 minutes) is determined by the ability to maintain a high, steady-rate level of oxygen uptake. This in turn is largely based on one's aerobic capacity. Using this rationale, a field performance test was devised to evaluate aerobic fitness in military personnel. The object of this test was to run-walk as far as possible in 15 minutes. In 1968, the run was shortened to 12 minutes.

In the original validation studies of the run-walk test, a strong correlation (r = 0.90) was found between the max $\dot{V}O_2$ of Air Force personnel and the distance covered in 12 minutes. The men, however, varied significantly in age, body mass, and max $\dot{V}O_2$. With more homogeneous groups, other investigators have been unable to demonstrate such a strong relationship between the run-walk scores and aerobic capacity. One study, for example, measured 11 to 14 year-old boys and reported a correlation of r = 0.65. For a group of 26 female athletes, the correlation between run-walk scores and max $\dot{V}O_2$ scores was r = 0.70, whereas for 36 untrained college women, the correlation was r = 0.67.

We would like to point out that a simple correlation of run-walk scores with max $\dot{V}O_2$ does not take into account age and body-weight factors unless they are included in the equa-

cal evaluation and formulae derivation must be performed.

The prediction of aerobic capacity should be approached with caution when using walking or running performance. The need to establish a consistent level of motivation and effective pacing is critical for inexperienced subjects. Some individuals may achieve an optimal pace so they do not run too fast in the early part of a run and are therefore forced to slow down or even stop due to lactic acid buildup as the test progresses. Other individuals, however, may begin too slowly and continue that way so that their final performance score reflects inappropriate pacing or motivation rather than physiologic and metabolic capacity. In addition, max $\dot{V}O_2$ is not the only variable that determines endurance walking-running performance. Factors such as body mass and body fatness, running economy, and the percentage of one's aerobic capacity that can be sustained without lactate buildup, all contribute significantly to successful running performance.

Predictions Based on Heart Rate.

Common tests to predict max $\dot{V}O_2$ use the exercise or postexercise heart rate with a standardized regimen of submaximal exercise performed either on a bicycle, treadmill, or step test. These tests make use of the essentially linear relationship between heart rate and oxygen uptake for various intensities of light to moderately heavy exercise. The slope of

Lower heart rate indicates a training effect. As the heart's stroke volume increases and the circulatory system becomes more efficient in delivering blood as a result of training, there will be a decrease in exercise heart rate as well as the heart rate in recovery.

this line (rate of heart rate increase) reflects the individual's aerobic fitness. The max $\dot{V}O_2$ can then be estimated by drawing a straight line through several submaximum points that relate heart rate and oxygen uptake (or exercise intensity) and then extending this line to some assumed maximum heart rate for the particular age group.

Figure 5-12 illustrates the application of this "extrapolation" procedure for trained and untrained subjects. The heart rate-oxygen uptake line was drawn from four submaximal measures during bicycle exercise. Although each person's heart rate-oxygen uptake line tends to be linear, the slope of the individual lines can differ considerably, largely due to the amount of blood the heart can pump with each beat. Consequently, a person with relatively high aerobic fitness can do more work and achieve higher oxygen uptake before reaching a heart rate of 140 or 160 beats per minute than a less "fit" person. Also, because the heart rate increases linearly with the intensity of exercise, the person with the smallest increase in heart rate tends to have the highest exercise capacity and hence the highest max $\dot{V}O_2$. For the two subjects illustrated in Figure 5-12 max $\dot{V}O_2$ was predicted by extrapolating the line to a heart rate of 195 beats per minute — the assumed maximum heart rate for subjects of college age.

The accuracy of predicting max $\dot{V}O_2$ from submaximal exercise heart rate is limited by the following assumptions:

- **Linearity of the heart rate-oxygen uptake (exercise intensity) relationship**. This assumption is met to a large degree, especially for various intensities of light to moderate exercise. In some subjects, the heart rate-oxygen uptake line curves or asymptotes at the heavier work loads in a direction that indicates a larger than expected increase in oxygen uptake per unit increase in heart rate. The oxygen uptake actually

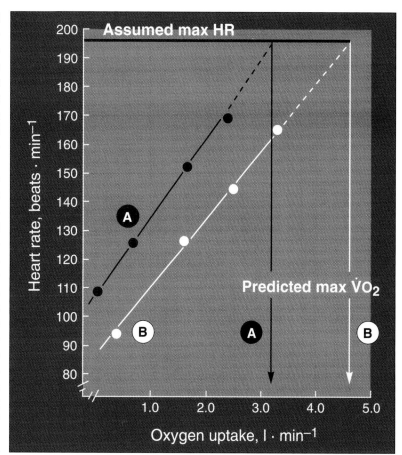

FIGURE 5-12. Prediction of max$\dot{V}O_2$ by extrapolating the linear relationship between submaximal heart rate and oxygen uptake during graded exercise. In an untrained (A) and aerobically trained (B) subject.

increases more than would be predicted through linear extrapolation of the heart rate-oxygen uptake line. Thus, the predicted max $\dot{V}O_2$ in these subjects would be underestimated.

- **Similar maximum heart rates for all subjects.** The standard deviation is approximately ± 10 beats per minute about the average maximum heart rate of individuals of the same age. Therefore, the max $\dot{V}O_2$ of a person with an actual maximum heart rate of 185 beats per minute would be overestimated if the heart rate-oxygen uptake line were extrapolated to 195 or 200 beats per minute. The opposite would be true for a subject with an actual maximum heart rate of 210 beats per minute. Maximum heart rate also decreases with age. Unless this age effect is considered, older subjects will be consistently overestimated by assuming a maximum heart rate of 195 beats per minute, which is the appropriate heart rate maximum for 25-year-olds. More is said in Chapter 18 concerning the effect of age on maximum heart rate.

- **Assumed constant economy.** In cases in which submaximal oxygen uptake is not measured, but is instead estimated from the exercise level, the predicted max $\dot{V}O_2$ may be in error by the magnitude of variability in exercise economy. A subject with poor economy (oxygen uptake at submaximal work higher than assumed) will be underestimated in terms of max $\dot{V}O_2$, because heart rate will be elevated due to the added oxygen cost of the uneconomical exercise. The variation among individuals in oxygen uptake during walking, stepping, or cycling does not usually exceed ± 6%. However, seemingly small modifications in test procedures can have profound effects on the metabolic cost of exercise. Allowing individuals to support themselves with the treadmill handrails, for example, can reduce the oxygen cost of exercise by as much as 30%!

- **Day-to-day variation in heart rate.** Even under highly standardized conditions, the variation in submaximal heart rate for an individual is about ± 5 beats per minute with day-to-day testing at the same exercise load.

Within the framework of these limitations, the max $\dot{V}O_2$ predicted from submaximal heart rate is generally within 10 to 20% of the person's actual value. Clearly, this is not acceptable accuracy for research purposes. These tests, however, may be well-suited for purposes of screening and classification in terms of aerobic fitness.

SUMMARY

1. The concepts of individual differences and specificity of exercise are important for understanding capacities for anaerobic and aerobic power. Individual differences refer to real differences among individuals, in contrast to the instability of a measure for any one individual. Specificity refers to metabolic and physiologic function that is not a general factor but one dependent on a host of factors.

2. The contribution of anaerobic and aerobic energy transfer depends largely on the intensity and duration of exercise. For strength and power-sprint activities, the primary energy transfer involves the immediate and short-term energy systems. The long-term aerobic energy system becomes progressively more important in activities that last longer than 2 minutes.

3. The capacity of each energy system can be estimated using appropriate physiologic measurements and performance tests; these can be used to evaluate a capacity at a particular time or to show changes consequent to specific training programs.

4. The stair-sprinting power test is commonly applied to measure power output generated by stored intramuscular high-energy phosphates. Peak power and average power capacity from the glycolytic pathway can be evaluated by the 30-second, all-out Wingate test. Interpretation of test results must be made within the framework of the exercise specificity principle.

5. Training status, motivation, and acid–base regulation are factors that may explain differences among individuals in the capacities of the immediate and short-term energy systems.

6. The maximal oxygen uptake provides reliable and important information on the power of the long-term energy system as well as the functional capacity of various physiologic support systems. Consideration for type and amount of exercise performed and related physiologic functioning is required to assure that a "true" score has been attained.

7. The maximal aerobic power is influenced by heredity, state and type of training, age, gender and body composition. Each factor contributes uniquely to an individual's max $\dot{V}O_2$.

8. Field methods to predict max $\dot{V}O_2$ should be viewed with caution; however, they may provide useful information in the absence of more valid laboratory methods.

SELECTED REFERENCES

Åstrand, P. O., and Rodahl, K.: *Textbook of Work Physiology*. New York, McGraw-Hill, 1986.

Bar-Or, O.: The Wingate anaerobic test: An update on methodology, reliability, and validity. *Sports Med.*, 4: 381, 1987.

Blomquist, C. G., et al.: Similarity of the hemodynamic responses to static and dynamic exercise of small muscle groups. *Circ. Res.*, 48(Suppl. I): 87, 1982.

Bouchard, C., et al.: Genetics of aerobic and anaerobic performances. In *Exercise and Sport Sciences Reviews*. Vol. 20. Edited by J. O. Holloszy. Baltimore, Williams & Wilkins, 1992.

Cain, S. M.: Mechanisms which control $\dot{V}O_2$ near $\dot{V}O_{2\ max}$: an overview. *Med. Sci. Sports Exerc.*, 27(1): 60, 1995.

Cooper, K.: Correlation between field and treadmill testing as a means for assessing maximal oxygen intake. *JAMA*, 203: 201, 1968.

Cureton, K. J., et al.: Body fatness and performance differences between men and women. *Res. Q.*, 50: 333, 1979.

Davis, J. A., et al.: Effect of ramp slope on measurement of aerobic parameters from the ramp exercise test. *Med Sci. Sports Exerc.*, 14: 339, 1982.

Eshjornsson, L. et al.: Fast-twitch Fibers may predict anaerobic performance in both females and males. *Int. J. Sports Med.*, 14: 257, 1993.

Franklin, B. A.: Exercise testing, training and arm ergometry, *Sports Med.*, 2; 109, 1985.

Gergley, T., et al.: Specificity of arm training on aerobic power during swimming and running. *Med. Sci. Sports Exerc.*, 16: 349, 1984.

Hagberg, J. M., et al.: Comparison of three procedures for measuring $\dot{V}O_2$ max in competitive cyclists. *Eur. J. Appl. Physiol.*, 39: 47, 1978.

Inbar, O., and Bar-Or, O.: Anaerobic characterisics in male children and adolescents. *Med. Sci. Sports Exerc.*, 18: 264, 1986.

Jacobs, I., et al.: Sprint training effects on muscle myoglobin, enzymes, fiber types, and blood lactate. *Med. Sci. Sports Exerc.*, 19: 368, 1987.

Joyner, M. J.: Physiological limiting factors and distance running: influence of gender and age on record performances. In *Exercise and Sport Sciences Reviews*. Vol. 21. Edited by J. O. Holloszy. Baltimore MD, Williams & Wilkins, 1993.

Karlsson, J., et al.: Relevance of muscle fibre type to fatigue in short intense and prolonged exercise in man. In *Human Muscle Fatigue: Physiological Mechanisms*. London, Pitman Medical, 1981.

Kasch, F. W., et al.: A longitudinal study of cardiovascular stability in active men aged 45 to 65 years. *Phys. Sportsmed.*, 16: 117, 1988.

Katch, V. L., et al.: Optimal test characteristics for maximal anaerobic work on the bicycle ergometer. *Res. Q.*, 48: 319, 1977.

Kline, G., et al.: Estimation of $\dot{V}O_2$ max from a one-mile track walk, gender, age, and body weight. *Med. Sci. Sports Exerc.*, 19: 253, 1987.

Magel, J. R., et al.: Specificity of swim training on maximum oxygen uptake. *J. Appl. Physiol.*, 38: 151, 1975.

Margaria, R., et al.: Measurement of muscular power (anaerobic) in man. *J. Appl. Physiol.*, 21: 1662, 1966.

McArdle, W. D., et al.: Comparison of continuous and discontinuous treadmill and bicycle tests for max $\dot{V}O_2$. *Med. Sci. Sports*, 5: 156, 1973.

McArdle, W. D., et al.: Specificity of run training on $\dot{V}O_2$ max and heart rate changes during running and swimming. *Med. Sci. Sports*, 10: 16, 1978.

Nindl, B.C., et al.: Lower and upper body anaerobic performance in male and female adolescent athletes. *Med. Sci. Sports Exerc.*, 27: 235, 1995.

Pelham, T. W., and Holt, L. E.: Testing for aerobic power in paddlers using sport-specific simulators. *J. Strength Cond. Res.*, 9(1): 52, 1995.

Rowland, T. W.: Aerobic response to endurance training in prepubescent children: a critical analysis. *Med. Sci. Sports Exerc.*, 17: 493, 1985.

Saavedra, C., et al.: Maximal anaerobic performance of the knee extensor muscles during growth. *Med. Sci. Sports Exerc.*, 23: 1083, 1991.

Sawka, M. N.: Physiology of upper body exercise, In *Exercise and Sport Sciences Reviews*. Vol. 14. Edited by K. B. Pandolf. New York, Macmillan, 1986.

Stamford, B. A.: Exercise in the elderly. In *Exercise and Sport Sciences Reviews*. Vol. 16. Edited by K. B. Pandolf. New York, Macmillan, 1988.

Sutton, J. R.: Limitations to maximal oxygen uptake. *Sports Med.*, 13: 127, 1992.

Toner, M. M., et al.: Cardiorespiratory responses to exercise distributed between the upper and lower body. *J. Appl. Physiol.*, 54: 1403, 1983.

Vogel, J. A., et al.: Analysis of aerobic capacity in a large United States population. *J. Appl. Physiol.*, 60: 494, 1986.

Wallick, M.E., et al.: Physiological responses to in-line skating compared to treadmill running. *Med. Sci. Sports Exerc.*, 27: 242, 1995.

Wasserman, K., et al.: *Principles of Exercise Testing and Interpretation*. Philadelphia, Lea & Febiger, 1987.

Wells, C. L., and Plowman, S. A.: Sexual differences in athletic performance: biological or behavioral? *Phys. Sportsmed.*, 11: 52, 1983.

Weltman, A., et al.: The lactate threshold and endurance performance. *Adv. Sports Med. Fitness*, 2: 91, 1989.

NUTRITION FOR PHYSICAL ACTIVITY

SECTION II

Proper nutrition forms the foundation for physical performance; it provides both the fuel for biologic work and the chemicals for extracting and using the potential energy contained within this fuel. Food also provides the essential elements for the synthesis of new tissue and the repair of existing cells.

Some may argue that adequate nutrition for exercise can easily be achieved through the intake of a well-balanced diet, and that, therefore, it is of little consequence in the study of exercise performance. We maintain, however, that the study of exercise when viewed within the framework of energy capacities must be based on an understanding of the sources of food energy and the role of nutrients in the process of energy release. With this perspective, it becomes possible for the exercise specialist to appreciate the importance of "adequate" nutrition and to evaluate critically the validity of claims concerning nutrient supplements and special dietary modifications for enhancing physical performance. Because various food nutrients provide energy and regulate physiologic processes associated with exercise, it is tempting to link dietary modification to improvement in athletic performance. Too often individuals spend considerable time and "energy" striving for the optimum in exercise performance, only to fall short due to inadequate, counterproductive, and sometimes harmful nutritional practices. Finally, it is now apparent that aspects of sound nutritional practice have an impact on a variety of disease conditions to which regular exercise can make a meaningful contribution.

After reading this chapter you should be able to:

- Define and give examples of monosaccharides, disaccharides, and poly-saccharides.

- Discuss the role of carbohydrates as an energy source, protein sparer, metabolic primer, and fuel for the central nervous system.

- Define and give one example of a triglyceride, saturated fatty acid, monounsaturated fatty acid, and polyunsaturated fatty acid.

- List the major characteristics of high- and low-density lipoproteins, and discuss the role of these lipoproteins in coronary heart disease.

- List the important functions of lipids in the body.

- Define essential and non-essential amino acids and give food sources for each.

- Describe how the factors of exercise intensity (low, moderate, and maxi-mal) and duration (short and long) influence the utilization of carbohy-drate, lipid, and protein in energy metabolism.

- Describe the alanine-glucose cycle and explain how protein is used for energy during exercise.

- List a function of each of the fat- and water-soluble vitamins, and the potential risks of excessive intake of these micronutrients.

- Outline the three broad roles of minerals in the body.

- Define the terms osteoporosis, exercise-induced anemia, sodium-induced hypertension, heat cramps, heat exhaustion, and heat stroke.

- Describe how physical activity affects (a) osteoporosis, and (b) the body's iron stores.

The carbohydrate, lipid, and protein nutrients consumed daily supply the necessary energy to maintain body functions both at rest and during various forms of physical activity. Aside from their role as biologic fuel, these nutrients (referred to as *macronutrients*) also play an important part in maintaining the structural and functional integrity of the organism. In Part 1, each of these nutrients is discussed in terms of its general structure, function, and source in specific foods in the diet. Emphasis is placed on the importance of the macronutrients in sustaining physiologic function during various intensities of physical activity.

CARBOHYDRATES

Carbohydrates are compounds constructed in a ratio of one atom of carbon and two atoms of hydrogen for each oxygen atom. The general formula for a simple carbohydrate is $(CH_2O)_n$, where n can be from three to seven carbon atoms.

Monosaccharides

The basic chemical structure of a simple sugar molecule consists of a chain of from three to seven carbon atoms with hydrogen and oxygen atoms attached by single bonds. The most common are the six-carbon sugar units *glucose, fructose,* and *galactose.* Glucose, also called dextrose or blood sugar, consists of 6 carbon, 12 hydrogen, and 6 oxygen atoms ($C_6H_{12}O_6$; Figure 6-1). It is formed as a natural sugar in food and can be produced in the body as a result of digestion of more complex carbohydrates, or it can be made by the process of gluconeogenesis where it is synthesized from the carbon skeletons of other compounds. After glu-

cose is absorbed by the small intestine, one of three things takes place:

- It is used directly by the cell for energy
- It is stored as glycogen in the muscles and liver
- It is converted to fats for energy storage

Fructose, also known as fruit sugar, is the sweetest of the monosaccharides and is present in large amounts in fruits and honey. Although some fructose is absorbed directly into the blood from the digestive tract, it is slowly converted to glucose in the liver. Galactose is not found freely in nature; rather, it must be produced from milk sugar in the mammary glands of lactating animals. In the body, galactose is converted to glucose for energy metabolism.

Disaccharides

The joining of two simple sugar molecules forms a double sugar or disaccharide of which sucrose, maltose, and lactose are examples. The

More of our carbohydrate from simple sugars. The average American consumes about 50% of dietary carbohydrate as simple sugars, mostly in the form of sucrose and high-fructose corn syrup. This amount includes more than 16 teaspoons of sucrose a day, or 60 pounds of table sugar and about 50 pounds of corn syrup each year, as contrasted to an average person's annual intake of only four pounds of table sugar 100 years ago!

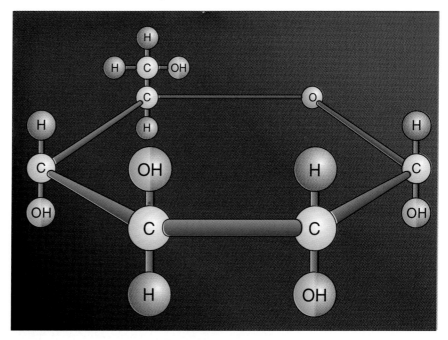

FIGURE 6-1. Three-dimensional ring structure of the simple sugar molecule glucose. The molecule resembles a hexagonal plate to which H and O atoms are attached.

monosaccharides and disaccharides collectively make up what are commonly referred to as the simple sugars. The three principal disaccharides are:

- **Sucrose** — glucose + fructose — the most common dietary disaccharide. It occurs naturally in most foods containing carbohydrate, especially in beet and cane sugar, brown sugar, sorghum, maple syrup, and honey.
- **Lactose** — glucose + galactose — found in natural form only in milk and is often called milk sugar.
- **Maltose** — glucose + glucose — occurs in malt products and in germinating cereals.

Polysaccharides

The term polysaccharide refers to the combination of three or more sugar molecules. There are generally two classifications of polysaccharides, plant and animal.

Plant Polysaccharides. Two common forms of plant polysaccharides are starch and fiber.

Starch. Hundreds to thousands of individual sugar molecules may join together to form a starch molecule. Starch, the most familiar form of plant polysaccharide, is found in seeds, corn, and in the various grains from which bread, cereal, spaghetti, and pastries are made. Large amounts are also present in peas, beans, potatoes, and roots, where it serves as an energy store for future use by plants.

Fiber. Cellulose and most other nonstarch fibrous materials that are generally resistant to human digestive enzymes are another form of polysaccharide. They are found exclusively in plants and make up the structural part of leaves, stems, roots, seeds, and fruit coverings. Other fibers such as mucilage and gums are found within the plant cell itself.

Fibers hold considerable water and thus give "bulk" to the food residues in the small intestine, often increasing stool weight and volume by 40 to 100%. This bulking action may aid gastrointestinal functioning and reduce the chances of contracting colon cancer and various other gastrointestinal diseases later in life. Fiber intake may also lower serum cholesterol in humans, especially the water-soluble mucilaginous fibers present in oats, beans, brown rice, peas, carrots, and a variety of fruits.

Table 6-1 gives the fiber content of some common foods. *Present nutrition-*

TABLE 6-1. Fiber content of some common foods listed in order of overall fiber content

	Serving Size	Total Fiber (g)	Soluble Fiber (g)	Insoluble Fiber (g)
100% bran cereal	1/2 cup	10.0	0.3	9.7
Peas	1/2 cup	5.2	2.0	3.2
Kidney beans	1/2 cup	4.5	0.5	4.0
Apple	1 small	3.9	2.3	1.6
Potato	1 small	3.8	2.2	1.6
Broccoli	1/2 cup	2.5	1.1	1.4
Strawberries	3/4 cup	2.4	0.9	1.5
Oats, whole	1/2 cup	1.6	0.5	1.1
Banana	1 small	1.3	0.6	0.7
Spaghetti	1/2 cup	1.0	0.2	0.8
Lettuce	1/2 cup	0.5	0.2	0.3
White rice	1/2 cup	0.5	0	0.5

al wisdom maintains that a dietary fiber intake of about 35 g per day is an important part of a well-structured diet.

Animal Polysaccharides. Glycogen is the large polysaccharide synthesized from glucose in the process of *glucogenesis* and stored in the tissues of animals. In well-nourished humans, approximately 375 to 475 g of carbohydrate are stored in the body. Of this, approximately 325 g are muscle glycogen (largest reserve), 90 to 110 g are liver glycogen (highest concentration), and only 15 to 20 g remain unstored and circulates as blood glucose. *As each gram of glycogen contains 4 calories of energy, the average person stores between 1,500 and 2,000 calories of energy within the bonds of the carbohydrate molecule.* This is about enough energy to power a 20-mile run.

During exercise, the carbohydrate stored as muscle glycogen is used as a source of energy for the specific muscle in which it is stored. In the liver, in contrast, glycogen is reconverted to glucose (under the control of a specific *phosphatase* enzyme) and transported in the blood for eventual use by the working muscles. The term glycogenolysis is used to describe this reconversion process that provides a rapid supply of glucose for muscular contraction during all forms of work. When liver and muscle glycogen are depleted through dietary restriction or exercise, glucose synthesis from the structural components of the other nutrients, especially proteins, tends to increase through *gluconeogenesis.* Hormones, particularly *insulin* that is secreted by the pancreas, play an important part in the regulation of liver and muscle glycogen stores by controlling the level of circulating blood sugar. If blood sugar level is high, the pancreas secretes additional insulin and excess circulating glucose is taken up by the cells. This type of "feedback" regulation maintains blood glucose at an appropriate and safe physiologic concentration. In contrast, if blood sugar falls below normal, insulin's opposing hormone,

glucagon, is immediately secreted to normalize the blood sugar level.

Because comparatively little glycogen is stored in the body, its quantity can be modified considerably through the diet. For example, a 24-hour fast or low-carbohydrate, normal-calorie diet results in a large reduction in glycogen reserves. Maintaining a carbohydrate-rich diet for several days enhances the body's carbohydrate stores to a level almost twice that obtained with a normal, well-balanced diet.

Functions of Carbohydrates

Carbohydrates serve several important functions related to exercise performance. These include:

Energy Source. The main function of carbohydrate is to serve as an energy fuel for the body. The energy derived from the breakdown of glucose and glycogen is ultimately used to power muscular contraction as well as all other forms of biologic work. Once the capacity of the cell for glycogen storage is reached, the excess sugars are converted and stored as fat. This helps to explain how body fat increases when excess calories are consumed in the form of carbohydrates.

Protein Sparer. Adequate carbohydrate intake helps to preserve tissue protein. Under normal conditions, protein serves a vital role in the maintenance, repair, and growth of body tissues, and to a considerably lesser degree, as a nutrient source of energy. However, when the body's carbohydrate reserves become reduced either through diets with inadequate caloric or carbohydrate content, or through participation in arduous endurance exercise programs, certain amino acids have carbon skeletons that can be rebuilt to glucose. This gluconeogenesis provides a metabolic option for augmenting carbohydrate availability in the face of depleted glycogen stores. However, there is a price to pay because gluconeogenesis can

Glucagon. Glucagon, termed the "insulin antagonist" hormone, is secreted by alpha cells of the pancreas. Glucagon's major function is to raise the blood glucose level by stimulating both glycogenolysis and gluconeogenesis in the liver.

The phosphatase enzyme is a "gatekeeper" for glucose. Liver cells contain the enzyme phosphatase that can change glycogen back to glucose which then exits the cell; muscles do not have this enzyme.

Insulin. Insulin is a peptide hormone, secreted by beta cells of the pancreas that aids the movement of nutrients — primarily glucose but also amino acids — into most cells by facilitated diffusion. Insulin also stimulates the synthesis of glycogen, protein, and fat.

cause a temporary reduction in the body's protein "stores," especially muscle protein. A chronic reduction in carbohydrate availability, either through diet or exercise, could definitely be counterproductive to training programs geared to increase muscle size and power.

Metabolic Primer. Carbohydrate serves as a "primer" for fat metabolism. Certain derivatives from the breakdown of carbohydrate (e.g., oxaloacetic acid) must be available to facilitate the breakdown of fat. With insufficient carbohydrate metabolism, either through limitation in the transport of glucose into the cell (which occurs in diabetes), or depletion of glycogen through improper diet or prolonged exercise, the body is unable to generate a sustained high level of aerobic energy transfer from lipid-only metabolism.

Fuel for the Central Nervous System. Carbohydrate is essential for the proper functioning of the central nervous system. Under normal conditions, the brain uses blood glucose almost exclusively as the preferred fuel because it essentially has no stored supply of this nutrient. The symptoms of a modest reduction in blood glucose, known as *hypoglycemia*, include feelings of weakness, hunger, and dizziness. This condition impairs exercise performance and may partially explain the fatigue associated with prolonged exercise. Because of the specific role played by glucose in the energy supply of nerve tissue, blood sugar is regulated within narrow limits. To this end, the liver provides a constant supply of blood glucose between meals.

Recommended Intake of Carbohydrates

Figure 6-2 illustrates the carbohydrate content of selected foods. Cereals, cookies, candies, breads, and cakes are rich carbohydrate sources. Because the values are based on carbohydrate percentage in relation to the total weight, including water content, fruits and vegetables appear to be less valuable sources of carbohydrates. The dried portion of these foods, however, is almost pure carbohydrate.

The typical American diet includes between 40 and 50% of its total calories in carbohydrate form. For a sedentary 70-kg person, this amounts to a daily intake of about 300 g of carbohydrate. For more active peo-

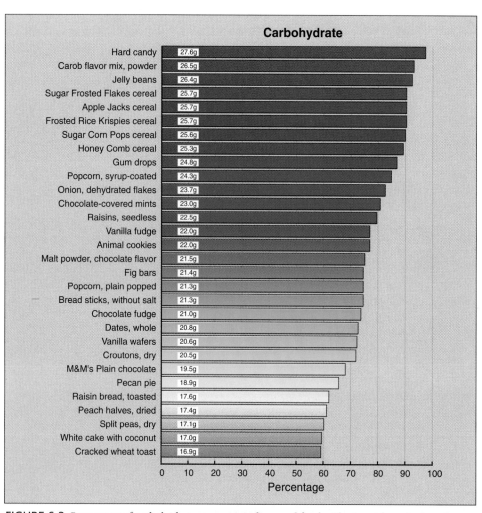

FIGURE 6-2. Percentage of carbohydrates in commonly served foods. The insert box displays the number of grams of carbohydrate per ounce of the food.

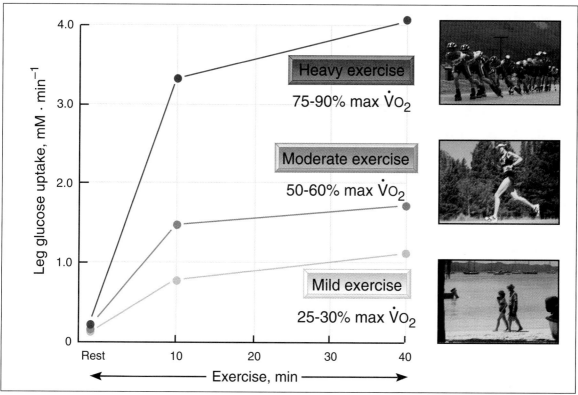

FIGURE 6-3. Blood glucose uptake by the leg muscles as affected by exercise duration and intensity. Exercise intensity is expressed as a percent of one's max $\dot{V}O_2$. (From Felig, P., and Wahren, J.: Fuel homeostasis in exercise. *N. Engl. J. Med.*, 293:1078, 1975.)

ple and those involved in exercise training, about 60% of the daily calories (400 to 600 g) should be in the form of carbohydrates, predominantly of the complex variety. This amount will be sufficient to replenish the carbohydrate used to power an increased level of physical activity.

Carbohydrate Utilization in Exercise

The fuel mixture during exercise depends on the intensity and duration of effort, as well as the fitness and nutritional status of the exerciser.

Intense Exercise. Stored muscle glycogen and blood-borne glucose are the prime contributors of energy in the early minutes of exercise and during high-intensity exercise, where the oxygen supply does not meet the demands for aerobic metabolism.

Figure 6-3 illustrates that during the initial stage of exercise, the uptake of circulating blood glucose by the muscles increases sharply and continues to increase as exercise progresses. After 40 minutes of exercise, the glucose uptake has risen to between 7 and 20 times the uptake at rest, depending on the intensity of the exercise. The increase in the percentage contribution of carbohydrate during intense exercise occurs because it is the only macronutrient that contributes energy under anaerobic conditions.

Moderate and Prolonged Exercise. Almost all of the energy is supplied from glycogen stored in the active muscles during the transition from rest to submaximal exercise. During the subsequent 20 minutes or so, liver and muscle glycogen provide about 40 to 50% of the energy requirement with the remaining requirement pro-

It depends on the exercise. In cycling exercise, glycogen is depleted mainly from the vastus lateralis muscle, while in running, it is the gastrocnemius and soleus muscle fibers that become depleted.

vided mainly by fat breakdown, with some utilization of blood glucose (Fig. 6-3). As exercise continues and glycogen stores become reduced, however, an increasingly greater percentage of energy is supplied through fat metabolism. Additionally, the glucose in blood becomes the major source of carbohydrate energy. Eventually, glucose output by the liver fails to keep pace with its use by the muscles and blood glucose concentration slowly begins to fall.

Fatigue may occur if exercise is performed to the point where the glycogen in the liver and specific muscles becomes severely lowered, even though sufficient oxygen is available to the muscles and the potential energy from stored fat remains almost unlimited. Endurance athletes commonly refer to this sensation of fatigue as "bonking" or "hitting the wall." It is unclear why carbohydrate depletion coincides with the point of fatigue in prolonged submaximal exercise. Part of the answer may relate to the important role of blood glucose in central nervous system function, and the use of muscle glycogen as a "primer" in fat metabolism.

Triglyceride, the most common fat. By far, triglycerides represent the most plentiful fat in the body. More than 95% of body fat is in this form.

LIPIDS

A lipid molecule possesses the same structural elements as the carbohydrate molecule except that the linking of the specific atoms is markedly different. Specifically, the ratio of hydrogen to oxygen is considerably higher in the lipid compound. For example, the common fat stearin has the chemical formula $C_{57}H_{110}O_6$. Whereas the H- to -O_2 ratio for carbohydrate is 2:1, for stearin it is 18.3:1 ($110 \div 6$).

According to common classification, lipids can be placed into one of three main groups: simple fats, compound fats, and derived fats.

Simple Fats

The simple fats are often called "neutral fats" and consist primarily of triglycerides, the major storage form of fat. A triglyceride molecule consists of two different clusters of atoms. One cluster is *glycerol,* a 3-carbon molecule. Attached to the glycerol molecule are three *clusters* of carbon-chained atoms termed *fatty acids.* The basic structures of the two kinds of fatty acid molecules, *saturated* and *unsaturated,* are shown in Figure 6-4. All foods with fat contain a mixture of saturated and unsaturated fatty acids.

Saturated Fatty Acids. A saturated fatty acid contains only single bonds between carbon atoms; the remaining bonds attach to hydrogen. The fatty acid molecule is said to be saturated because it holds as many hydrogen atoms as is chemically possible.

Saturated fats are found primarily in animal products including beef, lamb, pork, and chicken. Saturated fats are also present in egg yolk and in the dairy fats of cream, milk, butter, and cheese. Coconut and palm oil, vegetable shortening, and hydrogenated margarine are sources of saturated fat from the plant kingdom and are present to a relatively high degree

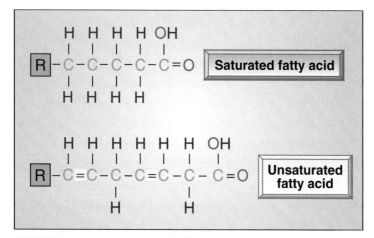

FIGURE 6-4. The major structural difference between saturated and unsaturated fatty acids is the presence or absence of double bonds between the carbon atoms. **R** represents the glycerol portion of the triglyceride molecule.

in commercially prepared cakes, pies, and cookies.

Unsaturated Fatty Acids. Fatty acids containing one or more double bonds along the main carbon chain are classified as unsaturated. In this case, each double bond in the carbon chain reduces the number of potential hydrogen-binding sites; therefore, the molecule is said to be unsaturated with respect to hydrogen. If only one double bond is present along the main carbon chain, as with canola, olive, and peanut oil, the fatty acid is said to be *monounsaturated.* If there are two or more double bonds along the main carbon chain, as with safflower, sunflower, soybean, and corn oil, the fatty acid is said to be *polyunsaturated.* In general, fats from plant sources are unsaturated.

Fatty Acids in the Diet. The amount of saturated fat consumed in the typical American diet has steadily increased to the point that the average person now consumes about 15% of total calories or over 50 lb of saturated fat per year, most of which is animal in origin. This is in contrast to nomadic groups like the Tarahumara Indians of Mexico whose high complex, unrefined carbohydrate diet contains only 2% of the total calories as saturated fat. Coinciding with the increased consumption of saturated fats in the more technologically advanced societies has been an increase in coronary heart disease. This relationship has led many nutritionists and medical personnel to suggest replacing at least a portion of the saturated fat in one's diet with fats that are unsaturated.

Compound Fats

Compound fats are composed of a neutral fat in combination with other chemicals such as phosphorus (*phospholipids*) and glucose (*glucolipids*). Another group of compound fats are the *lipoproteins,* formed primarily in the liver from the union of triglycerides, phospholipids, or cholesterol with protein. The lipoproteins are important because they constitute the main form of transport for fat in the blood. If blood lipids (Greek: *lipos* meaning fat) were not bound to protein or some other substance they would float to the top like cream in nonhomogenized milk.

High- and Low-Density Lipoproteins. There are basically three types of lipoproteins. *High-density lipoproteins (HDL)* are produced in the liver and small intestine and contain the largest amount of protein and correspondingly, the smallest amount of cholesterol. A *low-density lipoprotein (LDL)* is a remnant of a *very-low-density-lipoprotein (VLDL).* Of all the lipoproteins, the *VLDL* contains the greatest percentage of lipid (95%) of which about 60% is in the form of triglycerides. Once the VLDL is acted on by the enzyme *lipoprotein lipase,* it becomes a denser LDL because it now contains less lipid. The LDL and the VLDL fractions contain the greatest fat and least protein components.

"Bad" cholesterol. Among the lipoproteins, LDLs, which normally carry almost 50% of the total cholesterol, have the greatest affinity for the arterial wall. They help to carry cholesterol into arterial tissue where it is chemically modified and ultimately participates in the proliferation of smooth muscle cells and further unfavorable changes that damage and narrow the artery in the process of *coronary heart disease.* A high level of LDL cholesterol is considered undesirable because it is implicated in plaque formation on the inner walls of blood vessels.

"Good" cholesterol. Unlike LDL, HDL operates as so-called good cholesterol to protect against heart disease by acting as a scavenger of cholesterol. HDL removes cholesterol from the arterial wall and transports

Less is better. A prudent recommendation is that saturated fat should represent no more than 10%, and preferably only 5% , of total calories

Consider the monounsaturates. Increasing monounsaturated fatty acids in the diet helps to lower LDL cholesterol without also reducing the "good" HDL cholesterol.

High-density lipoproteins. HDL is composed of the greatest percentage of protein (about 50%), the least total lipid (about 20%), and the least cholesterol (about 20%) of all the lipoproteins. High levels of HDL relate to a low risk for heart disease.

The leaner the better. Recent research indicates that beef fat, and not the lean portion, is related to elevated blood cholesterol. If beef is trimmed of all visible fat and the diet is low in saturated fat, lean beef can be included in a cholesterol-lowering diet.

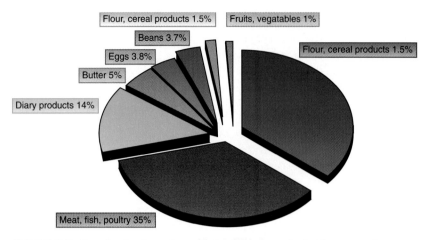

FIGURE 6-5. Contribution from the major food groups to the lipid content of the typical American diet.

including the building of cell membranes, and the synthesis of vitamin D and the adrenal gland hormones, and estrogen, androgen, and progesterone, the hormones responsible for male and female secondary sex characteristics. Cholesterol also plays an intimate role in the formation of the bile secretions that emulsify fat during digestion.

The richest source of cholesterol in foods is egg yolk. Cholesterol is also plentiful in red meats and organ meats such as liver, kidney, and brains, and in shellfish, especially shrimp, as well as in dairy products, such as ice cream, cream cheese, butter, and whole milk. *Cholesterol is not present in any foods of plant origin.*

Fats in Food

Figure 6-5 shows the approximate percentage contribution of some of the common food groups to the total fat content of the typical American diet. Vegetable fat generally contributes about 34% of the daily fat intake, whereas the remaining 66% is from animal fat.

Functions of Lipids

Lipids serve diverse yet essential functions in the body. Their roles include:

Energy Source and Reserve. Fat is an ideal cellular fuel because each lipid molecule carries large quantities of energy per unit weight, is easily transported and stored, and is readily converted into energy. One gram of lipid contains about 9 calories of energy, more than twice the energy storage capacity of an equal quantity of carbohydrate and protein. This is largely because of the greater quantity of hydrogen in the lipid molecule compared to hydrogen in a molecule of carbohydrate and protein. In addition, fat is a relatively water-free, concentrated fuel, whereas *2.7 g of water are stored with each gram of glycogen*

it to the liver where it is incorporated into bile and subsequently excreted via the intestine.

The quantity of LDL and HDL, as well as the specific ratio of these lipoproteins and subfractions, may provide a more meaningful signal of coronary heart disease risk than total cholesterol per se. Regular aerobic exercise and abstinence from cigarette smoking also increase the HDL level and can favorably affect the LDL:HDL ratio. This is discussed more fully in Chapter 18.

Derived Fats

This group of fats includes substances derived from the simple and compound fats. The most widely known of the derived fats is cholesterol, a sterol found only in animal tissue that contains no fatty acids but exhibits some of the physical and chemical characteristics of fat. Cholesterol is present in all cells and is either consumed in foods (*exogenous cholesterol*) or synthesized within the cell (*endogenous cholesterol*). Even when an individual maintains a "cholesterol-free diet," the rate of endogenous cholesterol synthesis may vary from 0.5 to 2.0 g per day. More can be produced, especially if the diet is high in saturated fat, which facilitates cholesterol synthesis by the liver.

Cholesterol is normally required in many complex bodily functions,

Carbohydrate loading and muscle girth. Body builders who think that the extra water stored with each gram of glycogen stored in skeletal muscle may add to muscle bulk will be disappointed by recent research findings. When body builders trained for 3 days on a carbohydrate loading diet (80% of total calories), there was no measureable difference in muscle girth compared to training on a diet low in carbohydrate (10% of total calories).

Quite a bit of energy! The per capita yearly fat consumption in the United States, extrapolated over a population of 250 million people, amounts to 16.5 billion total pounds of dietary fat, or the equivalent of 839 billion calories!

when glycogen is formed in the cell from glucose.

The fat content of the body constitutes approximately 15% of the body mass of males and 25% of females. Consequently, the potential energy stored in the fat molecules of an average size college-aged male who weights 70 kg is about 94,500 kcal (10,500 g of body fat x 9 kcal · g⁻¹). Most of this fat is available for energy, especially during prolonged exercise. The potential energy stored in this quantity of body fat would be sufficient to power the equivalent of walking three times from Boston to San Francisco (assuming that walking requires about 100 kcal energy expenditure per mile)! Contrast this to the limited 2,000 calorie energy reserve of stored carbohydrate in the body tissues that could provide energy only for about a 20-mile walk!

Protection and Insulation. Fat serves as a protective shield against trauma to the vital organs such as the heart, liver, kidneys, spleen, brain, and spinal cord. Body fat located in storage depots just below the skin serves an important insulating function that determines one's ability to tolerate extremes of cold exposure. In most instances, however, excess body fat is a liability in terms of temperature regulation, especially during sustained exercise in air when the body's heat production can be increased 20 times above the resting level. In this situation, heat flow from the body is retarded by the shield of insulation from subcutaneous fat.

Vitamin Carrier and Hunger Depressor. Dietary fat serves as a carrier and transport medium for the fat-soluble vitamins — vitamins A, D, E, and K. Ingesting about 20 g of fat daily is sufficient to supply the necessary fat-soluble vitamins. Because fat emptying from the stomach takes about 3.5 hours after ingestion, some fat in the diet helps delay the onset of "hunger pangs" and contributes to the feeling of satiety after a meal. This is one rea-

son why reducing diets containing moderate amounts of fat are considered more successful than some lower-fat diets.

RECOMMENDED INTAKE OF LIPIDS

In the United States, dietary fat represents approximately 38% of total calorie intake. Although standards for optimal fat intake have not been firmly established, medical personnel believe that to promote optimal health, fat intake should not exceed 30% of the energy content of the diet. Of this fat intake, at least 70% should be in the form of unsaturated fatty acids.

For dietary cholesterol, the American Heart Association recommends that no more than 300 mg (0.01 oz) of cholesterol be consumed each day, an intake equivalent to no more than 100 mg per 1000 calories of food ingested. Three hundred mg of cholesterol is almost the amount in the yolk of one large egg, and just about one-half the cholesterol ingested by the average American male. Reducing daily cholesterol intake to 150 to 200

Excessive fat storage. For some athletes such as football linemen, some additional fat storage provides an added cushion that may aid in protection from the normal hazards of the sport. This possible protective benefit, however, must be evaluated against the liability imposed by the excess "dead weight" in terms of both energy expenditures and thermal regulation and their possible detrimental effects on exercise performance.

The real dietary culprit. Saturated fatty acids in the diet may stimulate a greater rise in blood cholesterol than comes from dietary cholesterol itself.

TABLE 6-2. Cholesterol and saturated fat content for 100 g of common foods

Foods	Saturated fat (mg)	Cholesterol (mg)
Butter	50.7	219
Peanut butter	8.5	0
Chocolate fudge	7.3	4
French fries, McDonald's	6.8	13
Ice cream, vanilla	6.2	44
Taco, beef	6.2	57
Doritos, taco flavor	4.8	0
Kentucky Fried Chicken	4.2	76
Hamburger, Big Mac	3.6	36
Pizza, cheese	3.4	47
Egg, raw	3.0	410
Beef liver, fried	2.8	482
Chicken breast, fried with skin	2.5	90
Chocolate milkshake	2.3	13
Milk, whole	2.1	14
Swordfish, broiled	1.4	50
Chicken breast, fried, without skin	1.3	91
Milk, lowfat 2%	1.2	9
Yogurt, plain low-fat	1.0	6
Shrimp, raw	0.3	152

mg may be even more desirable. The cholesterol and saturated fat content of some common foods is presented in Table 6-2.

Lipid Utilization in Exercise

The energy requirements of exercise are met chiefly from the fatty acids released from triglycerides in the fat storage sites, and delivered in the circulation to muscle tissue as free fatty acids (FFA) bound to blood albumin. Energy is also derived from the triglycerides stored within the muscle cell

total energy requirements. This probably occurs by a small drop in blood sugar and subsequent decrease in insulin and increase in glucagon output by the pancreas. This ultimately reduces glucose metabolism and stimulates the liberation and subsequent breakdown of lipids for energy.

The data in Figure 6-6 show that the uptake of fatty acids by active muscles rises during 1 to 4 hours of moderate exercise. In the first hour of exercise, about 50% of the energy is supplied by fat. As exercise continues into the third hour, fat contributes up to 70% of the total energy requirement.

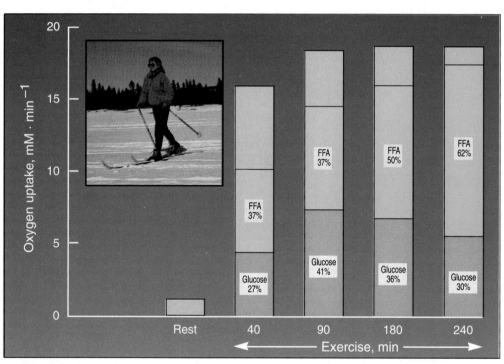

FIGURE 6-6. Uptake of oxygen and nutrients by the legs during prolonged exercise. (Orange and green areas represent the proportion of the total oxygen uptake caused by the oxidation of free fatty acids (FFA) and blood glucose. Blue areas indicate the oxidation of non-blood-borne fuels (muscle glycogen and intramuscular fats and proteins). (From Ahlborg, G., et al.: Substrate turnover during prolonged exercise in man. *J. Clin. Invest.,* 53:1080, 1974.)

Peptide bonds. Peptide bonding consists of a sequence of covalent chemical bonds between the carboxyl group of one amino acid and the amino group of the next amino acid. Amino acid bonding forms the backbone for building more complex protein compounds.

itself. During brief periods of relatively moderate exercise (such as jogging at a 10-minute per mile pace), energy is derived in approximately equal amounts from carbohydrate and lipid. As exercise continues for an hour or more and carbohydrates become depleted, there is a gradual increase on the reliance of fat for energy. In prolonged exercise, fat (mainly as FFA) may supply nearly 80% of the

PROTEINS

Proteins, from the Greek word meaning "of prime importance", are found in all living matter and function primarily in the growth and repair of body tissue. Proteins are similar to carbohydrates and lipids in that each molecule contains atoms of carbon, oxygen, and hydrogen. The major difference is that proteins also contain nitrogen, sulfur, phosphorus, and iron. Nitrogen makes up about 16% of a protein molecule.

Amino Acids

The basic units or building blocks of protein are amino acids. These are small organic compounds that contain at least one *amino radical* (NH_2) and one radical called an *organic acid* (COOH, technically termed a carboxyl group). *The difference between the various amino acids is their side chain.* The chemical structure of the amino acid alanine is illustrated at the top of Figure 6-7. Also depicted is the process of transamination.

Amino acids are joined together by *peptide bonds;* the joining of two amino acids produces a *dipeptide,* and three amino acids linked together form a *tripeptide.* A linkage of up to as many a 1000 amino acids is known as a *polypeptide.*

Essential and Nonessential Amino Acids. There are 20 different amino acids required by the body, although tens of thousands of the same amino acids may be present in a single protein compound. Of the different amino acids, nine cannot be synthesized in the body at a sufficient rate to prevent impairment of normal cellular function. These amino acids are called *essential* or indispensable amino acids because they must be obtained preformed in foods. The remaining 12 that can be manufactured by the body are termed *nonessential* or disposable amino acids. This does not mean they are unimportant, but simply that the body can synthesize them from ingested protein and non-protein nutrients at a rate to meet the demands for normal growth and tissue repair.

Sources of Proteins

Dietary Sources. The major sources of protein in the American diet are eggs, meat, milk, fish, and poultry. Sources of high-quality protein (i.e., protein containing a full complement of essential amino acids) are eggs, milk, meat, fish, and poultry. The mixture of essential amino acids present in eggs has been judged to be the best among food sources; hence, eggs are given the highest quality rating of 100 for comparison with other foods. Some common sources of dietary protein are rated in Table 6-3. It should be emphasized that all of the essential amino acids can be obtained by consuming a variety of plant foods (grains, fruits, and vegetables), each with a different quality and quantity of amino acids. Currently, almost two thirds of dietary protein comes from

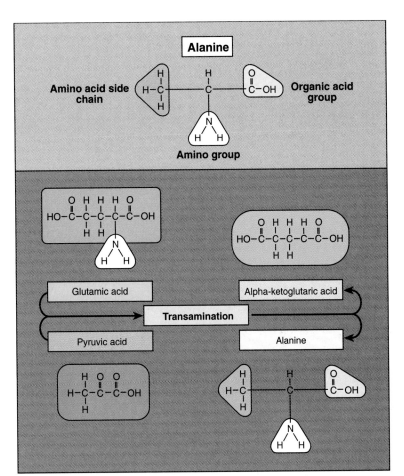

FIGURE 6-7. Chemical structure of alanine and the process of transamination in which an amino group from a donor group is transferred to an acceptor acid to form a new amino acid

animal sources, whereas 80 years ago protein came equally from both the plant and animal kingdoms. This present day reliance on animal protein is largely responsible for the relatively high intake of cholesterol and saturated fat.

Synthesis in the Body. Nonessential amino acids can be synthesized in the body from the carbon, oxygen, and hydrogen fragments of carbohydrates and lipids. This process, called *transamination,* is illustrated in the bottom of Figure 6-7 where a molecule of pyruvic acid combines with the amino group (NH_2) from the amino acid glutamic acid to create the amino acid alanine. As a result of transamination, the glutamic acid without its amino group becomes a different compound called alpha–ketoglutaric acid. This compound is

TABLE 6-3. Rating of common sources of dietary protein

Food	Protein Rating
Eggs	100
Fish	70
Lean beef	69
Cow's milk	60
Brown rice	57
White rice	56
Soybeans	47
Brewer's hash	45
Whole-grain wheat	44
Peanuts	43
Dry beans	34
White potato	34

A larger protein requirement in children. The protein demand per unit of body mass during infancy and childhood ranges between 2.5 and 5 times that required by adults.

For vegetarians, diversity is the key. The essential amino acids can be obtained in a vegan diet if the RDA for protein is consumed with 60% of the protein coming from grain products, 35% from legumes, and the remaining 5% from green leafy vegetables. For a 70-kg person who requires about 56 g of protein, the essential amino acids would be obtained by consuming approximately $1\frac{1}{4}$ cups of beans, $\frac{1}{4}$ cup of seeds or nuts, about 4 slices of whole-grain bread, 2 cups of vegetables (half being leafy green), and $2\frac{1}{2}$ cups from various grain sources such as brown rice, oatmeal, and cracked wheat.

Not found in the plant kingdom. Vitamin B_{12} is not available in plants because it is produced by bacteria in the digestive tract of animals. Only a small amount of this vitamin is needed (3 µg = RDA). Thus, vitamin B_{12} deficiency in nonvegetarians is usually caused by failure in intestinal absorption.

Mix and match. With a vegetarian diet complete proteins can be obtained with the following combinations:
  Beans and rice
  Peas and corn
  Bread and lentils
  Potatoes with milk or egg
  Cereals with milk or egg

now available to be metabolized for energy or to receive an amino group to rebuild an amino acid.

The process opposite to transamination is deamination. In this process, an amino group is removed from the amino acid molecule. The remaining carbon skeleton can then be converted into a carbohydrate or lipid or used for energy. The split-off amino group forms urea in the liver and is then excreted by the kidneys.

Functions of Proteins

Amino acids provide the major substance for the synthesis of cellular components in addition to the formation of new tissue. The amino acid requirement for these tissue-building or anabolic processes can vary considerably both within and among individuals. During periods of rapid growth, as occur in infancy and childhood, more than one-third of the protein intake is retained for tissue anabolism. As growth rate declines, so does the percentage of protein retained for growth-related processes. Even when growth stabilizes, there still is a continual turnover of tissue protein.

The protein content of cells is not always fixed. The protein in skeletal muscle, which represents about 65% of the body's total protein, can be increased dramatically with resistance training. Simply ingesting large amounts of dietary protein, however, does *not* cause a muscle cell to increase in size. If it did, then just eating an excess 100 g of protein daily, an amount consumed by many athletes, would theoretically increase the muscle mass by about 500 g a day! For the serious athlete who trained hard with resistance exercises for only 3 days a week for 1 year, such dietary practices would increase muscle mass by about 75,000 g or the equivalent of 75 kg (165 lb) of muscle tissue. Obvously, this is impossible to achieve!

Aside from their structural roles, proteins play an important role in reg-

ulating the acid-base quality of the body fluids. This buffering function is important during intense exercise when large quantities of acid metabolites are produced. Proteins are present in blood and assist with the body's fluid balance. Globulins and albumins, two plasma proteins, exert osmotic pressure within the bloodstream. This counters the tendency of the blood's fluid or serum component to seep out of the capillaries into the surrounding tissues from the force of arterial blood pressure. This helps to maintain plasma volume by preserving the serum within blood vessels.

The Vegetarian Approach to Sound Nutrition

The diets of numerous individuals, including champion athletes, consist predominately of nutrients from varied plant sources as well as some dairy products. For the active individual, one potential problem with a vegetarian-type diet is the difficulty in consuming sufficient calories to match energy output. With the exceptions of calcium, phosphorus, iron, and vitamin B_{12}, a strict vegetarian's nutritional problem is one of getting ample high-quality protein. This is easily resolved with a *lacto-vegetarian* diet that allows the addition of milk and related products such as ice cream, cheese, and yogurt. The lacto-vegetarian approach minimizes the problem of obtaining a sufficient intake of protein, calcium, phosphorous, and vitamin B_{12}. By adding an egg to the diet (referred to as *a lacto-ovovegetarian diet*), an intake of the indispensable essential amino acids is assured. The vegetarian approach has additional positive "spin-offs" because foods from the plant kingdom are (1) rich sources of vitamins and minerals, (2) high in fiber, and (3) generally low in calories and fat, especially saturated fatty acids — and they contain no cholesterol!

The contribution of various food groups to the protein content of the American diet is shown in Figure 6-8.

By far, the greatest intake of protein comes from animal sources, whereas only about 30% comes from vegetable sources.

Recommended Intake of Proteins

Despite the beliefs of many coaches and trainers, there is probably no exercise or training benefit from eating excessive amounts of protein. For athletes, muscle mass is not increased simply by eating high-protein foods. Additional calories in the form of protein are, after deamination, used directly for energy or converted to fat and stored in the subcutaneous depots. Excessive and prolonged protein intake may be harmful from a medical standpoint because the metabolism of large quantities of this nutrient can place an undue strain on liver and kidney function.

The Recommended Dietary Allowance

The *Recommended Dietary Allowance (RDA)* for protein, including the various vitamins and minerals required by the body, are standards for nutrient intake developed by the Food and Nutrition Board of the National Research Council/National Academy of Science. RDA levels are expressed as an average and are believed to represent a liberal, yet safe level of excess to meet the nutritional needs of practically all healthy people. The RDA should be viewed as a probability statement for adequate nutrition: as nutrient intake falls below the RDA, the probability for malnourishment for a particular person is increased, and this probability becomes progressively greater as the nutrient intake becomes lower. Malnutrition is the cumulative result of weeks, months, and even years of reduced nutrient intake.

Table 6-4 shows the RDAs for protein for adolescent and adult men and women. On the average, a daily intake of about

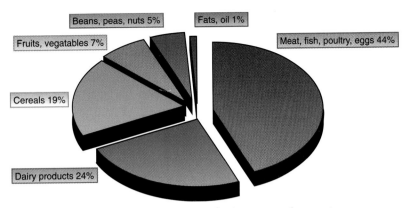

FIGURE 6-8. Contribution from the major food sources to the protein content of the typical American diet.

0.8 g of protein per kg body weight is recommended. (To determine your protein requirement, multiply your body weight in pounds by 0.37).

Although little experimental evidence supports the practice of protein supplementation, it is possible that growing athletes, athletes involved in strength development programs that enhance muscle tissue growth, and endurance programs that increase protein breakdown, and those subjected to recurring trauma, may need a slightly larger protein intake than the recommended 0.8 g · kg^{-1}. Any additional protein requirement is more than likely met by the generally increased food intake of these athletes to compensate for the increased energy expenditure associated with training. The result is that

> **Nitrogen balance and imbalance.** Nitrogen balance exists when the intake of nitrogen (protein) equals nitrogen excretion. The body is in positive nitrogen balance when nitrogen intake is greater than nitrogen excretion, as when new tissue is being synthesized and protein is retained (e.g., during childhood, pregnancy, recovery from illness, or muscle growth through training). A greater output of nitrogen relative to its intake (negative nitrogen balance) indicates the use of protein for energy and possible encroachment on the body's available amino acids, primarily those in skeletal muscle.

TABLE 6-4. Recommended dietary allowances of protein for adolescent and adult men and women

Recommended Amount	Men		Women	
	Adolescent	Adult	Adolescent	Adult
Grams of protein per kg body weight	0.9	0.8	0.9	0.8
Grams per day based on average weight[a]	59.0	56.0	50.0	44.0

[a]Average weight is based on a "Reference" man and woman. For adolescents (ages 14-18), average weight is approximately 65.8 kg (145 lb) for males and 55.7 kg (123 lb) for females. For adult men, average weight is 70 kg (154 lb); for adult women, average weight is 56.8 kg (125 lb).

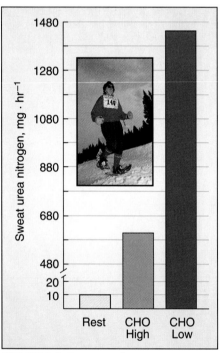

FIGURE 6-9. Excretion of urea in sweat at rest, and during exercise after carbohydrate loading (*CHO High*) and carbohydrate depletion (*CHO Low*). The largest utilization of protein (as reflected by sweat urea) occurs when glycogen reserves are low. (From Lemon, P. W. R., and Nagel, F.: Effects of exercise on protein and amino acid metabolism. *Med. Sci. Sports Exerc.,* 13:141, 1981.)

excess protein consumed will probably be stored as excess body fat!

Preparations of Simple Amino Acids

The common practice among some weight lifters, body builders, and other power athletes of consuming liquids, powders, or pills of predigested protein is a waste of money and may actually be counterproductive in terms of the desired outcome. For example, many of these preparations contain proteins that are predigested to simple amino acids through chemical action in the laboratory. The belief is that the simple amino-acid molecule is absorbed more easily and rapidly by the body and in some magical way is available rapidly to facilitate the expected muscle growth brought on by training. This, however, is not the case. Dietary proteins are also absorbed rapidly in the intestine by the healthy body when they are part of the more complex di- and tripeptide molecules as well as in simple amino-acid form. The intestinal tract is better able to handle protein in its more complex form, whereas a concentrated amino-acid solution draws water into the intestine. This process can cause irritation, cramping, and diarrhea. Simply stated, amino acid supplementation in any form much above the RDA has not been shown experimentally to improve strength, power, muscle mass, or endurance.

PROTEIN UTILIZATION IN EXERCISE AND TRAINING: IS THE RDA REALLY ENOUGH?

Nutritionists and exercise physiologists have long maintained that the RDA for protein offered a "margin of safety" liberal enough to provide for any amino acid molecules catabolized for energy during exercise or required for the augmented protein synthesis following exercise. Recent research on protein balance in exercise, however, presents a compelling argument that protein is used to a

greater extent than previously thought, particularly as an energy substrate during exercise of long-duration and into recovery. These conclusions were based on studies that expanded the classic method of determining protein breakdown through urea excretion as well as using radioactive tracers that "label" the CO_2 portion of the amino-acid molecule.

As shown in Figure 6-9, the sweat mechanism clearly is an important means for excreting the nitrogen from protein breakdown during exercise. Furthermore, the use of protein for energy in exercise was greatest when subjects exercised in the glycogen-depleted state. This emphasizes the important role of carbohydrate as a protein sparer and suggests that the demand on protein "reserves" in exercise is linked to carbohydrate availability. Certainly this would become an important factor in endurance exercise or in frequent heavy training in which glycogen reserves become greatly reduced.

These observations certainly support the importance of a high-carbohydrate diet as a means to conserve muscle protein for athletes who engage in protracted, hard training. The use of protein for energy and the depression of protein synthesis in heavy exercise in such cases may help to explain why individuals involved in resistance training to augment muscle size generally refrain from significant training involving endurance-type exercise.

The Alanine-Glucose Cycle

Certain proteins in the body are not readily available for energy. Proteins in muscle, however, are more labile; when the demand arises, they enter the process of energy metabolism, especially during long-duration exercise.

A model has been proposed in Figure 6-10 that the amino acid alanine indirectly serves the energy requirements of exercise. Amino acids within the muscle are converted to glutamate and then to alanine. The alanine released from the exercising muscle is transported to the liver where it is deaminated. The remaining carbon skeleton is converted to glucose by the process of gluconeogenesis and then is released to the blood and delivered to the working muscles. The carbon fragments from the amino acids that form alanine can then be oxidized for energy within the specific muscle cell. Energy derived from the *alanine-glucose cycle* may supply as much as 10 to 15% of the total exercise requirement, or as much as 60% of the liver's glucose output.

Little is known concerning the actual protein requirements of individuals who train 4 to 6 hours a day by resistance-type exercise to develop muscular size, strength, and power. Recent evidence suggests that their requirement may be greater than for sedentary individuals. It is also possible that despite an increased utilization of protein for energy during heavy training, adaptations occur within the muscle that augment the efficiency with which the body uses dietary protein to enhance amino acid balance. Whether there will be a modification of the current protein RDA for specific athletic groups awaits further research. Until such data become available, it seems reasonable to acknowledge the heretofore unrecognized significant role of protein as a potential energy fuel.

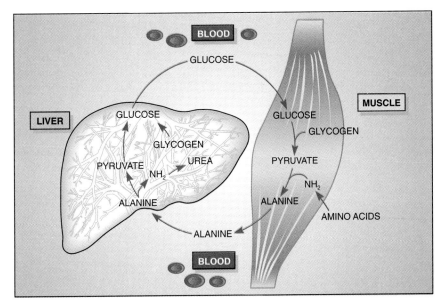

FIGURE 6-10. The alanine-glucose cycle. Alanine, which is synthesized in muscle from glucose-derived pyruvic acid, is released into the blood and converted to glucose and urea in the liver. This glucose is then released back into the blood and delivered to the muscle for energy. During exercise, the increased production and output of alanine from muscle helps maintain blood glucose for the needs of the nervous system and active muscles. (From Felig, P., and Wahren, J.: Amino acid metabolism in exercising man. *J. Clin. Invest.,* 50:2703, 1971).

A possible exception. Nitrogen balance studies suggest that endurance and strength athletes in heavy training may require protein at between 1.2 and 1.6 g · kg^{-1} body mass daily. This is usually met by the higher caloric intakes of such active men and women. Consequently, most athletes do not need protein supplements.

S U M M A R Y

PART 1

1. Simple sugars consist of a chain of from 3 to 7 carbon atoms with hydrogen and oxygen in the ratio of 2 to 1. Glucose, the most common simple sugar, contains a 6-carbon chain as $C_6H_{12}O_6$.

2. There are three kinds of carbohydrates: monosaccharides (sugars like glucose and fructose); disaccharides like sucrose, lactose, and maltose; and polysaccharides that contain three or more simple sugars to form starch, fiber, and glycogen.

3. Glycogenolysis refers to the process of reconverting glycogen to glucose, whereas gluconeogenesis refers to the process of glucose synthesis, especially from protein sources.

4. Americans typically consume 40 to 50% of their total calories as carbohydrates. This is generally in the form of fruits, grains, and vegetables, although greater sugar intake in the form of sweets (simple sugars) is common.

5. Carbohydrates, stored in limited quantity in liver and muscle, serve four functions: (1) as a major source of energy, (2) to spare the breakdown of proteins, (3) as a metabolic primer for fat metabolism, and (4) as the preferred fuel for the central nervous system.

6. During intense exercise, muscle glycogen and blood glucose are the primary fuels for exercise. The body's glycogen stores also serve an important role in energy balance in sustained, high levels of aerobic exercise such as marathon running, triathalon-type events, long-distance cycling, and endurance swimming.

7. Individuals involved in heavy training regimens should consume about 60% of their daily calories (amounting to approximately 400 to 600 g) as carbohydrates, predominantly in the complex form.

8. Lipids, like carbohydrates, contain carbon, hydrogen, and oxygen atoms, but the ratio of hydrogen to oxygen is much higher. Lipids are synthesized by plants and animals. They can be classified into three groups: simple fats (glycerol + 3 fatty acids), compound fats composed of simple fats in combination with other chemicals (phospholipids, glucolipids, and lipoproteins), and derived fats like cholesterol which are made from simple and compound fats.

9. Saturated fatty acids contain as many hydrogen atoms as is chemically possible; thus, the molecule is said to be saturated with respect to hydrogen. Saturated fats are present primarily in animal meat, egg yolk, dairy fats, and cheese. High intakes of saturated fats have been linked to elevated blood cholesterol and the development of coronary heart disease.

10. Unsaturated fatty acids contain fewer hydrogen atoms attached to the carbon chain. Instead, the carbon atoms are joined by double bonds, and they are said to be either mono– or polyunsaturated with respect to hydrogen. Increasing the proportion of these fats in the diet may offer protection against heart disease.

11. Lowering blood cholesterol, especially that carried by the LDL, may provide significant protection against coronary heart disease.

12. Lipids provide the largest nutrient store of potential energy to power biologic work. They protect vital organs and provide insulation from the cold. Fat also acts as the carrier of the fat-soluble vitamins A, D, E, and K.

13. During light and moderate exercise of about 10 minutes duration, fat contributes about 50% of the energy requirement. As exercise continues, the role of stored fat becomes more important during prolonged work where the fatty acid molecules may provide more than 80% of the energy needs of the body.

14. Proteins differ chemically from lipids and carbohydrates in that they contain nitrogen in addition to sulfur, phosphorous, and iron.

15. Proteins are formed from subunits called amino acids. The body requires 20 different amino acids, each containing an amino radical (NH_2) and an organic acid radical called a carboxyl group (COOH). In addition to NH_2 and COOH, amino acids contain a side-chain molecule that gives the amino acid its particular chemical characteristics.

16. Eight of the 20 amino acids cannot be synthesized in the body. These are called essential amino acids and they must be consumed in the diet.

17. Proteins are found in the cells of all animals and plants. Proteins containing all the essential amino acids are called complete (high-quality) proteins; the other proteins are referred to as incomplete or low-quality proteins. Animal proteins found in eggs, milk, cheese, meat, fish, and poultry are examples of high-quality, complete proteins.

18. All of the essential amino acids can be obtained by consuming a variety of plant foods, each with a different quality and quantity of amino acids.

19. Certain proteins, especially those in nervous and connective tissues, are not generally used in energy metabolism. The amino acids alanine and glutamic acid, however, play a key role in providing carbohydrate fuel for exercise. This is achieved through the process of gluconeogenesis. In prolonged exercise, the alanine-glucose cycle may account for as much as 60% of the total glucose released by the liver.

20. Protein breakdown during exercise becomes apparent when the body's carbohydrate reserves are low. Such findings further support the wisdom of maintaining optimal glycogen stores (by consuming high carbohydrate foods) during training.

21. Future research must determine whether the increased demand on body protein with heavy training is sufficient to increase the protein requirement above that provided by the RDA for individuals who maintain adequate energy intake.

The effective regulation of all metabolic processes requires a delicate blending of food nutrients in the watery medium of the cell. Of special significance in the metabolic mixture are the micronutrients — the small quantities of vitamins and minerals that play highly specific roles in facilitating energy transfer. *These substances are readily obtained in the foods consumed in well-balanced meals.* With proper nutrition from a variety of food sources, there is little need to consume vitamin and mineral supplements; such practices are both physiologically and economically wasteful.

VITAMINS

The Nature of Vitamins

The formal discovery of vitamins revealed that they were essential organic substances needed in minute amounts by the body to perform highly specific metabolic functions. The body requires only about 350 g (12 oz) of vitamins from the 820 kg (1820 lbs) of food consumed by the average adult during the year. Vitamins are often considered accessory nutrients because they do not supply energy, serve as basic building units for other compounds, or contribute substantially to the body's mass. Nonetheless, prolonged inadequate intake of a particular vitamin can trigger the symptoms of vitamin deficiency and lead to severe medical complications. For example, symptoms of thiamin deficiency can be observed after only 2 weeks on a thiamin-free diet, and symptoms of vitamin C deficiency can appear after 3 or 4 weeks. At the other extreme, consuming excessive quantities of some fat-soluble vitamins can cause a toxic overdose that is manifested as hair loss, irregularities in bone formation, fetal malformation,

hemorrhage, bone fractures, abnormal liver function, and even death.

Classification of Vitamins

Thirteen different vitamins have been isolated, analyzed, and synthesized, and their recommended dietary intakes established. The vitamins also have been classified into one of two groups depending on their particular chemical properties.

Fat-Soluble Vitamins. Vitamin A was the first of the vitamins to be classified as fat-soluble because it dissolves in the fat and oil in foods. Daily ingestion of the fat-soluble vitamins is unnecessary because they are stored in the liver and in the fat cells of adipose tissue, mainly the subcutaneous tissues. These vitamins are retained in the tissues for a relatively long time because there is no mechanism for them to leave the body other than as by-products of their eventual breakdown. Consequently, it may take years for symptoms of deficiency to become evident for a fat-soluble vitamin. However, because the fat-soluble vitamins are usually obtained in dietary fat, consuming a "fat-free" diet will speed up the development of a vitamin deficiency.

The four fat-soluble vitamins — composed entirely of the elements carbon, hydrogen, and oxygen — are vitamins A, D, E, and K. Each has a different chemical structure and performs different, highly specific functions. Table 6-5 lists the RDA, food sources, major bodily functions, and symptoms resulting from both excess and deficiency of fat-soluble vitamins.

Water-Soluble Vitamins. Certain vitamins are classified as water soluble because they are transported throughout the watery medium of the body;

The supplementers. The greatest use of vitamin supplements is among white female college graduates aged 25 to 40 who live in the western region of the United States.

Natural versus synthetic vitamins. There is no difference or advantage between a vitamin obtained naturally from food and a synthetic vitamin. Even among the various supplements, the huge profit gained by the manufacturer is the only advantage in consuming so-called natural or organically isolated vitamins compared to those synthesized in the laboratory.

Provitamin. Many vitamins are found in food in an inactive or precursor form. In the body, these provitamins are changed to the active form of the vitamin. In this regard, the vitamin content of a specific food is most accurately expressed in terms of the total potential vitamin activity available from both its actual vitamin content and its precursor provitamins.

Storage of fat-soluble vitamins. Vitamins A and D are stored predominantly in the liver, whereas vitamin E is distributed throughout the body's fatty tissues. Vitamin K is stored only in small amounts, mainly in the liver.

TABLE 6-5. Recommended dietary intake, food sources, major bodily functions, and symptoms of deficiency or excess of the fat-soluble vitamins for healthy adults (age 19–50)*

Vitamin	RDA (mg) Males	RDA (mg) Females	Dietary Sources	Major Body Functions	Deficiency	Excess
Vitamin A (retinol)	1.0	0.8	Provitamin A (beta-carotene) widely distributed in green vegetables. Retinol present in milk, butter, cheese, fortified margarine	Constituent of rhodopsin (visual pigment). Maintenance of epithelial tissues. Role in mucopolysaccharide synthesis	Xerophthalmia (keratinization) of ocular tissue), night blindness, permanent blindness	Headache, vomiting, peeling of skin, anorexia, swelling of long bones
Vitamin D	0.01†	0.01	Cod-liver oil, eggs, dairy products, fortified milk, and margarine	Promotes growth and mineralization of bones. Increases absorption of calcium	Rickets (bone deformities) in children. Osteomalacia in adults	Vomiting, diarrhea, loss of weight, kidney damage
Vitamin E (tocopherol)	10.0	8.0	Seeds, green leafy vegetables, margarines, shortenings	Functions as an antioxidant to prevent cell damage	Possibly anemia	Relatively nontoxic
Vitamin K (phylloquinone)	0.08	0.06	Green leafy vegetables. Small amount in cereals, fruits, and meats	Important in blood clotting (involved in formation of active prothrombin)	Conditioned deficiencies associated with severe bleeding; internal hemorrhages	Relatively nontoxic. Synthetic forms at high doses may cause jaundice

*Recommended Dietary Allowances. Revised 1989. Food & Nutrition Board, National Academy of Sciences-National Research Council, Washington, D.C.
† 0.005 mg for adults 25 and older.

Antioxidants and heart disease risk. The antioxidant vitamins A, C, and E (and ß-carotene) appear to reduce heart attack risk. The proposed mechanism for protection is that they prevent oxidation of LDL cholesterol. It is the oxidation of LDL — a process similar to butter turning rancid — that contributes to the plaque-forming artery-clogging process of atherosclerosis.

thus, they are not stored to any appreciable extent in the tissues. The water-soluble vitamins are normally voided in the urine because their amount in plasma exceeds the capacity for reabsorption by the kidneys. Consequently, these vitamins must be consumed regularly — usually daily or at least within a period of several days. The nine water-soluble vitamins are vitamin C (ascorbic acid) and the B-complex group: thiamin (B_1), riboflavin (B_2), niacin, pyridoxine (B_6), and B_{12}, pantothenic acid, folic acid, and biotin. The RDA, food sources, major bodily functions, and symptoms resulting from both excess and deficiency of the water-soluble vitamins are summarized in Table 6-6.

Toxicity of Vitamins. Once the enzyme systems that are catalyzed by specific vitamins become saturated, the excess vitamins function as chemicals in the body. In excess, these chemicals can be harmful. Although the potential for overdose is considerably less for the water-soluble than for the fat-soluble vitamins, prolonged excessive intake of vitamins of either type can produce toxic effects, and sometimes the outcome is fatal.

Functions of Vitamins

Vitamins perform diverse functions. They generally serve as essential links and regulators in the chain of

TABLE 6-6. Recommended dietary intake, food sources, major bodily functions, and symptoms of deficiency or excess of the water-soluble vitamins for healthy adults (age 19–50)*

Vitamin	RDA (mg) Males	RDA (mg) Females	Dietary Sources	Major Body Functions	Deficiency	Excess
Vitamin B$_1$ (thiamin)	1.5	1.1	Pork, organ meats, whole grains, legumes	Coenzyme (thiamin prophosphate) in reactions involving the removal of carbon dioxide	Beriberi (peripheral nerve changes, edema, heart failure)	None reported
Vitamin B$_2$	1.7	1.3	Widely distributed in foods	Constituent of two flavin nucleotide coenzymes involved in energy metabolism (FAD an FMN)	Reddened lips, cracks at mouth corner (cheilosis), eye lesions	None reported
Niacin	19	15	Liver, lean meats, grains, legumes (can be formed from tryptophan)	Constituent of two coenzymes in oxidation-reduction reactions (NAD$^+$ and NADP)	Pellagra (skin and gastro-intestinal lesions, nervous, mental disorders)	Flushing, burning and tingling around neck, face, and hands
Vitamin B$_6$ (pyridoxine)	2.0	1.6	Meats, vegetables, whole-grain cereals	Coenzyme (pyridoxal phosphate) involved in amino acid and glycogen metabolism)	Irritability, convulsions, muscular twitching, dermatitis, kidney stones	None reported
Pantothenic acid	4–7‡	4–7‡	Widely distributed in foods	Constituent of coenzyme A, which plays a central role in energy metabolism	Fatigue, sleep disturbances, impaired coordination, nausea	None reported
Folacin	0.2	0.2	Legumes, green vegetables, whole-wheat products	Coenzyme (reduced form) involved in transfer of single-carbon units in nucleic acid and amino acid metabolism	Anemia, gastro-intestinal disturbances, diarrhea, red tongue	None reported
Vitamin B$_{12}$	0.002	0.002	Muscle meats, eggs, dairy products, (absent in plant foods)	Coenzyme involved in transfer of single-carbon units in nucleic acid metabolism	Pernicious anemia, neuro-logic disorders	None reported
Biotin	0.03	0.10	Legumes, vegetables, meats	Coenzymes required for fat synthesis, amino acid metabolism, and glycogen (animal starch) formation	Fatigue, depression, nausea, dermatitis, muscular pains	None reported
Vitamin C (ascorbic acid)	60†	60	Citrus fruits, tomatoes, green peppers, salad greens	Maintains inter-cellular matrix of cartilage, bone, and dentine. Important in collagen synthesis.	Scurvy (degeneration of skin, teeth, blood vessels, epithelial hemorrhages)	Relatively nontoxic. Possibility of kidney stones

*Recommended Dietary Allowances. Revised 1989. Food and Nutrition Board, National Academy of Sciences-National Research Council, Washington, D.C.
† 100 for adults who smoke.
‡ Because there is less information on which to base allowances, these figures are given in the form of ranges.

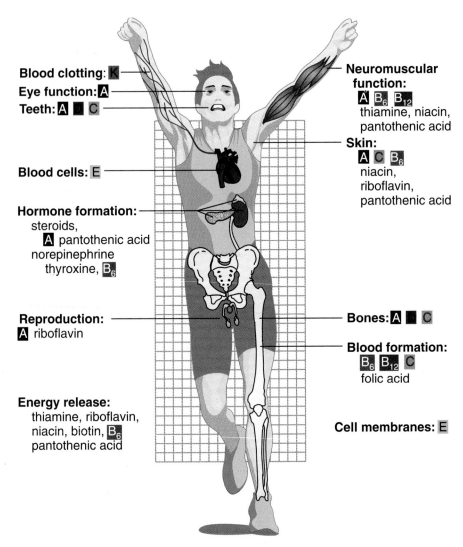

Blood clotting: K
Eye function: A
Teeth: A ▪ C

Blood cells: E

Hormone formation:
steroids,
A pantothenic acid
norepinephrine
thyroxine, B₆

Reproduction:
A riboflavin

Energy release:
thiamine, riboflavin,
niacin, biotin, B₆
pantothenic acid

Neuromuscular function:
A B₆ B₁₂
thiamine, niacin,
pantothenic acid

Skin:
A C B₆
niacin,
riboflavin,
pantothenic acid

Bones: A ▪ C

Blood formation:
B₆ B₁₂ C
folic acid

Cell membranes: E

FIGURE 6-11. Biologic functions of vitamins in the body.

Essential for energy transfer. Many vitamins serve as coenzyme components or precursors of coenzymes that regulate energy metabolism. These coenzymes, when united with a protein compound (apoenzyme), form an active enzyme that accelerates the interconversion of chemical compounds.

metabolic reactions that release energy within the food molecule. They are also intimately involved in the process of tissue synthesis as well as in many other biologic processes. Figure 6-11 summarizes many of the biologic functions of vitamins in the body.

The water-soluble vitamins play an essential role as part of coenzymes in the complex series of energy-generating reactions that occur within the body's cells. Figure 6-12 presents an overview of the various routes of the food nutrients in metabolism and the role of the water-soluble vitamins in these metabolic pathways. Because vitamins can be used repeatedly in metabolic reactions, the vitamin needs of physically active individuals are generally

no greater than for those who are sedentary.

Vitamins and Exercise Performance

An adequate quantity of all vitamins is usually available in the daily diet for individuals who consume well-balanced meals. This is true regardless of gender, age, and level of physical activity. Indeed, there is no need for the physically active person to consume extra vitamins in the form of special foods or supplements. Contrary to popular belief, vitamins themselves contain no usable energy and they cannot be a source of "quick energy" as touted by some vitamin manufacturers. Also, for individuals who participate regularly in physical activities that require a moderate to high level of caloric expenditure, food intake is generally increased to sustain the added energy requirements of exercise. If this added food is obtained through well-balanced meals, a proportionate increase is assured in micronutrient intake.

Supplements, A Competitive Edge?

Figure 6-12 illustrates that the B-complex vitamins play key roles as coenzymes in important energy-yielding reactions during carbohydrate, lipid, and protein breakdown.

Consequently, it is tempting to speculate that increasing the intake of these vitamins will "supercharge" energy release and improve physical performance. The belief that "if a little is good, more will be better" has led many coaches, athletes, and fitness enthusiasts either to advocate or use vitamin supplements. More than 45 years of research, however, has not supported the wisdom of using vitamin supplements to improve exercise performance or the trainability of nutritionally adequate, healthy people. *When vitamin intake is at recommended levels, supplements neither improve exercise performance nor necessarily increase the blood levels of these nutrients.* The facts have become clouded by the "testimonials" of some coaches and elite athletes to the effect that their success was due to a particular dietary modification that usually included vitamin supplements. This is a classic example of "buyer beware" in terms of trying to use testimonials to create the impression that a product "really is" effective.

MINERALS

The Nature of Minerals

In addition to the elements oxygen, carbon, hydrogen, and nitrogen, approximately 4% of the body's mass is composed of some 22 mostly metallic elements collectively called minerals. Important minerals are those found in enzymes, hormones, and vitamins. Minerals also appear in combination with specific compounds, for example, calcium phosphate in bone, or singularly, such as free calcium (Ca^{++}) and sodium (Na^{++}) in the intracellular fluids. In the body, minerals are classified as *minor minerals* (those requiring less than 100 mg a day), and *major minerals* (those required in amounts greater than 100 mg a day). Excess accumulation of minerals is useless to the body and could become toxic if allowed to build up through regular overconsumption.

Kinds and Sources of Minerals

Minerals occur freely in nature, mainly in the waters of rivers, lakes, and oceans, in topsoil, and beneath the earth's surface. Minerals are found in the root systems of plants and in the body structures of animals that consume these plants and water. The best sources of minerals are animal products. This is because minerals are more highly concentrated in animal tissues than they are in plants.

Focus on well balanced nutrition. Consuming daily vitamin supplements to improve the quality of an unbalanced, nutritionally inadequate diet is both naive and potentially harmful. Simply stated, "A poor diet plus a vitamin pill is still a poor diet."

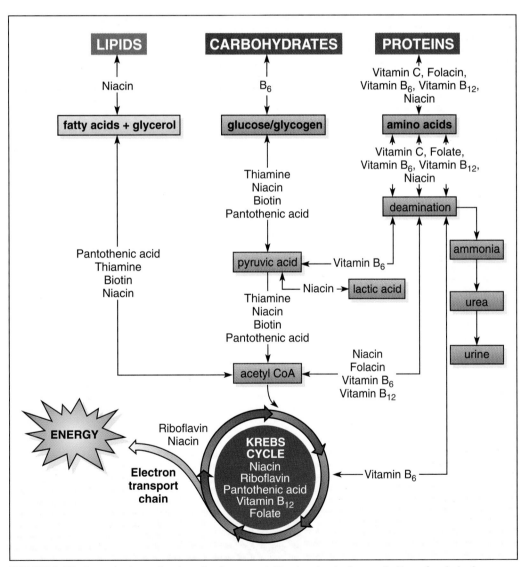

FIGURE 6-12. General schema for the role of water-soluble vitamins in the metabolism of carbohydrates, lipids, and proteins.

TABLE 6-7. The important major and trace minerals for healthy adults (age 19-50) and their dietary requirements, food sources, functions, and the effects of deficiencies and excesses*

Mineral	RDA For Males and Females[†] (mg)	Dietary Sources	Major Body Functions	Deficiency	Excess
Major					
Calcium	1200[‡] 1200	Milk, cheese, dark green vegetables, dried legumes	Bone and tooth formation Blood clotting Nerve transmission	Stunted growth Rickets, osteoporosis Convulsions	Not reported in humans
Phosphorus	1200[‡] 1200	Milk, cheese, yogurt, meat, poultry, grains, fish	Bone and tooth formation Acid-base balance	Weakness, demineralization of bone Loss of calcium	Erosion of jaw (phossy jaw)
Potassium	2000	Leafy vegetables, cantelope, lima beans, potatoes, bananas, milk, meats, coffee, tea	Fluid balance Nerve transmission Acid-base balance	Muscle cramps Irregular cardiac rhythm Mental confusion Loss of appetite Can be life-threatening	None if kidneys function normally Poor kidney function causes potassium build-up and cardiac arrythmias
Sulfur	Unknown	Obtained as part of dietary protein, and is present in food preservatives	Acid-base balance Liver function	Unlikely to occur if dietary intake is adequate	Unknown
Sodium	1100–3300	Common salt	Acid-base balance Body water balance Nerve function	Muscle cramps Mental apathy Reduced appetite	High blood pressure
Chlorine (chloride)	700	Chloride is part of salt-containing food Some vegetables and fruits	Important part of extracellular fluids	Unlikely to occur if dietary intake is adequate	Along with sodium, contributes to high blood pressure
Magnesium	350 280	Whole grains, green leafy vegetables	Activates enzymes Involved in protein synthesis	Growth failure Behavioral disturbances Weakness, spasms	Diarrhea
Minor					
Iron	10 15	Eggs, lean meats, legumes, whole grains, green leafy vegetables	Constituent of hemoglobin and enzymes involved in energy metabolism	Iron deficiency anemia (weakness reduced resistance to infection)	Siderosis Cirrhosis of liver
Fluorine	1.5–4.0	Drinking water, tea, seafood	May be important in maintenance of bone structure	Higher frequency of tooth decay	Mottling of teeth, increased bone density Neurologic disturbances
Zinc	15 12	Widely distributed in foods	Constituent of enzymes involved in digestion	Growth failure Small sex glands	Fever, nausea, vomiting, diarrhea
Copper	1.5–3.0[§] 1.5–3.0	Meats, drinking water	Constituent of enzymes associated with iron metabolism	Anemia, bone changes (rare in humans)	Rare metabolic condition (Wilson's disease)
Selenium	0.070 0.055	Seafood, meat, grains	Functions in close association with vitamin E	Anemia (rare)	Gastrointestinal disorders, lung irritation
Iodine (Iodide)	150	Marine fish and shellfish, dairy products, vegetables, iodized salt	Constituent of thyroid hormones	Goiter (enlarged thyroid)	Very high intakes depress thyroid activity
Chromium	0.075–0.25[§] 0.05–0.25[§]	Legumes, cereals, organ meats Fats, vegetable oils, meats, whole grains	Constituent of some enzymes Involved in glucose and energy metabolism	Not reported in humans Impaired ability to metabolize glucose	Inhibition of enzymes Occupational exposures: skin and kidney damage

*Recommended Dietary Allowances. Revised 1989. Food and Nutrition Board, National Academy of Sciences-National Research Council, Washington, D.C.
[†] First values are for males.
[‡] 800 mg for adults 25 and older.
[§] Because there is less information on which to base allowances, these figures are given in the form of ranges.

Functions of Minerals

Table 6-7 lists the important major and minor minerals, and their daily food sources, functions, and the effects of deficiencies and excesses. Whereas vitamins activate chemical processes without becoming part of the products of the reactions they catalyze, minerals are often incorporated within the structures and working chemicals of the body. Minerals serve three broad roles in the body:

- They provide *structure* in the formation of bones and teeth
- They are intimately involved in a *functional* role to maintain normal heart rhythm, muscle contractility, nerve conduction, and the acid-base balance of body fluids
- They play a *regulatory* role in cellular metabolism and serve as important parts of enzymes and hormones that modify and regulate cellular activity

Figure 6-13 lists the important minerals that participate in catabolic (breakdown) and anabolic (buildup) cellular processes.

Minerals: Their Relation to Physical Activity

The minerals required by the body can be readily obtained from food sources in a well-balanced diet. In the following sections, specific functions are described for several of the more important minerals found in foods, as well as their influence and significance during physical activity. Often, mineral metabolism is influenced by the stress of regular exercise.

Calcium. Approximately 1400 g of calcium are stored in the body, making it the body's most abundant mineral. When combined with phosphorus, it forms *hydroxyapatite,* the crystalline structure of bones and teeth. In its ionized form, calcium is important in muscle contraction, transmission of nerve impulses, activation of enzymes, blood clotting, and fluid movement across plasma membranes.

Osteoporosis: Calcium, Estrogen, and Exercise. More than 99% of the body's total calcium is contained in the skeleton. When calcium intake is deficient, the body draws on its calcium reserves in bone to replace the deficit. If the imbalance is prolonged, the condition of *osteoporosis* (literally meaning "porous bones") eventually sets in as the bones lose their mineral mass and progressively become porous and brittle. Among older individuals, especially women past the age of 60, osteoporosis has reached epidemic proportions. Nearly 25% of women over age 65 will suffer spontaneous bone fractures! The increased susceptibility to osteoporosis is closely related to the decrease in estrogen production that accompanies the menopause. Estrogen is believed to enhance calcium absorption and limit its resorption (withdrawal) from bone.

Dietary Calcium Is Crucial. The previous 800 mg RDA has been upgraded to 1200 mg for males and females aged 11 to 24 years. Many experts recommend a further increase to between 1200 and 1500 mg for estrogen-deprived women after menopause to ensure a positive calcium balance during this period. It is not clear, however, just how beneficial these calcium supplements are in the absence of adequate estrogen.

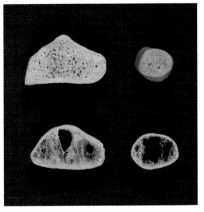

Normal radius and ulna (top), and radius and ulna in a patient with bone loss due to osteoporosis (bottom). Photos courtesy of Dr. Lisbeth Nilas, Department of Clinical Chemistry, Glostrup Hospital, Glostrup, Denmark.

Major Minerals	Trace Minerals
Sodium	Iron
Potassium	Zinc
Calcium	Copper
Phosphorus	Selenium
Magnesium	Iodine
Sulfur	Fluorine
Chlorine	Chromium
	Molybdenum
	Manganese

Research is continuing to discover how these minerals affect the body: boron, nickel, vanadium, arsenic, cobalt, lithium, silicon, tin, and cadmium.

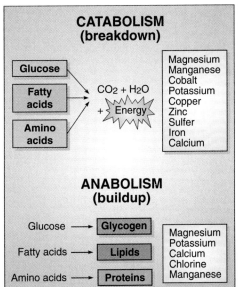

CATABOLISM (breakdown)

Glucose, Fatty acids, Amino acids → $CO_2 + H_2O$ + Energy

Magnesium, Manganese, Cobalt, Potassium, Copper, Zinc, Sulfer, Iron, Calcium

ANABOLISM (buildup)

Glucose → Glycogen
Fatty acids → Lipids
Amino acids → Proteins

Magnesium, Potassium, Calcium, Chlorine, Manganese

FIGURE 6-13. Minerals are involved in the catabolism (breakdown) and anabolism (build-up) of the macronutrients.

A bone disease of epidemic proportions. Osteoporosis accounts for more than 1.2 million fractures yearly, including 500,000 spinal fractures and 230,000 hip fractures. Each year, 1.3 million osteoporotic women will fracture one or more of their bones. About 1 of every 6 older men and 1 of 3 women will eventually sustain a hip fracture. Shockingly, death occurs in as many as 20% of these individuals; those who survive often require long-term nursing care. X-rays cannot detect decreases in bone mass until 30 to 50% of the bone mineral is lost!

Electrolyte concentrations in blood serum and sweat. Values are expressed in milliequivalents per liter (mEq/L).

	Na$^+$	K$^+$	Cl$^-$	Mg^{++}
Blood serum	140	4.0	110	1.5–2.1
Sweat	40–45	3.9	39	3.3

Young, fit women with middle-aged bones. Some amenorrheic young adult females have the bone mass of middle-aged women. In one study, bone density in the lumbar region was 14% lower in amenorrheic athletes who ran nearly twice the mileage compared to athletes with regular menstrual cycles. This is troubling because these amenorrheic athletes were actually losing bone mass during a period of potential bone growth. Further bad news was that intervention did not lead to resumption of normal ovarian function in all of the amenorrheic athletes.

Exercise Is Helpful. Men and women who maintain physically active lifestyles have significantly greater bone mass compared to sedentary counterparts. Even at ages 70 and 80, if former athletes keep physically active, their bone mass will be greater compared with *inactive* individuals of the same age. Exercise of moderate intensity provides a safe and potent stimulus to maintain and even increase bone mass. Especially beneficial is weight-bearing exercise; examples include walking, running, dancing, rope skipping, or resistance-training activities in which significant muscular force can be generated against the long bones of the body.

Muscular forces acting on specific bones appear to modify the dynamics of bone metabolism at the point of stress. For example, the leg bones of older cross-country runners show greater bone mineral content compared with the bones of less active counterparts. Likewise, the bones in the playing arm of a tennis player and the throwing arm of a baseball player are thicker compared with the less used, nondominant arm. Of course, all the benefits of exercise are predicated on adequate calcium being available for the bone-forming process.

Is Too Much Training Harmful? There is a paradox between exercise and bone dynamics for premenopausal women who train intensely and reduce their body mass and body fat to a point at which the menstrual cycle actually ceases, a condition termed *secondary amenorrhea.* The hormonal imbalances associated with menstrual cessation are likely to remove estrogen's protective effect on bone, making these women vulnerable to calcium loss and possible depletion in bone mass. Concurrently, nutritional factors (e.g., low protein and fat intake) magnify the problem. If amenorrhea persists, the benefits of exercise on bone mass are negated, the risk of musculoskeletal injuries during exercise increases, and significant osteoporosis sets in at an early age.

Sodium, Potassium, and Chlorine. The minerals sodium, potassium, and chlorine are collectively termed *electrolytes* because they are dissolved in the body as ions. The major function of the electrolytes is to modulate fluid exchange within the body's various fluid compartments. This allows for a well-regulated exchange of nutrients and waste products between the cell and its external fluid environment. Sodium and chlorine are the chief minerals in blood plasma and extracellular fluid, while potassium is the chief intracellular mineral.

Another important function of sodium and potassium is to establish the proper electrical gradient across cell membranes. This electrical difference between the interior and exterior of the cell is required for nerve impulse transmission, stimulation and contraction of muscle, and proper functioning of glands.

Sodium: How Much Is Enough? In general, if sodium intake is low, the hormone aldosterone acts on the kidneys to conserve sodium. Conversely, if sodium intake is high, the excess is excreted in the urine. Consequently, a normal balance for this electrolyte is usually maintained throughout a wide range of intakes. For some individuals, however, this is not always the case and excessive sodium intake is not adequately regulated. A chronic excess of dietary sodium can raise fluid volume and possibly increase peripheral vascular resistance; both of these factors could elevate blood pressure to levels that pose a health risk. This *sodium-induced hypertension* occurs in about one-third of the hypertensive people in the United States.

For decades, a first line of defense to treat high blood pressure has been to eliminate excess sodium from the diet. By decreasing the intake of sodium, sodium and fluid levels in the body may be concomitantly reduced to lower blood pressure favorably. Although the effectiveness of sodium restriction for controlling hypertension in the general population is presently debated among medical specialists, it does appear that certain individuals are "salt sensitive": they respond favorably to salt restriction with a lowering of blood pressure.

A person who consumes the typical Western diet ingests about 3000 to 7000 mg of sodium daily. This value is 6 to 14 times the 500 mg of sodium the body actually requires on a daily basis. Thus, the National Research Council recommendation of 1100 to 3300 mg per day is liberal in terms of actual sodium requirements. A large sodium intake results primarily from the heavy reliance placed on table salt in processing, curing, cooking, seasoning, and storing foods.

Iron. From 3 to 5 g or about 1/6 of an oz of iron is normally contained in the body. Approximately 80% of the body's iron is part of a functionally active molecule called *heme.* It is ferrous iron that makes heme chemically reactive to permit its rapid attachment and detachment with oxygen. Heme, when combined with the protein *globin,* forms *hemoglobin,* the major constituent of red blood cells. This iron-protein compound increases the oxygen-carrying capacity of blood about 65 times.

Iron serves other important functions besides its role in oxygen transport by red blood cells. Heme iron constitutes an important component of *myoglobin,* a compound similar to hemoglobin that aids in the storage and transport of oxygen within muscle cells. A third depot of heme iron is in specialized chains of enzymes called *cytochromes* whose function is to catalyze energy transfer within the mitochondria. Recall from Chapter 2 that the cytochromes, in conjunction with iron, operate by transferring electrons (hydrogens) during energy-generating oxidation-reduction cellular reactions. In essence, iron plays a pivotal role in oxygen transport and utilization in processes that power all forms of biologic work.

Iron Stores. Approximately 20% of iron in the body is not combined in functionally active compounds. This iron is stored in the liver, spleen, and bone marrow and is known as *hemosiderin* and *ferritin.* These storage reserves replenish the iron lost from the functional compounds and provide the "backup" iron reserves in periods of dietary insufficiency. Unfortunately, this is all too frequent for those consuming the typical Western diet, in which iron content averages only about 6 mg per 1000 calories of food intake. Thus, a young adult female who consumes 1700 calories daily takes in only about 10 mg of iron. Without supplementation, iron intake would remain at about 30% below her RDA of 15 mg.

Individuals who consume insufficient iron or who have limited iron absorption or high rates of iron loss often develop reduced concentrations of hemoglobin in the blood. In an extreme condition of iron insufficiency, commonly called *iron deficiency anemia,* hemoglobin is reduced to levels characterized by general sluggishness, loss of appetite, and reduced capacity for sustaining even mild exercise. With "iron therapy," both blood hemoglobin content and physiologic responses generally return to normal levels. Table 6-8 lists the RDA for iron for children and adults.

The Source of Iron is Important. While iron absorption from the intestine varies with iron need, a considerable difference in the bioavailability of iron occurs in relation to the composition of the diet. For example, only between 2 to 20% of the iron obtained from the plant kingdom is absorbed, compared with 10 to 35% of animal heme iron. Research indicates that vegetarian athletes have poorer iron status than their counterparts who consume the same quantity of iron from predominantly animal sources. Iron bioavailability from plants can be improved by consuming iron from both heme and nonheme sources. Thus, consuming red meat with grain and vegetable products increases

Regular exercise and increased muscle strength slow the aging of the skeleton. Moderate to high intensity aerobic exercise (walking, jogging, aerobic dancing, stair climbing) performed 3 days a week for 50 to 60 minutes a workout, builds bone and retards its rate of loss. Muscle-strengthening exercises are also beneficial. Individuals with greater back strength and those who train regularly with resistance exercise have a greater spinal bone mineral content than weaker and untrained individuals.

Hold the potassium. Although significant potassium is lost through sweating, this is usually not a problem for the athlete who consumes a diet rich in fruits, juices, vegetables, and whole grain products.

Iron insufficiency is a universal problem. More than 550 million people worldwide suffer from iron insufficiency, making it the most common nutritional deficiency in the world.

While the beneficial effects of physical activity are well known, possible negative side-effects have only recently appeared in the research literature. Research has focused on exercise-induced production of the "free radical" state of oxygen known as superoxide. A free radical is a molecule or molecular fragment containing an unpaired electron in the valence shell. Recall from Chapter 1 that oxidation occurs by either adding oxygen, removing hydrogen, or transferring electrons, the latter being the primary source of metabolic free radical production. While most of the oxygen consumed by the body during exercise combines with hydrogen to form water, up to 5% will form superoxides as electrons escape from the respiratory chain. When superoxide forms, it dismutates to hydrogen peroxide (H_2O_2). Superoxide is rapidly converted to O_2 and H_2O by the enzyme superoxide dismutase.

There are at least two ways that reactive oxygen or free radicals can be produced during exercise. The first is via an electron leak in the mitochondria, probably at the cytochrome level where superoxide radicals are produced. The second is during ischemia — underperfusion that often occurs during intense exercise. Oxidative damage will occur if free radical production is great enough to overcome the body's normal antioxidant defense system. Free radicals can damage practically every component of a cell including its proteins, nucleic acids, and in particular the fatty acid bilayer membrane.

The potential for free radical damage during exercise exists and seems to depend on exercise intensity and state of training. Intense or exhaustive exercise by untrained subjects is more likely to produce oxidative damage, and is more likely to be found in muscle than in blood. Antioxidant scavengers that react with radicals (and thus blunt their potential for damage) include vitamins E and C, the mineral selenium, coenzyme Q_{10} that occurs naturally in the body, and the provitamin beta-carotene. Because wheat germ oil contains large amounts of vitamin E, it has been used by athletes as a primary antioxidant supplement.

Limited research suggests that selenium, which probably plays a contributory role in free radical extinction, is not crucial in the protection against exercise induced oxidative damage. Vitamin E, however, may be the most important antioxidant related to exercise. Vitamin E-deficient animals begin an exercise program with cell membrane function compromised from oxidative damage, and thus reach exhaustion earlier than animals with normal levels of vitamin E. Vitamin E supplementation above normal levels may not necessarily give added protection against exercise-induced oxidative damage. Some evidence, however, is rather impressive. The insert graph shows the effects of three weeks of 200 mg of vitamin E supplementation on pentane elimination (pentane is a primary marker of free radical production). As can be seen, free radical production is dramatically reduced with vitamin E supplementation.

The research dealing with coenzyme Q_{10} and vitamin C antioxidant effects are less well defined. Coenzyme Q_{10} is thought to act as an antioxidant either by itself or as a recycler of vitamin E. There is little evidence that this substance has the same direct antioxidant effect as vitamin E. While vitamin C is known as a strong antioxidant, its effect in exercise is less well known. Clearly, more research will be forthcoming in this interesting and important area.

Pentane levels before and after 20 min of exercise at 100% max $\dot{V}O_2$ with and without vitamin E supplementation. Adapted from Pincemail, J., et al.: Pentane measurement in man as an index of lipoperoxidation. *Bioelectronchem. Bioenerg.* 18:117, 1987.

References

Alessio, H. M. Exercise-induced oxidative stress. *Med. Sci. Sports Exerc.* 25:218, 1993.

Jenkins, R. R., and A. Goldfarb. Introduction: oxidant stress, aging and exercise. *Med. Sci. Sports Exerc.* 25:210, 1993.

overall iron absorption. Iron absorption also can be increased by adding foods rich in vitamin C which converts the ferric form of iron to the ferrous state and makes it available for absorption at the alkaline pH of the intestine. In a practical sense, people who take an iron supplement should drink a large glass of orange juice with it.

Females: A Population At Risk. Inadequate iron intake frequently occurs among young children, teenagers, females of childbearing age, and groups of physically active females. A moderate iron deficiency anemia is common during pregnancy, when iron demand is increased for both the mother and fetus. In addition, females usually lose between 5 and 45 mg of iron during menstruation. This menstrual iron loss is the main source of variation in the iron requirements of menstruating women. This need for extra iron, coupled with a generally poor dietary intake of iron, accounts for the fact that 30 to 50% of American women exhibit significant dietary iron insufficiencies.

Exercise-Induced Anemia: Fact or Fiction? Because of the great interest in endurance activities combined with the increased participation of women in such sports, research has focused on the influence of hard training on the body's iron status. The term "sports anemia" is sometimes used to describe an assumed effect of training on reductions in hemoglobin to levels approaching clinical anemia, defined as 12 g and 13 g of hemoglobin per 100 ml blood for women and men, respectively. Some researchers maintain that exercise training creates an added demand for iron that outstrips its intake.

It is postulated that heavy training creates an increase in iron demand due to a loss of iron in sweat (probably minimal), as well as a loss of hemoglobin in urine that results from

TABLE 6-8. Recommended dietary allowances for iron*

	Age	Iron (mg)
Children	1–10	10
Males	11–18	12
	19+	10
Females	11–50	15
	51+	10
	Pregnant	30†
	Lactating	15†

*Recommended Dietary Allowances, Revised 1989, Food and Nutrition Board, National Academy of Sciences-National Research Council, Washington, D.C.
†Generally, this increased requirement cannot be met by ordinary diets; therefore, the use of 30 to 60 mg of supplemental iron is recommended.

the destruction of red blood cells. Iron loss also may occur from mechanical trauma during weight-bearing activity caused by repetitive pounding of the feet on the ground surface (footstrike hemolysis). There may be some gastrointestinal bleeding following long distance running that is unrelated to age, gender, or performance time. Such increases in iron loss would certainly stress the body's iron reserves needed for the synthesis of new red blood cells.

To support the possibility that exercise can induce anemia, some studies indicate that suboptimal hemoglobin concentration and hematocrit are more prevalent among endurance athletes. On closer scrutiny, however, it appears that any reduction in hemoglobin concentration is transient and occurs in the early phase of training, with hemoglobin then returning to pretraining values. This general response is illustrated in Figure 6-14 for a group of high-school female cross-country runners during a competitive season.

The decrease in hemoglobin generally parallels the disproportionately large expansion in plasma volume with training. For example, just 4 days of submaximal exercise training increases

Bioavailability of Iron. Two main factors influence iron absorption from the gut: present iron status and the composition of the diet, especially in terms of heme and nonheme iron. On average, about 17% of iron consumed in the typical American diet is absorbed.

Vegetarian athletes at greater risk. Research indicates that vegetarian athletes have a poorer iron status than their counterparts who consume the same quantity of iron from predominantly animal sources.

plasma volume by 20%, whereas the red blood cell volume remains unchanged. Consequently, total hemoglobin may actually increase with training, yet its concentration in plasma decreases. Despite this apparent dilution of hemoglobin, aerobic capacity and exercise performance consistently increase during training. Although there may be some mechanical destruction of red blood cells with vigorous exercise and some loss of iron in sweat, it is unclear whether these factors are of sufficient magnitude to strain an athlete's iron reserves and precipitate anemia if iron intake is normal.

Iron supplementation in a person whose diet is sufficient in this mineral does *not* lead to an increase in hemoglobin, hematocrit, or other measures of iron status. Even in instances of mild iron deficiency without anemia, iron supplementation may not enhance exercise capacity or aerobic perfor-

mance. When supplements are administered they should not be used indiscriminately because excessive iron can accumulate to toxic levels in the body and cause serious side effects.

MINERALS AND EXERCISE PERFORMANCE

For normal individuals receiving the RDA of minerals, there is no evidence that supplementation benefits exercise performance. An important consequence of prolonged exercise, especially in hot weather, is the loss of water and mineral salts, primarily sodium and some potassium chloride in sweat. These losses impair heat regulation and exercise performance, and can lead to severe dysfunction related to heat disorders. The yearly toll of heat-related deaths during spring and summer football practice provides a tragic illustration of the importance of fluid and electrolyte replacement. It is not uncommon for an athlete to lose anywhere from 1 to 5 kg of water each practice session or during a game as a result of sweating. This fluid loss also corresponds to a depletion of 1.5 to 8.0 g of salt because each kilogram (1 liter) of sweat generally contains about 1.5 g of salt. *The crucial and immediate need in these situations, however, is to replace the water lost through sweating.*

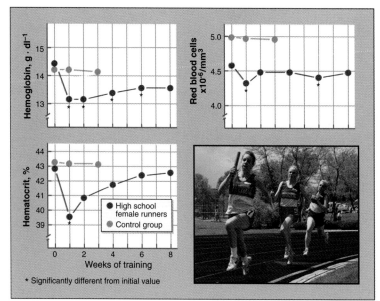

FIGURE 6-14. Hemoglobin, red blood cell count, and hematocrit in high-school female cross-country runners and a comparison group during the competitive season. (Adapted from Puhl, J. L., et al.: Erythrocyte changes during training in high school women cross-country runners. *Res. Q. Exerc. Sport,* 52:484, 1981.)

SUMMARY

1. Vitamins are organic substances that neither supply energy nor contribute to the body's mass; instead, they serve crucial functions in almost all body processes. Vitamins must be obtained from food or from dietary supplementation.

2. There are 13 known vitamins classified as either water- or fat-soluble. The fat-soluble vitamins are vitamins A, D, E, and K; vitamin C and the B-complex vitamins are water-soluble.

3. Fat-soluble vitamins taken in excess accumulate in the tissues and eventually can be toxic. Except in relatively rare and specific instances, excesses of water-soluble vitamins are generally nontoxic and are eventually excreted in the urine.

4. Vitamins regulate metabolism, facilitate energy release, and are important in the process of bone and tissue synthesis.

5. Research generally shows that vitamin supplementation (above that obtained in a well-balanced diet) is not related to improved exercise performance or potential for training. In fact, excessive dosages of fat-soluble, and in some instances water-soluble vitamins, can result in serious illness.

6. About 4% of the body's mass is composed of 22 elements called minerals. Minerals are a part of enzymes, hormones, and vitamins; they are found in muscles, connective tissues, and all body fluids.

7. A primary function of minerals is in metabolism where they serve as important parts of regulatory enzymes. Minerals provide structure in the formation of bones and teeth and are also important for the synthesis of the biologic nutrients, carbohydrate, lipid, and protein.

8. With a balanced diet, there is generally adequate mineral intake, except perhaps in geographic regions where there is an absence of certain minerals in the soil such as iodine.

9. Among older individuals, particularly women, the disease of osteoporosis has reached almost epidemic proportions. Adequate calcium intake and regular exercise of a weight bearing nature seem to provide an effective defense against bone loss at any age.

10. Women who train intensely and reduce body weight to the point where menstruation is adversely affected often show advanced bone loss at an early age.

11. About 40% of women of childbearing age in the United States suffer from iron insufficiency. This could lead to iron deficiency anemia, a condition that could significantly affect exercise performance.

12. It is not clear whether regular physical activity creates a significant drain on the body's iron reserves. If this proves to be the case, females who, as a group, have the greatest iron requirements and lowest intake, could be at risk of developing anemia. Assessment of the body's iron status should include an evaluation of both hematological characteristics and iron reserves.

WATER IN THE BODY

From 40 to 60% of an individual's body mass is water. Water constitutes 65 to 75% of the weight of muscle and less than 25% of the weight of fat. There are two main water "compartments in the body": *intracellular,* referring to inside the cell, and *extracellular,* referring to outside the cell. The extracellular fluid includes the blood plasma and lymph, saliva, fluids in the eyes, fluids secreted by glands and the intestines, fluids that bathe the nerves of the spinal cord, and fluids excreted from the skin and kidneys. Of the total body water, an average of 62% is located intracellularly and 38% is located extracellularly.

Functions of Body Water

Water is truly a remarkable nutrient that is essential to life. Its functions are as follows:

- Water serves as the body's transport and reactive medium
- Diffusion of gases always takes place across surfaces moistened by water
- Nutrients and gases are transported in aqueous solution and waste products leave the body through the water in urine and feces
- Water has tremendous heat-stabilizing qualities because it absorbs a considerable quantity of heat with only a small change in temperature
- Water is part of fluids that lubricate the joints, keeping bony surfaces from grinding against each other
- Because it is noncompressible, water provides structure and form to the body through the turgor it gives body tissues

Water compartments. Of the total water content of the body, about 62% exists as intracellular fluid (ICF) and 38% as extracellular fluid (ECF). For a 70 kg person, total body water is about 42 liters. Thus, ICF volume is 26 liters (0.62 x 42) and ECF volume equals 16 liters (0.38 x 42). Blood plasma accounts for 20% of the ECF, or a volume of about 3 liters. Much of the fluid lost through sweating is ECF, predominantly from the blood plasma.

WATER BALANCE: INTAKE VERSUS OUTPUT

The body's water content remains relatively stable over time. Although water output frequently exceeds water intake, the imbalance is quickly adjusted with appropriate ingestion of fluid. The sources of water intake and output at normal ambient temperatures are shown in the top panel of Figure 6-15. The bottom panel of the figure indicates that fluid balance can change dramatically during exercise, especially in a hot, humid environment.

Water Intake

Normally, about 2.5 liters (2.7 quarts) of water are required each day for a sedentary adult living within the normal range of environmental temperatures. This water is supplied from three sources: liquids, foods, and metabolism.

From Liquids. On a typical day, the average person consumes 1200 ml of water. This amount changes drastically during exercise and thermal stress, when fluid intake can increase five or six times above normal. There is a report of a male endurance runner who lost 13.6 kg (30 lb) of water weight during a 2 day, 17 hour, 55-mile run across Death Valley, California. This highly conditioned athlete was able to maintain fluid intake to a reasonable degree, so weight loss at the completion of this unusual event was only 1.4 kg. Fluid loss and replenishment amounted to between 3.5 and 4 gallons of liquid!

In Foods. Most foods contain varying quantities of water. Fruits and vegetables (lettuce, pickles, green beans, broccoli) are high in water content, whereas the water contained in butter, oils, dried meats, chocolate, cookies, and cakes is quite low. Generally, about 1000 ml of water is contained in the foods consumed in the daily diet.

Metabolic Water. Carbon dioxide and water are formed in varying amounts when food nutrients are degraded for energy. This metabolic water provides about 25% of the daily water requirement for a sedentary person. For example, the complete breakdown of 100 g of carbohydrate produces 55 g of metabolic water and protein produces 100 g, while the combustion of a similar quantity of lipid produces 107 g of water. Because each gram of glycogen is hydrated with 2.7 g of water, this water also becomes available when glycogen is used as the fuel for biologic work. For a sedentary person, about 350 ml of water is provided through the daily metabolic processes.

Water Output

Water is lost from the body in urine, through the skin, as water vapor in the expired air, and in feces.

In Urine. Under normal conditions, the kidneys reabsorb about 99% of the 140 to 160 liters of filtrate formed each day. Consequently, the daily urine volume excreted by the kidneys ranges from 1000 to 1500 ml or about 1.5 quarts.

Water is always being lost from the body by urine formation. About 15 ml of water are required to eliminate 1 g of solute by the kidneys. This portion of water in urine is "obligated" in order to rid the body of metabolic by-products such as urea (an end product of protein breakdown), uric acid (a breakdown product of nucleic acids), the electrolytes sodium and potassium, sulfate ions, and creatinine. The ingestion and subsequent energy metabolism of large quantities of protein (as would occur with a high-protein diet) facilitates water loss through urea production and subsequent excretion. This increased urine

flow could actually speed up the body's dehydration.

Through the Skin. A small quantity of water, perhaps 350 ml, continually seeps from the deeper tissues through the skin to the body's surface; this water loss is called *insensible perspiration.*

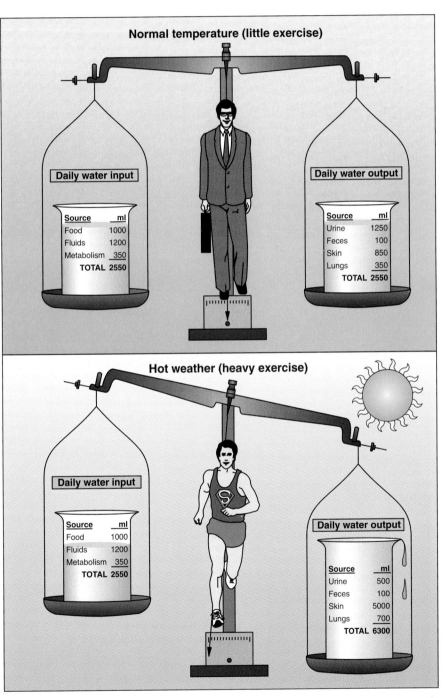

FIGURE 6-15. Water balance in the body. *Top:* Exercise in normal ambient temperature and humidity. *Bottom:* Moderate to heavy exercise in a hot, humid environment.

Water is also lost through the skin in the form of sweat produced by specialized sweat glands located beneath the skin. *Evaporation of sweat provides the refrigeration mechanism to cool the body.* Under normal conditions, 500 to 700 ml of sweat are secreted each day. This by no means reflects sweating capacity, because 8 to 12 liters of sweat (about 10 kg at a rate of 1 liter per hour) can be produced during prolonged exercise in a hot environment.

As Water Vapor. The amount of insensible water loss through small water droplets in exhaled air is about 250 to 350 ml per day. Exercise significantly affects this source of water loss. For physically active persons, about 3.5 ml of water is lost from the respiratory passages each minute during strenuous exercise. This amount varies considerably with climate, being less in hot, humid weather and greater at cold temperatures where the inspired air contains little moisture.

In Feces. Between 100 and 200 ml of water are lost through intestinal elimination because approximately 70% of fecal matter is water. With diarrhea or vomiting, the water loss can increase to 1,500 to 5,000 ml. This can create significant dehydration and electrolyte loss.

WATER REQUIREMENT IN EXERCISE

The most serious consequence of profuse sweating is the loss of body water. During a vigorous workout, sweating frequently causes a person to lose between 1 and 2 kg of body fluid. For endurance athletes, a fluid loss equivalent to 4% of body weight is not uncommon in a training session. Of course, the amount of water lost depends on the severity and duration of physical activity as well as environmental conditions. The *relative humidity* of the ambient air is also important, as this greatly affects the cooling efficiency of sweating. The term relative humidity refers to the water content of the air. During conditions of 100% relative humidity, the air is completely saturated with water vapor. Thus, evaporation of fluid from the skin is impossible, and this important avenue for body cooling is closed. Under such conditions, sweat beads on the skin and eventually rolls off. On a dry day, the air can hold considerable moisture, and fluid evaporates rapidly from the skin. This enables the sweating mechanism to function at optimal efficiency and body temperature is more easily controlled.

Heat Disorders

Even a moderate loss of fluid through sweating is not without consequences. *Blood volume becomes reduced when sweating causes a fluid loss of about 2% of body mass.* This places a strain on circulatory function that ultimately impairs capacity for both exercise and thermoregulation.

The three important heat disorders can be described as follows:

- **Heat cramps.** Involuntary muscle spasms that occur during or after intense physical activity and are easily observed in the specific muscles exercised. This form of heat illness is probably caused by an imbalance in the body's fluid and electrolyte concentrations.
- **Heat exhaustion.** Usually characterized by a weak, rapid pulse, low blood pressure in the upright position, headache, dizziness, and general weakness. Sweating may be reduced, but body temperature is not elevated to dangerous levels. Heat exhaustion is caused by ineffective circulatory adjustments compounded by depletion of extracellular fluid, especially blood volume due to excessive sweating. The person should stop exercising and move to a cooler environment, and fluids should be administered.
- **Heat stroke.** This is the most serious and complex of the heat

maladies and requires immediate medical attention. Heat stroke is a failure of the body's heat-regulating mechanisms caused by excessively high body temperature. When thermoregulation fails, sweating usually ceases, the skin becomes dry and hot, body temperature rises to dangerous levels, and excessive strain is placed on the circulatory system. If left untreated, the disability progresses and death ensues from circulatory collapse and eventual damage to the central nervous system. Immediate aggressive steps to lower body temperature while awaiting medical treatment include alcohol rubs, ice packs, and whole-body immersion in cold or even ice water.

Practical Recommendations for Fluid Replacement.

The primary aim of fluid replacement is to maintain plasma volume so that circulation and sweating progress at optimal levels. Ingesting "extra" water before exercising in the heat provides some thermoregulatory protection. It delays the development of dehydration, increases sweating during exercise, and brings about a smaller rise in body temperature compared to exercising without prior fluids. In this regard, it is wise to consume 400 to 600 ml (13 to 20 oz) of cold water 10 to 20 minutes before exercising. Doing this, however, does not eliminate the need for *continual fluid replacement* during exercise.

Gastric Emptying

Fluids must be emptied from the stomach before being absorbed in the small intestine. There are several factors that influence gastric emptying.

- **Fluid temperature.** Cold fluids (5°C; 41°F) are emptied from the stomach at a faster rate than fluids at body temperature
- **Fluid volume**. Ingesting a volume of about 250 ml (8.5 oz) at

15-minute intervals is a realistic goal for fluid intake during exercise because larger volumes tend to produce feelings of a "full stomach."

- **Fluid osmolarity.** Gastric emptying is slowed when the ingested fluid is concentrated with electrolytes or simple sugars, whether in the form of glucose, fructose, or sucrose. For example, a 40% sugar solution is emptied from the stomach at a rate only one-fifth that of plain water.

During exercise in a cold environment, fluid loss from sweating may not be so great. Here, a reduction in gastric emptying and subsequent fluid uptake can be tolerated and a more concentrated sugar solution (15 to 20 g per 100 ml of water) may be beneficial. The trade-off between the composition of the ingested fluid and the rate of gastric emptying must be evaluated on the basis of both environmental stress and energy demands. In terms of survival, fluid replacement is the *primary concern* during prolonged exercise in the heat. More is said concerning the desirable composition of "sports drinks" and their effects on fluid replacement in Chapter 7.

Adequacy of Rehydration

Preventing dehydration and its consequences, especially a dangerously elevated body temperature, or *hyperthermia,* can be achieved only with an adequate water replacement schedule. This is often "easier said than done" because some individuals feel that ingesting water hinders exercise performance. For wrestlers, dehydration is a way of life. Young boys and men will lose considerable fluid so they can wrestle in a lower weight class. This is also the case for many ballet dancers who are continually preoccupied with their weight so as to appear thin. Many individuals on weight loss programs incorrectly believe that by restricting fluid intake, body fat loss will in some way occur at a more rapid rate.

Heat stroke does happen. During U.S. Marine Corps recruit training, between 10 to 30 cases of heat stroke occur annually.

Defend against dehydration. Water that beads and drips off the skin is of no benefit to body cooling. It is only when sweat evaporates that a cooling effect is noted. The only effective way to prevent dehydration is to drink water regularly during exercise. As a practical guide, it is a good idea to wear loose-fitting white workout clothes during hot-weather exercise (a loose fit permits air circulation between skin an environment, and white reflects heat more effectively than other colors). Also, do not remove soaked clothing: changing to dry clothes hinders evaporative cooling.

Fluid replacement is critical. Sweat loss during a marathon run at world record pace (2 hr, 6 min, 50 s) averages about 5.3 liters (12 lb), depending on environmental conditions. This fluid loss corresponds to an overall reduction of about 6 to 8% in body mass. To avoid exercise-induced dehydration, it is important to consume fluids regularly during physical activity.

Drink early and often. Fluids are normally emptied from the stomach at a rate of about 800–1200 ml per hour. However, when a person is already dehydrated, gastric emptying is significantly delayed and symptoms of GI disturbance increase. The important lesson is to drink sufficiently early on during exercise before a state of dehydration is reached.

Changes in body weight before and after exercising should be used to indicate water loss during exercise and the adequacy of rehydration in subsequent recovery. Coaches often have their athletes "weigh in" before and after practice, and insist that weight loss be minimized by periodic water breaks during activity. The thirst mechanism is an imprecise guide to water needs after exercising. In fact, if rehydration were left entirely to a person's thirst, it could take several days to reestablish fluid balance, especially after severe dehydration.

Volume of Fluid to Ingest Each Hour to Obtain the Noted Amount of Carbohydrate

CHO concentration in drink, g · 100 ml⁻¹	30 gm/hr	40 gm/hr	50 gm/hr	60 gm/hr	
2%	1500 ml	2000 ml	2500 ml	3000 ml	Volume too large; greater than 1200 ml/hr
4%	750	1000	1250	1500	
6%	500	667	833	1000	Adequate fluid replacement 600-1250 ml/hr
8%	375	500	625	750	
10%	300	400	300	600	
15%	200	267	333	400	Low fluid replacement; less than 600 ml/hr
20%	150	200	250	300	
25%	120	160	200	240	
50%	60	80	100	120	

Modified from Coyle, E.F., and S.J.Montain. Benefits of fluid replacement. Med. Sci Sports Exerc. 24:S324, 1992.

SUMMARY

PART 3

1. Water makes up 40 to 60% of the total body mass. Muscle is 72% water by weight, whereas water represents only about 20 to 25% of the weight of body fat.

2. Of the total body water, roughly 62% is located intracellularly and 38% extracellularly in the plasma, lymph, and other fluids outside the cell.

3. Food and oxygen are always supplied in aqueous solution and waste products always leave by a watery medium. Water also helps give structure and form to the body and plays a vital role in temperature regulation.

4. Normal daily water intake of about 2.5 liters is supplied from (1) liquid intake (1.2 liters), (2) food (1.0 liters), and (3) metabolic water produced during energy-yielding reactions (0.3 liters).

5. Water is lost from the body each day (1) in the urine (1 to 1.5 liters), (2) through the skin as insensible perspiration (0.50 to 0.70 liters), (3) as water vapor in expired air (0.25 to 0.30 liters), and (4) in feces as about 70% of fecal matter is water (0.10 liters).

6. Exercise in hot weather greatly increases the body's water requirement. In extreme conditions the fluid needs can increase five or six times above normal.

7. Several factors affect the rate of gastric emptying: cold fluids are emptied from the stomach more rapidly than fluids at body temperature; when the stomach is partially filled with fluid, the rate of gastric emptying increases; and concentrated sugar solutions impair gastric emptying and fluid replacement.

8. The primary aim of fluid replacement is to maintain plasma volume so that circulation and sweating progress at optimal levels. For the ideal replacement schedule during exercise, fluid intake should match fluid loss. The effectiveness of this replacement can be evaluated by monitoring changes in body weight before, during, and following workouts.

Aloia, J.F., et al.: Calcium supplementation with and without hormone replacement therapy to prevent post-menopausal bone loss. *Ann. Inter. Med.,* 120: 97, 1994.

Antioxidant vitamins and ß-carotene in disease prevention. Proceedings of a conference held in London, UK. *Am. J. Clin. Nutr.,* 53(Suppl.): 189S, 1991.

Barr, S. L., et al.: Reducing total dietary fat without reducing saturated fatty acids does not significantly lower total plasma cholesterol concentrations in normal males. *Am. J. Clin. Nutr.,* 55:682, 1992.

Bønaa, K. H., et al.: Effect of eicosapentaenoic and docosahexaenoic acids on blood pressure in hypertension. *N. Engl. J. Med.,* 322:795, 1990.

Brooks, G. A.: Amino acid and protein metabolism during exercise and recovery. *Med. Sci. Sports Exerc.,* 19:S150, 1987.

Butterfield, G. E.: Amino acids and high protein diets. In *Perspectives in Exercise Science and Sports Medicine, Ergonomics - The Enhancement of Exercise and Sport Performance.* Vol. 4. Edited by M. Williams, and D. Lamb, Indianapolis, Benchmark Press, 1991.

Clarkson, P. M.: Minerals: exercise performance and supplementation in athletes. *J. Sports Sci.,* 9:91, 1991.

Clevidence, B. A.: Plasma lipid and lipoprotein concentrations of men consuming a low-fat, high-fiber diet. *Am. J. Clin. Nutr.* 55:689, 1992.

Conroy, B.P., et al.: Bone mineral density in elite junior Olympic weight lifters. *Med. Sci. Sports Exerc.,* 25:1103, 1993.

Coyle, E. F., and Montain, S. J.: Carbohydrate and fluid ingestion during exercise: are there trade-offs? *Med. Sci. Sports Exerc.,* 24:671, 1992.

Drinkwater, B.L.: C.H. McCloy Research Lecture: Does physical activity play a role in preventing osteoporosis? *Res. Q. Exerc. Sport.* 65: 197, 1994.

Drinkwater, B. L., et al.: Menstrual history as a determinant of current bone density in young athletes. *JAMA,* 263:545, 1990.

Eichner, E.R.: Sports anemia, iron supplements, and blood doping. *Med. Sci. Sports Exerc.,* 24:S315, 1992.

Faulkner, R.A., et al.: Comparison of bone mineral content and bone mineral density of dominant and non-dominant limbs in children 8–16 years of age. *Am. J. Biol.,* 5:491,1993.

Gisolfi, C. V., and Duchman, S. M.: Guidelines for optimal replacement beverages for different athletic events. *Med. Sci. Sports Exerc.,* 24:679, 1992.

Hamdy, R.C., et al.: Regional differences in bone density of young men involved in different exercises. *Med. Sci. Sports Exerc.,* 26: 884, 1994.

Haymes, E. M.: Vitamin and mineral supplementation to athletes. *Int. J. Sports Nutr.,* 1:146, 1991.

Jacobs, I., et al.: Effects of prior exercise or ammonium chloride ingestion on muscular strength and endurance. *Med. Sci. Sports Exerc.,* 25: 809, 1993.

Jenkins, R.R.: Oxidation stress and antioxidants: A review. *Int. J. Sports Nutr.,* 3: 356, 1993.

Kanter, M.M.: Free radicals, exercise, and antioxidant supplementation. *Int. J. Sports Nutr.,* 4: 205, 1994.

Kashtan, H., et al.: Wheat bran and oat bran supplements' effects on blood lipids and lipoproteins. *Am. J. Clin. Nutr.,* 55:976, 1992.

Katch, F.I.: U.S. government raises serious questions about reliability of U.S. Department of Agriculture's food composition database. *Int. J. Sports Nutr.,* 5: 62, 1995.

Lemon, P. W. R.: Effect of exercise on protein requirements. In *Foods, Nutrition and Sports Performance.* Edited by C. Williams, and J. T. Devlin. London, E. & F. N. Spon , 1992.

Lemon, P. W. R., et al.: Protein requirements and muscle mass/strength changes during intensive training in novice bodybuilders. *J. Appl. Physiol.,* 73:767, 1992.

Levy, D., et al.: Stratifying the patient at risk for coronary disease: new insights from the Framingham Heart Study. *Am. Heart J.,* 119:712, 1990.

Marcus, R., et al.: Osteoporosis and exercise in women. *Med Sci. Sports Exerc.,* 24:S301, 1992.

Noakes, T. D.: Fluid replacement during exercise. In *Exercise and Sport Sciences Reviews.* Vol. 21. Edited by J. O. Holloszy. Baltimore, MD, Williams & Wilkins, 1993.

Lipid Research Clinics Program: The Lipid Research Clinics Coronary Primary Prevention Trial results: I. Reduction in incidence of coronary heart disease. *JAMA,* 251:351, 1984.

Position of the American Dietetic Association: Nutrition for physical fitness and athletic performance of adults. *ADA Rep.,* 81:933, 1987.

Recker, R. R., et al.: Bone gain in young adult women. *JAMA,* 268:2403, 1992.

Rimm, E.B., et al.: Vitamin E consumption and the risk of coronary heart disease in men. *N. Engl. J. Med.,* 328: 1450, 1993.

Saltin, B., and Gollnick, P. D.: Fuel for muscular exercise: role of carbohydrate. In *Exercise, Nutrition, and Human Performance,* Edited by E. S. Horton, and R. L. Terjung. New York, Macmillan, 1988.

Sawka, M.N.: Physiological consequences of hypohydration: exercise performance and thermal regulation. *Med. Sci. Sports Exerc.,* 24:657, 1992.

Selby, G. B.: When does an athlete need iron? *Phys. Sportsmed.,* 19:97, 1991.

Sharon, N. : Carbohydrates. *Sci. Am.,* 243:90, 1980.

Sherman, W. A., and Wimer, G. S.: Insufficient dietary carbohydrate during training: does it impair athletic performance? *Int. J. Sport Nutr.,* 1:28, 1991.

Singh, A., et al.: Chronic multivitamin-mineral supplementation does not enhance physical performance. *Med. Sci. Sports Exerc.,* 24:726, 1992.

Snow-Harter, C., and Marcus, R.: Exercise, bone mineral density, and osteoporosis. In *Exercise and Sport Sciences Reviews.* Vol. 19. Edited by J. O. Holloszy. Baltimore, Williams & Wilkins, 1991.

Tarnopolsky, M. A.: Protein, caffeine, and sports. *Phys. Sportsmed.,* 21(3):137, 1993.

Telford, R. D., et al.: The effect of 7 to 8 months of vitamin/mineral supplementation on athletic performance. *Int. J. Sport Nutr.,* 2:135, 1992.

Trice, I., Haymes, E.M.: Effects of caffeine ingestion on exercise-induced changes curing high-intensity, intermittent exercise. *Int. J. Sports Nutr.,* 5: 37, 1995.

Use of vitamin and mineral supplements in the United States. *Nutr. Rev.,* 70:43, 1990.

Yaspelkis, B. B., and Ivy, J. L.: Effect of carbohydrate supplements and water on exercise metabolism in the heat. *J. Appl. Physiol.,* 71:680, 1991.

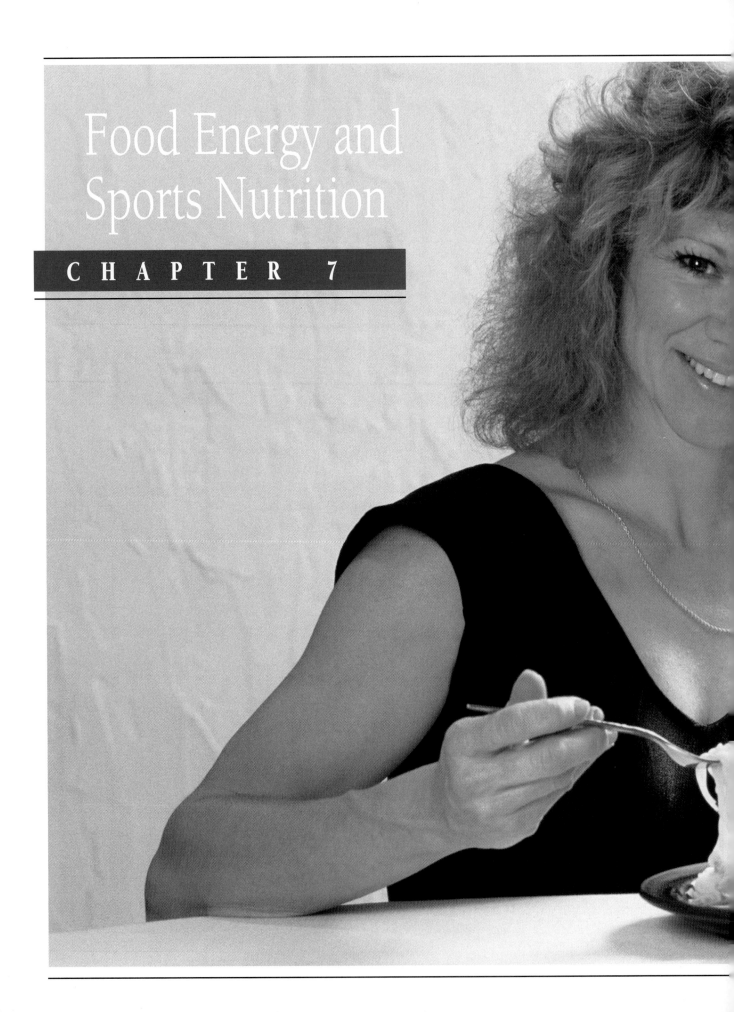

Food Energy and Sports Nutrition

CHAPTER 7

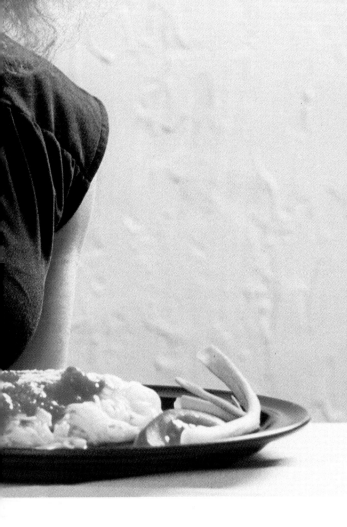

After reading this chapter, you should be able to:

- Define the following: (a) heat of combustion, (b) digestive efficiency, and (c) Atwater factors.

- Compare the nutrient and energy intake of physically active men and women and sedentary counterparts.

- Contrast the recommendations of the Four-Food-Group Plan and the Eating-Right Pyramid.

- Advise an athlete concerning the timing and composition of the pre-event or precompetition meal. Defend your reasons for limiting lipid and protein intake.

- Summarize the effects of low, normal, and high carbohydrate intake on glycogen reserves and subsequent endurance performance.

- Advise endurance athletes about (a) the potential negative effects of consuming a drink with a high sugar content 30 to 60 minutes before competition and (b) the ideal composition of a "sports drink."

- Define the term "glucose polymer" and give the reason why these compounds are often added to a sports drink.

- Make a general recommendation concerning carbohydrate intake for athletes involved in heavy endurance training.

- Give advice on how to replenish carbohydrate reserves after a hard bout of training or competition.

- Compare the classic procedure for carbohydrate loading to the modified loading procedure.

All biologic functions require energy. Because the carbohydrate, lipid, and protein food nutrients contain the energy that ultimately powers biologic work, it is possible to classify both food and physical activity in terms of energy. Part 1 deals with the quantification of food energy.

Part 1 MEASUREMENT OF FOOD ENERGY

GROSS ENERGY VALUE OF FOODS

Many laboratories throughout the world have used a bomb calorimeter similar to that shown in Figure 7-1 to measure the gross or total energy value of the various food nutrients. The principle behind this method of *direct calorimetry* is simple — the food is burned and the heat liberated measured. The bomb calorimeter works as follows. A weighed portion of food is placed inside a small chamber filled with oxygen under pressure. The food is ignited and literally explodes and burns when an electric current ignites a fuse inside the chamber. The heat released as the food burns, termed the *heat of combustion*, is absorbed by a surrounding water bath. Because the calorimeter is fully insulated, no heat escapes to the outside. The precise amount of heat absorbed by the water is determined by measuring the increase in water temperature with a sensitive thermometer. For example, when one 4.7 oz, 4-inch sector of apple pie is completely burned in the calorimeter, 350 kcal of heat energy is released. This raises 3.5 kg, or 7.7 lbs, of ice water to the boiling point.

Caloric Value of Foods

Heat of Combustion. The burning of 1 g of pure carbohydrate yields a heat of combustion of 4.20 kcal, 1 g of pure protein releases 5.65 kcal, and 1 g of pure lipid yields 9.45 kcal. Because most foods in the diet consist of various proportions of these three nutrients, the caloric value of a given food such as a hamburger or french fries is determined by the macronutrient content of an average serving. It is evident from the heats of combustion that the energy content will be greater for a food high in fat than in one that is relatively fat free. For example, the number of calories in 1 cup of whole milk is 160 kcal, whereas the same amount of skimmed milk contains 90 kcal. If someone who normally consumes 1 quart of milk each day switches to skimmed milk, the quantity of calories ingested each year would be reduced by the amount equal to about 11.4 kg (25 lb) of body fat!

When a gram of carbohydrate or lipid is "burned" within the cell, the body liberates the same value of 4.20 kcal for carbohydrate and 9.45 kcal for lipid as did the bomb calorimeter. The energy yield from lipid is more than *twice* that of carbohydrate because of the difference in the structural composition between the two nutrients. As noted in Chapter 6, the chemical formula for a simple carbohydrate always has a ratio of two

Kilojoule. The accepted international standard for expressing energy is the joule. To convert kcal to kilojoule (kJ), multiply the kcal value by 4.2.

Heat of combustion. The heat liberated by the burning or oxidation of food in the bomb calorimeter is referred to as its heat of combustion and represents the total energy value of the food.

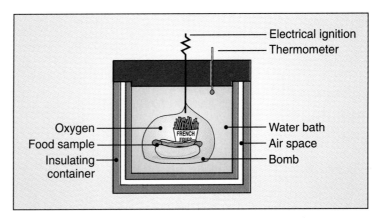

FIGURE 7-1. A bomb calorimeter is used to directly measure the energy value of food.

hydrogen atoms for each atom of oxygen. Lipid molecules, on the other hand, contain significantly more hydrogen than oxygen. The fatty acid palmitic acid, for example, has the structural formula $C_{16}H_{30}O_2$. This means there are more hydrogen atoms that can be cleaved away and oxidized to produce energy during the breakdown of a lipid.

The energy available to the body from protein breakdown is less than that released in the bomb calorimeter. In addition to carbon, hydrogen, and oxygen, proteins contain nitrogen. Because the body cannot use nitrogen, it combines with hydrogen to form urea (NH_2CONH_2) that is excreted in the urine. This elimination of hydrogen represents a loss of potential energy. For this reason, the energy yield from 1 g of protein in the body is 4.35 kcal instead of the 5.65 kcal released during its complete oxidation in the bomb calorimeter.

Digestive Efficiency. An important consideration in determining the ultimate caloric yield of ingested macronutrients is the efficiency of their availability to the body. Efficiency in this sense refers to completeness of digestion and absorption. Normally about 97% of carbohydrates, 95% of lipids, and 92% of proteins are digested and absorbed. When these digestive efficiencies are considered,

the net kcal value per gram for carbohydrate is 4.0, for lipid it is 9.0, and for protein it is 4.0. These corrected heats of combustion are called the *"Atwater Factors"* after the scientist who first investigated the energy released from food in the calorimeter and in the body.

Caloric Value of a Meal

By use of net Atwater kcal values, the caloric content of any food can be determined as long as its composition and weight are known. Suppose, for example, we wished to determine the kcal value for $1/_2$ cup of creamed chicken. The weight of this portion is equivalent to 3.5 oz or about 100 g. Based on laboratory analysis of a standard recipe, the macronutrient composition of 1 g of creamed chicken contains 0.2 g or protein, 0.12 g of lipid, and 0.06 g of carbohydrate. Using the net kcal values, 0.2 g of protein contains 0.8 kcal (0.20 x 4.0), 0.12 g of lipid equals 1.08 kcal (0.12 x 9.0), and 0.06 g of carbohydrate yields 0.24 kcal (0.06 x 4.0). The total caloric value of 1 g of creamed chicken would therefore equal 2.12 kcal (0.80 + 1.08 + 0.24). Consequently, a 100 g serving would contain 100 times as much, or 212 kcal. An example of these computations is presented in Table 7-1. Although this table shows the method for calculating the kcal value of ice

---

Digestive efficiency. The average percentage for digestive efficiency varies somewhat depending on the particular food. This is especially true for protein, where digestive efficiency ranges from a high of 97% for animal protein to a low of 78% for dried legumes. Furthermore, the available energy from a meal is reduced when it has a high fiber content.

TABLE 7-1. Method of calculating the caloric value of a food from its composition of macronutrients

Food: Ice cream (vanilla)
Weight: three-fourths cup = 100 grams

	Composition		
	Protein	Lipid	Carbohydrate
Percentage	4%	13%	21%
Total grams	4	13	21
In one gram	0.04 g	0.13 g	0.21 g
Calories per gram	0.16	1.17	0.84
	(0.4 x 4.0 kcal)	(0.13 x 9.0 kcal)	(0.21 x 4.0 kcal)

Total calories per gram: 0.16 + 1.17 + 0.84 = 2.17 kcal
Total calories per 100 grams: 2.17 x 100 = 217 kcal

cream, the same method can be used for a serving of any food. Reducing the portion size by half would of course reduce caloric intake by 50%.

Fortunately, there is seldom need to compute the kcal value of foods as shown in the previous example. This is because the United States Department of Agriculture has already made these determinations for almost all foods. What we have done in Section II of the *Student Study Guide and Workbook* is to present a list of the energy and nutritive values for approximately 2000 foods from the *Food and Diet Analyzer* computer program that accompanies the workbook. The specific values for each food are expressed per ounce or 28.4 g of the food item. The specific values for each food (including specialty and fast-food items) include calories in an average portion as well as its content of protein, lipid, carbohydrate, calcium, sodium, iron, vitamins B_1, B_2, C, and A, fiber, and cholesterol.

A Calorie is a Calorie is a Calorie

When examining the energy value of various foods, a rather striking yet reasonable observation is noted with regard to a food's energy value. Consider, for example, five common foods: raw celery, cooked cabbage, cooked asparagus spears, mayonnaise, and salad oil. To consume 100 kcal of each of these foods, a person must eat 20 stalks of celery, 4 cups of cabbage, 30 asparagus spears, but only 1 tablespoon of mayonnaise or $4/_5$ tablespoon of salad oil. The point is that a small serving of some foods contains the equivalent energy value as a large quantity of other foods. Viewed from a different perspective, one would have to consume more than 4000 stalks of celery, 800 cups of cabbage, or 30 eggs to supply the daily energy needs of a fairly sedentary individual, whereas the same energy would be supplied by ingesting only $1 1/_2$ cups of mayonnaise or about 8 oz of salad oil! The major difference in these foods is that high-fat foods exist as relatively concentrated sources of energy and contain little water. In contrast, foods low in fat or high in water tend to contain relatively little energy. An important concept, however, is that 100 kcal from mayonnaise and 100 kcal from celery are exactly the same in terms of energy. Simply stated, *a calorie is a calorie is a calorie*. The number of calories contained in foods is additive: the more you eat, the more calories you consume. If the food has a high concentration of calories, as in the case of fatty foods, and you consume even a moderate portion, you will of course consume a large number of calories.

Energy is energy. There is no difference between calories from an energy standpoint, a calorie being a unit of heat regardless of the food source.

S U M M A R Y

PART 1

1. A calorie or kilocalorie (kcal) is a measure of heat used to express the energy value of food. This food energy is directly measured in a bomb calorimeter.
2. The heat of combustion represents the heat liberated by the complete oxidation of food. The gross energy values are 9.4 for lipids, 4.2 for carbohydrates, and 5.65 kcal per gram for proteins.
3. The coefficient of digestibility is the proportion of ingested food actually digested and absorbed for use by the body. This represents about 97% for carbohydrates, 95% for lipids, and 92% for proteins. Thus, the net kcal values per gram (Atwater Factors) are 4 (carbohydrate), 9 (lipid), and 4 (protein).
4. With appropriate calorific values, it is possible to compute the caloric content of any meal as long as the carbohydrate, lipid, and protein composition is known.
5. From an energy standpoint, a calorie is a unit of heat energy regardless of the food source. Thus, it is incorrect to consider 300 kcal of chocolate ice cream any more energy rich than 300 kcal of watermelon, 300 kcal of pepperoni pizza, or 300 kcal of bagels and sour cream.

An optimal diet is defined as one in which the supply of required nutrients is adequate for tissue maintenance, repair, and growth without an excess energy intake. Only in the last few years has it been possible to make a reasonable estimate of the specific nutrient needs for individuals of different ages and body sizes, with considerations for individual differences in digestion, storage capacity, nutrient metabolism, and daily levels of energy expenditure. Dietary recommendations for athletes may be further complicated by the specific energy requirements of a particular sport as well as by the athlete's dietary preferences. *Truly, there is no one diet for* *optimal exercise performance.* Sound nutritional guidelines must be followed, however, in planning and evaluating food intake.

NUTRIENT REQUIREMENTS

Many coaches make dietary recommendations based on their own "feelings" and past experiences rather than rely on available research evidence. This problem is compounded because athletes often have either inadequate or incorrect information concerning prudent dietary practices or the role of specific nutrients in the diet. Although research in this area is far from complete, the general consensus is that active people and athletes do not require additional nutrients beyond those obtained in a balanced diet. This is important because a large number of adult Americans exercise regularly to keep fit. In fact, *research indicates that active Americans, including those involved in exceptional endurance activities, consume typical diets that are remarkably similar in composition to those consumed by their more sedentary counterparts.* As shown in Table 7-2, the main difference in dietary habits between athletes and nonathletes is that athletes eat more of the same foods which results in a larger total quantity of food consumed to support the extra energy required by training. *In essence, sound nutrition for athletes is sound human nutrition.* For the endurance athlete and other athletes involved in arduous training, special consideration must be given to maintaining adequate and regular carbohydrate intake.

Recommended Nutrient Intake

Figure 7-2 shows the recommended basic nutrient intake for protein, lipid, and carbohydrate, expressed both in grams and as a

TABLE 7-2. Comparison of carbohydrate, lipid, protein, and caloric intake of middle-aged male and female runners and sedentary controls[a]

	Runners	Sedentary Controls
Males		
Calories (kcal·day⁻¹)	2959.0*	2361.0
Protein (g·day⁻¹)	102.1	93.6
Protein (%)	13.8*	15.8
Lipid (g·day⁻¹)	134.4*	109.0
Lipid (%)	40.8	41.5
Carbohydrate (g·day⁻¹)	294.6*	225.7
Carbohydrate (%)	39.8	38.6
Cholesterol (mg·1000 kcal⁻¹)	175.0	190.0
Saturated fat (g·1000 kcal⁻¹)	16.2	16.0
Polyunsaturatd fat (g·1000 kcal⁻¹)	9.0	9.3
Females		
Calories (kcal·day⁻¹)	2386.0*	1871.0
Protein (g·day⁻¹)	82.2	76.7
Protein (%)	14.2*	17.4
Lipid (g·day⁻¹)	110.7	83.0
Lipid (%)	41.1	40.3
Carbohydrate (g·day⁻¹)	234.3*	174.7
Carbohydrate (%)	39.5	39.1
Cholesterol (mg·1000 kcal⁻¹)	190.0	205.0
Saturated fat (g·1000 kcal⁻¹)	16.8	16.5
Polyunsaturatd fat (g·1000 kcal⁻¹)	8.5	7.9

[a] % calories do not total 100% because alcohol calories constitute the difference.
* Values for runners are significantly different from controls.
(From: Blair, S.N., et al.: Comparisons of nutrient intake in middle-aged men and women runners and controls. *Med. Sci. Sports. Exerc.*, 13:310, 1981.)

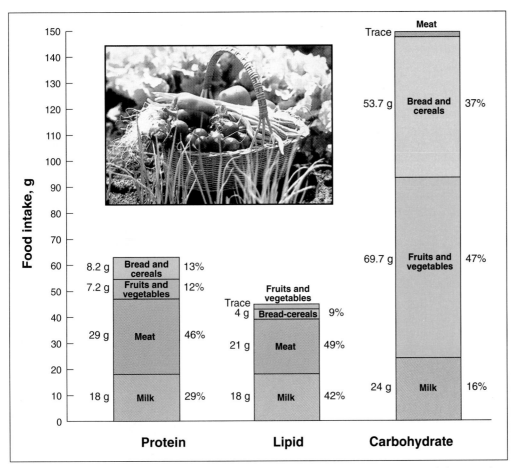

FIGURE 7-2. Basic recommendations for carbohydrate, lipid, and protein components, and the general categories of food sources in a balanced diet.

percent of the total intake, as well as the general category of food sources for these nutrients. These guidelines provide for the necessary vitamin, mineral, and protein requirements even though the energy content of this food intake amounts to only about 1200 kcal per day. In terms of average values for young adult Americans, the total daily energy requirement is about 2100 kcal for women and 2700 kcal for men. Once the basic nutrient requirements are met (as recommended in Figure 7-2), the extra energy needs of the person can be supplied for a variety of food sources based on individual preference.

For a physically active person, the "prudent diet" should contain about 60% of its calories in the form of carbohydrates, predominantly as unrefined starches. Because glycogen synthesis in liver and muscle is related to

dietary carbohydrate, some researchers in exercise physiology recommend increasing the daily carbohydrate intake to 70% of total calories (400 to 600 g) to prevent a gradual depletion of glycogen stores with successive days of hard training.

The Four-Food-Group Plan

A practical approach to sound nutrition is to categorize foods that make similar nutrient contributions and then provide servings from each category in the daily diet. A key to achieving success with such an approach is variety. This can be readily achieved by use of the Four-Food-Group Plan described in Table 7-3.

Adequate nutrition is assured as long as the recommended number of servings from the variety provided in each group is supplied, and cooking

Active men and women need carbohydrate. Stored muscle glycogen and blood-borne glucose are prime contributors of energy when the oxygen supplied to muscles is insufficient in relation to oxygen needs. In addition to this anaerobic role of carbohydrate, glycogen also provides substantial energy during high levels of aerobic exercise. Consequently, dietary carbohydrate is of utmost importance to individuals maintaining a physically active lifestyle.

and handling are proper. For individuals on meatless diets, a small amount of milk, milk products, or eggs should be included because vitamin B_{12} is available *only* in foods of animal origin. In fact, if milk and eggs are included in a vegetarian diet ("lacto-ovovegetarian" diet), nutritional quality will be approximately equivalent to the typical recommended diet that contains meat, fish, and poultry.

Table 7-4 presents examples of three daily low calorie menus formulated from the guidelines of the basic diet plan shown in Table 7-3. Provided the foods are stored and prepared in a proper manner, these menus provide all of the essential nutrients, even though the energy value of each is well below the average adult requirement. In fact, these menus serve as excellent nutritional models for reducing diets. For active individuals whose daily energy requirement may be as large as 5000 calories, all that need be done once the essentials are provided is to increase the quantity of food consumed with greater emphasis given to carbohydrate-rich food sources. This is achieved either by increasing the size of portions, the frequency of meals or snacks, or the variety of nutritious foods consumed at each meal.

The Eating Right Pyramid

The Four-Food-Group Plan developed in 1958 by the U.S. Department of Agriculture (USDA) was greatly influenced by lobbyists of the beef and dairy industries. Based on findings from research in cancer, heart disease, and nutrition over the past 35 years, the shortcomings of the "basic four" (with its overemphasis on meat and milk products) as a guide to healthful eating became apparent. To reflect the current state of nutritional knowledge

---

TABLE 7-3. The Four-Food Group Plan

Food Category	Examples	Recommended Daily Servings[c]
I. Milk and milk products[a]	Milk, cheese, ice cream, sour cream, yogurt	2[e]
II. Meat and high protein[b]	Meat, fish, poultry, eggs—with dried beans, peas, nuts, or peanut butter as alternatives	2
III. Vegetables and fruits[d]	Dark green or yellow vegetables; citrus fruits or tomatoes	4
IV. Cereal and grain food	Enriched breads, cereals, flour, baked goods, or whole-grain products	4

[a] If large quantities of milk are normally consumed, *fortified* skimmed milk should be substituted to reduce the quantity of saturated fats.

[b] Fish, chicken, and high-protein vegetables contain significantly less saturated fats than other protein sources.

[c] A basic serving of meat or fish is usually 100 g or 3.5 oz of edible food; 1 cup (8 oz) milk; 1 oz cheese; 1/2 cup fruit, vegetables, juice; 1 slice bread; 1/2 cup cooked cereal or 1 cup ready-to-eat cereal.

[d] One should be rich in vitamin C; at least one every other day rich in vitamin A.

[e] Children, teenagers, and pregnant and nursing women—4 servings.

TABLE 7-4. Three daily menus formulated from guidelines established by the Four-Food-Group Plan[a]

3 Meals a Day	5 Meals a Day	6 Small Meals a Day
Breakfast	**Breakfast**	**Breakfast**
1/2 cup unsweetened grapefruit juice 1 poached egg; 1 slice toast 1 tsp butter or margarine tea or coffee, black	1/2 grapefruit 2/3 cup bran flakes 1 cup skim or low-fat milk or other beverage	1/2 cup orange juice 3/4 cup ready-to-eat cereal 1/2 cup skim milk tea or coffee, black
Lunch	**Snack**	**Mid-Morning Snack**
2 oz lean roast beef[b] 1/2 cup cooked summer squash 1 slice rye bread 1 tsp butter or margarine 1 cup skim milk 10 grapes	1 small package raisins 1/2 bologna sandwich	1/2 cup low-fat cottage cheese
Dinner	**Lunch**	**Lunch**

3 oz poached haddock[b]
1/2 cup cooked spinach
tomato and lettuce salad
1 tsp oil + vinegar or lemon
1 small biscuit
1 tsp butter or margarine
1/2 cup canned drained
  fruit cocktail
1/2 cup skim milk
	1 slice pizza
	carrot sticks
	1 apple
	1 cup skim or low-fat milk
		2 oz sliced turkey on
		  1 slice white toast
		1 tsp butter or margarine
		2 canned drained peach halves
		1/2 cup skim milk

	Snack	**Mid-afternoon Snack**
	1 banana	1 cup fresh spinach and lettuce salad 2 tsp oil + vinegar or lemon 3 saltines
	Dinner	**Dinner**

	baked fish with
	  mushrooms (3 oz)[b]
	baked potato
	2 tsp margarine
	1/2 cup tomato juice or skim or
	  low-fat milk
		1 cup clear broth
		3 oz broiled chicken breast[b]
		1/2 cup cooked rice with
		  1 tsp butter or margarine
		1/4 cup cooked mushrooms
		1/2 cup cooked broccoli
		1/2 cup skim milk

		Evening Snack
		1 medium apple 1/2 cup skim milk
Total Calories: about 1200	**Total Calories: about 1400**	**Total Calories: about 1200**

[a] Each menu provides *all* essential nutrients; the energy or caloric value of the diet can be easily increasd by increasing the size of the portions, the frequency of meals, or the variety of foods consumed at each sitting.

[b] Cooked weight

more clearly, the USDA developed a new model for good nutrition as illustrated in Figure 7-3. The result was the "Eating-Right Pyramid" that maintains the concept of the basic four food groups but refocuses emphasis on grains, vegetables, and fruits as the basis of the diet and downplays food sources high in animal protein, lipids, and dairy products.

Exercise and Food Intake

For individuals who engage regularly in moderate to intense physical activity, it is relatively easy to match

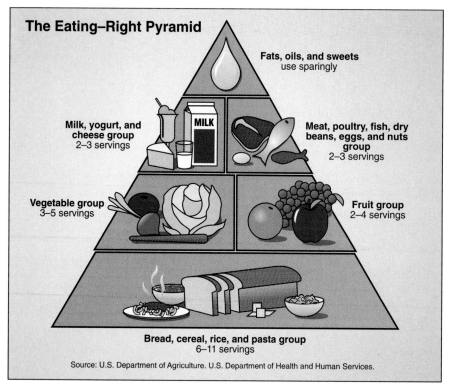

The Eating–Right Pyramid

Fats, oils, and sweets
use sparingly

Milk, yogurt, and
cheese group
2–3 servings

MILK

Meat, poultry, fish, dry
beans, eggs, and nuts
group
2–3 servings

Vegetable group
3–5 servings

Fruit group
2–4 servings

Bread, cereal, rice, and pasta group
6–11 servings

Source: U.S. Department of Agriculture. U.S. Department of Health and Human Services.

FIGURE 7-3. The Eating-Right Pyramid emphasizes grains, vegetables, and fruits as important sources for nutrients.

Dieting can hinder exercise performance and optimal nutrition.
Reliance on starvation diets or other potentially harmful practices such as high-fat, low-carbohydrate diets, "liquid-protein" diets, or water diets is counterproductive for weight control, exercise performance, and optimal nutrition for good health. Reliance on low-carbohydrate diets compromises the energy supply required for vigorous physical activity or regular training.

Caloric intake of athletes. With the exception of the relatively high daily energy intake of athletes at extremes of performance and training, such as triathletes and Tour de France cyclists (5880 kcal), daily caloric intake for athletes generally does not exceed 4000 kcal for men and 3000 kcal for women.

food intake with the daily level of energy expenditure. Lumbermen, for example, who expend about 4500 kcal daily, unconsciously adjust their caloric intake to balance closely their energy output. Consequently, body weight remains stable despite an extremely large food intake. The balancing of food intake to meet a new level of energy output takes about a day or so, during which time a new energy equilibrium is attained. Apparently, this fine balance between energy expenditure and food intake is not maintained in sedentary people. Here, the caloric intake generally exceeds the daily energy expenditure. This lack of precision in regulating food intake at the low end of the physical activity spectrum probably accounts for the "creeping obesity" commonly observed in highly mechanized and technically advanced societies.

The daily food intake of athletes in the 1936 Olympics reportedly averaged more than 7000 kcal, or roughly three times the average daily intake of a non-athlete. These values are often quoted and used to justify what appears to be an enormous food requirement of athletes in training. However, these figures, are only estimates because objective dietary data were not presented in the original research report. In all likelihood, the results are inflated estimates of the energy expended (and required) by the athletes. For example, research has shown that distance runners who train upward to 100 miles per week (6 min per mile pace at about 15 kcal per minute) probably do not expend more than 800 to 1300 "extra" kcal each day above their normal energy requirement. For these endurance athletes, the daily food intake should supply about 4000 kcal to balance the increased energy expenditure. Figure 7-4 presents data on energy intake from a large sample of elite male and female endurance, strength, and team sport athletes in the Netherlands. For male athletes energy intake ranged between 2900 and 5900 kcal per day, while the daily intake of female competitors ranged between 1600 and 3200 kcal.

Eat More, Weigh Less. As was shown in Table 7-2, the caloric intake of 61 middle-aged men and women who ran an average of 60 km per week amounted to about 40 to 60% more kcal per kg of body mass compared with sedentary controls. This larger daily caloric intake for the runners was accounted for by the extra energy required to run between 8 and 10 kilometers daily. Paradoxically, the active men and women who ate considerably more on a daily basis weighed considerably less than subjects who were less physically active. Such data are generally consistent with other studies of active people and add further evidence to the strong argument that *regular exercise of moderate intensity provides an effective means by which a person can actually "eat more yet weigh less" and maintain a lower per-*

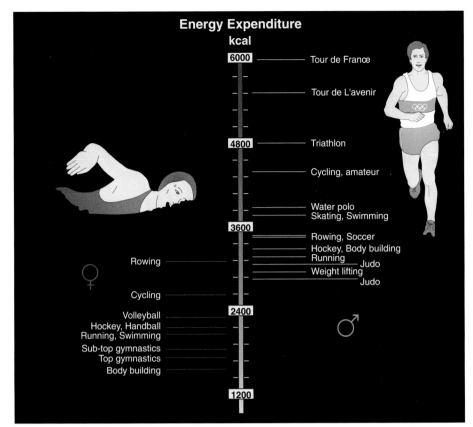

Energy Expenditure
kcal

6000 —— Tour de France

—— Tour de L'avenir

4800 —— Triathlon

—— Cycling, amateur

Water polo
Skating, Swimming

3600

Rowing, Soccer
Hockey, Body building
Running
Judo
Weight lifting
Judo

Rowing ——

Cycling ——

Volleyball ——
Hockey, Handball ——
Running, Swimming ——

Sub-top gymnastics ——
Top gymnastics ——
Body building ——

2400

1200

FIGURE 7-4. Daily energy intake in kcal per day in elite male and female endurance, strength, and team sport athletes. (From van Erp-Baart, A. M. J., et al.: Nationwide survey on nutritional habits in elite athletes. *Int. J. Sports Med.,* 10:53, 1989.)

centage of body fat. The key is increased daily physical activity. Active people maintain a lighter and leaner body and a healthier heart disease risk profile despite an increased intake of the typical American diet. Table 7-5 presents a general model for food intake for active male and female athletes as well as an example of a 2500 kcal menu containing 350 g of carbohydrate.

THE PRECOMPETITION MEAL

Carbohydrate is favored as the main nutrient source for intense exercise, and also is crucial as an energy source in prolonged exercise. The precompetition meal must therefore provide adequate quantities of this nutrient to assure normal levels of blood glucose and sufficient glycogen "energy reserves." This, of course, presumes that the person has maintained a nutritionally sound diet throughout training. As a general rule, foods that are high in lipid and protein content should be eliminated from the diet on the day of competition. These foods are digested slowly and remain in the digestive tract for a longer time than carbohydrate-rich foods of similar energy content. Furthermore, with the increased stress and tension that usually accompany competition, there may be significant diversion of blood from the intestines and an accompanying decrease in absorption from the digestive tract. *A three-hour period generally is adequate for the meal to be digested and absorbed.*

Good sources of carbohydrate. Mix and match some good souces of carbohydrate for the pre-exercise meal.

Carbohydrate Content
1 slice whole wheat bread (12 g)
1 tablespoon jelly (13 g)
1 apple and banana (20 g)
1 cup orange or apple juice (28 g)
1 cup yogurt (43 g)

What to eat before competing. The main purpose of the precompetition or pregame meal is to provide the athlete with adequate food energy and assure optimal hydration. A precompetition meal containing 200–350 g of carbohydrate 3 to 6 hours before exercising has the potential for improving performance by maximizing muscle and liver glycogen storage as well as providing glucose for intestinal absorption during exercise.

TABLE 7-5. An active athlete needs about 50 kcal of food per kg (23 kcal per lb) of body weight each day to provide enough calories for "optimal" athletic performance. A sample training diet would ideally consist of 60% carbohydrate, 15 to 20% protein, and less than 25% fat.

Body Weight	110 lbs (50 kg)	132 lbs (60 kg)	154 lbs (70 kg)	176 lbs (80 kg)
Total kcal*	2500	3000	3500	4000
Milk group (90 kcal) Skim milk, 1 cup Plain, low-fat yogurt, 1 cup	4	4	4	4
Meat group (55-75 kcal) Cooked, lean meat (fish, poultry), 1 oz Egg, 1 Peanut butter, 1 tbl. Low-fat cheese, 1 oz. Cottage cheese, 1/4 cup	5	5	6	6
Fruits	7	9	10	12
Vegetables	3	5	6	7
Grains	16	18	20	24
Fat	5	6	8	10

Sample high carbohydrate 2500 kcal menu (350 g)

Breakfast	Lunch	Dinner	Snack #1	Snack #2
1 cup bran cereal 8 oz low fat milk 1 english muffin 1 tsp margarine 4 oz orange juice	3 oz lean roast beef 1 hard roll 2 tsp. mayonnaise or mustard lettuce and tomato 1/2 cup cole slaw 2 fresh plums 2 oatmeal cookies 8 oz seltzer water with lemon	Chicken Stir-fry: 3 oz chicken 1 cup diced vegetables 2 tsp. oil 2 cups rice 1 cup orange and grapefruit sections 1 cup vanilla yogurt Iced tea with lemon	3 cups popcorn	8 oz apple cider

Modified from Carbohydrates and Athletic Performance. *Sports Science Exchange.* Vol. 7. Gatorade Sports Science Institute, Chicago, 1988.

Replenishing carbohydrate. To replenish carbohydrate after a hard bout of training or competition, it is wise to start consuming carbohydrate rich foods as soon as possible after exercising. A good idea is to eat about 50 to 75 g of carbohydrate every two hours until about 500 g are consumed. Legumes (peas, beans), fructose, and milk products should be avoided due to their slow rate of intestinal absorption.

The glycogen supply is limited. High-intensity excercise for an hour can decrease liver glycogen by about 55%. A 2-hour strenuous workout can just about deplete the glycogen content of the liver and specifically exercised muscles.

High Protein is Not the Best Choice

Many athletes are psychologically accustomed to and even dependent on the "classic" pregame meal of steak and eggs. Although this meal may be satisfying to the athlete, coach, and restaurateur, its benefits have never been demonstrated in terms of improved exercise performance. In fact, a meal so low in carbohydrates may actually hinder optimal performance. For one thing, carbohydrates are digested and absorbed more rapidly than either proteins or lipids. Thus, carbohydrates are available for energy faster and may also reduce the feeling of fullness following a meal. A high-protein meal can also elevate the resting metabolism more than a high-carbohydrate meal. Added heat production may place a further strain on temperature regulation that could be detrimental to exercise performance in hot weather. Concurrently, the breakdown of protein for energy facilitates dehydration because the by-products of amino acid breakdown demand water for urinary excretion.

Liquid Meals

Commercially prepared liquid meals offer an alternate, effective approach to pre-event meal feeding. These foods are generally well balanced in nutritive value; they are high in carbohydrate yet contain enough lipid and protein to contribute to a feeling of satiety. Because they are in liquid form, they also contribute to the athlete's fluid needs. Another advantage is more rapid digestion and they leave essentially no residue in the intestinal tract. The liquid meal approach to nutrition on the day of competition is effective during day-long activities such as swimming and track meets, or tennis and basketball tournaments. In these situations, an athlete may have relatively little time for or interest in food. Liquid meals are also practical for supplementing the caloric intake of athletes who have difficulty maintaining their body weight or who wish to increase it.

DIET AND EXERCISE PERFORMANCE

Carbohydrate Needs in Intense Training

Repeated days of strenuous endurance workouts for activities such as distance running, swimming, cross-country skiing, and cycling can induce a state of fatigue in which continued hard training becomes progressively more difficult. Often referred to as "staleness," this physiologic state is caused by a gradual depletion of the body's glycogen reserves, even though the person's diet may contain the typical percentage of carbohydrate. In one experiment, after three successive days of running 16.1 km (10 miles) a day, runners had nearly depleted the glycogen in the thigh muscles even though their diet contained about 45% carbohydrates. By the third day, the quantity of glycogen used during the run was less than on the first day and the energy for exercise was supplied predominantly from lipid breakdown. However, no further glycogen depletion occurred when daily dietary carbohydrate was increased to 500 to 600 g (70% of caloric intake). This demonstrates the importance of maintaining adequate carbohydrate intake during training.

Glycogen is not rapidly replenished when it becomes severely depleted. At least 24 hours are needed to restore muscle glycogen levels after prolonged, exhaustive exercise. Unmistakably, during periods of heavy training, daily carbohydrate allowances must be increased to balance glycogen utilization and permit optimal glycogen resynthesis.

Diet, Glycogen Stores, and Endurance

In the late 1930s, scientists observed that endurance performance was significantly improved simply by consuming a carbohydrate-rich diet for three days prior to exercising. Conversely, endurance was drastically reduced if the diet consisted predominantly of lipids. Researchers have evaluated different methods to increase the glycogen content of muscle because of the crucial relationship between diet composition and optimal physical performance. In one series of experiments, subjects consumed one of three diets. The first maintained normal caloric intake but supplied the major quantity of calories from lipids and only 5% of calories from carbohydrate. The second diet was normal for calories and contained the average percentages of macronutrients. The third diet pro-

vided 80% of calories as carbohydrates. The results, illustrated in Figure 7-5 reveal that the glycogen content of leg muscles, expressed as grams of glycogen per 100 g of muscle, averaged 0.6 for subjects fed the high-fat diet, 1.75 for the normal diet, and 3.75 for the high-carbohydrate diet. Furthermore, the subjects' endurance capacity varied greatly depending on the pre-exercise diet. When the subjects were fed the high-carbohydrate diet, endurance was more than three times greater than when they consumed the high-fat diet!

These findings highlight the important role that nutrition plays in establishing appropriate energy reserves for exercise and training. A diet deficient in carbohydrate rapidly depletes muscle and liver glycogen. This subsequently affects performance in both maximal, short-term anaerobic exercise and in high intensity, prolonged aerobic activities. These observations are pertinent for the athlete as well as for moderately active people who modify their diets and consume

Optimizing glycogen reserves. Gradually reducing or tapering the intensity of workouts several days prior to competition while maintaining a high carbohydrate intake is a sound approach for establishing optimal energy reserves.

It takes time. When carbohydrate intake is optimal, the body's glycogen stores are replenished at a rate of about 5% per hour. Thus, under the best of circumstances it will take at least 20 hours to reestablish glycogen stores after a glycogen-depleting bout of exercise.

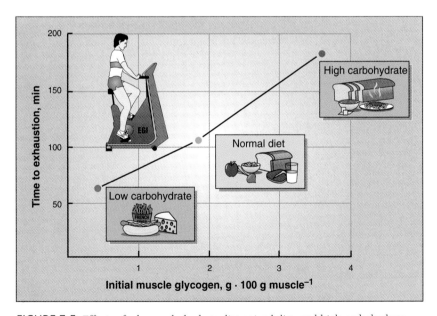

FIGURE 7-5. Effects of a low-carbohydrate diet, mixed diet, and high-carbohydrate diet on the glycogen content of the quadriceps femoris muscle and the duration of endurance exercise on a bicycle ergometer. With a high-carbohydrate diet, endurance time was 3 times greater compared to a diet low in carbohydrate. (Adapted from Bergstrom, J., et al.: Diet, muscle glycogen and physical performance. *Acta Physiol. Scand.,* 71:140, 1967.)

less than the recommended quantity of carbohydrate.

Sugary Drinks: A Wise Solution?

Although research has firmly established the important role of carbohydrate during various intensities of physical activity, carbohydrate supplements are not always beneficial.

During Exercise. Performance during high-intensity aerobic exercise is improved by consuming carbohydrate-laden drinks at regular intervals. Supplementary carbohydrate may spare muscle glycogen because the ingested glucose is used as fuel, or it helps to maintain a more optimal level of blood glucose that prevents headache, lightheadedness, nausea, and other symptoms of central nervous system distress. Maintaining a status quo for blood glucose also supplies the needs of muscles when glycogen reserves become depleted in the later stages of prolonged exercise. During less intensive exercise, the beneficial effect of carbohydrate feeding is negligible because moderate exercise is fueled mainly by the breakdown of lipid with little drain on carbohydrate reserves.

What to Drink? Commercially available carbohydrate drinks are not necessarily more effective than a liquid mixture of glucose or sucrose. Such a drink (5% solution) can be prepared by adding 50 g of either glucose or sucrose to 1 liter of water. For prolonged, high-intensity aerobic exercise in cool weather, a practical recommendation is to ingest a strong 50% sugar solution (70 g of sugar in 140 ml of water) 20 to 30 minutes after the start of exercise, followed by less concentrated solutions that contain about 24 g of carbohydrate (8 oz of a 5% solution every 15 minutes) over 30-minute intervals during exercise.

Glucose Feedings and Water Uptake. An important property of sugar drinks

is their potential *negative effect* on water absorption from the digestive tract. This is because the emptying of fluid from the stomach into the small intestine where it is absorbed is inhibited by the concentration of particles in solution. This effect could be detrimental during exercise in the heat, when adequate fluid intake and absorption are crucial to the athlete's health and safety. Researchers have devised a strategy to counter the negative effects of sugar molecules on gastric emptying so that plasma volume is preserved during exercise in the heat. This is accomplished by formulating the drink with *glucose polymers* that greatly reduce the number of particles in solution while increasing the drink's carbohydrate content. Polymerized glucose may facilitate the movement of water and glucose from the stomach to the small intestine for absorption compared to a drink of similar carbohydrate content of simple sugar. An added bonus is that once glucose is in the intestine, its absorption stimulates both sodium and water uptake.

Before Exercise. Drinking a strong sugar solution 30 to 60 minutes prior to exercise actually hinders endurance capacity. For example, the riding time of young men and women on an exercise bicycle was reduced nearly 20% when they consumed a 25% glucose solution 30 minutes before exercising compared with similar exercise preceded by drinking the same volume of plain water. Consuming concentrated sugar drinks before exercise causes blood sugar to rise dramatically within 5 to 10 minutes. This leads to an overshoot in insulin release from the pancreas that actually produces a decline in blood sugar (hypoglycemia) as glucose moves rapidly into the muscle cells. At the same time, insulin inhibits the mobilization of lipids for energy. Consequently, carbohydrate is metabolized during subsequent exercise to a much greater degree than under normal conditions. This results in a more

OPTIMAL REPLACEMENT OF FLUID AND CARBOHYDRATE DURING PROLONGED EXERCISE

Intense aerobic exercise can be performed for an extended time as long as core temperature is regulated and plasma volume maintained, and if there is adequate carbohydrate available for energy.

Heat produced during exercise is primarily dissipated by evaporation of sweat from the body's surface. Dehydration, a consequence of water loss due to sweating, impairs heat dissipation and reduces endurance performance. Fluid ingestion prior to and during exercise attenuates the detrimental effects of dehydration on temperature regulation and exercise performance. By adding carbohydrate to the fluid replacement beverage, additional energy for exercise is provided as the endogenous carbohydrate becomes depleted. To reduce fatigue and prevent dehydration, it is important to determine the optimal fluid and carbohydrate mixture for an endurance activity. This mixture of fluid and food energy is important because of the possibility that the intake of large fluid volumes may impair carbohydrate uptake, and concentrated sugar solutions may impair fluid replacement.

The purpose of carbohydrate ingestion during endurance exercise is to maintain blood glucose concentration and sustain carbohydrate oxidation during the latter stages of exercise. Research has shown that there is little difference between liquid glucose or sucrose, or starch as the ingested fuel source during exercise. The optimal carbohydrate replacement rate is between 30 to 60 g (about 1 to 2 oz) per hour, ingested at least 30 min prior to the time when fatigue would normally occur without a carbohydrate supplement.

Fluid replacement depends on the rate of gastric emptying (determined by the volume of the fluid ingested) and the fluid's carbohydrate concentration. There is a trade-off between carbohydrate ingestion and amount of gastric emptying. It is possible, however, to empty up to 1700 ml of water per hour from the stomach, even when drinking an 8% solution of carbohydrate. However, 1000 ml (about 1 quart) of fluid ingestion per hour is probably optimal to offset dehydration, as larger amounts of fluid often result in gastrointestinal discomfort.

Practical Recommendations

- The magnitude of dehydration can be evaluated by closely monitoring changes in body weight. Each one pound of weight loss corresponds to 450 ml (15 fluid oz) of dehydration.

- During prolonged exercise an accompanying dehydration, drink fluids at the rate they are being depleted, or at least drink at a rate close to 80% of the rate of sweating.

- The endurance athlete can meet both carbohydrate (up to 30 to 60 $g \cdot hr^{-1}$) and fluid needs by drinking 625 to 1250 ml $\cdot hr^{-1}$ of a beverage containing 4 to 8% carbohydrate.

Reference

Coyle, E.F., and S.J. Montain. Benefits of fluid replacement with carbohydrate during exercise. *Med Sci Sports Exerc.*, 24:S324, 1992.

Volume of Fluid to Ingest Each Hour to Obtain the Noted Amount of Carbohydrate

CHO concentration in drink, $g \cdot 100\ ml^{-1}$	30 gm/hr	40 gm/hr	50 gm/hr	60 gm/hr	
2%	1500 ml	2000 ml	2500 ml	3000 ml	Volume too large; greater than 1200 ml/hr
4%	750	1000	1250	1500	
6%	500	667	833	1000	Adequate fluid replacement 600-1250 ml/hr
8%	375	500	625	750	
10%	300	400	300	600	
15%	200	267	333	400	Low fluid replacement; less than 600 ml/hr
20%	150	200	250	300	
25%	120	160	200	240	
50%	60	80	100	120	

Modified from: Coyle, E. F., and S. J. Montain. Benefits of fluid replacement with carbohydrate during exercise. *Med Sci. Sports Exerc.* 24: S324, 1992.

TABLE 7-6. Two-stage dietary plan for increasing muscle glycogen storage

Stage 1 — Depletion
> Day 1: Exhausting exercise performed to deplete muscle glycogen in specific muscles
>
> Days 2, 3, 4: Low-carbohydrate food intake (high percentage of protein and lipid in the daily diet

Stage 2 — Carbohydrate Loading
> Days 5, 6, 7: High carbohydrate food intake (normal percentage of protein in the daily diet)

Competition Day
> Follow high-carbohydrate pre-competition meal.

Fructose is not optimal. Fructose is not the optimal carbohydrate for a sports drink because it takes longer to become converted to useful glucose for energy. Fructose delivers only about 0.2 g of glucose to active muscles each minute, whereas glucose, sucrose, and maltodextrins can deliver up to 1.0 g.

Strategy for carbohydrate loading. Because carbohydrate loading occurs only in the specific muscles exercised, the person must engage the muscles involved in his or her sport during the depletion phase of the loading procedure. In preparation for a marathon, a 15- or 20-mile run is usually necessary; for swimming and bicycling, 90 minutes of moderately intense exercise in the specific activity would be required.

Athlete beware! Don't confuse carbohydrate-loading drinks like *Exceed, High Carbohydrate Source,* or *Gator Lode* with sports drinks to be consumed during exercise. These more concentrated drinks (up to 40% carbohydrate in solution) will blunt the intestinal absorption of water. They are, however, ideal for carbohydrate replenishment after exercise that has depleted glycogen reserves.

rapid glycogen depletion and causes fatigue to occur sooner than would normally be the case.

Fructose is absorbed more slowly from the gut than either glucose or sucrose and causes only a minimal insulin response with essentially no decline in blood glucose. This has prompted some to suggest that fructose would be beneficial for immediate pre-exercise carbohydrate feeding. Although the theoretical rationale for this use of fructose appears sound, the ergogenic benefits are inconclusive. What is important is that consuming high-fructose beverages is, because of its slow rate of absorption, often accompanied by significant *gastrointestinal distress* that in itself can negatively affect exercise performance.

CARBOHYDRATE LOADING: A WAY TO INCREASE GLYCOGEN RESERVES

Research has shown that a particular combination of diet and exercise results in significant "packing" of muscle glycogen. This procedure is termed *carbohydrate loading* and is commonly used by endurance athletes. The end result of carbohydrate loading is an even greater increase in muscle glycogen than would occur with simply consuming a carbohydrate-rich diet.

Classic Procedure

The classic procedure for carbohydrate loading, outlined in Table 7-6, is accomplished as follows:

- Glycogen stores are reduced with a period of relatively long (about 60 to 90 min) high intensity, aerobic exercise.
- Muscle glycogen is further depleted by maintaining a high-fat, low-carbohydrate diet (60 to 120 g carbohydrate) for several days while continuing a moderate exercise program.
- Activity level is reduced for the next several days; at the same time, a switch is made to a carbohydrate-rich diet (400 to 600 g carbohydrate).

With this procedure, the muscle glycogen increases to a new, higher level. Of course, adequate protein, minerals, vitamins, and abundant water also must be part of the daily diet.

The combination of diet and exercise to produce glycogen packing or "supercompensation" should be of considerable interest to the serious endurance athlete whose success can be influenced by the body's carbohydrate reserves. For nonathletes or those involved in activities lasting less than 75 minutes, normal levels of muscle glycogen are more than adequate to sustain exercise. Normal levels of glycogen can be assured by ingesting approximately 60% of the daily caloric intake as carbohydrates. This should be increased if the energy requirements are consistently high, as occurs during intensive training.periods.

Table 7-7 lists sample meal plans for carbohydrate depletion (*Stage 1*) and carbohydrate loading (*Stage 2*) that precede the endurance event.

Negative Aspects. The wisdom of repeated bouts of carbohydrate loading has yet to be verified. A severe carbohydrate overload interspersed with periods of high lipid or protein intake may increase blood cholesterol and urea nitrogen levels and could pose problems in people susceptible to adult-onset diabetes or heart disease, or for those who have certain muscle enzyme deficiencies or kidney disease. During the low-carbohydrate phase of the loading procedure, the potential exists for a marked ketosis that is often observed among individuals who exercise in the carbohydrate-depleted state. Failure to eat a balanced diet may eventually lead to deficiencies in some minerals and vitamins, particularly water-soluble vitamins. Furthermore, the glycogen-depleted state certainly reduces a person's capability to engage in hard training and may result in an actual detraining effect. The elimination of dietary carbohydrate for three days could also set the stage for a loss of lean tissue because the muscles' amino acids are used in gluconeogenesis to maintain blood glucose. For this reason, the less stringent *modified approach* to carbohydrate loading outlined in the next section is an attractive option.

Modified Loading Procedure

Many negative aspects of the classic carbohydrate loading sequence can be

Maintain blood glucose. Maintaining plasma glucose for use by active muscles later in long term exercise can be accomplished by ingesting 30 to 60 g of carbohydrate per hour throughout exercise or by ingesting about 200 g late (at about 90–120 min) in exercise. Ingested supplemental carbohydrate at the point of fatigue is not absorbed rapidly enough to be of value.

Carbohydrate loading is not a panacea. Carbohydrate loading should only be considered for physical activities that last longer than one hour and are performed at high intensity. For activities of shorter duration, a well balanced diet with about 60% carbohydrate (7 g per kg body weight) is all that's required.

TABLE 7-7. Sample meal plan for carbohydrate depletion and carbohydrate loading diets preceding an endurance event*

Meal	Stage 1 Depletion	Stage 2 Carbohydrate Loading
Breakfast	1/2 cup fruit juice 2 eggs 1 slice whole-wheat toast 1 glass whole milk	1 cup fruit juice 1 bowl hot or cold cereal 1 to 2 muffins 1 tbsp butter coffee (cream/sugar)
Lunch	6-oz hamburger 2 slices bread salad 1 tbsp mayonnaise and salad dressing 1 glass whole milk	2–3 oz hamburger with bun 1 cup juice 1 orange 1 tbsp mayonnaise pie or cake
Snack	1 cup yogurt	1 cup yogurt, fruit, or cookies
Dinner	2 to 3 pieces chicken, fried 1 baked potato with sour cream 1/2 cup vegetables iced tea (no sugar) 2 tbsp butter	1–1 1/2 pieces chicken, baked 1 baked potato with sour cream 1 cup vegetables 1/2 cup sweetened pineapple iced tea (sugar) 1 tbsp butter
Snack	1 glass whole milk	1 glass chocolate milk with 4 cookies

*During Stage 1, the intake of carbohydrate is approximately 100 g or 400 kcal; in Stage 2, the carbohydrate intake is increasd to 400 to 625 g or about 1600 to 2500 kcal.

FIGURE 7-6. Recommended combination of diet and exercise for overloading muscle glycogen stores during the week before an important endurance contest. Exercise is gradually reduced during the week, and the carbohydrate content of the diet is increased for the last three days. (From Sherman, W. M., et al.: Effect of exercise-diet manipulation on muscle glycogen and its subsequent utilization during performance. *Int. J. Sports Med.,* 2:114, 1981.)

eliminated by following the less stringent, modified carbohydrate-loading dietary protocol outlined in Figure 7-6. This six-day protocol is achieved without prior exercise to exhaustion. The athlete trains at a high aerobic intensity for 1.5 hours and gradually reduces or tapers the duration of exercise on successive days. Carbohydrates represent about 50% of the total calories during the first three days; they are then increased to about 70% of total calories for the last three days before competition. This results in an increase in glycogen reserves to about the same level as is achieved with the classic protocol.

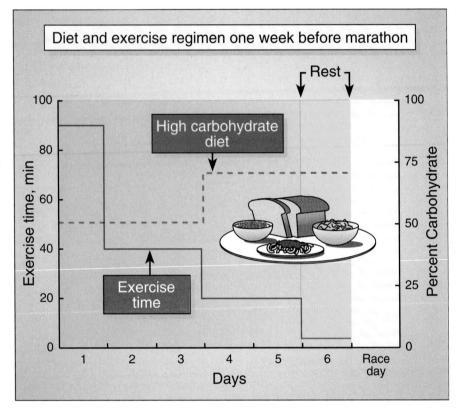

SUMMARY

PART 2

1. Within rather broad limits, the nutrient requirements of athletes and other individuals engaged in training programs can be achieved with a balanced diet.
2. With well-planned menus, the necessary vitamin, mineral, and protein requirements can be met with a food intake of about 1200 kcal a day. Additional food can then be consumed to meet the energy needs that fluctuate, depending on the daily level of physical activity.
3. For people who are physically active, 60% or more of the calories should come from carbohydrates, particularly polysaccharides. This will generally represent between 400 and 600 g on a daily basis.
4. Successive days of prolonged, hard training may gradually deplete the body's carbohydrate reserves, even if the recommended carbohydrate intake is maintained. This could lead to a "training staleness" because muscle glycogen may take several days to return to normal levels following a single session of prolonged exercise.
5. In all likelihood, the caloric requirements of athletes in the most strenuous sports do not exceed 4000 kcal per day unless body mass is considerable.

Such a high caloric intake usually supplies well above the RDA requirements for protein, vitamins, and minerals.

6. The pre-event meal should include foods that are readily digested and contribute to the energy and fluid requirements of exercise. For this reason, the meal should be high in carbohydrate and relatively low in lipid and protein.

7. Commercially prepared liquid meals offer a practical approach to pregame nutrition and caloric supplementation. These "meals" are well balanced in nutritive value, contribute to fluid needs, are absorbed rapidly, and leave practically no residue in the digestive tract.

8. Two or three hours should be sufficient time to permit digestion and absorption of the pre-event meal.

9. Many of the negative aspects of the classic carbohydrate loading sequence can be eliminated by following the less stringent, modified carbohydrate-loading dietary protocol.

SELECTED REFERENCES

Applegate, E.A.: Nutritional consideration for ultra-endurance performance. *Int. J. Sport Nutr.*, 2:118, 1991.

Bacharrach, D.W., et al.: Carbohydrate drinks and cycling performance. *J. Sports Med. Phys. Fitness.* 34:161, 1994.

Beek, E.J. van der.: Vitamin supplementation and physical exercise performance. In *Foods, Nutrition and Sports Performance.* Edited by C. Williams, and J. T. Devlin., London, E. and F. N. Spon, 1992.

Berning, J.R., et al.: The nutritional habits of young adolescent swimmers. *Int. J. Sport Nutr.*, 1:240, 1991.

Brouns, F., and Beckers, E.: Is the gut an athletic organ? *Sports Med.* 15:242, 1993.

Brownell, K.D., et al. (Eds.): *Eating, Body Weight, and Performance in Athletes.* Phila., Lea & Febiger, 1992.

Burke, L.M., et al.: Muscle glycogen storage after prolonged exercise: effect of the glycemic index on carbohydrate feedings. *J. Appl. Physiol.*, 1019, 1993.

Burke, L.M., et al.: Dietary intakes and food use groups of elite Australian male athletes. *Int. J. Sports Med.*, 1:378, 1991.

Burstein, R., et al: Glucose polymer ingestion-effect on fluid balance and glycemic state during a 4-d march. *Med. Sci. Sports Exerc.*, 26: 360, 1994.

Carter, J.E., and Gisolfi, C.V.: Fluid replacement during and after exercise in the heat. *Med. Sci. Sports Exerc.*, 21:532, 1989.

Coggan, A.R., and Coyle, E.F.: Carbohydrate ingestion during prolonged exercise: Effects on metabolism and performance. In *Exercise and Sport Science Reviews.*. Vol. 19. Edited by J. O. Holloszy. Baltimore, Williams & Wilkins, 1991.

Coggan, A.R., et al.: Plasma glucose kinetics in a well-trained cyclist fed glucose throughout exercise. *Int. J. Sport Nutr.*, 1:279, 1991.

Coyle, E.F., et al.: Introduction to physiology and nutrition for competitive sport. In: *Physiology and Nutrition for Competitive Sport.* (Eds) Lamb, D.R., et al. Volume 7. Cooper Publishing Group. Carmel, IN. 1994. Pg. xv.

Coyle, E. F., and Coyle, E.: Carbohydrates that speed recovery from training. *Phys. Sportsmed.*, 21:111, 1993.

Davis, J. M., et al.: Fluid availability of sports drinks differing in carbohydrate type and concentration. *Am. J. Clin. Nutr.*, 51:1504, 1990.

Deuster, P. A., et al.: Nutritional survey of highly trained women runners. *Am. J. Clin. Nutr.*, 44:954, 1986.

Eilmore, J. A.: Eating and weight disorders in the female athlete. *Int. J. Sport Nutr.*, 1:104, 1991.

Erp-Baart, A. M. J. van, et al.: Nationwide survey on nutritional habits in elite athletes, Part I. Energy, carbohydrate, protein, and fat intake. *Int. J. Sports Med.*, 10:53, 1989.

Felig, P., et al.: Hypoglycemia during prolonged exercise in normal men. *N. Engl. J. Med.*, 306:895, 1967.

Fujisawa, T., et al.: The effects of exercise on fructose absorption. *Am. J. Clin. Nutr.*, 58: 75, 1993.

Gisolfi, C.V., et al.: Intestinal water absorption from select carbohydrate solutions is humans. *J. Appl. Physiol.*, 7: 2142, 1992.

Grandjean, A. C.,: Macronutrient intakes of US athletes compared with the general population and recommendations made for athletes. *Am. J. Clin. Nutr.*, 49:1070, 1989.

Hargreaves, M., and Briggs, C. A. Effect of carbohydrate ingestion on exercise metabolism. *J. Appl. Physiol.*, 65:1553, 1988.

Hawley, J.A., et al., Carbohydrate, fluid, and electrolyte requirements of the soccer player: a review. *Int. J. Sports Med.*, 4: 221, 1994.

Hickson, J. F., Jr., and Wolinsky, I. (Eds.): *Nutrition in Exercise and Sport.* Boca Raton, FL, CRC Press, 1989.

Horowitz, J.F., and Coyle, E.F.: Metabolic responses to pre-exercise meals containing various carbohydrates and fats. *Am. J. Clin. Nutr.*, 58:235, 1993.

Kleiner, S. M., et al.: Metabolic profiles, diet, and health practices of championship male and female bodybuilders. *J. Am. Diet. Assoc.*, 90:962, 1990.

Kovisto, V. A., et al.: Glycogen depletion during prolonged exercise: influence of glucose, fructose, or placebo. *J. Appl. Physiol.*, 58:731, 1985.

Lindeman, A. K.: Eating for endurance or ultraendurance. *Phys. Sportsmed.*, 20:87, 1992.

Lugo, M., et al.: Metabolic responses when different forms of carbohydrate energy are consumed during cycling. *Int. J. Sports Nutr.*, 3: 398, 1993.

Maughan, R.: Physiology and nutrition for middle distance and long distance running. In: *Physiology and Nutrition for Competitive Sport.* (Eds) Lamb, D.R., et al. Volume 7. Cooper Publishing Group. Carmel, IN. 1994. Pg. 329.

Miles, D.S., et al.: Effect of dietary fiber on the metabolizable energy of human diets. *J. Nutr.*, 118:1075, 1988.

Mitchell, J. B., et al.: Effects of carbohydrate ingestion on gastric emptying and exercise performance. *Med. Sci. Sports Exerc.,* 20:110, 1988.

Murray, R., et al.: The effects of glucose, fructose, and sucrose ingestion during exercise. *Med. Sci. Sports Exerc.,* 21:275, 1989.

Rauch, L.H.G., et al.: The effects of carbohydrate loading on muscle glycogen content and cycling performance. *Int. J. Sports Nutr.,* 5: 25, 1995.

Reed, M. J., et al.: Muscle glycogen storage post-exercise: effect of mode of carbohydrate administration. *J. Appl. Physiol.,* 67:720, 1989.

Rokitzki, L., et al.: α-tocopherol supplementation in racing cyclists during extreme endurance training. *Int. J. Sports Nutr.,* 4: 255, 1994.

Sawka, M.N.: Physiological consequences of hypohydration: exercise performance and thermoregulation. *Med. Sci. Sports Exerc.,* 24:657, 1992.

Schedl, H.P., et al. Intestinal absorption during rest and exercise: implications for formulating an oral rehydration solution (ORS). *Med. Sci. Sports Exerc.,* 26: 267, 1994.

Scott, C. B., et al.: Effect of macronutrient composition of an energy-restrictive diet on maximal physical performance. *Med. Sci. Sports Exerc.,* 24:814, 1992.

Sherman, W. M., and Wimer, G. S.: Insufficient carbohydrate during training: does it impair performance? *Int. J. Sport Nutr.,* 1:28, 1991.

Sherman, W. M., et al.: Effect of exercise-diet manipulation on muscle glycogen and its subsequent utilization during performance. *Int. J. Sports Med.,* 1:114, 1981.

Sjodin, A.M., et al.: Energy balance in cross-country skiers: a study using doubly labeled water. *Med. Sci. Sports Exerc.,* 26: 720, 1994.

Sole, C. C., and Noakes, T. D.: Faster emptying for glucose-polymer and fructose solutions than for glucose in humans. *Eur. J. Appl. Physiol.* 58:605, 1989.

Tessier, F., et al.: Selenium and training effects on the glutathione system and aerobic performance. *Med. Sci. Sports Exerc.,* 27(3): 390, 1995.

Vist, G.E., and Maughn, R.J.: Gastric emptying of dilute glucose solutions in man. *Med. Sci. Sports Exerc.,* 22: S70, 1992.

Vist, G.E., and Maughn, R.J.: Gastric emptying of dilute glucose solutions in man; effect of beverage glucose concentration. *Med. Sci. Sports Exerc.,* 26: 1269, 1994.

Williams, C. and Devlin, J. T. (Eds.): *Foods, Nutrition and Sports Performance.* London, E. & F.N. Spon, 1992.

Wilmore, J. H.: Eating and weight disorders in the female athlete. *Int. J. Sport Nutr.,* 1:104, 1991.

Yaspelkis, B.B. III, and Ivy, J.L.: Effects of carbohydrate supplements and water on exercise metabolism in the heat. *J. Appl. Physiol.,* 71: 680, 1991.

THE PHYSIOLOGIC SUPPORT SYSTEMS

SECTION III

Most sport, recreational, and occupational activities require a moderately intense yet sustained energy release. This energy for the phosphorylation of ADP to ATP is provided by the aerobic breakdown of carbohydrates, lipids, and proteins. If a steady rate cannot be achieved between oxidative phosphorylation and the energy requirements of the activity, an anaerobic-aerobic energy imbalance develops, lactic acid accumulates, tissue acidity increases, and fatigue quickly develops. The ability to sustain a high level of physical activity without undue fatigue depends on two factors: (1) the capacity and integration of the various physiologic systems for oxygen delivery and (2) the capacity of the specific muscle cells to generate ATP aerobically.

Understanding the role of the ventilatory, circulatory, muscular, and endocrine systems during exercise enables us to appreciate individual differences in exercise capacity. Knowing the energy requirements of exercise and the corresponding physiologic adjustments to meet these requirements also provides a sound basis to develop a fitness program as well as to evaluate one's status before and during such a program.

The Pulmonary System and Exercise

After reading this chapter, you should be able to:

- Diagram the ventilatory system showing the glottis, trachea, bronchi, bronchioles, and alveoli.

- Discuss the process of inspiration and expiration at rest and during exercise.

- Define the term "Valsalva" and discuss the physiologic consequences of this maneuver.

- Describe what triggers exercise-induced asthma and the factors that modify its severity.

- Define the terms minute ventilation, alveolar ventilation, ventilation-perfusion ratio, and anatomic and physiologic dead space.

- Discuss the Bohr effect and its benefit during physical activity.

- List the means by which carbon dioxide is transported in the blood.

- Identify the major factors that regulate pulmonary ventilation at rest and during exercise.

- Describe how hyperventilation extends breath-holding time but could be dangerous in sport diving.

- Draw the relationship between ventilation, blood lactate, and oxygen uptake during incremental exercise indicating the point for the OBLA. What changes in the ventilatory equivalent can detect the OBLA?

Part 1 PULMONARY STRUCTURE AND FUNCTION

I f the oxygen supply of humans depended only on diffusion through the skin, it would be impossible to sustain the basal energy requirement, let alone the 3- to 4-liter gas exchange each minute necessary to run at a 5-minute per mile pace in a 26.2-mile marathon. Within the compact human body, the needs for gas exchange are met by the remarkably effective *ventilatory system*. This system, depicted in Figure 8-1, regulates the gaseous state of the body's "external" environment to provide aeration of body fluids of the "internal" environment during rest and exercise.

ANATOMY OF VENTILATION

The process by which ambient air is brought into and exchanged with the air in the lungs is termed pulmonary ventilation. Air entering through the nose and mouth flows into the conductive portion of the ventilatory system where it is adjusted to body temperature, filtered, and almost completely humidified as it passes through the *trachea*. This air-conditioning process continues as the inspired air passes into two *bronchi*, the large tubes that serve as primary conduits in each of the two lungs. The bronchi further subdivide into numerous *bronchioles* that conduct the inspired air through a tortuous, narrow route until it eventually mixes with the existing air in the *alveoli*, the terminal branches of the respiratory tract.

Lungs

The lungs provide the surface between the blood and the external environment. Although the lung volume varies between 4 and 6 liters (about the amount of air contained in a basketball), its moist surface area is considerable. The lungs of an average-sized person weigh about 1 kg, yet if spread out as in Figure 8-2, this tissue would cover a surface of 60 to 80 m². This is about 35 times greater than the surface of the person and would be sufficient to cover almost half a tennis court or an entire badminton court! The interface for the aeration of blood is considerable because during any second of maximal exercise, there is probably no more than 1 pint of blood in the fine network of blood vessels within the lung tissue.

Alveoli

There are more than 300 million alveoli. These elastic, thin-walled,

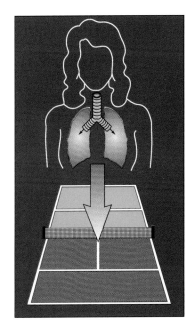

FIGURE 8-2. The lungs provide a large surface for gas exchange.

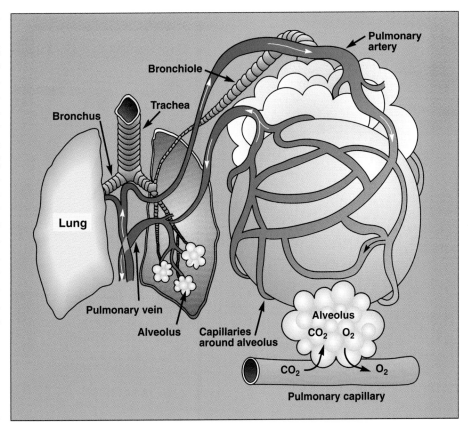

FIGURE 8-1. A general view of the ventilatory system that shows the respiratory passages, alveoli, and gas exchange function in an alveolus.

membranous sacs provide the vital surface for gas exchange between the lungs and the blood. Alveolar tissue has the largest blood supply of any organ in the body. Millions of short, thin-walled capillaries and alveoli lie side by side with air moving on one side and blood on the other. Diffusion occurs through the extremely thin barrier of these alveolar and capillary cells.

During each minute at rest, approximately 250 ml of oxygen leave the alveoli and enter the blood, and about 200 ml of carbon dioxide diffuse in the reverse direction into the alveoli. During heavy exercise in trained endurance athletes, about 20 times this quantity of oxygen is transferred across the alveolar membrane. *The primary function of ventilation during rest and exercise is to maintain a fairly constant, favorable concentration of oxygen and carbon dioxide in the alveolar chambers.*

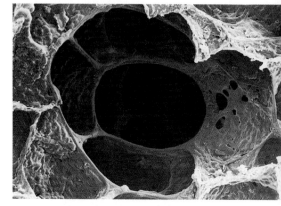

Looking down a human alveolar duct. The openings of the alveoli are framed by connective tissue.

This ensures effective gaseous exchange before the blood leaves the lungs to be transported throughout the body.

MECHANICS OF VENTILATION

Figure 8-3 illustrates the physical principle that underlies breathing.

Two lung-shaped balloons are suspended in a jar whose glass bottom has been replaced by a thin rubber membrane. The jar's volume increases when the membrane is pulled down, and the air pressure within the jar becomes less than the air outside the jar so air rushes in causing the balloons to inflate. Conversely, if the elastic membrane is allowed to recoil, the pressure in the jar temporarily increases and air rushes out. A considerable volume of air can be exchanged within the balloons in a given time period if the distance and rate of the descent and ascent of the rubber membrane are increased. This is essentially how ambient and alveolar air are exchanged in the lungs.

The lungs are not merely suspended in the chest cavity as in the example with the balloons. Rather the difference in pressure within the lungs and the lung-chest wall interface causes the lungs to adhere to the interior of the chest wall and literally follow its every movement. Thus any change in the volume of the thoracic cavity causes a corresponding change in lung

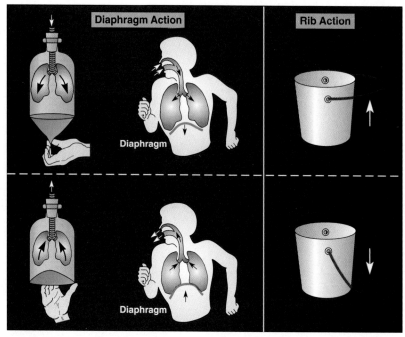

FIGURE 8-3. Mechanics of breathing. During *inspiration*, the chest cavity increases in size because of the raising of the ribs and lowering of the muscular diaphragm. During *exhalation*, the ribs swing down and the diaphragm returns to a relaxed position. This reduces the volume of the thoracic cavity and air rushes out. The movement of the jar's rubber bottom causes air to enter and leave the two balloons and simulates the action of the diaphragm. The movement of the bucket handle simulates the action of the ribs.

volume. The lungs depend on accessory means for altering their volume because they contain no muscles. Changes in lung volume during inspiration and expiration occur by the action of voluntary muscles.

Inspiration

A large dome-shaped sheet of muscle called the *diaphragm* serves the same purpose as the rubber membrane of the jar. This muscle makes an airtight separation between the abdominal and thoracic cavities. During *inspiration,* the diaphragm muscle contracts, flattens out, and moves downward toward the abdominal cavity by as much as 10 cm. This movement causes the chest cavity to enlarge and become more elongated. Consequently the air in the lungs expands, and its pressure, referred to as *intrapulmonic pressure,* becomes reduced slightly below atmospheric pressure. When this happens, air is literally sucked in through the nose and mouth, causing the lungs to inflate with air. The degree of filling depends on the magnitude of inspiratory movements. Inspiration is complete when thoracic cavity expansion ceases and intrapulmonic pressure increases to equal atmospheric pressure.

During exercise, the contraction of the *scaleni* and *external intercostal* muscles between the ribs causes the ribs to rotate and lift up and away from the body. This action is similar to the movement of the handle lifted up and away from the side of the bucket at the right in Figure 8-3. The descent of the diaphragm, the upward swing of the ribs, and the outward thrust of the sternum all cause the volume of the chest cavity to increase with a subsequent inhalation of ambient air.

Expiration

Expiration, the process of air movement from the lungs, is predominantly a passive process during rest and light intensity exercise. Expiration results from the recoil of the stretched lung tissue and the relaxation of the inspiratory muscles. This causes the sternum and ribs to swing down and the diaphragm to move back toward the thoracic cavity. These movements decrease the size of the chest cavity and compress alveolar gas so that air moves out through the respiratory tract into the atmosphere. During ventilation in moderate to heavy exercise, the internal intercostal muscles and abdominal muscles act powerfully on the ribs and abdominal cavity to cause a reduction in thoracic dimensions. Exhalation occurs more rapidly and to a greater depth in this way.

Valsalva Maneuver. During quiet breathing, the intrapulmonic pressure may fall only about 2 or 3 mm Hg during the inspiratory cycle and increase a similar amount above atmospheric pressure during exhalation. If, however, the *glottis* is closed following a full inspiration and the expiratory muscles are maximally activated, the compressive forces of exhalation can increase the intrathoracic pressure by more than 150 mm Hg above atmospheric pressure, with somewhat higher pressures generally noted within the abdominal cavity. This forced exhalation against a closed glottis, termed the *Valsalva maneuver,* commonly occurs in weightlifting and in other activities that require a rapid and maximum application of force for a short duration. The fixation of the abdominal and chest cavities with this maneuver probably enhances the action of muscles that are attached to the chest.

Physiologic Consequences of the Valsalva.

With the onset of the Valsalva maneuver at the start of lifting a heavy object (Fig. 8-4), blood pressure rises abruptly as the elevated intrathoracic pressure forces blood from the heart into the arterial system. Subsequently, because venous blood is under relatively low pressure, these veins are compressed, and blood flow is significantly reduced into the heart. A reduction in venous return and sub-

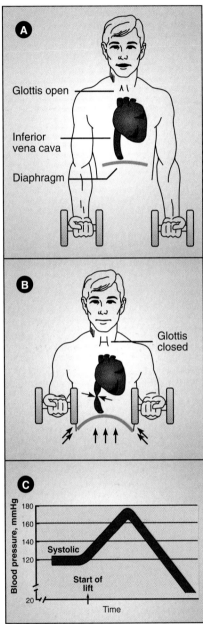

FIGURE 8-4. The Valsalva maneuver significantly reduces the return of blood to the heart. This occurs because the increase in intrathoracic pressure collapses the vein (inferior vena cava) that passes through the chest cavity. (*A*) Normal breathing. (*B*) Straining exercise with accompanying Valsalva. (*C*) Blood pressure response before and during straining-type exercise.

sequent fall in arterial blood pressure can diminish the blood supply to the brain and frequently produces dizziness, "spots before the eyes," and even fainting with straining-type exercises. Normal blood flow is re-established (with perhaps even an "overshoot" in flow) once the glottis is opened and intrathoracic pressure is released.

LUNG VOLUMES AND CAPACITIES

The various lung volume measures that reflect one's ability to increase the depth of breathing are illustrated in Figure 8-5. Average values for these volumes for men and women are also represented. The subject breathes from a calibrated recording spirometer used for measuring oxygen uptake

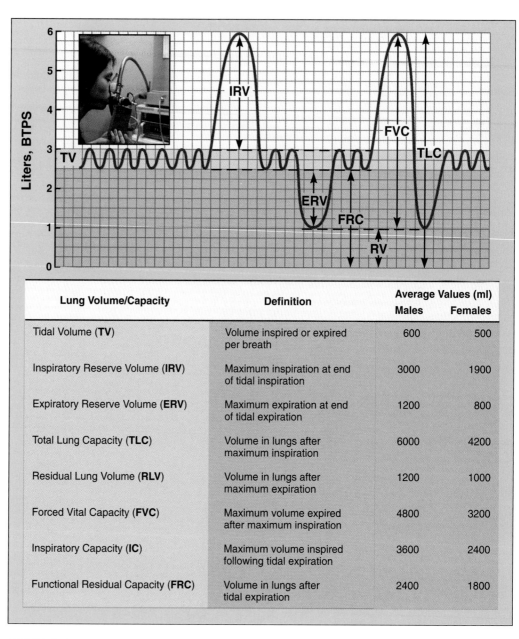

Lung Volume/Capacity	Definition	Average Values (ml)	
		Males	Females
Tidal Volume (**TV**)	Volume inspired or expired per breath	600	500
Inspiratory Reserve Volume (**IRV**)	Maximum inspiration at end of tidal inspiration	3000	1900
Expiratory Reserve Volume (**ERV**)	Maximum expiration at end of tidal expiration	1200	800
Total Lung Capacity (**TLC**)	Volume in lungs after maximum inspiration	6000	4200
Residual Lung Volume (**RLV**)	Volume in lungs after maximum expiration	1200	1000
Forced Vital Capacity (**FVC**)	Maximum volume expired after maximum inspiration	4800	3200
Inspiratory Capacity (**IC**)	Maximum volume inspired following tidal expiration	3600	2400
Functional Residual Capacity (**FRC**)	Volume in lungs after tidal expiration	2400	1800

FIGURE 8-5. Static measures of lung volume.

by the closed-circuit method (Chapter 4).

Static Lung Volumes

The bell of the spirometer falls and subsequently rises as air is inhaled and exhaled from it. This provides a record of the ventilatory volume and breathing rate. The volume of air moved during either the inspiratory or expiratory phase of each breath is termed *tidal volume (TV)*. The TV for healthy men and women under resting conditions usually ranges between 0.4 and 1.0 liters of air per breath.

After several tracings are recorded for TV, the subject breathes in normally and then inspires as deeply as possible. This additional volume of about 2.5 to 3.5 liters above the inspired tidal air represents a reserve for inhalation and is termed the *inspiratory reserve volume (IRV)*. After measuring the IRV, the normal breathing pattern is once again established. Following a normal exhalation, the subject continues to exhale and forces as much air as possible from the lungs. This additional volume is the *expiratory reserve volume (ERV);* it ranges between 1.0 and 1.5 liters for an average-sized man. During exercise, there is a considerable increase in TV because of the encroachment on both inspiratory and expiratory reserve volumes, particularly the inspiratory volume.

The total volume of air that can be voluntarily moved in one breath, from full inspiration to maximum expiration, or vice versa, is termed the *forced vital capacity (FVC)*. Although values for FVC vary considerably with body size and body position during the measurement, average values are usually 4 to 5 liters in healthy young men and 3 to 4 liters in healthy young women. FVCs of 6 to 7 liters are not uncommon for tall individuals, and a value of 7.6 liters has been reported for a professional football player and 8.1 liters for an Olympic gold medal-

ist in cross-country skiing. The large lung volumes of some athletes probably reflect genetic influences because static lung volumes *do not* change appreciably with training.

Residual Lung Volume. After a forced, maximal exhalation, there still is a volume of air remaining in the lungs that cannot be expelled. This volume is referred to as the *residual lung volume (RLV)*; it averages between 1.0 and 1.2 liters for women and 1.2 and 1.4 liters for men. RLV tends to increase with age, but the IRV and ERV become proportionally smaller.

Changes in the various lung volumes with aging are generally attributed to a decrease in the elastic components of the lung tissue and a decline in pulmonary muscle power. These factors, however, are probably not entirely an aging phenomenon per se. Recent evidence indicates that endurance training in older athletes may slow the decline in lung functions associated with aging.

Dynamic Lung Volumes

Dynamic ventilation depends on two factors: the volume of air moved per breath and the speed at which this air can be moved.

The speed of airflow depends on the resistance offered by the respiratory passages to the smooth flow of air as well as the resistance offered by the chest and lung tissue to a change in shape during breathing.

FEV-to-FVC Ratio. Normal values for vital capacity can be achieved even with severe lung disease if no time limit is placed on the ventilatory maneuver. For this reason, physicians usually obtain a more "dynamic" measure of lung function, such as the percentage of the FVC that can be expired in 1 second. This measure, termed *forced expiratory volume-to-forced vital capacity ratio ($FEV_{1.0}$/FVC)*, provides an indication of expiratory power and

Glottis. The glottis is the narrowest part of the larynx where air passes into and out of the trachea. Normally, its action covers the trachea during swallowing to prevent food from entering the "windpipe."

Evaluating lung volumes. Lung volumes vary with age, gender, and body size, especially stature. For this reason, these factors must be considered when comparing lung volumes among individuals.

An impressive system. Pulmonary reserve is so great that when lung disease is present, patients rarely show symptoms of distress until a large part of their ventilatory capacity is lost. In fact, distance running can be engagd in regularly and successfully even in the presence of mild airway obstruction.

ity to sustain high levels of submaximal ventilation. For example, 20 weeks of regular run training improved the ventilatory muscle endurance approximately 16% in healthy adult men and women. Less lactic acid was produced during submaximal breathing exercise, probably because of the increase in the aerobic enzyme levels of the ventilatory muscles that occurred with endurance training. This would reduce the feeling of "breathlessness" and pulmonary discomfort frequently observed in untrained persons who perform prolonged submaximal exercise.

PULMONARY VENTILATION

Minute Ventilation

During quiet breathing at rest, the breathing rate averages 12 breaths per minute, whereas the tidal volume averages about 0.5 liter of air per breath. Under these conditions, the volume of air breathed each minute, or *minute ventilation* ($\dot{V}_E$), is 6 liters.

$$\text{Minute ventilation } (\dot{V}_E) = \text{Breathing rate x Tidal volume}$$
$$6 \text{ liters} \cdot \text{min}^{-1} = 12 \times 0.5 \text{ liter}$$

Significant increases in minute ventilation result from an increase in either the depth or rate of breathing or both. During strenuous exercise, the breathing rate of healthy young adults usually increases to 35 to 45 breaths per minute, although elite athletes achieve rates as high as 60 to 70 breaths per minute during maximal exercise. Tidal volumes of 2.0 liters and larger are also common during maximal exercise. Consequently, with increases in breathing rate and tidal volume, the minute ventilation in adults can easily reach 100 liters or about 17 times the resting value. In well-trained male endurance athletes, ventilation may increase to 160 liters per minute during maximal exercise. In fact, ventilation volumes of 200 liters per minute

have been reported in several research studies, and a high of 208 liters was observed for a professional football player during maximal exercise. *Even with these large minute ventilations, the tidal volume rarely exceeds 55 to 65% of the vital capacity for both trained and untrained individuals.*

Alveolar Ventilation

Alveolar ventilation refers to that portion of the minute ventilation that enters into and mixes with the air in the alveolar chambers. A portion of the air breathed during inspiration does not enter the alveoli and thus is not involved in gaseous exchange with the blood. This air that fills the nose, mouth, trachea, and other nondiffusible conducting portions of the respiratory tract is contained within the *anatomic dead space.* In healthy people, this volume averages 150 to 200 ml or about 30% of the resting tidal volume. The composition of dead-space air is almost identical to that of ambient air except that it is fully saturated with water vapor.

Because of the dead-space volume, approximately 350 ml of the 500 ml of ambient air inspired in the tidal volume at rest enters into and mixes with the existing alveolar air. This does not mean that only 350 ml of air enter and leave the alveoli with each breath. On the contrary, if the tidal volume is 500 ml, 500 ml of air enter the alveoli but only 350 ml is fresh air. This represents about one-seventh of the total air in the alveoli. Such a relatively small, seemingly inefficient alveolar ventilation prevents drastic changes in the composition of alveolar air and ensures a consistency in arterial blood gases throughout the entire breathing cycle.

The minute ventilation does not always reflect the actual alveolar ventilation. This is shown in Table 8-2. In the first example of shallow breathing, the tidal volume is reduced to 150 ml, yet it is still possible to achieve a 6-liter per minute ventilation if the breathing rate is increased to 40 breaths per minute. The same 6-liter minute volume can also be achieved by decreasing the breathing rate to 12 breaths per minute and increasing the tidal volume to 500 ml. By doubling tidal volume and halving the ventilatory rate, as in the example of deep breathing, the 6-liter minute ventilation is again achieved. Each of these ventilatory adjustments, however, drastically affects alveolar ventilation. In the example of shallow breathing, all that has been moved is the dead-space air: No alveolar ventilation has taken place. In the other examples, the breathing is deeper, and a larger portion of each breath enters into and mixes with the existing alveolar air. *It is this alveolar ventilation that determines the gaseous concentrations at the alveolar-capillary membrane.*

Dead Space Versus Tidal Volume. The preceding examples for alveolar ventilation were oversimplified because a constant dead space was assumed despite changes in tidal volume. Actually, the anatomic dead space increases somewhat as tidal volume becomes larger as a result of some stretching of the respiratory passages with a fuller inspiration. This increase in dead space is still proportionately less than the increase in tidal volume. Consequently deeper breathing provides for more effective alveolar ventilation than does similar minute ventilation achieved only through an increase in breathing rate.

Ventilation-Perfusion Ratio. Adequate gas exchange between the alveoli and the blood requires ventilation that is well matched to the quantity of blood perfusing the pulmonary capillaries. For example, at rest approximately 4.2 liters of air ventilate the alveoli each minute, whereas an average of 5.0 liters of blood flow through the pulmonary capillaries. In this instance, the ratio of alveolar ventilation to pulmonary blood flow, termed the *ventilation-perfusion ratio,* is approximately 0.8 (4.2 ÷ 5.0). This ratio means that each liter of pulmonary blood is matched by an alveolar ventilation of 0.8 liter. In light exercise, the ventilation-perfusion ratio is maintained at about 0.8, whereas in heavy exercise, there is a disproportionate increase in alveolar ventilation. For healthy subjects, the ventilation-perfusion ratio may increase above 5.0 to ensure adequate aeration of the blood returning in the venous circulation.

Physiologic Dead Space. In certain instances, a portion of the alveoli may not function adequately in gas exchange due to either an underperfusion of blood or an inadequate ventilation relative to the size of the alveoli. This portion of the

Warm-up benefits. Light warm-up exercise is beneficial to the asthmatic because it puts the broncho-sensitive individual in a "refractory period" where the subsequent intense exercise may not trigger bronchoconstriction. This benefit may last up to 2 hours.

Post-Exercise Coughing. Exercise is frequently associated with dryness in the throat and coughing during the recovery period. This is common after exercise in cold weather. The phenomenon of post-exercise coughing is directly related to the overall rate of water loss from the respiratory tract (rather than respiratory heat loss) associated with the large ventilatory volumes during exercise.a

TABLE 8-2. Relationship between tidal volume, breathing rate, and both minute and alveolar ventilation

Condition	Tidal Volume (ml)	x	Breathing Rate (breaths · min^{-1})	=	Minute Ventilation (ml · min^{-1})	−	Dead Space Ventilation (ml · min^{-1})	=	Alveolar Ventilation (ml · min^{-1})
Shallow breathing	150		40		6000		(150 ml x 40)		0
Normal breathing	5000		12		6000		(150 ml x 12)		4200
Deep breathing	1000		6		6000		(150 ml x 6)		5100

alveolar volume with a poor ventilation-perfusion ratio is termed the *physiologic dead space*. As illustrated in Figure 8-6, the physiologic dead space in the healthy lung is small and can be considered negligible.

Physiologic dead space, however, can increase to as much as 50% of the tidal volume. This occurs with inadequate perfusion during hemorrhage or blockage of the pulmonary circulation with an embolism or with inadequate alveolar ventilation that occurs in emphysema, asthma, and pulmonary fibrosis. Adequate gas exchange becomes impossible when the total dead space of the lung exceeds 60% of the lung volume.

Depth versus Rate. Alveolar ventilation during increasing intensities of exercise is maintained through an increase in both the rate and depth of breathing. In moderate exercise, well-trained athletes achieve adequate alveolar ventilation by increasing tidal volume with only a small increase in breathing rate. With deeper breathing, alveolar ventilation may increase from 70% of the minute ventilation at rest to over 85% of the total exercise ventilation Figure 8-7 shows that the increase in tidal volume in exercise is due largely to encroachment on the inspiratory reserve volume with an accompanying but smaller decrease in the end-expiratory level. With more intense exercise, increases in tidal volume begin to plateau at about 60% of vital capacity, and minute ventilation is further increased through an increase in breathing frequency. These adjustments occur unconsciously; each individual develops a "style" of breathing in which the respiratory frequency and tidal volume are blended to provide effective alveolar ventilation. Conscious attempts to modify breathing during general physical activities such as running are usually doomed to failure and probably are of no benefit in terms of performance. In fact, conscious manipulation of breathing would be detrimental to the exquisitely regulated physiologic adjustments to exercise. *At rest and in exercise, each individual should breathe in the manner that seems most natural.*

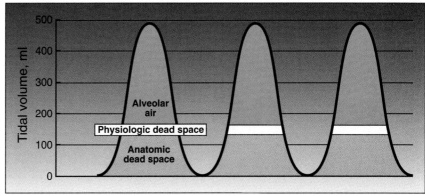

FIGURE 8-6. Distribution of tidal volume in a healthy subject at rest. Tidal volume includes about 350 ml of ambient air that mixes with alveolar air, 150 ml of air in the larger air passages (anatomic dead space), and a small portion of air distributed to either poorly ventilated or poorly perfused alveoli (physiologic dead space).

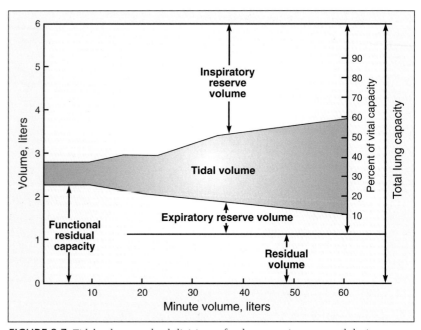

FIGURE 8-7. Tidal volume and subdivisions of pulmonary air at rest and during exercise. (Adapted from Lambertsen, C.J.: Physical and mechanical aspects of respiration. In *Medical Physiology*. Edited by V.B. Mountcastle. St. Louis, C.V. Mosby Co., 1968.)

PART 1

1. The lungs provide a large interface between the body's internal fluid environment and the gaseous external environment. At any one second, there is probably no more than a pint of blood in the pulmonary capillaries.

2. Pulmonary ventilation is geared to maintain favorable concentrations of alveolar oxygen and carbon dioxide to ensure adequate aeration of the blood flowing through the lungs.

3. Pulmonary airflow depends on small pressure differences between ambient air and air within the lungs. These differences are brought about by the action of various muscles that act to alter the dimensions of the chest cavity.

4. A forced exhalation against a closed glottis is called a Valsalva maneuver. It can cause a large increase in pressure within the chest and abdominal cavities that compresses the thoracic veins, thereby significantly reducing venous return to the heart.

5. Lung volumes vary with age, gender, and body size, especially stature, and should be evaluated only in relation to norms based on these factors.

6. Tidal volume is increased during exercise by encroachment on both the inspiratory and the expiratory reserve volumes. Even when a person breathes to vital capacity, air still remains in the lungs at maximal exhalation. This residual lung volume allows for an uninterrupted exchange of gas during all phases of the breathing cycle.

7. Forced expiratory volume in 1 second and maximum voluntary ventilation give a dynamic picture of one's ability to sustain high levels of airflow. They serve as excellent screening tests to detect possible lung disease.

8. Tests of static and dynamic lung function are of little use in predicting fitness and exercise performance, provided that the values fall within a normal range.

9. Exercise-induced bronchospasm is an obstructive phenomenon that depends on both the rate and magnitude of airway cooling and subsequent rewarming. This response is essentially eliminated when humidified air is breathed during the exercise task.

10. Minute ventilation is a function of breathing rate and tidal volume. It averages 6 to 10 liters at rest, whereas in maximum exercise, increases in breathing rate and depth may produce ventilations as high as 200 liters per minute.

11. Alveolar ventilation is the portion of the minute ventilation that enters the alveoli and is involved in gaseous exchange with the blood.

12. The ratio of alveolar ventilation to pulmonary blood flow is termed the ventilation-perfusion ratio. At rest and in light exercise, this ratio is maintained at about 0.8. This indicates that each liter of pulmonary blood is matched by an alveolar ventilation of 0.8 liters. In heavy exercise, alveolar ventilation in healthy individuals increases disproportionately, and the ratio may reach 5.0.

13. At rest and in exercise, a healthy person has his or her own breathing style. It is futile to try to coach individuals to breathe differently than their own style.

Our supply of oxygen depends on the oxygen concentration in ambient air and its pressure. Ambient or atmospheric air remains relatively constant in terms of composition. It is composed of approximately 20.93% oxygen, 79.04% nitrogen (this includes small quantities of other inert gases that behave physiologically like nitrogen), 0.03% carbon dioxide, and usually small quantities of water vapor. The gas molecules move at relatively great speeds and exert a pressure against any surface with which they come in contact. At sea level, the pressure of the gas molecules in air is sufficient to raise a column of mercury to a height of 760 mm, or 29.9 inches. These barometric readings vary somewhat with changing weather conditions and are considerably lower at higher altitude.

. . . .

RESPIRED GASES: CONCENTRATIONS AND PARTIAL PRESSURES

The molecules of a specific gas in a mixture of gases exert their own *partial pressure*. The total pressure of the mixture is the sum of the partial pressures of the individual gases. Partial pressure is computed as:

$$\textbf{Partial Pressure = Percent concentration x Total pressure of gas mixture}$$

Ambient Air

The volume, percentage, and partial pressure of the gases in dry, ambient air at sea level are presented in Table 8-3. The partial pressure of oxygen is 20.93% of the total pressure of 760 mm Hg exerted by air, or 159 mm Hg (0.2093 x 760 mm Hg); the random movement of the minute quantity of carbon dioxide exerts a pressure of only 0.2 mm Hg (0.0003 x 760 mm Hg), whereas nitrogen molecules exert a pressure that would raise the mercury in a manometer about 600 mm (0.7904 x 760 mm Hg). Partial pressure is usually denoted by a *P* in front of the gas symbol; in ambient air at sea level, the Po_2 is 159 mm Hg, for Pco_2 it is 0.2 mm Hg, and for Pn_2 it is 600 mm Hg.

Tracheal Air

As air enters the nose and mouth and passes down the respiratory tract, it becomes completely saturated with water vapor. This vapor dilutes the inspired air mixture somewhat. At a body temperature of 37°C, for example, the pressure of water molecules in humidified air is 47 mm Hg; this leaves 713 mm Hg (760–47) as the total pressure exerted by the inspired dry air molecules. Consequently, the effective Po_2 in tracheal air is lowered by about 10 mm Hg from its ambient value of 159 mm Hg to 149 mm Hg (0.2093[760–47 mm Hg]). Because carbon dioxide is almost negligible in inspired air, the humidification process has little effect on the inspired Pco_2.

Alveolar Air

The composition of alveolar air differs considerably from the incoming breath of moist ambient air because

TABLE 8-3. Partial pressure and volume of the gases in dry ambient air at sea level

Gas	Percentage	Partial Pressure (at 760 mm Hg)	Volume of Gas (ml · l⁻¹)
Oxygen	20.93	159 mm Hg	209.3
Carbon dioxide	0.03	0.2 mm Hg	0.4
Nitrogen	79.04[a]	600 mm Hg	790.3

[a] Includes 0.93% argon and other trace rare gases.

carbon dioxide is continually entering the alveoli from the blood, whereas oxygen is leaving the lungs to be carried throughout the body. Table 8-4 shows that alveolar air contains approximately 14.5% oxygen, 5.5% carbon dioxide, and about 80.0% nitrogen.

After subtracting the vapor pressure of moist alveolar gas, the average alveolar P_{O_2} is 103 mm Hg (0.145 [760–47 mm Hg]) and 39 mm Hg (0.055 [760–47 mm Hg]) for P_{CO_2}. *These values represent the average pressures exerted by oxygen and carbon dioxide molecules against the alveolar side of the alveolar-capillary membrane.* They are not physiologic constants but vary somewhat with the phase of the ventilatory cycle as well as with the adequacy of ventilation in various portions of the lung. Recall that a relatively large volume of air remains in the lungs after each normal exhalation. This functional residual capacity serves as a damper so each incoming breath of air has only a small effect on the composition of alveolar air. In the alveoli, therefore, the partial pressure of gases remains relatively stable.

· · · · · · · · · · · · · · ·

MOVEMENT OF GAS IN AIR AND FLUIDS

In accord with *Henry's law*, the amount of gas that dissolves in a fluid is a function of two factors: the *pressure* of the gas above the fluid and the *solubility* of the gas in the fluid.

Pressure

Oxygen molecules continually strike the surface of the water in the three chambers illustrated in Figure 8-8. Because the pure water in container A contains no oxygen, a large number of oxygen molecules enter the water and

TABLE 8-4. Partial pressure and volume of alveolar gases at sea level (37°C)

Gas	Percentage	Partial Pressure (at 760–47 mm Hg)	Volume of Gas (ml · l⁻¹)
Oxygen	14.5	103 mm Hg	145
Carbon dioxide	5.5	39 mm Hg	55
Nitrogen	80.0	571 mm Hg	800
Water Vapor		47 mm Hg	

become dissolved. Because dissolved gas molecules are also in random motion, some oxygen molecules leave the water. In chamber B, the net movement of oxygen is still into the fluid from the gaseous state. Eventually, the number of molecules entering and leaving the fluid becomes equal as in chamber C. When this occurs, the gas pressures are in equilibrium, and there is no net diffusion of oxygen. Conversely, if the pressure of dissolved oxygen molecules exceeds the pressure of the gas in the air, oxygen leaves the fluid until a new pressure equilibrium is reached.

Solubility

For two different gases at identical pressures, the number of molecules moving into or out of a fluid is determined by the solubility of each gas. For each unit of pressure favoring dif-

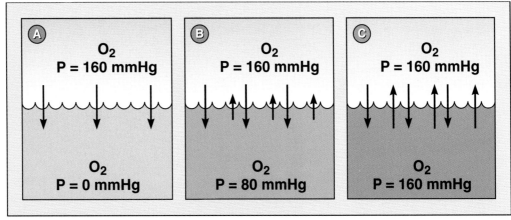

FIGURE 8-8. Solution of oxygen in water: (*A*) When oxygen first comes in contact with pure water. (*B*) After the dissolved oxygen is halfway to equilibrium with gaseous oxygen. (*C*) Equilibrium is established between the oxygen in air and water.

fusion, approximately 25 times more carbon dioxide than oxygen will move into (or from) a fluid. Viewed another way, equal quantities of oxygen and carbon dioxide will enter or leave a fluid under significantly different pressure gradients for each gas. This is precisely what takes place in the body.

· · · · · · · · · · · · · · ·

GAS EXCHANGE

The exchange of gases between the lungs and the blood as well as their movement at the tissue level is due entirely to the passive process of diffusion. Figure 8-9 illustrates the pressure gradients favoring gas transfer in the body.

In the Lungs

At rest, the pressure of oxygen molecules in the alveoli is about 60 mm Hg greater than in the venous blood that enters the pulmonary capillaries. Consequently oxygen dissolves and

diffuses through the alveolar membrane *into* the blood. Carbon dioxide exists under a slightly greater pressure in returning venous blood than it does in the alveoli. Thus there is net diffusion of carbon dioxide *from* the blood into the lungs. Although the pressure gradient of 6 mm Hg for carbon dioxide diffusion is small compared with that for oxygen, adequate transfer of this gas is achieved rapidly as a result of its high solubility. Nitrogen, which is neither utilized nor produced in metabolic reactions, remains essentially unchanged in alveolar-capillary gas.

Even during intense exercise in most individuals, the speed at which red blood cells pass through the pulmonary capillaries does not increase by more than 50% of the speed at rest. An important reason for this is that with increasing exercise intensity, the pulmonary capillaries can increase the volume of blood contained within them to about three times the resting value. Thus the velocity of pulmonary blood flow during exercise does not compromise its aeration. As a result, blood leaving the lungs to be delivered throughout the body contains oxygen at a pressure of approximately 100 mm Hg and carbon dioxide at 40 mm Hg; these values do not change much during vigorous exercise.

In the Tissues

In the tissues where oxygen is consumed in energy metabolism and an almost equal amount of carbon dioxide is produced, gas pressures can differ considerably from those in arterial blood. At rest, the average P_{O_2} in the fluid immediately outside a muscle cell rarely drops below 40 mm Hg, and the cellular P_{CO_2} averages about 46 mm Hg. In heavy exercise, however, the pressure of oxygen molecules in the mus-

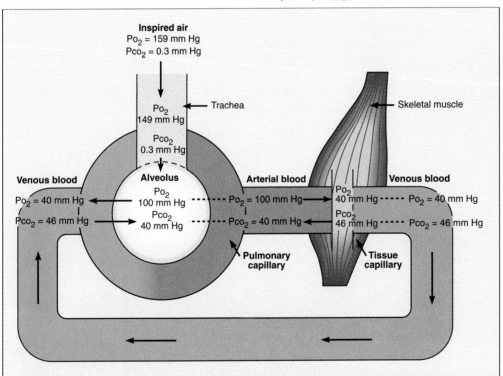

FIGURE 8-9. Pressure gradients for gas transfer in the body at rest. Indicated are the P_{O_2} and P_{CO_2} of ambient, tracheal, and alveolar air as well as these gas pressures in venous and arterial blood and muscle. Movement of gases at the alveolar-capillary and tissue-capillary membranes is always from an area of higher partial pressure to one of lower partial pressure. (From Mathews, D.K., and Fox, E.L.: *The Physiological Basis of Physical Education and Athletics.* Philadelphia. W.B. Saunders Co., 1976.)

> **Gas exchange occurs rapidly.** The process of diffusion in the healthy lung is so rapid that an equilibrium of blood gas with alveolar gas takes less than 1 second, or at about the midpoint of the blood's transit through the lungs.

cle tissue may fall to about 3 mm Hg, whereas the pressure of carbon dioxide approaches 90 mm Hg. The pressure differences between gases in the plasma and tissues establishes the gradients for diffusion. Oxygen leaves the blood and diffuses toward the metabolizing cell, while carbon dioxide flows from the cell to the blood. The blood then passes into the veins and is returned to the heart to be pumped to the lungs. As the blood enters the dense capillary network of the lungs, diffusion rapidly begins once again.

If it were not for our capacity to breathe, some average pressure would be reached between alveolar and blood gases, and diffusion would cease. By bringing in another breath of air, however, the oxygen content of the alveoli is increased, whereas the carbon dioxide content is diluted. By adjusting alveolar ventilation to metabolic demands, the composition of alveolar gas remains remarkably constant, even during strenuous exercise that increases oxygen uptake and carbon dioxide output as much as 25 times.

Not all CO_2 is "bad." The body does not attempt to rid itself completely of carbon dioxide. On the contrary, as the blood leaves the lungs with a Pco_2 of 40 mm Hg, it still contains about 50 ml of carbon dioxide in each 100 ml of blood. This "background level" of carbon dioxide is vital because it provides a chemical signal for the control of breathing through its effect on the respiratory center in the medulla.

SUMMARY

PART 2

1. The partial pressure of a specific gas in a mixture of gases is proportional to the concentration of the gas and the total pressure exerted by the mixture.

2. The quantity of gas that dissolves in a fluid is determined by pressure and solubility. Because carbon dioxide is about 25 times more soluble in plasma than oxygen, large amounts of this gas move into and out of body fluids down a relatively small diffusion or pressure gradient.

3. In the lungs and tissues, gas molecules diffuse down their concentration gradients from an area of higher concentration or higher pressure to one of lower concentration or lower pressure.

4. At rest and during increasing intensities of exercise, adjustments in alveolar ventilation occur so the composition of alveolar gas remains constant. Oxygen pressure is maintained at about 100 mm Hg, and carbon dioxide pressure is maintained at about 40 mm Hg. Because venous blood contains oxygen at lower and carbon dioxide at higher pressure than alveolar gases, oxygen diffuses into the blood, and carbon dioxide diffuses into the lungs.

5. Gas exchange is so rapid in the healthy lung that equilibrium occurs at about the midpoint of the blood's transit through the pulmonary capillaries. Even with vigorous exercise, the velocity of blood flow through the lungs generally does not restrict the full loading of oxygen and unloading of carbon dioxide.

6. At the tissues, the diffusion gradient favors the movement of oxygen from the capillary to the tissues and carbon dioxide from the cells into the blood. In exercise, these gradients are expanded, and oxygen and carbon dioxide diffuse rapidly.

OXYGEN TRANSPORT IN THE BLOOD

Oxygen is carried in the blood in two ways:

- In physical solution: Dissolved in the fluid portion of the blood
- Combined with hemoglobin: In loose combination with the iron-protein hemoglobin molecule in the red blood cell.

In Physical Solution

Oxygen is not particularly soluble in fluids. In fact, at an alveolar Po_2 of 100 mm Hg only about 0.3 ml of gaseous oxygen dissolves in each 100 ml of plasma; this is equivalent to 3 ml of oxygen per liter of plasma. Because the average blood volume is about 5 liters, 15 ml of oxygen are carried dissolved in the fluid portion of the blood (3 ml per liter x 5). This is enough oxygen to sustain life for about four seconds. Viewed from a somewhat different perspective, if oxygen alone in physical solution were available to the body, about 80 liters of blood would have to be circulated each minute simply to supply the resting oxygen requirements. This rate is about two times higher than the maximum blood flow ever recorded for an exercising human!

The small quantity of oxygen transported in physical solution, however, does serve several important physiologic functions. The random movement of dissolved oxygen molecules establishes the Po_2 of the blood and tissue fluids. This pressure of dissolved oxygen plays a role in the regulation of breathing; it also determines the loading of hemoglobin with oxygen in the lungs and its subsequent unloading in the tissues.

Combined with Hemoglobin

Metallic compounds are present in the blood of many species of animals and serve to augment the blood's oxygen-carrying capacity. In humans, this compound is *hemoglobin,* an iron-containing protein pigment. Hemoglobin, a main component of the body's 25 trillion red blood cells, increases the blood's oxygen-carrying capacity 65 to 70 times above that normally dissolved in plasma. Thus, for each liter of blood, about 197 ml of oxygen are temporarily "captured" by hemoglobin. Each of the four iron atoms in the hemoglobin molecule can loosely bind one molecule of oxygen in the reversible reaction:

$$Hb_4 + 4O_2 \longrightarrow Hb_4O_8$$

This "oxygenation" reaction requires no enzymes, and it occurs without a change in the valance of Fe^{++}, which would occur in the more permanent process of oxidation. The oxygenation of hemoglobin to oxyhemoglobin depends entirely on the partial pressure of oxygen in solution.

Oxygen-Carrying Capacity of Hemoglobin. In men, there are approximately 15 to 16 g of hemoglobin in each 100 ml of blood. The value is between 5 and 10% less for women and averages about 14 g per 100 ml of blood. This apparent gender difference accounts to some degree for the lower aerobic capacity of women, even after considering differences in body mass and body fat.

Each gram of hemoglobin can combine loosely with 1.34 ml of oxygen. Thus if the hemoglobin content of the

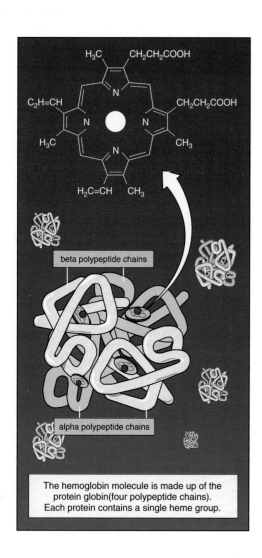

The hemoglobin molecule is made up of the protein globin(four polypeptide chains). Each protein contains a single heme group.

blood is known, its oxygen-carrying capacity can be calculated as follows:

oxygen are carried in each 100 ml of blood leaving the lungs; 19.7 ml are

$$\text{Blood's oxygen capacity} = \frac{\text{Hemoglobin}}{\text{g} \cdot 100 \text{ ml}^{-1} \text{ blood}} \times \text{Oxygen capacity of hemoglobin}$$

On average, approximately 20 ml of oxygen would be carried with the hemoglobin in each 100 ml of blood when the hemoglobin is fully saturated with oxygen; that is, when all the hemoglobin is converted to Hb_4O_8.

Po$_2$ and Hemoglobin Saturation. Thus far, it has been assumed that hemoglobin becomes fully saturated with oxygen when exposed to alveolar gas. Figure 8-10 illustrates the *oxyhemoglobin dissociation curve* that shows the saturation of hemoglobin with oxygen at various Po$_2$ values, including that of normal alveolar-capillary gas (Po$_2$ = 100 mm Hg).

Shown on the right ordinate of this dissociation curve is the quantity of oxygen carried in each 100 ml of normal blood at a particular plasma Po$_2$. Percent saturation of hemoglobin (Hb) is calculated as follows:

bound to hemoglobin, and 0.3 ml are dissolved in plasma. The percentage composition of centrifuged whole blood for plasma and red blood cells (hematocrit) as well as representative values for the quantity of oxygen carried in each component is shown in Figure 8-11.

Figure 8-10 also shows that the saturation of hemoglobin changes little until the pressure of oxygen falls to about 60 mm Hg. The flat, upper portion of the oxyhemoglobin curve provides a margin of safety to ensure that the blood is adequately loaded with oxygen. Even if the alveolar Po$_2$ is reduced to 75 mm Hg, as could occur with certain lung diseases or when one travels to a higher altitude, the saturation of hemoglobin is only lowered about 6%. At an alveolar Po$_2$ of 60 mm Hg, hemoglobin is still 90% saturated with oxygen. Below this

$$\text{Percent saturation} = [\text{O}_2 \text{ combined with Hb} \div \text{O}_2 \text{ capacity of Hb}] \times 100$$

Po$_2$ in the Lungs. Hemoglobin is about 98% saturated with oxygen at the normal alveolar Po$_2$ of 100 mm Hg. By applying this partial pressure value to the right ordinate of Figure 8-10, it can be seen that for each 100 ml of blood leaving the lungs, hemoglobin carries about 19.7 ml of oxygen. Clearly, any additional increase in alveolar Po$_2$ contributes little to the quantity of oxygen already combined with hemoglobin. In addition to the oxygen bound to hemoglobin, the plasma of each 100 ml of arterial blood contains about 0.3 ml of oxygen in solution. Thus for healthy individuals who breathe ambient air at sea level, approximately 20.0 ml of

pressure, however, the quantity of oxygen that will combine with hemoglobin drops sharply.

Po$_2$ in the Tissues. At rest, the Po$_2$ in the cell fluids is approximately 40 mm Hg. Dissolved oxygen from the plasma diffuses across the capillary membrane through the tissue fluids into the cells. This reduces the plasma Po$_2$ below the Po$_2$ in the red blood cell, and hemoglobin is unable to maintain its high oxygen saturation. The released oxygen ($HbO_2 \longrightarrow Hb + O_2$) moves out of the blood cells through the capillary membrane and into the tissues.

At the tissue-capillary Po$_2$ at rest (Po$_2$= 40 mm Hg), hemoglobin holds

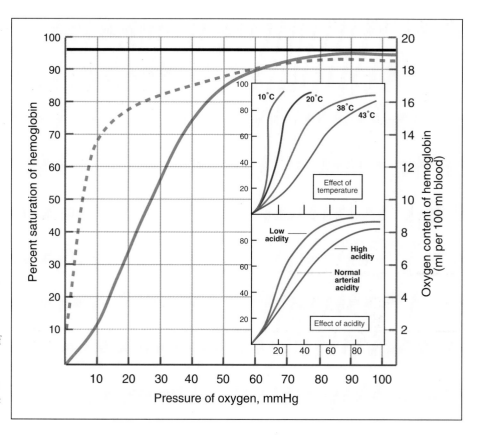

FIGURE 8-10. The *oxyhemoglobin* dissociation curve. Percent saturation of hemoglobin (*solid line*) and myoglobin (*dashed line*) in relation to oxygen pressure. The right ordinate shows the quantity of oxygen carried in each 100 ml of blood under normal conditions. The insert curves illustrate the effects of temperature and acidity in altering the affinity of hemoglobin for oxygen. The bold horizontal line at the top indicates percent saturation of hemoglobin at the sea level alveolar P_{O_2}.

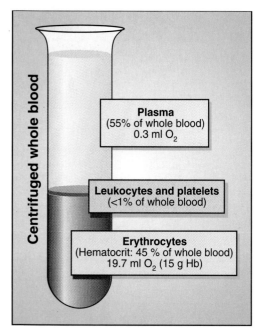

FIGURE 8-11. Major components of whole blood, including the quantity of oxygen carried in each 100 ml of blood (Hb = hemoglobin).

about 75% of its total oxygen (see Figure 8-10). Blood leaving the tissues, therefore, carries about 15 ml of oxygen in each 100 ml of blood; nearly 5 ml of oxygen have been released to the tissues. This difference in the oxygen content of arterial and mixed venous blood is termed the *arteriovenous oxygen difference* or *a-v̄ O_2 difference* and is expressed in milliliters of oxygen per 100 ml blood.

The a-v̄ O_2 difference at rest normally averages 4 to 5 ml of oxygen per 100 ml of blood. The large quantity of oxygen still remaining with hemoglobin provides an "automatic" reserve by which cells can immediately obtain oxygen should the metabolic demands suddenly increase. As the cell's need for oxygen increases in exercise, the tissue P_{O_2} becomes reduced and a larger quantity of oxygen is rapidly released from hemoglobin. During vigorous exercise, for

example, when the extracellular P_{O_2} decreases to about 15 mm Hg, only about 5 ml of oxygen remain bound to hemoglobin. As a result, the a-v̄ O_2 difference increases to 15 ml of oxygen per 100 ml of blood. When tissue P_{O_2} falls to 3 mm Hg during exhaustive exercise, virtually all of the oxygen is released from the blood that perfuses the active tissues. Clearly without any increase in local blood flow, the amount of oxygen released to the muscles can increase almost three times above that normally supplied at rest — just by a more complete unloading of hemoglobin.

The Bohr Effect. The solid line in Figure 8-10 shows the oxyhemoglobin dissociation curve under resting physiologic conditions at an arterial pH of 7.4 and tissue temperature of 37°C. The insert curves depict other important characteristics of hemoglobin. Any increase in acidity, temperature, or concentration of carbon dioxide causes the dissociation curve to shift significantly downward and to the right. This phenomenon is called the

Bohr effect after its discoverer Nils Bohr and is a consequence of an alteration in the molecular structure of hemoglobin. The Bohr effect describes the reduced effectiveness of hemoglobin to hold oxygen, especially in the P_{O_2} range of 20 to 50 mm Hg. This is particularly important in vigorous exercise because even more oxygen is released to the tissues with the accompanying increase in metabolic heat, carbon dioxide, and lactic acid. At the P_{O_2} in the alveoli, the Bohr effect in pulmonary capillary blood is negligible. This is important because it allows hemoglobin to load completely with oxygen as blood passes through the lungs, even during maximal exercise.

The compound *2,3-diphosphoglycerate* (2,3-DPG) produced in the red blood cell during the anaerobic reactions of glycolysis also facilitates the dissociation of oxygen from hemoglobin. Individuals with cardiopulmonary disorders and those who live at higher altitudes have an increased level of this metabolic intermediate. Studies also suggest that high intensity exercise elevates red blood cell 2,3-DPG. Under each of these conditions, this response would represent a compensatory adjustment to facilitate oxygen release to the cell. In general, the effects of 2,3 DPG are relatively slow compared with the almost immediate response caused by temperature, acidity, and CO_2.

Myoglobin, the Muscle's Oxygen Store

Myoglobin is an iron-protein compound found in skeletal and cardiac muscle. Myoglobin is similar to hemoglobin because it also combines reversibly with oxygen; however, each myoglobin molecule contains only one iron atom in contrast to hemoglobin that contains four atoms. Myoglobin adds additional oxygen to the muscle in the reaction:

$$Mb + O_2 \longrightarrow MbO_2$$

Oxygen Released at Low Pressures. Aside from its function as an "extra" source of oxygen in muscle, myoglobin facilitates the transfer of oxygen to the mitochondria, especially in the beginning of exercise and during intense exercise when there is a considerable drop in cellular P_{O_2}. It can be noted from the dissociation curve for myoglobin shown in Figure 8-10 (dashed line) that the line is not s-shaped, as is the case with hemoglobin, but instead forms a rectangular hyperbola. This shows that myoglobin binds and retains oxygen at low pressures more readily than hemoglobin. During rest and moderate levels of exercise, therefore, myoglobin retains a high saturation with oxygen. For example, at a P_{O_2} of 40 mm Hg, myoglobin retains 95% of its oxygen. The greatest quantity of oxygen is released from MbO_2 when the tissue P_{O_2} drops to 5 mm Hg or less. Unlike hemoglobin, myoglobin does not demonstrate a Bohr effect.

Effects of Training. As might be expected, slow-twitch muscle fibers with a high capacity to generate ATP aerobically contain relatively large quantities of myoglobin. In animals, the myoglobin level of muscle appears to be related to the animal's level of physical activity. The leg muscles of active hunting dogs contain more myoglobin than the muscles of sedentary house pets; this is also the case for grazing cattle compared with cattle that are penned. Whether myoglobin levels can be enhanced in humans as part of the adaptive response to training remains unclear.

CARBON DIOXIDE TRANSPORT IN THE BLOOD

Once carbon dioxide is formed in the cell, its only means for "escape" is through the diffusion and subsequent transport to the lungs in the venous blood. Carbon dioxide is carried:

Oxygen breathing. Breathing oxygen-enriched (hyperoxic) mixtures prior to or in recovery from exercise may give a psychological lift, but its physiological contribution is trivial at best.

Myoglobin contributes color. Reddish muscle fibers have a high concentration of this respiratory pigment, whereas fibers deficient in myoglobin appear pale or white.

- In physical solution (small amount) in the blood plasma
- Combined with hemoglobin
- Combined with water (large amount) in bicarbonate form

Figure 8-12 illustrates the various ways carbon dioxide is transported from the tissues to the lungs.

Carbon Dioxide in Solution

Approximately 5% of the carbon dioxide produced during energy metabolism is carried as free carbon dioxide in solution in the plasma. Although this quantity is relatively small, it is the random movement of dissolved carbon dioxide molecules that establishes the Pco_2 of the blood.

Carbon Dioxide as Bicarbonate

Carbon dioxide in solution combines with water in a reversible reaction to form carbonic acid.

$$CO_2 + H_2O \longleftrightarrow H_2CO_3$$

This reaction is slow, and little carbon dioxide would be carried in this form if it were not for the action of *carbonic anhydrase,* a zinc-con-

taining enzyme in the red blood cell. This catalyst accelerates the interaction of CO_2 and water about 5,000 times.

Once carbonic acid is formed in the tissues, most of it ionizes to hydrogen ions (H^+) and bicarbonate ions (HCO_3^-) as follows:

In the tissues

$$CO_2 + H_2O \xrightarrow{\text{carbonic anhydrase}} H_2CO_3 \longrightarrow H^+ + HCO_3^-$$

The H^+ is then buffered by the protein portion of hemoglobin to maintain the pH of the blood within relatively narrow limits (see "Acid-Base Concentration and pH," Chapter 1). Because HCO_3^- is quite soluble in blood, it diffuses from the red blood cell into the plasma in exchange for the chloride ion (Cl^-) that moves into the blood cell to maintain ionic equilibrium. This is known as the "chloride shift" and it causes the Cl^- content of the erythrocytes in venous blood to be higher than the arterial blood cells, especially during exercise.

Sixty to eighty percent of the total carbon dioxide is carried as plasma bicarbonate. As tissue Pco_2 increases, carbonic acid is formed rapidly. Conversely, in the lungs, carbon dioxide leaves the blood and this lowers the plasma Pco_2 and disturbs the equilibrium between carbonic acid and the formation of bicarbonate ions. As a result, H^+ and HCO_3^- recombine to form carbonic acid. In turn, carbon dioxide and water reform and carbon dioxide exits through the lungs as follows:

In The Lungs

$$H^+ + HCO_3^- \longrightarrow H_2CO_3 \xrightarrow{\text{carbonic anhydrase}} CO_2 + H_2O$$

Because the plasma bicarbonate is lowered in the pulmonary capillaries, the Cl^- moves from the red blood cell back into the plasma.

Carbon Dioxide as Carbamino Compounds

At the tissue level, carbon dioxide reacts directly with the amino acid molecules of blood proteins to form carbamino compounds. This is particularly true for the globin portion of hemoglobin that carries about 20% of the body's carbon dioxide as follows:

$$CO_2 + HbNH \longrightarrow HbNHCOOH$$
$$\text{(Hemoglobin)} \qquad \text{(Carbaminohemoglobin)}$$

The formation of carbamino compounds is reversed as the plasma P_{CO_2} is lowered in the lungs. This causes carbon dioxide to move into solution and enter the alveoli. Concurrently the oxygenation of hemoglobin reduces its binding ability for carbon dioxide. The interaction between oxygen loading and carbon dioxide release is termed the *Haldane effect*; this phenomenon facilitates the removal of carbon dioxide in the lung.

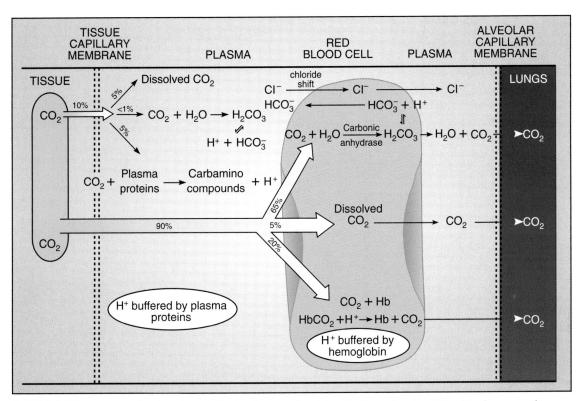

FIGURE 8-12. Transport of carbon dioxide in the plasma and red blood cells as dissolved CO_2, bicarbonate, and carbamino compounds. By far, the greatest amount of carbon dioxide is carried in combination with water to form carbonic acid.

PART 3

1. Hemoglobin, the iron-protein pigment in the red blood cell, increases the oxygen-carrying capacity of whole blood about 65 times that carried in physical solution dissolved in the plasma.

2. The small amount of oxygen dissolved in plasma exerts molecular movement and establishes the partial pressure of oxygen in the blood. This determines the loading at the lungs (oxygenation) and unloading at the tissues (deoxygenation) of hemoglobin.

3. The blood's oxygen transport capacity varies only slightly with normal variations in hemoglobin content. Iron deficiency anemia, however, significantly decreases the blood's oxygen-carrying capacity and consequently reduces aerobic exercise performance.

4. The s-shaped nature of the oxyhemoglobin dissociation curve shows that hemoglobin saturation changes very little until the P_{O_2} falls below 60 mm Hg. Because such low pressures occur in the tissues, the quantity of oxygen bound to hemoglobin falls sharply. Thus, oxygen is released rapidly from capillary blood and flows into the tissues in response to the cells' metabolic demands.

5. At rest, only about 25% of the blood's total oxygen is released to the tissues; the remaining 75% returns to the heart in the venous blood. This is the arteriovenous oxygen difference and indicates that an "automatic" reserve of oxygen exists so cells can rapidly obtain oxygen should the metabolic demands increase suddenly.

6. Increases in acidity, temperature, and carbon dioxide concentration cause an alteration in the molecular structure of hemoglobin, thereby reducing its effectiveness to hold oxygen. Because these factors are accentuated in exercise, the release of oxygen to the tissues is further facilitated.

7. In skeletal and cardiac muscle, the iron-protein pigment myoglobin acts as an "extra" oxygen store. It releases its oxygen at low oxygen pressures. This probably facilitates oxygen transfer to the mitochondria during strenuous exercise, when there is a considerable decrease in cellular P_{O_2}.

8. A small amount of carbon dioxide is carried as free carbon dioxide in solution in the plasma. This dissolved carbon dioxide establishes the P_{CO_2} of the blood.

9. The major quantity of carbon dioxide is transported in chemical combination with water and is carried as bicarbonate as follows:

$$CO_2 + H_2O \longrightarrow H_2CO_3 \longrightarrow H^+ + HCO_3^-$$

In the lungs, this reaction is reversed, and carbon dioxide leaves the blood and moves into the alveoli.

10. About 20% of the body's carbon dioxide combines with blood proteins, including hemoglobin to form carbamino compounds.

CONTROL OF VENTILATION

The rate and depth of breathing are exquisitely adjusted in response to the body's metabolic needs. In healthy individuals, the arterial gas pressures of oxygen and carbon dioxide and pH are essentially regulated at the resting value independent of exercise intensity. Ventilation is controlled by intricate neural circuits that relay information from higher centers in the brain, from the lungs themselves, and from other sensors throughout the body. In addition, the gaseous and chemical state of the blood that bathes the medulla and chemoreceptors in the aorta and carotid arteries acts to mediate alveolar ventilation. As a result, relatively constant alveolar gas pressures are maintained even during exhaustive exercise. A schematic representation of the input for ventilatory control is shown in Figure 8-13.

Neural Factors

The normal respiratory cycle results from inherent automatic activity of inspiratory neurons whose cell bodies are located in the medial portion of the medulla. These neurons activate the diaphragm and intercostal muscles, and the lungs inflate. The inspiratory neurons cease firing because of their own self-limitation as well as to the inhibitory influence from expiratory neurons also located in the medulla. As the lungs inflate, stretch receptors in lung tissue are also stimulated, especially in the bronchioles. These receptors act to inhibit inspiration and stimulate expiration.

As the inspiratory muscles relax, exhalation occurs by the passive recoil of the stretched lung tissue and raised ribs. The activation of expiratory neurons and associated muscles that further facilitate expiration is synchronized with this passive phase. As expiration proceeds, the inspiratory center is progressively released from inhibition and once again becomes active.

The inherent activity of the respiratory center cannot itself account for the smooth pattern of breathing in response to the metabolic demands of exercise. The controlling influence of neurons in the cerebral hemispheres, the pons, and other regions of the brain also plays an important role in establishing the duration and intensity of the inspiratory cycle. For example, activation of the inspiratory center stimulates the pons region of the hindbrain, especially during labored breathing. The pons, in turn, relays excitatory impulses to the expiratory center, which hastens the exhalation phase of the breathing cycle.

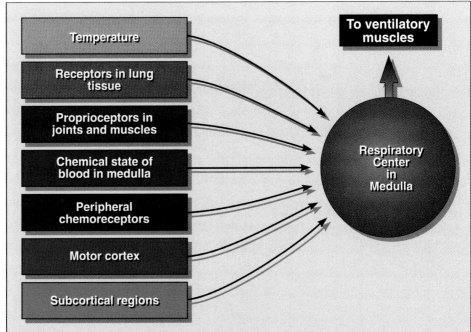

FIGURE 8-13. Schematic representation of various factors that affect the control of pulmonary ventilation by the medulla.

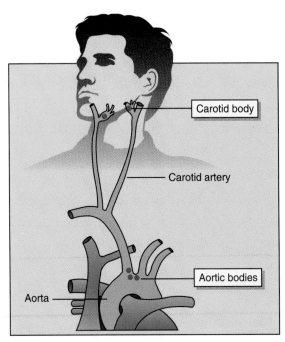

FIGURE 8-14. Aortic and carotid cell bodies sensitive to a reduced plasma Po_2 are located in the aortic arch and bifurcation of the carotid arteries. These peripheral receptors provide the body's first line of defense against arterial hypoxia.

Our immediate defense at altitude. A decrease in arterial Po_2, as would occur when one ascends to high altitudes, activates the aortic and carotid receptors to increase alveolar ventilation, thus increasing alveolar Po_2. The chemoreceptors alone protect the organism against a reduced oxygen pressure in inspired air.

Humoral Factors

Pulmonary ventilation at rest is largely regulated by the chemical state of the blood. Variations in arterial Po_2, Pco_2, acidity, and temperature activate sensitive neural units in the medulla and arterial system that adjust ventilation to maintain arterial blood chemistry within narrow limits.

Plasma Po_2 and Chemoreceptors. Inhalation of a gas mixture that contains 80% oxygen greatly increases alveolar Po_2 and causes about a 20% reduction in minute ventilation. Conversely, if the inspired oxygen concentration is reduced, the minute ventilation increases, especially if the alveolar Po_2 falls below 60 mm Hg. Recall that at 60 mm Hg, there is a dramatic fall in hemoglobin oxygen saturation.

Sensitivity to reduced oxygen pressures does not appear to reside in the respiratory center. Rather it is more a result of the stimulation of peripheral *chemoreceptors*. As illustrated in Figure 8-14, these specialized neurons are located in the arch of the aorta and at the branching of the carotid arteries in the neck.

Aside from providing an early warning system against reduced oxygen pressure, peripheral chemoreceptors also act to stimulate ventilation in response to increases in carbon dioxide, temperature, metabolic acidosis, and a fall in blood pressure.

Plasma Pco_2 and H^+ Concentration. At rest, the most important respiratory stimulus is the carbon dioxide pressure in arterial plasma. Small increases in Pco_2 in the inspired air cause large increases in minute ventilation. The resting ventilation is almost doubled, for example, by increasing the inspired Pco_2 to just 1.7 mm Hg (0.22% CO_2 in inspired air).

The regulation of ventilation by arterial Pco_2 is probably not related to molecular carbon dioxide. Rather, ventilation appears to be controlled by plasma acidity that varies directly with the blood's CO_2 content. Recall that carbonic acid formed from carbon dioxide and water rapidly dissociates to bicarbonate ions (HCO_3^-) and hydrogen ions (H^+). The increase in hydrogen ions, especially in the cerebrospinal fluid that bathes the respiratory areas, stimulates inspiratory activity. Then, as ventilation increases, CO_2 is eliminated, this lowers the arterial H^+ concentration.

Hyperventilation and Breath-Holding

If a person holds his or her breath after a normal exhalation, it takes about 40 seconds before the urge to breathe becomes so strong that the person is forced to inspire. The desire to breathe is due mainly to the stimulating effects of increased arterial Pco_2 and H^+ concentration and not to the decreased Po_2 in the breathhold condition. The "break point" for breathhold corresponds to an increase in arterial Pco_2 to about 50 mm Hg.

If this same person before breathhold consciously increases ventilation above the normal level, the composition of alveolar air changes and becomes more like that of ambient air. With overbreathing or *hyperventilation*, alveolar Pco_2 may decrease to 15 mm Hg. This decrease creates a considerable diffusion gradient for the run-off of CO_2 from the venous blood that enters the pulmonary capillaries. Consequently, a larger than normal quantity of CO_2 leaves the blood, and arterial Pco_2 becomes reduced significantly below normal levels. This extends the breathhold until the arterial Pco_2 and/or the H^+ concentration rise to the level to stimulate ventilation.

Hyperventilation and subsequent breath-hold have been used by swimmers and divers to try to improve physical performance. In sprint swimming, for example, it is undesirable from a mechanical viewpoint to roll the body and turn the head during the breathing phase of the stroke. Consequently many swimmers hyperventilate on the starting blocks to prolong breath-hold time during the swim. In sport diving, the intention of hyperventilation is the same as in competitive swimming — to extend breath-hold time. In this sport, however, the results can be tragic. As the length and depth of the dive increase, the oxygen content of the blood may be reduced to critically low values before arterial P_{CO_2} reaches the level to stimulate breathing and signal ascent to the surface. The reduction in arterial P_{O_2} can cause the diver to lose consciousness before reaching the surface.

REGULATION OF VENTILATION IN EXERCISE

Chemical Control

Chemical stimuli probably cannot entirely explain the increased ventilation (*hyperpnea*) during physical activity. For example, even when artificial changes are made in P_{O_2}, P_{CO_2}, and acidity, increases in minute ventilation are not nearly as large as those observed in vigorous exercise.

During exercise, arterial P_{O_2} is not reduced to an extent that would increase ventilation due to chemoreceptor stimulation. In fact, in vigorous exercise, the large breathing volumes may cause the alveolar P_{O_2} to rise above the average resting value of 100 mm Hg. This rise is illustrated in Figure 8-15 where venous and alveolar P_{CO_2} and alveolar P_{O_2} are plotted in relation to oxygen uptake during a progressive exercise test.

During light and moderate exercise, pulmonary ventilation is closely coupled to the metabolic rate in a manner that is proportional to both carbon dioxide production and oxygen uptake. Under these conditions, the alveolar (and arterial) P_{CO_2} is generally maintained at about 40 mm Hg.

In strenuous exercise, there is an increase in acidity and subsequent hydrogen ion concentration. This provides an additional ventilatory stimulus that usually reduces alveolar P_{CO_2} below this value, sometimes to as low as 25 mm Hg. This would actually result in a decrease in arterial P_{CO_2} to facilitate carbon dioxide elimination.

Nonchemical Control

As exercise begins, ventilation increases so rapidly that it occurs almost within a single ventilatory cycle. This immediate change is followed by a plateau that lasts about 30 seconds and then gradually increases as the ventilation approaches a steady state. When exercise is terminated, ventilation decreases exponentially to a point about 40% of the steady-state value and then slowly returns to a resting level. The rapidity of the ventilatory response at the onset and cessation of exercise strongly suggests that this portion of exercise hyperpnea is mediated by input other than changes in arterial P_{CO_2} and H^+ content.

Neurogenic Factors. Neurogenic factors include both cortical and peripheral influences.

A dangerous practice. In a report of 23 cases of drowning and 35 near drownings, the individuals (98% males) were attempting to achieve a prolonged breathhold. All were good swimmers and 80% were in pools with lifeguards.

Alveolar P_{O_2} rises in heavy exercise. The slight increase in alveolar P_{O_2} in heavy exercise may hasten the equilibrium of alveolar blood gases; this facilitates the oxygenation of blood in the alveolar capillaries.

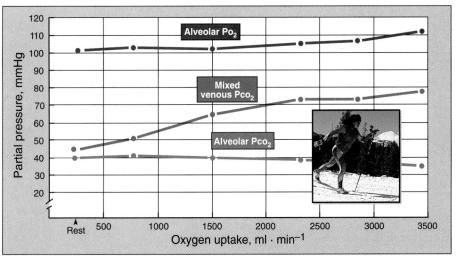

FIGURE 8-15. Values for P_{CO_2} in mixed venous blood that enters the lungs and the alveolar P_{O_2} and P_{CO_2} in relation to oxygen uptake during graded exercise. Note that despite the increased metabolic demands of exercise, alveolar P_{O_2} and P_{CO_2} remain at near resting levels. (Data from the Laboratory of Applied Physiology, Queens College.)

- **Cortical Influence.** Neural outflow from regions of the motor cortex as well as cortical activation in anticipation of exercise stimulates the respiratory neurons in the medulla. Cortical outflow may act in concert with the demands of exercise to contribute to the abrupt increase in ventilation when exercise begins.
- **Peripheral Influence.** Ventilatory adjustments to exercise also arise from sensory input from joints, tendons, and muscles. Although such peripheral receptors have not been identified, experiments involving passive limb movements, electrical stim-

ulation of muscles, and voluntary exercise with the muscle's blood flow occluded, support the existence of such *mechanoreceptors* that produce a reflex hyperpnea.

Influence of Temperature. An increase in body temperature has a direct stimulating effect on the neurons of the respiratory center, and probably exerts some control over ventilation in prolonged exercise. The changes in ventilation at the beginning and end of exercise, however, are much more rapid than can be accounted for by changes in the body's core temperature.

Integrated Regulation

The control of breathing in exercise is not the result of a single factor but rather is the combined and perhaps simultaneous result of several chemical and neural stimuli.

The model for respiratory control illustrated in Figure 8-16 suggests that neurogenic stimuli from the cerebral cortex or the exercising limbs cause the initial, abrupt increase in breathing when exercise begins. After this initial change, minute ventilation gradually rises to a steady level that adequately meets the demands for metabolic gas exchange. Then, the regulation of alveolar gas pressures is probably maintained by central and reflex chemical stimuli, especially those stimuli provided by temperature, carbon dioxide, and hydrogen ions.

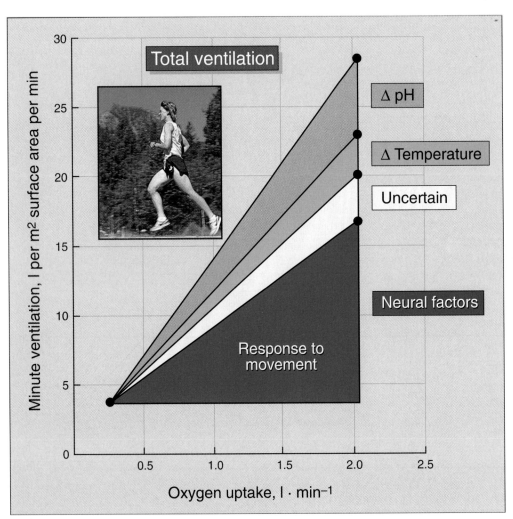

FIGURE 8-16. Composite of the factors that influence ventilatory response to exercise. The contribution of changes in acidity (ΔpH) and temperature (Δt) as well as the effects of neurogenic stimuli from the cerebral regions and/or joints and muscles is estimated. The yellow-shaded wedge represents the ventilatory change not quantitatively accounted for by the other three factors. (From Lambertson, C. J.: Interactions of physical, chemical, and nervous factors in respiratory control. In *Medical Physiology.* Edited by V.B. Mountcastle. St. Louis, C.V. Mosby Co., 1974.)

PART 4

1. The normal respiratory cycle results from the inherent activity of neurons in the medulla. Superimposed on this neural output are intricate neural circuits that relay information from higher brain centers, from the lungs themselves, and from other sensors throughout the body.

2. At rest, several chemical factors act directly on the respiratory center or modify its activity reflexly through chemoreceptors to control alveolar ventilation. The most important factors are the level of arterial P_{CO_2} and acidity. A drop in arterial oxygen pressure, as would occur during ascent to high altitude or in severe pulmonary disease, will also provide a breathing stimulus.

3. Hyperventilation significantly lowers arterial P_{CO_2} and H^+ concentration. This prolongs breath-hold time until normal levels of carbon dioxide and acidity are reached to stimulate breathing. Extended breath-hold by hyperventilation should not be practiced during underwater swimming because the consequences can be deadly.

4. Ventilatory adjustments to exercise are augmented by nonchemical regulatory factors. These factors include (a) cortical activation in anticipation of exercise as well as outflow from the motor cortex when exercise begins, (b) peripheral sensory input from mechanoreceptors in joints and muscles, and (c) elevation in body temperature.

5. Effective alveolar ventilation in exercise is the result of many neural and chemical factors that operate singularly and in combination. Each factor probably takes on greater importance at a particular phase of the adjustment to exercise.

Part 5 PULMONARY VENTILATION DURING EXERCISE

VENTILATION AND ENERGY DEMANDS

Physical activity affects oxygen uptake and carbon dioxide production more than any other form of physiologic stress. With exercise, large amounts of oxygen diffuse from the alveoli into the venous blood returning to the lungs. Conversely, considerable quantities of carbon dioxide move from the blood into the alveoli. Concurrently ventilation increases to maintain the proper alveolar gas concentrations to allow for this increased exchange of oxygen and carbon dioxide.

Ventilation in Steady-Rate Exercise

Figure 8-17 illustrates the relationship between oxygen uptake and minute ventilation during various levels of exercise up to the maximal oxygen uptake.

During light and moderate steady-rate exercise, ventilation increases linearly with oxygen uptake and carbon dioxide production and averages between 20 and 25 liters of air for each liter of oxygen consumed. Under these conditions, ventilation is mainly increased by increasing tidal volume, whereas at higher exercise levels breathing frequency takes on a more important role. With this adjustment in ventilation, there is complete aeration of blood because the alveolar P_{O_2} and P_{CO_2} remain at near resting values and the transit time for the blood flowing through the pulmonary capillaries is slow enough to allow for complete gas exchange.

The ratio of minute ventilation to oxygen uptake is termed the *ventilatory equivalent* and is symbolized $\dot{V}_E/\dot{V}_{O_2}$. In healthy young adults, the $\dot{V}_E/\dot{V}_{O_2}$ ratio is usually maintained at about 25 to 1 (that is, 25 liters of air breathed per liter of oxygen consumed) during submaximal exercise up to about 55%

Less breathing during swimming. Because of the restrictive nature of prone swimming on breathing, the ventilatory equivalents are significantly lower at all levels of energy expenditure. This restriction may pose a problem in providing for adequate gas exchange during maximal swimming, and may partly contribute to the generally lower maximal oxygen uptake during swimming compared to running.

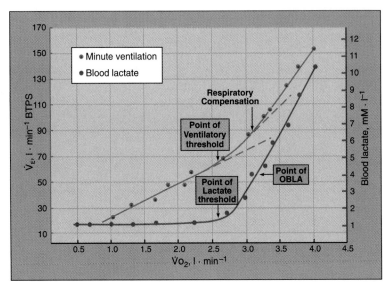

FIGURE 8-17. Pulmonary ventilation, blood lactate, and oxygen uptake during graded exercise to maximum. The dashed line represents the extrapolation of the linear relationship between $\dot{V}_E$ and $\dot{V}O_2$ during submaximal exercise. The lactate threshold is that point where blood lactate begins to increase above the resting value. It is detected by the point where the relation between $\dot{V}_E$ and $\dot{V}O_2$ deviates from linearity. (OBLA represents the point of lactate increase above a 4 mM · L^{-1} baseline.) Respiratory Compensation is a further increase in ventilation to counter the falling pH in heavy anaerobic exercise.

of the maximal oxygen uptake. The $\dot{V}_E/\dot{V}O_2$ ratio is higher in younger children and averages about 32 to 1 in children 6 years old.

there is no increase in blood lactate. The exercise level or level of oxygen uptake where blood lactate begins to show a systematic increase above a baseline level of about 4 mM · L^{-1} is termed the point of *onset of blood lactate accumulation* (OBLA). The OBLA normally occurs between 55 and 65% of the maximal oxygen uptake in healthy, untrained subjects, and often is more than 80% in more highly trained endurance athletes.

The lactic acid generated during anaerobic metabolism is buffered in the blood by sodium bicarbonate, as demonstrated in the following reaction:

$$\text{Lactic acid} + \text{NaHCO}_3 \longrightarrow \text{Na lactate} + \text{H}_2\text{CO}_3 \longrightarrow \text{H}_2\text{O} + \text{CO}_2$$

Ventilation in Non-Steady-Rate Exercise

In more intense submaximal exercise, the minute ventilation takes a sharp upswing and increases disproportionately with increases in oxygen uptake. As a result, the ventilatory equivalent is greater than during steady-rate exercise and may increase to 35 or 40 liters of air per liter of oxygen consumed.

Onset of Blood Lactate Accumulation. Sufficient oxygen is supplied to and used by the working muscles during steady-rate exercise. Under these conditions, lactic acid production does not exceed lactic acid removal; thus,

The excess, nonmetabolic carbon dioxide released in this buffering reaction stimulates an increase in pulmonary ventilation, and as a consequence CO_2 is exhaled into the atmosphere. This additional exhaled CO_2 causes an increase in the respiratory exchange ratio to values that exceed 1.00.

The exact cause of the OBLA is controversial. It is often assumed that OBLA represents muscle hypoxia and therefore anaerobiosis. Muscle lactic acid accumulation, however, is not necessarily linked to muscle hypoxia and anaerobiosis and the oxygen deficit. For example, lactic acid can accumulate in the presence of adequate muscle oxygenation. This implies an imbalance between lactic acid appearance in the blood and its subsequent rate of disappearance. This imbalance may not be a result of muscle hypoxia but rather the result of decreased lactic acid clearance in total, or increased lactic acid production only in specific muscle fibers. Thus, caution is urged in interpreting too broadly the specific metabolic significance of the OBLA and its possible relationship to tissue hypoxia.

The OBLA during exercise is directly assessed by measuring the lactate level in the blood. Because blood lactate accumulation is associated with changes in carbon dioxide production, blood pH, bicarbonate and hydrogen ion concentration, and respiratory exchange ratio, it has been suggested that these variables also can be used to assess OBLA indirectly. Although these measures are related to OBLA, it is doubtful that each can be used to denote the onset of anaerobic metabolism precisely. Nevertheless, it is common practice to use "bloodless" techniques, such as changes in the respiratory exchange ratio or ventilatory equivalent during incremental exercise to signal the onset of metabolic acidosis within exercising muscle. Even if the association between ventilatory dynamics and metabolic events is fortuitous, much useful information about exercise performance has resulted with application of these indirect prediction procedures.

OBLA and Endurance Performance. As was discussed in Chapter 3 in comparisons of trained and untrained individuals, lactate begins to accumulate in the blood of a trained individual at both a higher level of oxygen uptake and a higher percentage of the maximal aerobic capacity. *In fact, the point of OBLA can be increased in training without a concomitant increase in max $\dot{V}O_2$.* It appears that the point of OBLA and max $\dot{V}O_2$ are determined by different factors and that muscle fiber type, capillary density, and the

alterations in skeletal muscle's oxidative capacities with training play a major role in establishing the percentage of one's aerobic capacity that can be sustained in endurance exercise.

Traditionally exercise physiologists have used the max $\dot{V}O_2$ as the yardstick to gauge one's capacity for endurance exercise. Although this measure generally relates to long-term exercise performance, it does not fully explain success in such performances. Experienced distance athletes generally compete at an exercise intensity just slightly above the point of OBLA. Consequently the exercise intensity at the point of OBLA is a consistent and powerful predictor of performance in aerobic exercise. This was clearly illustrated in a study of competitive race-walkers. Here, the race-walking velocity and oxygen uptake at which blood lactate began to increase were highly correlated to 20-km performance. In fact, the race-walking velocity at OBLA predicted performance in the race to within 0.6% of the actual time! A subject's max $\dot{V}O_2$ was a poor predictor of actual performance. Changes in endurance performance with training are often more closely related to the training-induced changes in the exercise level for OBLA than to the changes in max $\dot{V}O_2$.

Three Important Factors That Determine Endurance Performance
- Maximal oxygen uptake
- Lactate threshold or OBLA
- Economy of effort

An added stimulus to breathing. Overbreathing occurs in heavy exercise because the lactic acid produced places an added demand on pulmonary ventilation. This happens when lactic acid is buffered to produce the weaker carbonic acid. In the lungs, carbonic acid splits into its components, water and carbon dioxide. Carbon dioxide provides an additional stimulus to increase ventilation.

DOES VENTILATION LIMIT AEROBIC CAPACITY?

If one's ability to breathe during exercise were inadequate, the line relating pulmonary ventilation and oxygen uptake would curve in a direction opposite to that indicated in Figure 8-17, and the ventilation equivalent would decrease. Such a response would indicate a failure for ventilation to keep pace with increasing oxygen demand; in this instance, we would truly "run out of wind." Actually a healthy individual tends to overbreathe in relation to oxygen uptake during heavy exercise. This overbreathing was clearly illustrated in

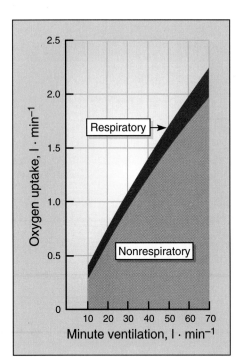

FIGURE 8-18. Relationship between minute ventilation and total oxygen uptake and its respiratory and nonrespiratory components during submaximal exercise in healthy subjects. (From Levison, H., and Cherniack, R.: Ventilatory cost of exercise in chronic obstructive pulmonary disease. *J. Appl. Physiol.*, 25:21, 1968.)

Cigarette smoke constricts airways. The increase in peripheral airway resistance with smoking is mainly due to the vagal reflex (possibly triggered from sensory stimulation of minute particles in the smoke) and partially by stimulation of parasympathetic ganglia by nicotine.

Ventilation capacity is rarely taxed. Even during maximal exercise, a considerable breathing reserve exists because pulmonary minute ventilation at this level of exercise represents only about 60 to 85% of a healthy person's maximum capacity for breathing.

Figure 8-15, which demonstrated that the ventilatory adjustment to strenuous exercise generally results in a decrease in alveolar P_{CO_2} with a concomitant small increase in alveolar P_{O_2}. Within this framework, it does not appear that pulmonary function is the "weak link" in the oxygen transport system of healthy individuals with an average to moderately high aerobic capacity.

An Exception. In the elite endurance athlete, in whom the cardiovascular and muscular adaptations to training have reached exceptional levels, the pulmonary system may be taxed maximally or even lag behind the functional capacity of the other "aerobic systems." If such a condition occurs, complete aeration of blood will not take place, and pulmonary ventilation or pulmonary gas exchange can limit maximal exercise performance.

Energy Cost of Breathing

Figure 8-18 shows the relationship between pulmonary ventilation and oxygen uptake during rest and submaximal exercise and its division into ventilatory and nonventilatory components. At rest and in light exercise in healthy subjects, the oxygen requirement of breathing is small, averaging 1.9 to 3.1 ml of oxygen per liter of air breathed, or about 4% of the total energy expenditure. As the rate and depth of breathing increase, the cost of breathing rises to about 4 ml of oxygen per liter of ventilation and may rise to as high as 9 ml of oxygen when ventilation exceeds 100 $1 \cdot min^{-1}$, or between 10 to 20% of the exercise oxygen uptake.

In Respiratory Disease. A healthy person rarely senses the effort of breathing, even during moderate exercise. In respiratory disease, however, the work of breathing in itself may become exhaustive. In patients who have obstructive pulmonary disease, the cost of ventilation at rest may be three times that of normal patients,

and during light exercise, it may increase to as much as 10 ml of oxygen for each liter of air breathed. In severe pulmonary disease, the energy cost of breathing may easily reach 40% of the total exercise oxygen uptake. This would encroach on the oxygen available to the exercising, nonrespiratory muscles; this seriously limits the exercise capabilities of patients with obstructive pulmonary disease.

Effects of Cigarette Smoking. The research relating smoking habits to exercise performance is meager, although most endurance athletes avoid cigarettes for fear of hindering performance due to a "loss of wind." The chronic cigarette smoker tends to show a decrease in dynamic lung function that in severe instances is manifested in obstructive lung disorders. Such pathologic processes usually take years to develop. Thus with young smokers, *chronic* alterations in lung function may be minimal and insignificant in terms of their effect on physical performance. Other more *acute* effects of cigarette smoking may adversely affect exercise capacity. For example, airway resistance at rest is increased as much as threefold in both chronic smokers and nonsmokers following 15 puffs on a cigarette during a 5-minute period. This added resistance to breathing lasts an average of 35 minutes and probably has only a minor effect in light exercise where the oxygen cost of breathing is small. In vigorous exercise, however, this residual effect of smoking could be detrimental because the additional cost of breathing might become prohibitive.

In one study of habitual cigarette smokers who exercised at 80% of maximal aerobic power, the energy requirement of breathing averaged 14% of the exercise oxygen uptake after smoking but only 9% in the "nonsmoking" trials for the heaviest smokers. Also, heart rates averaged 5 to 7% lower during exercise following 1 day of cigarette abstinence, and all subjects reported that they felt better exercising in the nonsmoking condition. It appears that a *substantial reversibility* of the increased oxygen cost of breathing with smoking can occur in chronic smokers with only 1 day of abstinence. Thus if athletes are unable to eliminate smoking completely, they should at least stop on the day of competition.

VENTILATORY ADAPTATIONS WITH TRAINING

Aerobic training brings about several changes in pulmonary ventilation during maximal and submaximal exercise.

- **Maximal Exercise:** Maximal exercise ventilation increases with improvements in maximal oxygen uptake. This makes sense physiologically because an increase in aerobic capacity results in a larger oxygen utilization and correspondingly larger production of carbon dioxide that must be eliminated through increased alveolar ventilation.

- **Submaximal Exercise:** After only 4 weeks of training, a considerable reduction in the ventilatory equivalent is observed in submaximal exercise. Consequently a smaller amount of air is breathed at a particular rate of submaximal oxygen uptake; this reduces the percentage of the total oxygen cost of exercise attributable to breathing. Theoretically, this would be important in endurance exercise for two reasons: (1) It would reduce the fatiguing effects of exercise on the ventilatory musculature, and (2) any oxygen freed from use by the respiratory muscles becomes available to the exercising muscles.

The mechanism is unknown for the training adaptations in ventilation in submaximal exercise. These changes, however, have been consistently observed in studies of adolescents and in both young and older men and women. In general, tidal volume becomes larger, breathing frequency is considerably reduced, and air remains in the lungs for a longer period of time between breaths. The result is an increase in the amount of oxygen extracted from the inspired air. The exhaled air of trained individuals often contains only 14 to 15% oxygen during submaximal exercise, whereas the expired air of untrained persons may contain 18% oxygen at the same intensity of exercise. Obviously the untrained person must ventilate proportionately more air to achieve the same submaximal oxygen uptake.

Specificity of the Ventilatory Response. Ventilatory adaptations appear to be specific to the type of exercise used in training. For subjects who performed either arm or leg exercise, the ventilation equivalent was always greater during arm exercise than during leg work (Fig. 8-19). After training, the ventilatory equivalent was significantly reduced. This finding was noted, however, *only* during exercise that used the specifically trained muscle groups. For the group trained by arm ergometry, the ventilation equivalent was reduced only in arm exercise and vice versa for the leg-trained group. This training adaptation was closely related to a less pronounced rise in blood lactate and heart rate in the specific training exercise. It is likely that the ventilatory adjustment to training results from neural and chemical adaptations in the specific muscles trained through exercise.

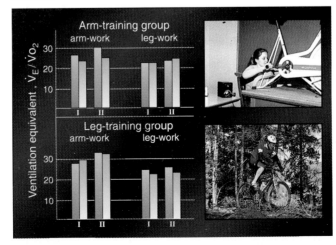

FIGURE 8-19. Ventilatory equivalents during light (I) and heavy (II) submaximal arm and leg exercise before and after arm training (*top*) and leg training (*bottom*). Yellow-green bars indicate posttraining values. (From Rasmussen, B., et al.: Pulmonary ventilation, blood gases, and blood pH after training of the arms and the legs. *J. Appl. Physiol.*, 38:250, 1975.)

PART 5

1. In light to moderate exercise, ventilation increases linearly with oxygen uptake. The ventilatory equivalent is maintained at about 20 to 25 liters of air breathed per liter of oxygen consumed.

2. In non-steady-rate exercise, ventilation increases disproportionately with increases in oxygen uptake, and the ventilatory equivalent may reach 35 or 40 liters.

3. The eventual sharp upswing in ventilation during incremental exercise provides a means for establishing a person's level for the onset of blood lactate accumulation or OBLA. This fitness measure relates to the onset of anaerobiosis and can be evaluated without a significant degree of metabolic acidosis or cardiovascular strain.

4. For healthy people, the oxygen cost of breathing is relatively small, even during the most severe exercise. In respiratory disease, however, the work of breathing becomes excessive and alveolar ventilation often becomes inadequate during exercise.

5. For most individuals, pulmonary ventilation is not taxed to a degree that would limit optimal alveolar gas exchange in maximal exercise. For the elite endurance athlete, improvements in pulmonary dynamics may lag behind the exceptional adaptations in cardiovascular and muscle function, and aeration may be compromised.

6. Airway resistance is greatly increased following cigarette smoking. This increases the oxygen cost of breathing which can be detrimental during prolonged, high intensity exercise.Reversibility of these smoking effects can occur with just one day of abstinence.

7. Training generally reduces the ventilatory equivalent in submaximal exercise. This "conserves" oxygen because the energy cost of breathing is lowered for a particular exercise task.

8. Ventilatory adjustments with training follow the principle of training specificity. A more efficient breathing pattern is generally observed only during the type of exercise used in training.

Aaron, E.A., et al.: Oxygen cost of exercise hyperpnea: Implications for performance. *J. Appl. Physiol.*, 75: 1818, 1992.

Babcock, M.A., and Dempsey, J.A.: Pulmonary system adaptations: limitations to exercise. In *Physical Activity, Fitness, and Health.* Edited by Bouchard, C., et al., Champaign, IL, Human Kinetics, 1994.

Bar-Or, O., and Inbar, O.: Swimming and asthma—benefits and deleterious effects. *Sports Med.*, 14: 397, 1992.

Bender, P.R., and Martin, B.J.: Maximal ventilation for exhausting exercise. *Med. Sci. Sports Exerc.*, 17:164, 1985.

Berk, J.L., et al.: Cold-induced bronchoconstriction: Role of cutaneous reflexes vs. direct airway effects. *J. Appl. Physiol.*, 63: 659, 1987.

Brooks, G.A.: Anaerobic threshold: Review of the concept and directions for future research. *Med. Sci Sports Exerc.*, 17:22, 1985.

Carter, R., et al.: Exercise training in patients with chronic obstructive pulmonary disease. *Med. Sci. Sports Exerc.*, 24:281, 1992.

Chevrolet, J.C., et al.: Alterations in inspiratory and leg muscle force and recovery pattern after a marathon. *Med. Sci. Sports Exerc.*, 25: 501, 1993.

Coast, J.R., et al.: Ventilatory work and oxygen consumption during exercise and hyperventilation. *J. Appl. Physiol.*, 74: 793, 1993.

Cordain, L., et al.: Lung volumes and maximal respiratory pressures in collegiate swimmers and runners. *Res. Q. Exerc. Sport,* 61:70, 1990.

Cunningham, D.A., et al.: Gas exchange dynamics with sinusoidal work in young and elderly women. *Respir. Physiol.*, 91: 43, 1993.

Davis, J.A.: Anaerobic threshold: Review of the concept and directions for future research. *Med. Sci, Sports Exerc.*, 17:6, 1985.

Dempsey, J.A.: Is the lung built for exercise? *Med. Sci. Sports Exerc.,* 18:143, 1986.

Eldridge, F.L.: Central integration of mechanisms in exercise hyperpnea. *Med. Sci. Sports Exerc.*, 26: 319, 1994.

Haas, F., et al.: Effect of aerobic training on forced expiratory airflow in exercising asthmatic humans. *J. Appl. Physiol.,* 63:1230, 1987.

Hagberg. J.M., et al.: Pulmonary function in young and older athletes and untrained men. *J. Appl Physiol.,* 65:101, 1988.

Harmon. E.A., et al.: Intra-abdominal and intra-thoracic pressures during lifting and jumping. *Med. Sci. Sports Exerc.,* 20:198, 1988.

Hopkins, S.R., and McKenzie, D.C.,: Hypoxic ventilatory response and arterial desaturation during heavy work. *J. Appl. Physiol.,* 67:1119, 1989.

Hough, D.O., and Dec, K.L.: Exercise-induced asthma and anaphylaxis. *Sports Med.,* 18: 162, 1994.

Johnson, B.D., et al.: Exercise induced diaphragmatic fatigue in healthy humans. *J. Physiol. (Lond.)* 460: 385, 1993.

Loat, C.E., and Rhodes, E.C.: Relationship between the lactate and ventilatory thresholds during prolonged exercise. *Sports Med.,* 15:104, 1993.

Luetkemeier, M.J., and Thomas, E.L.: Hypervolemia and cycling time trial performance. *Med. Sci. Sports Exerc.,* 26: 503, 1994.

Mador, M.J., and Acevedo, F.A.: Effect of respiratory muscle fatigue on breathing pattern during incremental exercise. *Am. Rev. Respir. Dis.,* 143:462, 1991.

Mahler, D. A.: Exercise-induced asthma. *Med. Sci. Sports Exerc.,* 25: 554, 1993.

McFadden, E.R., Jr., and Gilbert, I.A.: Current concepts in exercise-induced asthma. *N. Engl. J. Med.,* 330: 1362, 1994.

McKenzie, D.C., et al.: The protective effects of continuous and interval exercise in athletes with exercise-induced asthma. *Med. Sci. Sports Exerc.,* 26: 951, 1994.

Nye, P.C.G.: Identification of peripheral chemoreceptor stimuli. *Med. Sci. Sports Exerc.,* 26: 311, 1994.

Paek, D., et al.: Breathing patterns during varied activities. *J. Appl. Physiol.,* 73:887, 1992.

Powers, S.K., et al.: Effects of incomplete pulmonary gas exchange on $\dot{V}O_2$ max. *J. Appl. Physiol.,* 66:2491, 1989.

Prfaut, C., et al.: Exercise-induced hypoxemia in older athletes. *J. Appl. Physiol.,* 76: 120, 1994.

Reiff, D.B., et al.: The effect of prolonged submaximal warm-up on exercise-induced asthma. *Am. Rev. Respir. Dis,.* 139:479, 1989.

Schapira, R.M., et al.: The value of expiratory time in the physical diagnosis of obstructive airway disease. *JAMA,* 270: 731, 1993.

Smith, M.A., et al.: Assessment of beat to beat changes in cardiac output during the Valsalva maneuver using bioimpedience cardiology. *Clin. Sci.,* 74:423, 1987.

Voy, R.O.: The US Olympic Committee experience with exercise-induced bronchospasm, 1984. *Med. Sci. Sports Exerc.,* 18:328, 1986.

Ward, S.: Assessment of peripheral chemoreflex contributions to exercise hyperpnea in humans. *Med. Sci. Sports Exerc.,* 26: 303, 1994.

Wasserman, K., and Koike, A.: Is the anaerobic threshold truly anaerobic? *Chest, 101:*211S, 1992.

Whipp, B.J.: Peripheral chemoreceptor control of exercise hyperpnea in humans. *Med. Sci. Sports Exerc.,* 26: 337, 1994.

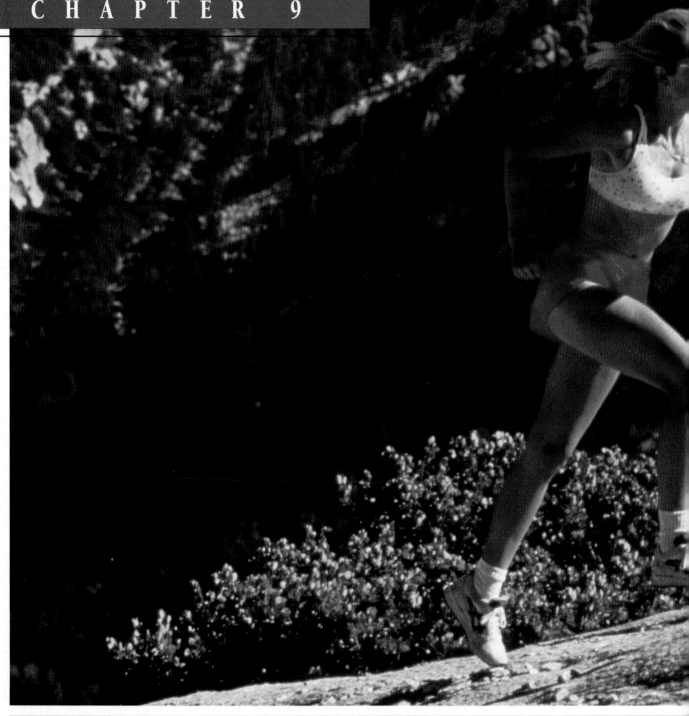

The Cardiovascular System and Exercise

After reading this chapter, you should be able to:

- List the important functions of the cardiovascular system.

- Describe how to measure blood pressure by the auscultatory method and give average values for systolic and diastolic blood pressure at rest and during aerobic exercise.

- Discuss blood pressure response during (a) resistance exercise, (b) upper body exercise, and (c) exercise in the inverted position.

- Discuss the potential benefits of aerobic exercise for a person with moderate hypertension.

- Identify intrinsic and extrinsic factors that regulate heart rate at rest and during exercise.

- Identify local and neural factors that regulate blood flow at rest and during exercise.

- Describe how cardiac output is measured. Compare average values of cardiac output at rest and maximal exercise for an endurance-trained athlete and sedentary person.

- Discuss the two physiologic mechanisms that can affect the stroke volume of the heart.

- Describe the relationship between maximal cardiac output and maximal oxygen uptake.

- Explain the meaning of the term, "athlete's heart."

The highly efficient ventilatory system is complemented by a rapid transport and delivery system consisting of the blood, the heart, and more than 60,000 miles of blood vessels that integrate the body as a unit. The circulatory system serves four important functions during physical activity:

- It delivers oxygen to the exercising muscles
- It returns blood to the lungs for aeration
- It transports heat, a byproduct of cellular metabolism, from the body's core to the skin
- It delivers fuel nutrients to the active tissues.

Part 1 THE CARDIOVASCULAR SYSTEM

COMPONENTS OF THE CARDIOVASCULAR SYSTEM

The cardiovascular system is a continuous vascular circuit that consists of a pump, a high-pressure distribution circuit, exchange vessels, and a low-pressure collection and return circuit. A schematic view of this system is presented in Figure 9-1.

Heart

Within the confines of the closed circulatory system, the force to propel blood is provided by the heart. This four-chambered organ, a fist-sized pump, beats at rest about 70 times a minute, 100,800 times a day, and 36.8 million times a year. Even for a person of average fitness, the maximum output of blood from this remarkable organ is greater than the fluid output from a household faucet turned wide open!

The heart muscle, or *myocardium*, is a form of striated muscle similar to skeletal muscle. The individual fibers, however, are interconnected in a latticework fashion. Consequently, when one cell is stimulated or depolarized, the action potential speeds through the myocardium to all cells, causing the heart to function as a unit.

Figure 9–2 shows the details of the heart as a pump. Functionally, the heart may be viewed as two separate pumps. The hollow chambers that compose the right side of the heart (right heart) perform two important functions:

- Receive blood returning from all parts of the body
- Pump blood into the lungs for aeration by way of the *pulmonary circulation*

The left side of the heart (left heart) also performs two important functions:

- Receive oxygenated blood from the lungs
- Pump blood into the thick-walled, muscular aorta for distribution throughout the body in the *systemic circulation*

A thick, solid muscular wall or septum separates the left and right sides of the heart.

The *atrioventricular valves* situated in the heart provide for a one-way passage of blood from the *right atrium* to the *right ventricle (tricuspid valve)* and from the *left atrium* to the *left ventricle* (*mitral* or *bicuspid valve*). The semilunar valves located in the arterial wall just outside the heart prevent blood from flowing back into the heart between contractions.

The relatively thin-walled, saclike atrial chambers serve as primer pumps to receive and store blood during the period of ventricular contraction. About 70% of the blood that returns to the atria flows directly into the ven-

The heart is a remarkable pump. At rest, the heart's output of blood is equivalent to 1400 gallons a day, or about 37 million gallons over a 72-year lifetime.

One powerful muscle. By the nature of the spiral and circular arrangement of bands of cardiac muscle, blood is virtually "wrung out" of the heart with each contraction.

tricle before the atria contract. Simultaneous contraction of both atria then forces the remaining blood into their respective ventricles directly below. Almost immediately after atrial contraction, the ventricles contract and force blood into the arterial system.

As pressure builds in the left ventricle, the atrioventricular valves snap closed. The heart valves remain closed for 0.02 to 0.06 seconds. This brief interval of rising ventricular tension during which the heart volume and fiber length remain unchanged represents the heart's *isovolumetric contraction period*. Blood is ejected from the heart when the ventricular pressure exceeds arterial pressure.

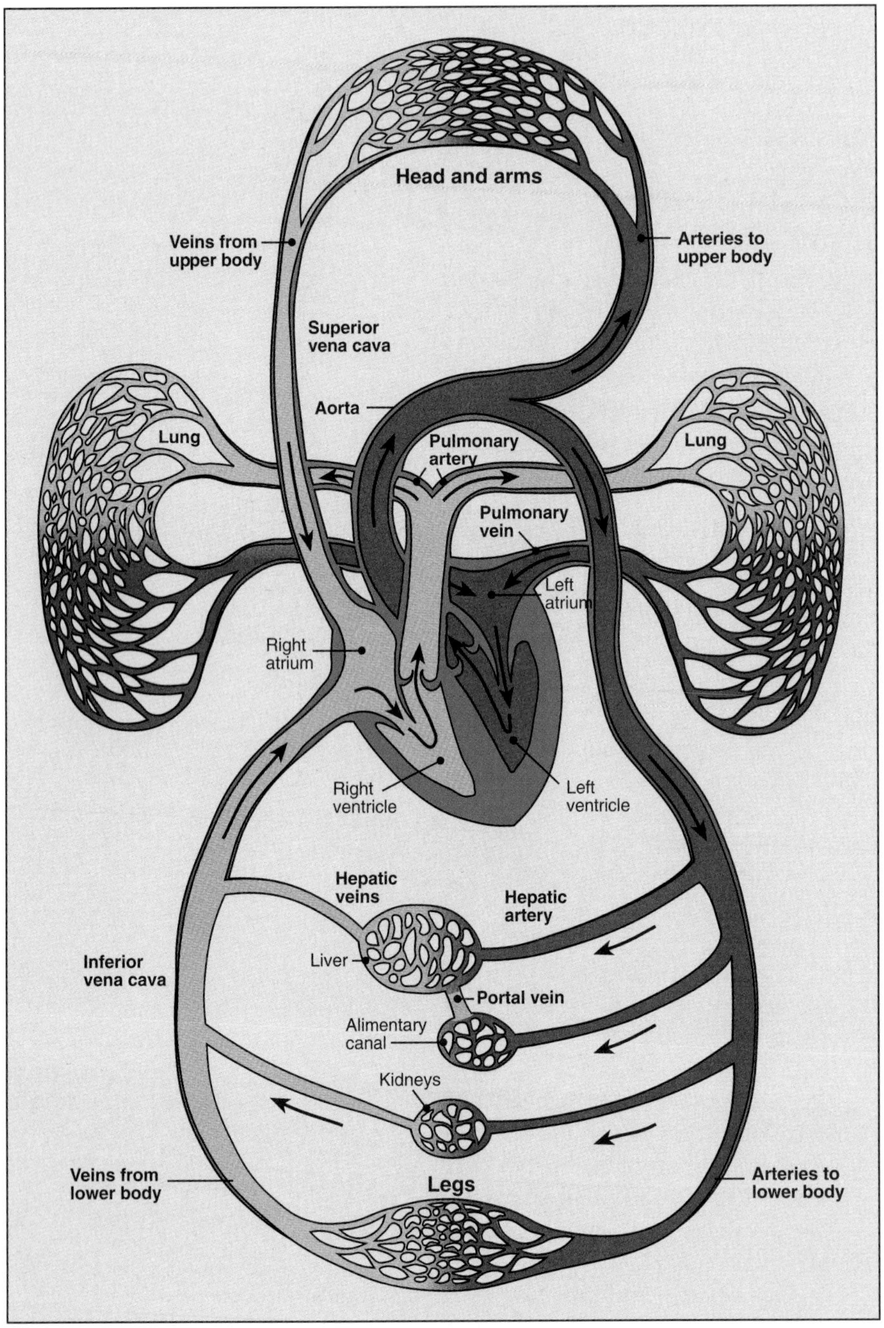

FIGURE 9-1. Schematic view of the cardiovascular system that consists of the heart and the pulmonary and systemic vascular circuits. The dark shading shows the oxygen-rich arterial blood, whereas the deoxygenated venous blood is somewhat paler. In the pulmonary circuit, the situation is reversed, and oxygenated blood returns to the heart in the right and left pulmonary veins.

Arteries

The arteries are the high-pressure tubing that conducts oxygen-rich blood to the tissues. As depicted in Figure 9-3, the arteries are composed of layers of connective tissue and smooth muscle. The walls of these vessels are so thick that no gaseous exchange takes place between arterial blood and the surrounding tissues. Blood pumped from the left ventricle into the highly muscular yet elastic aorta is eventually distributed throughout the body by smaller arterial branches called *arterioles*. The walls of arterioles are composed of circular layers of smooth muscle that either constrict or relax to regulate peripheral blood flow. As is discussed in a following section, it is the capacity of these "resistance vessels" to alter dramatically their internal diameter that provides a rapid and effective means for regulating blood flow through the vascular circuit. This redistribution function is particularly important during exercise because blood can be diverted to working muscles from areas that temporarily can compromise their blood supply.

Capillaries

The arterioles continue to branch and form smaller and less muscular vessels called *metarterioles*. These tiny vessels end in a network of microscopic blood vessels called *capillaries*. These vessels generally contain about 5% of the total blood volume. As was shown in Figure 9-3, the capillary wall consists of only a single layer of

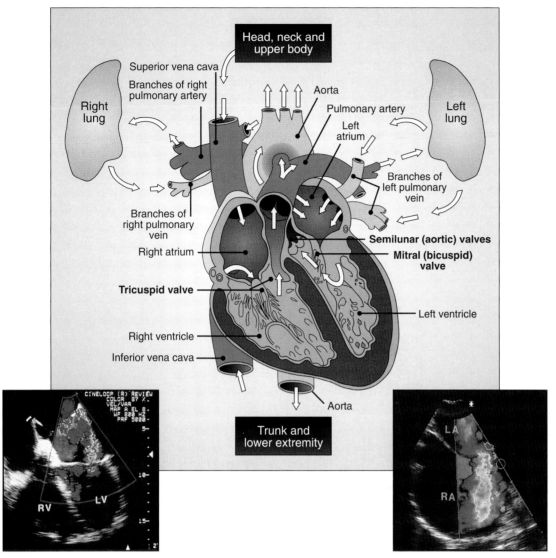

FIGURE 9-2. The heart. The heart's valves provide for the one-way flow of blood as indicated by the arrows. The insert photos are echocardiograms (pictures generated from sound waves) of blood flow through the atrium and ventricles of a 12 year-old child. (Echocardiograms courtesy of Dr. Achi Ludomirsky, Echocardiography Laboratory, Section of Pediatric Cardiology, CS Mott Children's Hospital, University of Michigan.)

endothelial cells. Some capillaries are so narrow that they provide room for only one blood cell to squeeze through, single file. The diameter of the capillary opening is controlled by a ring of smooth muscle called the *precapillary sphincter* that encircles the vessel at its origin. The action of this sphincter is extremely important in exercise because it provides a localized means for regulating capillary blood flow within a specific tissue to meet its metabolic requirements.

Branching of the microcirculation results in an increase in the cross-sectional area of these peripheral vessels that is about 800 times greater than that of the 1-inch diameter aorta. *Because the velocity of blood flow is inversely proportional to the cross section of the vasculature, there is a progressive decrease in velocity as blood moves toward and into the capillaries.* Thus, about 1.5 seconds are required for a blood cell to pass through an average capillary.

Veins

The continuity of the vascular system is maintained as the capillaries feed deoxygenated blood at almost a

A considerable surface. The total surface of the body's capillary walls is more than 100 times greater than the external surface of an average male adult. This translates into an extremely effective means for exchange between the blood and tissues when this tremendous surface is combined with a slow rate of blood flow.

trickle into the *venules* or small veins. Blood flow then increases somewhat because the cross-sectional area of the venous system is now less than the capillaries. The smaller veins in the lower portion of the body eventually empty into the body's largest vein, the *inferior vena cava,* that travels through the abdominal and chest cavities toward the heart. Venous blood coming from the head, neck, and shoulder regions empties into the *superior vena cava* and moves downward to join the inferior vena cava at heart level. This mixture of blood from the upper and lower body then enters the right atrium where it descends into the right ventricle and is pumped through the pulmonary artery to the lungs. Gas exchange takes place in the alveolar-capillary network of the lungs, and the blood returns in the pulmonary veins to the left side of the heart to begin once again its journey throughout the body.

As illustrated in Figure 9-4, blood pressure and blood flow vary considerably in the systemic circulation. In the aorta and the large arteries, blood pressure fluctuates between 120 and 80 mm Hg during the cardiac cycle. The pressure then falls in direct proportion to the resistance encountered in the vascular circuit. The blood at the arteriole end of the capillaries exerts an average pressure of only 30 mm Hg. As blood enters the venules, the impetus for blood flow is almost entirely lost. By the time blood reaches the right atrium, the pressure has decreased to approximately zero. Because the venous system operates under relatively low pressure, the walls of the veins are much thinner and less muscular than the thicker-walled and less distensible arteries (see Figure 9-3).

Venous Return. The low pressure of venous blood poses a special problem

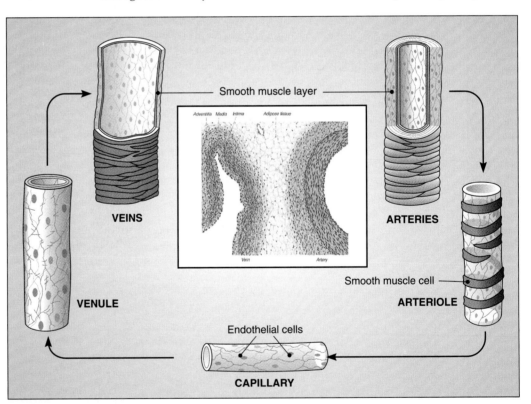

FIGURE 9-3. Blood vessel walls. Each vessel is lined by a single layer of endothelial cells. Arterial walls are surrounded by fibrous tissue and are wrapped in several layers of smooth muscle. The arterioles are sheathed in a single layer of muscle cells; capillaries consist only of one layer of endothelial cells. In the venule, endothelial cells are sheathed in fibrous tissue, and veins also possess a layer of smooth muscle.

that is partly solved by a unique characteristic of veins. Figure 9-5 shows that thin, membranous, flaplike valves spaced at short intervals within the vein permit a one-way blood flow back to the heart. Because venous blood is under relatively low pressure, veins are easily compressed by the smallest muscular contractions or even by minor pressure changes within the chest cavity during the act of breathing. This alternate compression and relaxation of the veins, as well as the one-way action of their valves provides a "milking" action similar to the action of the heart. Compression of the veins imparts considerable energy for blood flow, whereas the "diastole" (or relaxation) of these vessels enables them to refill as blood moves toward the heart. If valves were not present in these vessels, the blood would tend to pool, as it sometimes does in the veins of the extremities, and people would faint every time they stood up because of a reduction in blood flow to the brain.

A Significant Blood Reservoir. The veins are not merely passive conduits. At rest, the venous system normally contains about 65% of the total blood volume; hence, the veins are considered capacitance vessels and serve as blood reservoirs. A slight increase in the tension or tone of the smooth muscle layer alters the diameter of the venous tree and produces a significant and rapid redistribution of blood from the peripheral venous circulation toward the central blood volume returning to the heart. This gives the venous system an important role as an *active blood reservoir* either to retard or to deliver blood to the systemic circulation.

Varicose Veins. Sometimes the valves within a vein become defective and fail to maintain the one-way flow of blood. This condition is called *varicose veins* and usually occurs in the superficial veins of the lower extremities owing to the force of gravity that

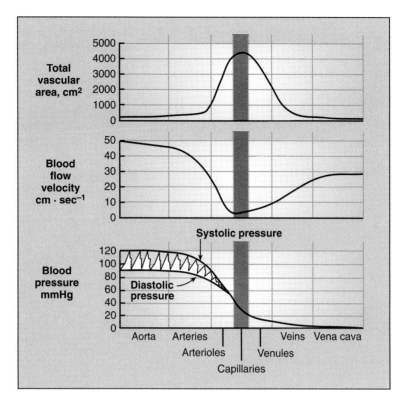

FIGURE 9-4. Blood flow and blood pressure in the systemic circulatory system. Note that blood pressure within the arterial system is inversely related to the total vascular area (resistance) in that section of the vascular tree.

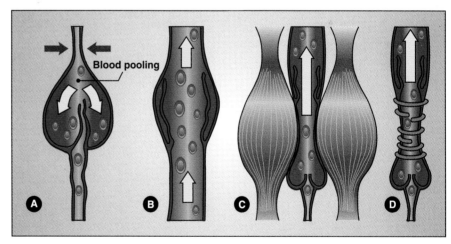

FIGURE 9-5. The valves in veins (*A*) prevent the backflow of blood, but in (*B*) do not hinder the normal one–way flow of blood. Blood can be pushed through veins by nearby active muscle (*C*), or by contraction of smooth muscle bands within the veins (*D*). (From Elias, H., and Pauly, J. E.: *Human Microanatomy.* Philadelphia, F. A. Davis, 1966.)

retards blood flow in an upright posture. Blood gathers in these veins, they become excessively distended and painful, and circulation from the affected area is actually impaired. In severe cases, the venous wall becomes inflamed and may degenerate—a condition called *phlebitis* — and the vessel must be removed surgically.

Individuals who have varicose veins should probably avoid excessive straining exercises often used in resistance training. During such sustained, nonrhythmic muscular contractions, both the muscle and the ventilatory "pumps" are unable to contribute significantly to venous return. The increased abdominal pressure associated with straining also impedes venous return. All of these factors act to cause blood to pool in the veins of the lower body and could aggravate an existing varicose-vein condition. Although exercise cannot prevent the occurrence of varicose veins, regular, rhythmic physical activity may minimize complications because muscle action keeps blood moving toward the heart.

Venous Pooling. The rhythmic action of muscular contraction and consequent compression of the vascular tree is so important to venous return that many people faint when forced to maintain an upright posture without movement. The classic "tilt table" experiment demonstrates this point. A subject lays supine on a table that can pivot to different positions. As long as the table remains horizontal, the subject's heart rate and blood pressure remain relatively unchanged. Once the table is tilted vertically, an uninterrupted column of blood exists from the subject's heart to toes. This creates a hydrostatic force of about 80 to 100 mm Hg and causes blood to pool in the lower extremities. This results in a backup of fluid in the capillary bed that then seeps into the surrounding tissues and causes swelling or *edema*. Consequently, venous return is reduced and blood pressure declines; at the same time, heart rate accelerates and venoconstriction occurs to counter the effects of venous pooling. If the upright position is still maintained, however, the subject eventually faints due to insufficient

cerebral blood supply. Tilting the person either horizontally or head down immediately restores circulation and consciousness.

The Active Cool-Down. The preceding discussion of venous pooling can be used to justify the action of those who continue to walk or jog at a slow pace after strenuous exercise. Such moderate exercise, or "cooling down," would certainly facilitate blood flow through the vascular circuit (including the heart) during recovery. Recall from Chapter 3 that this "active recovery" also aids in removing lactic acid from the blood. The pressurized suits worn by test pilots and special support stockings also aid in reducing the hydrostatic shift of blood to the veins of the lower extremities in the upright position. A similar supportive effect can be achieved in upright exercise in a swimming pool because the external support of the water facilitates the blood's return to the heart.

BLOOD PRESSURE

A surge of blood enters the aorta with each contraction of the left ventricle, distending the vessel and creating pressure within it. The stretch and subsequent recoil of the vascular wall travels as a wave through the entire arterial system. This wave of pressure can readily be felt as the characteristic pulse in the superficial radial artery on the thumb side of the wrist, in the temporal artery (on the side of the head at the temple), or at the carotid artery along the side of the trachea (near the "Adam's apple") in the neck. Each site is convenient for counting the heart rate at rest and after exercise because in healthy persons the pulse rate and heart rate are identical. Figure 9-6 illustrates the pulse taken at these three convenient locations.

At Rest. Figure 9-7 illustrates the measurement of blood pressure by the

Blood pressure = cardiac output x total peripheral resistance. This represents the forces exerted by the blood against the walls of the arteries during a cardiac cycle and is written as systolic/diastolic or, for example, 120/80 mm Hg (stated as 120 over 80).

Hypertension and race. American blacks overall have twice the incidence of high blood pressure as whites and nearly seven times the rate of severe hypertension. Compounding the issue of race and hypertension is the fact that blacks in the United States have a much greater incidence of elevated blood pressure than blacks in Africa. This has led researchers to focus on the possible causative role of diet, stress, cigarette smoking, and other lifestyle and environmental factors in triggering this chronic blood pressure response in genetically susceptible blacks.

auscultatory method. At rest, the highest pressure generated by the heart to move blood through a healthy, resilient vascular system is usually about 120 mm Hg during the contraction of the left ventricle or systole. As the heart relaxes and the aortic valves close, the natural elastic recoil of the aorta and other arteries provide for a continuous head of pressure to maintain a steady flow of blood to the periphery until the next surge of blood is received from the contraction of the heart. During this *diastole* or relaxation phase of the cardiac cycle, blood pressure in the arterial system decreases to about 70 to 80 mm Hg. In people with arteries "hardened" by deposits of minerals and fatty materials within their walls, or with excessive resistance to blood flow in the periphery resulting from kidney malfunction or nervous strain, systolic

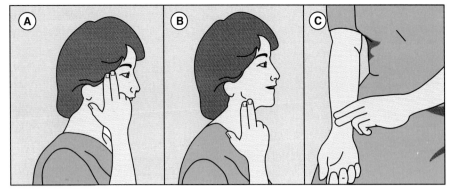

FIGURE 9-6. Pulse rate taken at the *(A)* temporal, *(B)* carotid, and *(C)* radial arteries.

pressure may increase from 120 to as high as 300 mm Hg and diastolic pressures may exceed 120 mm Hg.

High blood pressure, or *hypertension,* imposes a chronic and excessive strain on the normal function of the cardiovascular system. Chronic

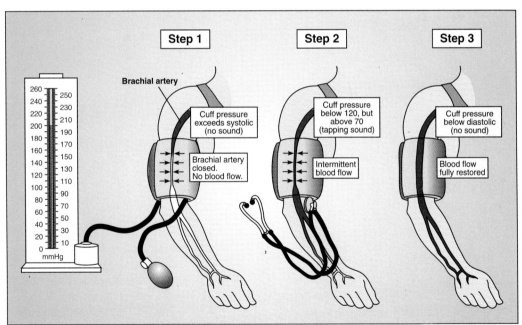

FIGURE 9-7. Measurement of blood pressure at the brachial artery by the auscultatory method. *Step 1.* A pressure cuff or sphygmomanometer is inflated so its pressure exceeds the systolic pressure or highest pressure within the artery. Blood flow is occluded and a brachial pulse (at the elbow fossa) cannot be felt (palpated) or heard (auscultated). Note the restriction of blood through the brachial artery. *Step 2.* The pressure within the cuff is reduced by small increments and the examiner listens until a faint sound occurs. This sound represents blood flowing through the brachial artery. The systolic pressure is the pressure exerted on the walls of the artery when the first soft tapping sounds occur. *Step 3.* As the pressure in the cuff is lowered further, distinct sounds continue to be heard as blood flows through the artery for longer portions of the cardiac cycle. Diastolic pressure refers to the pressure in the artery when the sounds disappear.

FIGURE 9-8. The relationship
between blood flow (cardiac
output) and systemic arterial
pressures measured at the
brachial artery during exercise.
(From Ekelund, L. G., and
Holmgaren, A.: Central hemodynamics during exercise. *Am.
Heart Assoc. Monograph,* No. 15:
33, 1967.)

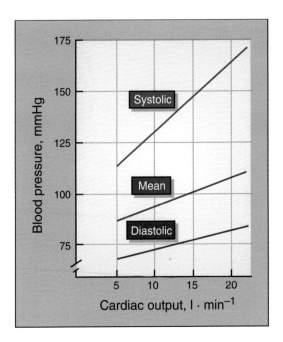

blood vessels in the active muscles
enhances blood flow through a large
portion of the body. The alternate
contraction and relaxation of the muscles themselves also provides significant pumping force to propel blood
through the vessels and return it to
the heart. Increased blood flow during moderate exercise causes systolic
pressure to rise rapidly in the first few
minutes of exercise and level off, usually between 140 and 160 mm Hg,
while diastolic pressure remains relatively unchanged.

Figure 9-8 illustrates the blood
pressure during exercise of progressively increasing intensity in relation
to the quantity of blood ejected into
the arterial circuit each minute
(*cardiac output*). As can be seen, the
various indices of arterial blood
pressure increase linearly with cardiac output. The greatest increases
in exercise blood pressure are
observed during cardiac systole,
whereas the diastolic pressure increases by only about 12% during
the full range of exercise. This
response is similar for both physically conditioned and sedentary
subjects. During maximum exercise
performed by healthy endurance athletes, however, the systolic blood
pressure may increase to 200 mm
Hg, a response most likely due to
the large cardiac outputs of these
athletes.

> **Higher blood pressures in arm exer-
> cise.** Not only is systolic blood pres-
> sure higher when comparing small
> muscle mass exercise to exercise
> using a larger quantity of muscle
> (e.g., arm vs. leg exercise), but the
> diastolic blood pressure is also greatly
> elevated.

hypertension that is not corrected can
eventually lead to heart failure, in
which the heart muscle weakens and
is unable to maintain its pumping
ability. In a stroke, brittle vessels
become obstructed or burst to cut off
the blood supply to vital brain tissue.

During Exercise

Rhythmic Exercise. During rhythmic
muscular activities such as jogging,
swimming, or bicycling, dilation of

Resistance Exercise. With straining-
type exercises (see insert box figure)
such as the various forms of resistance
training (including lifting of barbells),
the blood pressure responses are dramatic as the sustained muscular forces
compress the peripheral arteries causing significant resistance to blood flow.
The additional workload for the heart
could be dangerous for those with
existing high blood pressure or heart
disease. For these people, more rhythmic forms of moderate exercise are
desirable.

Upper Body Exercise. As shown in
Table 9-1, at a given percentage of the
maximal oxygen uptake, systolic and

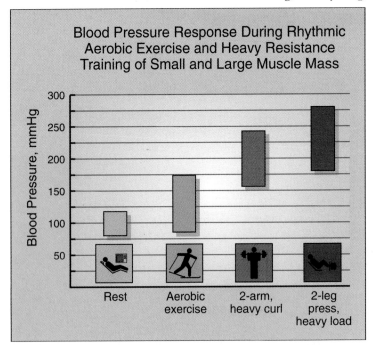

**Blood Pressure Response During Rhythmic
Aerobic Exercise and Heavy Resistance
Training of Small and Large Muscle Mass**

diastolic blood pressures are considerably higher when exercise is performed with the arms than with the legs. It is likely that the smaller muscle mass and vasculature of the arms offer greater resistance to blood flow than the larger muscle mass and vasculature of the legs. Blood flow to the arms during exercise therefore requires a much larger systolic head of pressure. Clearly, this form of exercise represents greater cardiovascular strain because the work of the heart is increased considerably. (See the section on Rate-Pressure Product, later in this chapter.) For individuals who have cardiovascular dysfunction, these observations support the use of exercise that requires larger muscle groups, such as walking, bicycling, and running, in contrast to unregulated exercises that engage a rather limited muscle mass such as shoveling, overhead hammering, or even arm ergometry. *If a systematic program of arm exercise is used, the training levels must be established based on the person's response to this form of exercise and not from some graded exercise test prescription that employs bicycling or running.*

Body Inversion. Inversion devices that allow a person to hang upside-down have become popular. The belief is that this position can offer relaxation, facilitate a strength-training response, or relieve lower back pain. No one has yet demonstrated with careful research that inverting the body is of any practical medical or physiologic significance, and the maneuver can trigger significant increases in blood pressure both at the start and throughout the inversion period. This raises concern about the possible consequences of inversion for people with high blood pressure, or the wisdom of performing exercises in the upside-down position which magnifies the normal rise in blood pressure with exercise. Furthermore, a brief period of inversion doubles pressure within the eye (intraocular pressure) in healthy

TABLE 9-1. Comparison of systolic and diastolic blood pressure during arm and leg exercise at similar percentages of the maximal oxygen uptake*

Percent of max $\dot{V}O_2$	Systolic Pressure (mm Hg)		Diastolic Pressure (mm Hg)	
	Arms	Legs	Arms	Legs
25	150	132	90	70
40	165	138	93	71
50	175	144	96	73
75	205	160	103	75

*From Åstrand, P. O., et al.: Intra-arterial blood pressure during exercise with different muscle groups. *J. Appl. Physiol.*, 20:253, 1965.

young adults. Clearly, individuals with eye disorders should refrain from prolonged periods of inverted posture.

In Recovery

After a bout of sustained submaximal exercise, systolic blood pressure is temporarily reduced below pre-exercise levels for both normotensive and hypertensive subjects. *This hypotensive response to previous exercise lasts about 2 to 3 hours into recovery.* Such findings further support the use of exercise as an important nonpharmacologic therapy in treating hypertension. Thus, it would be justified to recommend that individuals participate in several bouts of light to moderate physical activity interspersed throughout the day.

Effects of Exercise Training

Although the degree to which regular exercise can benefit a hypertensive condition is still unclear, it does appear that both systolic and diastolic blood pressure can be lowered to a modest degree with a program of exercise training. Such results have been observed with normotensive and hypertensive subjects.

Aerobic Exercise Training. In patients with documented coronary-artery disease and in young, middle-aged and

Post-exercise hypotension. In one study of hypertensive men, moderate aerobic exercise caused blood pressure in recovery to fall below the pre-exercise value for an average of 12.7 hours.

TABLE 9-2. Measures of blood pressure at rest and during submaximal exercise prior to and following 4 to 6 weeks of training in seven middle-aged patients with coronary heart disease[a]

Measure[b]	Rest			Submaximal Exercise		
	Mean Value		Difference (%)	Mean Value		Difference (%)
	Before	After		Before	After	
Systolic blood pressure (mm Hg)	139	133	− 4.3	173	155	−10.4
Diastolic blood pressure (mm Hg)	78	73	− 6.4	92	79	−14.1
Mean blood pressure (mm Hg)	97	92	− 5.2	127	109	−14.3

[a] Modified from Clausen, J. P., et al.: Physical training in the management of coronary artery disease. *Circulation* 40:143, 1969.
[b] Blood pressure was measured directly by a pressure transducer inserted into the brachial artery.

Resistance exercise and resting blood pressure. Contrary to popular belief, body builders, power lifters, and Olympic weight lifters do not have resting blood pressures higher than observed for the general population.

---

elderly "borderline" hypertensive patients, the effects of exercise training on blood pressure are the most impressive. As indicated in Table 9-2, the average resting systolic pressure of seven middle-aged male patients decreased from 139 to 133 mm Hg after 4 to 6 weeks of interval training. In addition, at similar submaximal exercise levels, systolic pressure fell from 173 to 155 mm Hg, and diastolic pressure was also reduced from 92 to 79 mm Hg. Similar findings were observed for an apparently healthy yet borderline hypertensive group of 37 middle-aged men after a 6-month exercise program.

The precise mechanism for the exercise-lowering effect on blood pressure is not known, although it may occur because of a reduction of the sympathetic nervous system hormones (catecholamines) with training. This response would contribute to a decrease in peripheral resistance to blood flow and a subsequent reduction in blood pressure. Exercise training may also facilitate the elimination of sodium by the kidneys to subsequently reduce fluid volume and blood pressure. At present, it is prudent to recommend regular exercise as a first line of defense in most therapeutic programs to manage borderline hypertension. For more severe elevations in blood pressure, a com-

bination of diet, weight loss, exercise, and pharmacologic therapies may be required.

Resistance Exercise Training. Resistance training exercises cause a greater rise in blood pressure compared with lower-intensity dynamic movement. However, it does not seem this form of training causes any long-term increase in resting blood pressure. In fact, a regular program of resistance training blunts the blood pressure response to this form of exercise. Trained bodybuilders, for example, show *smaller increases* in systolic and diastolic blood pressure with resistance exercise than both novice and untrained groups. Regular resistance training also benefits the resting blood pressure of borderline hypertensive adolescents.

THE HEART'S BLOOD SUPPLY

Although literally tons of blood may flow through the heart's chambers each day, none of its nourishment passes directly into the myocardium. This is because there are no direct circulatory channels within the heart's chambers leading to its tissues. Instead, the heart muscle has an elaborate circulatory network of its own. As shown inFigure 9-9 these vessels

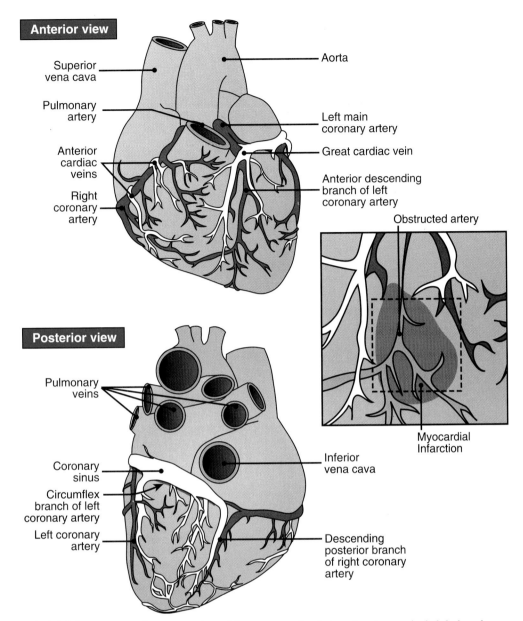

FIGURE 9-9. Anterior and posterior view of the coronary circulation. Arteries are shaded dark and veins are unshaded. The insert figure illustrates a myocardial infarction resulting from the blockage of a coronary vessel.

form a visible, crown-like network that arises from the top portion of the heart called the *coronary circulation.*

The openings for the left and right coronary arteries are situated in the aorta just above the semilunar valves at a point where the oxygenated blood leaves the left ventricle. These arteries then curl around the heart's surface; the right coronary supplies predominantly the right atrium and ventricle, whereas the greatest volume of blood flows in the left coronary artery to the left atrium and ventricle and a small

part of the right ventricle. These vessels divide and eventually form a dense capillary network within the heart muscle. Blood then leaves the tissues of the left ventricle through the *coronary sinus;* blood from the right ventricle exits through the anterior cardiac veins, which then empty directly into the right atrium.

Myocardial Oxygen Utilization

At rest, the oxygen utilization of the myocardium is high in relation to its blood flow. About 70 to 80% of the oxygen is extracted from the blood that flows in the coronary vessels. This is in contrast to most other tissues at rest that use only about one-fourth of the available oxygen. The increased myocardial oxygen demands during exercise can only be met, therefore, by a proportionate increase in coronary blood flow. In vigorous exercise, coronary blood flow may increase four to six times above the resting level as a result of increased myocardial metabolism and increased aortic pressure:

- **Increased myocardial metabolism:** Exercise has a direct effect on the coronary vessels causing them to dilate. For example, hypoxia has an extremely potent dilating effect for increasing blood flow through the myocardium. In addition to localized factors, hormones of the sympathetic nervous system are released during exercise and cause coronary dilatation
- **Increased aortic pressure:** The increased arterial pressure during exercise forces a proportionately greater quantity of blood into the coronary circulation. The ebb and flow of blood in the coronary vessels fluctuates with each phase of the cardiac cycle. On the average, coronary blood flow is about 2.5 times greater during diastole than during systole.

The blood supply to the heart is so profuse that at least one capillary supplies each of the heart's muscle fibers. Impairment in coronary blood flow usually results in chest pains or a condition known as *angina pectoris.* These pains become pronounced during exercise. In fact, the stress of exercise is often used to document or evaluate this condition. A blood clot, or thrombus, lodged in one of the coronary vessels may severely impair normal heart function. Although this form of "heart attack," or more specifically *myocardial infarction,* may be mild, a more complete blockage causes severe damage to the myocardium and could be fatal.

The Rate-Pressure Product: An Estimate of Myocardial Work

Myocardial oxygen uptake is determined by interactions between several mechanical factors — most important, the development of tension within the myocardium and its contractility, and heart rate. With increases in each of these factors during exercise, myocardial blood flow increases to balance oxygen supply with demand. One commonly used estimate of myocardial workload and resulting oxygen uptake is the product of peak systolic blood pressure (SBP), as measured at the brachial artery, and heart rate (HR). This index of relative cardiac work, termed the *double product* or *rate-pressure product* (RPP), is highly related to directly measured myocardial oxygen uptake and coronary blood flow in healthy subjects over a wide range of exercise intensities. The RPP is computed as:

$$RPP = SBP \times HR$$

The RPP has been used extensively in exercise studies of coronary heart disease patients to provide a physiologic correlate to either the onset of angina or electrocardiographic abnormalities. Once this is established, various clinical, surgical, or exercise interventions can be evaluated to determine their effect on cardiac performance. For one thing, the well-documented lowering of exercise heart rate and systolic blood pressure (and hence myocardial oxygen uptake) with training helps explain the improved exercise capacity of cardiac patients with regular exercise. Furthermore, several research studies have shown that prolonged and intense aerobic training can result in a significant increase in the RPP achieved by cardiac patients. In nine patients followed over a 7-year training period, the RPP increased by

11.5% before the appearance of ischemic symptoms. Such findings are important because they provide indirect evidence for an improved level of myocardial oxygenation, perhaps caused by greater coronary vascularization or reduced obstruction, as part of the training adaptation.

Energy for the Heart

As with all tissue, the heart uses the chemical energy stored in food nutrients to reform the ATP to power its work. The heart, however, relies almost exclusively on energy released in aerobic reactions. As such, myocardial fibers have the greatest mitochondrial concentration of all of the body's tissues.

Glucose, fatty acids, and the lactic acid formed in skeletal muscle during glycolysis provide the energy for proper myocardial functioning. At rest, these three substrates are used to resynthesize ATP. In essence, the heart uses for energy whatever substrate it "sees" on a physiologic level — so during heavy exercise, when the efflux of lactic acid from skeletal muscle into the blood increases significantly, the heart may derive more than 50% of its total energy from the oxidation of circulating lactate. During prolonged submaximal physical activity as in distance running, skiing, swimming, skating, hiking, and bicycling, the myocardial metabolism of free fatty acids rises to almost 70% of its total energy requirement.

SUMMARY

PART 1

1. The striated fibers of the myocardium are interconnected so that large portions of the heart contract in a unified manner. Functionally, the heart may be viewed as two separate pumps: One pump receives blood that returns from the body and pumps it to the lungs for aeration (pulmonary circulation), and the other receives oxygenated blood from the lungs and pumps it throughout the body (systemic circulation).

2. Pressure changes created during the cardiac cycle act on the heart's valves to provide a one-way flow of blood through the vascular circuit.

3. The dense capillary network provides a large, effective surface for exchange between the blood and tissues. These minute vessels adjust blood flow in response to

the tissue's metabolic activity.

4. Compression and relaxation of the veins by the action of skeletal muscles impart considerable energy to facilitate venous return. This provides additional justification for the use of active recovery after vigorous exercise.

5. Nerves and hormones act on the smooth muscle layer in the venous walls causing them to constrict or stiffen. This alteration in venous tone can profoundly affect the distribution of total blood volume.

6. The surge of blood with the contraction of the ventricles (and subsequent run-off during relaxation) creates pressure changes within the arterial vessels. The systolic pressure, or highest pressure generated during the cardiac cycle, occurs during ventricular contraction. The diastolic pres-

sure is the lowest pressure reached before the next ventricular contraction.

7. Hypertension imposes a chronic stress on cardiovascular function. Regular aerobic training brings about modest reductions in systolic and diastolic blood pressure at rest and during submaximal exercise.

8. Systolic blood pressure increases in proportion to oxygen uptake and cardiac output during graded exercise, whereas diastolic pressure remains relatively unchanged or increases slightly. At the same relative exercise load, systolic pressures are greater when exercise is performed with the arms than with the legs.

9 After exercise, blood pressure falls below pre-exercise levels and may remain lower for several hours or longer.

10. During resistance exercise, peak systolic and diastolic blood pressures mirror the hypertensive state and may pose a risk to individuals who have existing hypertension. However, regular training with resistance exercise appears to blunt this hypertensive response.

11. At rest, about 80% of the oxygen flowing through the coronary arteries is extracted by the myocardium. This high extraction means that the increased myocardial oxygen demands in exercise can be met only by a proportionate increase in coronary blood flow.

12. Because the myocardium is essentially aerobic tissue, it must continually be supplied with oxygen. Impairment of coronary blood flow causes angina pectoris, and blockage of a coronary artery (myocardial infarction) can cause irreversible damage to the heart muscle.

13. The product of heart rate and systolic blood pressure is called the rate-pressure product; it provides a convenient estimate of the relative workload on the myocardium. This index has been used to study the effects of exercise training on cardiac performance in heart disease patients.

14. The main substrates used by the heart for energy are glucose, fatty acids, and lactic acid. The percentage utilization of these substrates varies with the severity and duration of exercise.

The potential for the vessels of the skin, viscera, and skeletal muscles to conduct blood exceeds by *three or four times* the capacity of the normal heart to pump blood. Consequently, complex mechanisms continually interact to maintain systemic blood pressure and blood flow to various tissues under diverse conditions. Nerves and chemicals regulate both the speed of the pumping heart and the internal opening of various blood vessels. This regulation provides for rapid and effective control of the heart as well as for the distribution of blood throughout the body. When a person is resting comfortably, about 5% or 250 ml of the 5 liters of blood pumped each minute from the heart goes to the skin. This is in contrast to exercise performed in a hot, humid environment in which as much as 20% of the total blood flow is diverted to the body's surface for the purpose of heat dissipation. This "shunting" with appropriate maintenance of blood pressure can occur only within a closed vascular system that can redistribute blood immediately to meet the body's metabolic and physiologic requirements.

REGULATION OF HEART RATE

Cardiac muscle is unique because it has the capability of maintaining its own rhythm. If left to this inherent rhythmicity, the heart would beat steadily between 50 and 80 times each minute. Nerves, however, that go directly to the heart as well as chemicals that circulate in the blood, can rapidly change the heart rate. These *extrinsic* controls of cardiac function cause the heart to speed up in "anticipation," even before the start of exercise. To a large extent, extrinsic regulation provides for heart rates that may be as slow as 30 beats per minute at rest in highly trained endurance athletes, and as fast as 220 beats per minute in maximum exercise.

Intrinsic Regulation

Situated within the posterior wall of the right atrium is a mass of specialized muscle tissue called the *sinoatrial (S-A) node*. This node spontaneously depolarizes and repolarizes to provide the "innate" stimulus to the heart. For this reason, the S-A node is referred to as the *"pacemaker."* The normal route for the transmission of the impulse across the myocardium is shown in Figure 9-10.

The Heart's Electric Impulse. Rhythms originating at the S-A node spread across the atria to another small knot of tissue, the *atrioventricular (A-V) node*. Here the impulse is delayed about 0.10 seconds to provide sufficient time for the atria to contract and force blood into the ventricles. The

Vascular dilation and constriction. If fully dilated, the body's blood vessels could hold about 20 liters of blood even though the actual total blood volume is only about 5 to 6 liters. Thus, a fine regulation of vascular dilation and constriction is required to maintain blood flow and blood pressure.

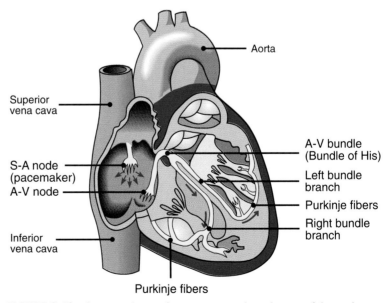

FIGURE 9-10. The normal route for excitation and conduction of the cardiac impulse. This impulse originates at the S-A node and then travels to the A-V node. The impulse is then propagated throughout the ventricular mass.

A-V node gives rise to the *A-V bundle (bundle of His)* that transmits the impulse rapidly through the ventricles over specialized conducting fibers referred to as the *Purkinje system.* These fibers form distinct branches that penetrate the right and left ventricles. Each ventricular cell is stimulated within about 0.06 seconds from the passage of the impulse into the ventricles; this permits a unified and simultaneous contraction of the entire musculature of both ventricles. The transmission of the cardiac impulse can be summarized as follows:

actually becomes more positive than the outside. During the diastolic phase of the cardiac cycle, the membranes repolarize and the resting membrane potential is re-established.

The electrical activity about the heart creates an electrical field throughout the body. Because the salty body fluids provide an excellent conducting medium, the sequence of electrical events before and during each cardiac cycle can be detected as voltage changes by electrodes placed on the skin's surface. The graphic record of the heart's electric activity is

> **The heart's period of rest.** The heart's relatively long period of depolarization of approximately 0.20 to 0.30 second is required before it can receive another impulse and contract again. This "rest" or refractory period serves an important function because it provides sufficient time for ventricular filling between beats.

S-A node ⟶ Atria ⟶ A-V node ⟶ A-V bundle (Purkinje fibers) ⟶ Ventricles

The Electrocardiogram (ECG). Similar to all nerve and muscle tissue, the outer surface of the myocardial cells is electrically more positive than the inside. This polarity is reversed just before contraction when the heart is stimulated and the inside of the cell

called the *electrocardiogram (ECG)*. A characteristic, normal ECG is presented in Figure 9-11. Also indicated are the important sequences that represent the major electrical activity of the heart muscle.

The *P wave* represents the depolarization of the atria. It lasts about 0.15 seconds and heralds atrial contraction. The P wave is then followed by the relatively large *QRS complex*. This reflects the electrical changes caused by the depolarization of the ventricles; at this point, the ventricles contract. Atrial repolarization that follows the P wave produces a wave so small that it is usually obscured by the large QRS complex. The *T wave* represents repolarization of the ventricles. This occurs during ventricular diastole.

The ECG serves useful purposes for the cardiologist and exercise specialist. It provides an effective means for monitoring heart rate objectively during exercise. Radiotelemetry makes it possible to transmit the ECG while the person is free to perform various types of exercise including football, weightlifting, basketball, ice hockey, dancing, and even swimming. Electrocardiography also serves as an extremely valuable tool for

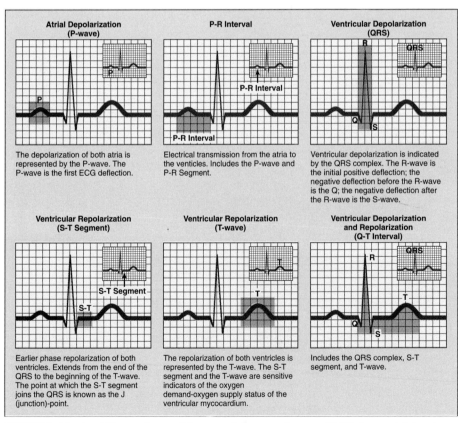

FIGURE 9-11. The different phases of the normal electrocardiogram (ECG) from atrial depolarization (*upper left*) to the repolarization of the ventricles (*lower right*).

uncovering abnormalities in heart function, especially those related to cardiac rhythm, electrical conduction, myocardial oxygen supply, and actual tissue damage. (See Chapter 18).

Extrinsic Regulation

Neural influences are superimposed on the inherent rhythmicity and conductivity of the myocardium. These influences originate in the cardiovascular center in the medulla and are transmitted through the sympathetic and parasympathetic components of the autonomic nervous system. As shown in Figure 9-12, the atria are supplied with large numbers of sympathetic and parasympathetic neurons, whereas the ventricles receive sympathetic fibers almost exclusively.

Sympathetic Influence. Stimulation of the sympathetic cardioaccelerator nerves releases the *catecholamines, epinephrine* and *norepinephrine.* These neural hormones act to accelerate the depolarization of the sinus node that causes the heart to beat faster. This acceleration in heart rate is termed *tachycardia.* The catecholamines also significantly increase myocardial contractility. Epinephrine released from the medullary portion of the adrenal glands in response to a general sympathetic activation also produces a similar, although slower-acting effect on cardiac function.

Parasympathetic Influence. Acetylcholine, the hormone of the parasympathetic nervous system, retards the rate of sinus discharge and slows the heart. This slowing of heart rate is termed *bradycardia.* The effect is largely mediated through the action of the vagus nerve whose cell bodies originate in the cardioinhibitory center in the medulla. Vagal stimulation has essentially no effect on myocardial contractility.

Training Effects. Exercise training creates an imbalance between the tonic

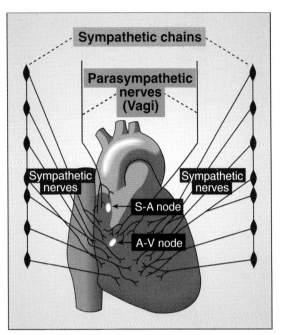

FIGURE 9-12. Distribution of sympathetic and parasympathetic nerve fibers to the heart.

activity of the sympathetic accelerator and parasympathetic depressor neurons in favor of greater vagal dominance. This is mediated primarily by an increase in parasympathetic activity and perhaps a decrease in sympathetic discharge. In addition, training may also decrease the intrinsic rate of firing of the S-A node. These adaptations account for the significant bradycardia often observed in highly conditioned endurance athletes or in sedentary subjects following aerobic training.

Peripheral Input. The cardiovascular center in the *medulla* receives sensory input from peripheral receptors in blood vessels, joints, and muscles. Stimuli from these mechanical and chemical receptors that monitor the state of active muscle modify either vagal or sympathetic outflow to bring about the appropriate cardiovascular response. Receptors in the aortic arch and carotid sinus respond to changes in arterial blood pressure. As blood pressure increases, the stretch of the arterial vessels activates these baroreceptors and brings about a reflex slowing of the heart, as well as a com-

Neural control of heart rate. In moderate exercise, the increase in heart rate is brought about by removal of parasympathetic stimulation; in more strenuous exercise, heart rate acceleration occurs by direct activation of the sympathetic cardioaccelerator nerves.

pensatory dilation of the peripheral vasculature. This causes blood pressure to decrease toward more normal levels. To some degree, this particular feedback mechanism is over-ridden during exercise because heart rate and blood pressure are both increased considerably. More than likely, the baroreceptors act as a brake to prevent abnormally high blood pressure levels in exercise.

Carotid Artery Palpation. In some individuals, strong external pressure against the carotid artery produces a slowing effect on the heart rate. This effect is probably mediated by direct stimulation of the baroreceptors at the bifurcation of the carotid artery. An accurate measure of heart rate is important for training when specific "target" heart rates are assigned to regulate training intensity (see Chapter 12). If the target heart rate method used to monitor the heart rate consistently gave low values (as could be the case with carotid artery palpation), the person would be pushed to a higher exercise level. This method would certainly be undesirable in exercise prescription for cardiac patients.

Generally, for both healthy adults and cardiac patients, carotid artery palpation causes little or no alteration in heart rate at rest or during exercise and recovery, and thus is an appropriate technique to gauge heart rate. However, various forms of vascular disease affect the sensitivity of the carotid sinus. With disease, palpation could give a falsely low reading for the heart rate. When this is of concern, an excellent substitute method is to determine pulse rate at the radial artery or temporal artery (see page 245) because palpation of these vessels causes no change in heart rate.

Cortical Input. Impulses from the cerebral cortex pass via small afferent nerves through the cardiovascular center in the medulla. Consequently, variations in one's emotional state significantly affect cardiovascular responses and make it difficult to obtain "true" resting values for heart rate and blood pressure. Cerebral impulses also cause the heart rate to rise rapidly in anticipation of exercise. The *anticipatory heart rate* probably results from both an increase in sympathetic discharge and reduction of vagal tone.

The extent of the anticipatory response is clearly demonstrated in Figure 9-13. The heart rate of trained sprint runners was telemetered at rest, at the starting commands, and during a 60-, 220-, and 440-yard race. Heart rate averaged 148 beats per minute at the starting commands in anticipation of the 60-yard sprint; this represented 74% of the total heart rate adjustment to the run! The magnitude of the anticipatory heart rate was greatest in the short sprint events and successively lower before the longer sprint distances.

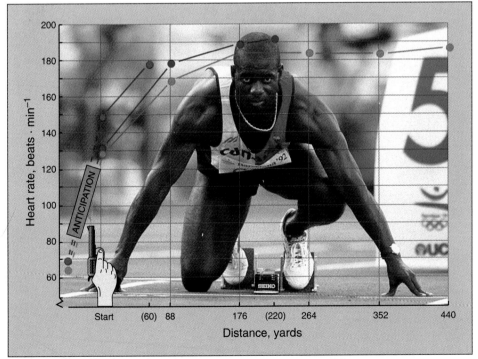

FIGURE 9-13. Heart rate response of sprint-trained runners. The greatest increase in anticipatory heart rate (heart rate prior to exercising) occurred in the short sprint events and became successively lower prior to the longer sprint distances. (From McArdle, W. D., et al.: Telemetered cardiac response to selected running events. *J. Appl. Physiol.*, 23: 566, 1967.)

The pattern of anticipatory heart rate was also demonstrated in events of longer duration. For example, the anticipatory heart rate of four athletes trained for the 880-yard run averaged 122 beats per minute, whereas heart rate averaged 118 beats, during the starting commands of the 1-mile run and 108 beats for the 2-mile run. The initial neural outflow in anticipation of exercise is desirable before intense activity of short duration (such as sprinting) to provide for the rapid mobilization of bodily reserves. On the other hand, this mechanism for "revving the body's engine" might be wasteful in events of longer duration.

In essence, the heart is "turned on" during exercise by an increase in sympathetic and decrease in parasympathetic activity combined with input from the central command in the brain. More than likely, considerable accelerator input is also provided by activating receptors in joints and muscles as exercise begins. Even in the so-called nonsprint events, heart rate is approximately 180 beats per minute within 30 seconds of 1- and 2-mile runs. Further increases in heart rate are gradual, with several plateaus being reached during the run.

DISTRIBUTION OF BLOOD

Effect of Exercise

Increased energy expenditure usually requires rapid adjustments in blood flow that affect the entire cardiovascular system. For example, nerves and local metabolic conditions act on the smooth muscular bands of arteriole walls and cause them to alter their internal diameter almost instantaneously. In addition, stimulation of nerves to the venous capacitance vessels causes them to "stiffen." Such venoconstriction permits large quantities of blood to move from peripheral veins into the central circulation.

During exercise, the vascular portion of active muscles is increased considerably by the dilation of local arte-

rioles. Concurrently, other vessels that can temporarily compromise their blood supply constrict or "shut down." Kidney function vividly illustrates this regulatory capacity for adjusting regional blood flow. Renal blood flow at rest is normally about 1100 ml per minute; this blood flow is about 20% or 1000 ml of the 5000 ml cardiac output. In maximal exercise, renal blood flow may be reduced to only 250 ml per minute or about 1% of a 25 liter exercise cardiac output!

Regulation of Blood Flow

Blood flow through the vascular circuit is in general accord with the physical laws of hydrodynamics as applied to rigid, cylindrical vessels. The volume of flow in any vessel is:

- Directly proportional to the pressure gradient between the two ends of the vessels and not to the absolute pressure within the vessel
- Inversely related to the resistance encountered to the flow

Resistance, which is the force impeding blood flow, is determined by three factors: (1) the thickness or viscosity of the blood, (2) the length of the conducting tube, and, most important, (3) the diameter of the blood vessel. The relationship between pressure, resistance, and flow can be expressed by an equation referred to as *Poiseuille's law:*

$$\text{Flow} = \text{Pressure gradient} \times \text{Vessel radius}^4 \div \text{Vessel length} \times \text{Viscosity}$$

In the body, the viscosity of the blood and the length of the transport vessel remain relatively constant under most circumstances. *Therefore, the most important factor that affects blood flow is the diameter of the conducting tube.* In fact, the resistance to flow changes with the vessel diameter raised to the fourth power; if the diameter is reduced by one-half, flow through the vessel decreases 16 times! Conversely, doubling the vessel's diameter increas-

Blood flow regulation. In a physiologic sense, constriction and dilation provide the most important mechanisms for regulating regional blood flow.

A responsive vasculature. The capacity of large portions of the vasculature to either constrict or dilate provides for a rapid redistribution of blood to meet the tissue's metabolic requirements while maintaining an appropriate blood pressure throughout the entire system.

es the volume 16 fold. If the pressure within the vascular circuit were to remain relatively constant, a considerable alteration in blood flow would be achieved with only a small change in vessel diameter.

Local Factors. At rest, only 1 of every 30 to 40 capillaries is actually open in muscle tissue. The opening of dormant capillaries in exercise serves three important functions:

- It provides for a significant increase in muscle blood flow
- Because more channels are open, the increased blood volume can be delivered with only a minimal increase in the velocity of flow
- The enhanced vascularization increases the effective surface for exchange between the blood and the muscle cells

A decrease in a tissue's oxygen supply produces a potent local stimulus for vasodilatation in skeletal and cardiac muscle. Furthermore, local increases in temperature, carbon dioxide, acidity, adenosine, and magnesium and potassium ions enhance regional blood flow. These *autoregulatory mechanisms* for blood flow make sense from a physiologic standpoint because they reflect elevated tissue metabolism and an increased need for oxygen. Rapid and local vasodilatation is the most effective immediate step for increasing a tissue's oxygen supply.

Neural Factors. Superimposed on the vasoregulation afforded by local factors is a central vascular control mediated by the sympathetic, and to a minor degree, the parasympathetic portions of the autonomic nervous system. For example, muscles contain small sensory nerve fibers that are highly sensitive to substances released in local tissue during exercise. When these fibers are stimulated, they provide input to the central nervous system to bring about an appropriate cardiovascular response. With central regulation, blood flow in one area cannot dominate when a concurrent oxygen need exists in other more "needy" tissues.

Figure 9-14 is a schematic view of the distribution of sympathetic outflow. These nerve fibers end in the muscular layers of small arteries, arterioles, and precapillary sphincters.

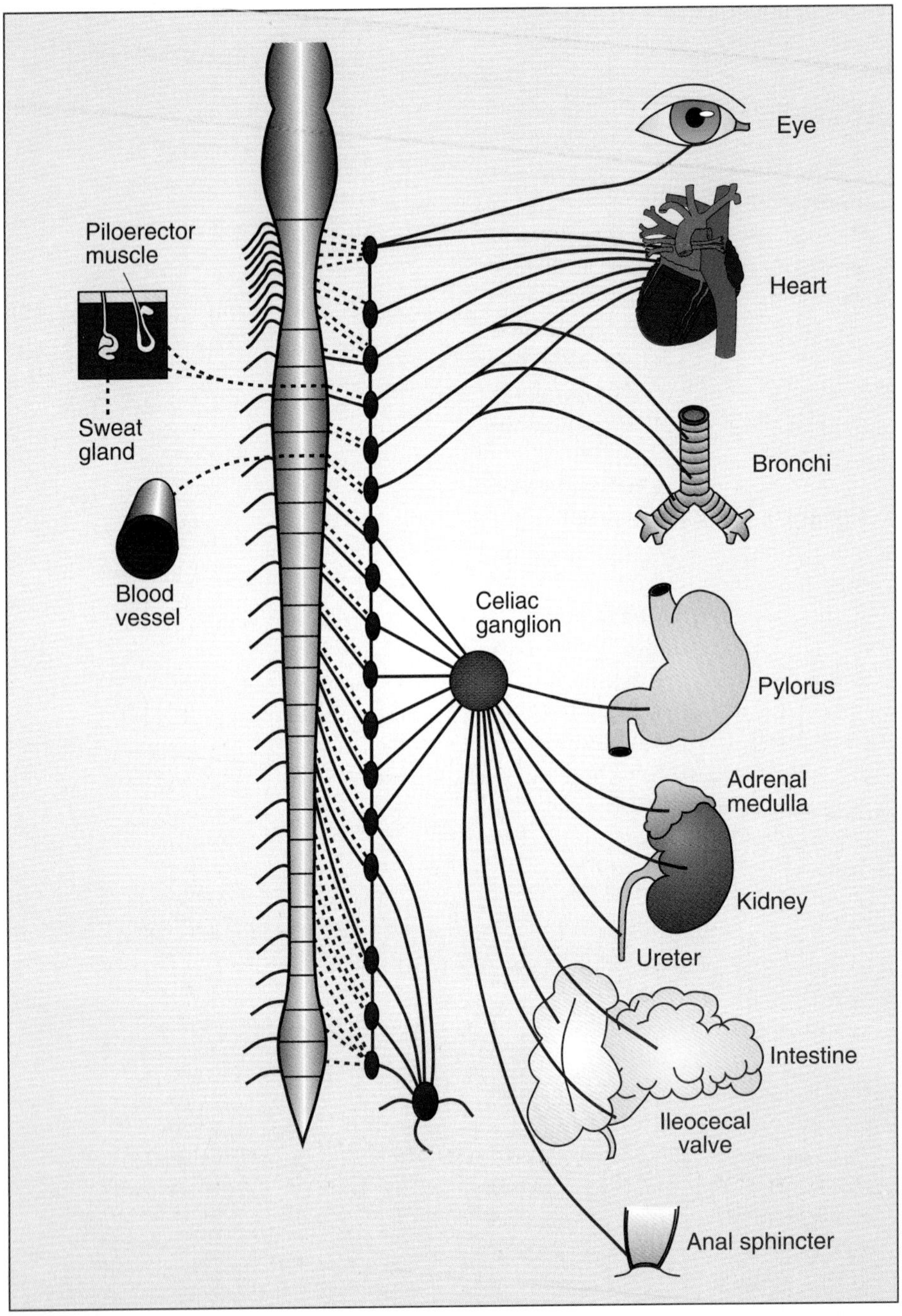

FIGURE 9-14. Schematic view of vascular regulation via sympathetic outflow to various organs and tissues.

Norepinephrine acts as a general vasoconstrictor and is released at certain sympathetic nerve endings. These sympathetic constrictor fibers are called *adrenergic fibers*. Other sympathetic neurons in skeletal and heart muscle release acetylcholine; these are the *cholinergic fibers* and their action is vasodilatation.

The sympathetic nervous system consists of both adrenergic constrictor and cholinergic dilator fibers. The constrictor nerves are constantly active; consequently some blood vessels are always in a state of constriction. The relative degree of this constrictor activity is referred to as *vasomotor tone*. Dilatation of blood vessels under the influence of adrenergic neurons is due more to a reduction in vasomotor tone than to an increase in the action of either sympathetic or parasympathetic dilator fibers. In addition, whatever sympathetically-activated vasoconstriction is present in active tissue is rapidly over-ridden by the powerful local vasodilation induced by metabolism.

Hormonal Factors. Sympathetic nerves also terminate in the medullary portion of the adrenal glands. In response to sympathetic activation, this glandular tissue secretes large quantities of epinephrine and a smaller amount of norepinephrine into the blood. These hormones then act as chemical messengers to bring about a generalized constrictor response, except in the blood vessels of the heart and skeletal muscles. During exercise, the hormonal control of regional blood flow is relatively minor compared with the more local, rapid, and powerful sympathetic neural drive.

INTEGRATED RESPONSE IN EXERCISE

The chemical, neural, and hormonal adjustments before and during exercise are summarized in Table 9-3.

At the onset of exercise (or even slightly before exercise begins), car-

TABLE 9-3. Summary of integrated chemical, neural, and hormonal adjustments prior to and during exercise

Condition	Activator	Response
Preexercise "anticipatory" response	Activation of motor cortex and higher areas of brain causes increase in sympathetic outflow and reciprocal inhibition of parasympathetic activity.	Acceleration of heart rate; increased myocardial contractility; vasodilation in skeletal and heart muscle (cholinergic fibers); vasoconstriction in other areas, especially skin, gut, spleen, liver, and kidneys (adrenergic fibers); increase in arterial blood pressure.
Exercise	Continued sympathetic cholinergic outflow; alterations in local metabolic conditions due to hypoxia, ↓ph, ↑ Pco$_2$, ↑ ADP, ↑ Mg^{++}, ↑Ca^{++}, and ↑ temperature.	Further dilation of muscle vasculature.
	Continued sympathetic adrenergic outflow in conjunction with epinephrine and norepinephrine from the adrenal medullae.	Concomitant constriction of vasculature in inactive tissues to maintain adequate perfusion pressure throughout the arterial system. Venous vessels stiffen to reduce their capacity. This venoconstriction facilitates venous return and maintains the central blood volume.

diovascular changes are initiated from nerve centers above the medullary region. These adjustments significantly increase the rate and pumping strength of the heart, as well as cause predictable alterations in regional blood flow that are proportional to exercise intensity. As exercise continues and becomes more intense, sympathetic cholinergic outflow plus local metabolic factors that act on chemosensitive nerves as well as directly on the blood vessels, cause dilatation of resistance vessels in the active musculature. This reduced peripheral resistance permits the active areas to accommodate greater blood flow. There are further constric-tor adjustments in less active tissues; thus, an adequate perfusion pressure is maintained even with the large dilatation of the muscle's vasculature. This constrictor action provides for the appropriate redistribution of blood to meet the metabolic requirements of active muscles.

Factors that affect venous return are equally as important as those that regulate arterial blood flow. The action of the muscle and ventilatory pumps, and the stiffening of the veins themselves, immediately increase blood flow back to the right ventricle. With these adjustments, a balance is maintained between cardiac output and venous return.

SUMMARY

PART 2

1. The cardiovascular system provides for rapid regulation of heart rate, as well as for the effective distribution of blood in the vascular circuit while maintaining blood pressure in response to the body's metabolic and physiologic needs.

2. The cardiac rhythm is initiated at the S-A node. The impulse then travels across the atria to the A-V node where it is delayed and then rapidly spreads across the large ventricular mass. With this normal conduction pattern, the atria and ventricles contract effectively to provide impetus for blood flow.

3. The ECG provides a record of the sequence of the heart's electrical events during the cardiac cycle. Electrocardiography is important for detecting various abnormalities in heart function at rest and during exercise.

4. Epinephrine and norepinephrine, the sympathetic catecholamines, act to accelerate heart rate and increase myocardial contractility. Acetylcholine, the parasympathetic neurotransmitter, acts through the vagus nerve to slow the heart.

5. The heart is "turned on" in the transition from rest to exercise by an increase in sympathetic activity and a decrease in parasympathetic activity. Both of these events are integrated with input from the brain's central command centers.

6. Neural and hormonal extrinsic factors modify the heart's inherent rhythmicity, enabling it to speed up rapidly in anticipation of exercise, and to increase to 200 beats per minute or higher in maximum exercise.

7. Palpation of the carotid artery is generally an appropriate means for determining the actual heart rate during and immediately after exercise.

8. A large part of the heart rate adjustment to exercise is probably due to cortical influence before and during the initial stages of the activity.

9. Nerves, hormones, and local metabolic factors act on the smooth muscle bands in various blood vessels. This causes them to alter their internal diameter to regulate blood flow. Adrenergic sympathetic fibers release norepinephrine that causes vasoconstriction; cholinergic sympathetic neurons secrete acetylcholine that brings about vasodilation.

Part 3 CARDIOVASCULAR DYNAMICS DURING EXERCISE

CARDIAC OUTPUT

Cardiac output is the primary indicator of the functional capacity of the circulation to meet the demands of physical activity. The output from the heart, as with any pump, is determined by its rate of pumping (*heart rate*) and the quantity of blood ejected with each stroke (*stroke volume*). Cardiac output is computed as:

> Cardiac output =
> Heart rate x Stroke volume

Measurement of Cardiac Output

It is a relatively simple task to measure the output from a hose, pump, or faucet. One need only open the valve, and collect and measure the volume of fluid ejected during a specified time period. This, however, is not the case with the measurement of cardiac output. Even if such a direct technique were applied, the disruption of the main output vessel in a closed circulatory system would in itself dramatically alter the output. Several methods are commonly used to measure cardiac output in humans; these include the Fick, CO_2 rebreathing, and indicator dilution methods.

Fick Method. Cardiac output can be computed if one knows a person's oxygen uptake during a minute, and the average difference between the oxygen content of arterial and mixed venous blood (a-v̄ O_2 difference). The question then to be answered is: How much blood must have circulated during the minute to account for the observed oxygen uptake, given the observed a-v̄ O_2 difference? The formula that expresses the relationship between cardiac output, oxygen uptake, and a-v̄ O_2 difference

embodies the principle set forth by Fick in 1870 and is termed the *Fick equation.*

> Cardiac output (ml · min⁻¹) = [O_2 uptake (ml · min⁻¹) ÷ a-v̄ O_2 difference (ml per 100 ml blood)] x 100

The Fick principle for determining cardiac output is illustrated in Figure 9-15. In this example, a person consumes 250 ml of oxygen during a minute at rest, and the a-v̄ O_2 difference during this time averages 5 ml of oxygen per 100 ml of blood. These values are substituted in the Fick equation:

> Cardiac output (ml · min⁻¹) = [250 ml O_2 ÷ 5 ml O_2] x 100 = 5,000 ml blood

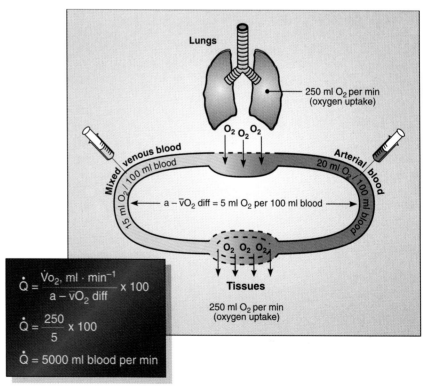

$$\dot{Q} = \frac{\dot{V}O_2, \text{ml} \cdot \text{min}^{-1}}{a - \overline{v}O_2 \text{ diff}} \times 100$$

$$\dot{Q} = \frac{250}{5} \times 100$$

$$\dot{Q} = 5000 \text{ ml blood per min}$$

FIGURE 9-15. Application of the Fick principle for measuring cardiac output (Q̇).

Although the Fick principle is straightforward, actual measurement by this technique is complex and is usually limited to a clinical setting where the benefits of measurement exceed any potential risk. The measurement of oxygen uptake involves the methods of open-circuit spirometry summarized in Chapter 4. A more difficult aspect is obtaining the a-v̄ O_2 difference. A representative sample of arterial blood can be obtained from any convenient systemic artery such as the femoral, radial, or brachial artery. Although these arteries are easily located, an arterial puncture can be traumatic to the patient. To obtain

bon dioxide substituted in the Fick equation. It is possible to obtain valid estimates of venous and arterial carbon dioxide levels by using a rapid carbon dioxide gas analyzer that measures the concentration of this gas throughout the ventilatory cycle. The technique is noninvasive or "bloodless" and requires only a breath-by-breath analysis of carbon dioxide. Carbon dioxide production is measured by the open-circuit method.

Once venous and arterial carbon dioxide concentrations are estimated, cardiac output is calculated in accordance with the Fick principle as follows:

$$\text{Cardiac output} = CO_2 \text{ production} \div \bar{v}\text{-a } CO_2 \text{ difference}$$

an accurate estimate of the average oxygen content of mixed venous blood, it is necessary to sample from an anatomic "mixing chamber" such as the right atrium, right ventricle, or even the pulmonary artery. This is achieved by threading a flexible tube (catheter) through the antecubital vein in the arm up into the superior vena cava and into the right heart. Arterial and mixed venous blood are then sampled during the same period of measurement as oxygen uptake.

The direct Fick technique has been used in numerous studies of cardiovascular dynamics under a variety of experimental conditions including exercise. In fact, this method generally provides the criterion to validate other techniques for cardiac output measurement. The main criticism of the Fick method is that its invasive nature may alter the measurement of cardiovascular dynamics. Thus, although the obtained value for cardiac output may be accurate, it may not reflect a person's "normal" cardiovascular response pattern.

Other Less Invasive Methods

CO₂ Rebreathing. Cardiac output also can be determined from values of car-

The advantages seem obvious for the CO_2 rebreathing method over the direct Fick technique. The method is bloodless, involves minimal interference with the subject, and does not require close medical supervision. Because the method is noninvasive, it may provide more accurate estimates of the cardiovascular dynamics during exercise than would be obtained by more invasive techniques. One limitation of the method requires the subject to exercise at a steady rate. This may place some restrictions on its use during maximal and "supermaximal" exercise or during the transition from rest to exercise.

Dye Dilution. Cardiac output also can be determined by injecting a known quantity of an inert dye into a large vein. The indicator material remains in the vascular stream usually bound to plasma proteins or red blood cells. It is then mixed as the blood travels to the lungs and back to the heart before being ejected into the systemic circuit. Arterial blood samples are continuously measured and the area under the dilution-concentration curve indicates the average concentration of indicator material as blood is pumped from the heart. The cardiac output is computed based on the dilution of a known quantity of dye in an unknown quantity of blood.

. . . .
CARDIAC OUTPUT AT REST

On the average, the entire blood volume, of approximately 5 liters (5,000 ml) is pumped from the left ventricle each minute. This value is similar for trained as well as untrained subjects.

Untrained Subjects

For the average person, a 5-liter cardiac output is usually sustained with a heart rate of about 70 beats per minute. If this heart rate value is substituted in the cardiac output equation (see following equation), the calculated stroke volume of the heart equals 71 ml per beat. Stroke volumes for women usually average 25% below values for men. This "gender difference" is essentially due to the smaller body size of the average woman compared to a male counterpart.

Endurance Athletes

For the endurance athlete, resting heart rate generally averages about 50 beats per minute at rest. Because the resting cardiac output of the athlete also averages 5 liters per minute, blood is circulated with a proportionately larger stroke volume of 100 ml per beat. Average values for cardiac output, heart rate, and stroke volume of trained and untrained individuals at rest are summarized as follows:

Although the calculations are straightforward, the underlying physiologic mechanisms are not fully understood. It is not clear whether the bradycardia that occurs with endurance training "causes" a larger stroke volume or vice versa, because the myocardium itself is strengthened through aerobic exercise. Two factors are probably operative with training:
- Endurance training increases vagal tone that slows the heart
- The heart muscle strengthened through endurance training is capable of a more forceful stroke with each contraction

. . . .
CARDIAC OUTPUT DURING EXERCISE

Blood flow increases in proportion to the intensity of exercise. In progressing from rest to steady-rate exercise, cardiac output undergoes a rapid increase followed by a gradual rise until it reaches a plateau. At this point, blood flow is sufficient to meet the metabolic requirements of exercise.

In relatively sedentary, college-aged men, cardiac output during strenuous exercise increases by about four times the resting level to an average maximum of 20 to 22 liters of blood per minute. Maximum heart rate for these young adults averages about 195 beats per minute. Consequently, stroke volume is generally between 103 and 113 ml of blood per beat during maximal exercise. In contrast, world-class endurance athletes have maximum cardiac outputs of 35 to 40 liters per minute. This is even

Stroke volume makes the difference. A significantly large stroke volume is the key factor that enables an endurance athlete to pump more blood from the heart each minute than an untrained counterpart.

	Rest					
	Cardiac output	=	**Heart rate**	x	**Stroke volume**	
Untrained:	5000 ml	=	70 b·min^{-1}	x	71 ml	
Trained:	5000 ml	=	50 b·min^{-1}	x	100 ml	

more impressive if one considers that the trained person may have a slightly lower maximum heart rate than the sedentary person of similar age. *Thus, the endurance athlete achieves a large cardiac output compared with his or her sedentary counterpart because of a considerably larger stroke volume.* For example, the cardiac output of an Olympic medal winner in cross-country skiing increased almost 8 times above rest to 40 liters per minute in maximum exercise with an accompanying stroke volume of 210 ml per beat. This is nearly twice the volume of blood pumped per beat compared with the maximum stroke volume of a healthy, sedentary person of the same age.

The functional capacity of the heart during maximum exercise in trained and untrained men is summarized as follows:

increasing intensity. One group of six highly trained endurance athletes had trained for several years; there were three sedentary college students in the other group. The students' exercise responses were evaluated before and after a 55-day training program designed to improve aerobic fitness.

Several important conclusions can be drawn from these data:

- The heart of the endurance athlete has a considerably larger stroke volume during rest and exercise than an untrained person of the same age
- For both trained and untrained individuals, the greatest increase in stroke volume in upright exercise occurs in the transition from rest to moderate exercise. As exercise becomes more intense, there are only small further increases in stroke volume

Maximum Exercise						
	Cardiac output	=	Heart rate	x	Stroke volume output	
Untrained:	22,000 ml · min⁻¹	=	195 b · min⁻¹	x	113 ml	
Trained:	35,000 ml · min⁻¹	=	195 b · min⁻¹	x	179 ml	

Stroke Volume During Exercise: Training Effects

Figure 9-16 illustrates the stroke volume response for two groups of men during upright exercise of

- Maximum stroke volume is reached at 40 to 50% of the maximal oxygen uptake; in young adults, this usually represents a heart rate of 120 to 140 beats per minute
- For untrained individuals, there is only a small increase in stroke volume in the transition from rest to exercise. For these individuals, the major increase in cardiac output is brought about by an acceleration in heart rate. For the trained endurance athletes, both heart rate and stroke volume increase to augment cardiac output, with the increase in the athlete's stroke volume generally being 50 to 60% above resting values

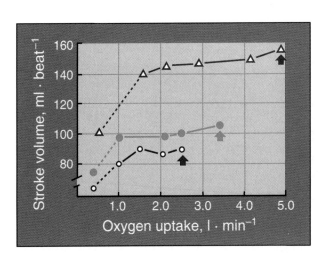

FIGURE 9-16. Stroke volume in relation to oxygen uptake during upright exercise in endurance athletes (▲) and sedentary college students prior to (○) and following (●) 55 days of aerobic training; (◆ = maximal values). (From Saltin, B.: Physiological effects of physical conditioning. *Med. Sci. Sports,* 1: 50, 1969.)

For previously sedentary subjects, 8 weeks of aerobic training substantially increases stroke volume, but these values are still well below values observed for elite athletes. The precise factor to account for this difference has yet to be determined. It probably reflects more prolonged training, genetics, or a combination of both.

Stroke Volume and max $\dot{V}O_2$. The importance of stroke volume in differentiating people who have high and low values for max $\dot{V}O_2$ is amplified in Table 9-4.

These data were obtained from three groups: athletes, healthy but sedentary men, and patients who had mitral stenosis, a valvular disease of the heart that results in inadequate emptying of the left ventricle. The differences in max $\dot{V}O_2$ between groups are closely related to differences in maximal stroke volume. Patients who had mitral stenosis had an aerobic capacity and maximum stroke volume that was half that of the sedentary subjects. This relationship was also apparent in comparisons between healthy subjects. The maximal oxygen uptake of the athletes averaged 62% larger than the sedentary group, and this was paralleled by a 60% larger stroke volume. Because the maximal heart rate in both groups was similar, the difference in cardiac output (and max $\dot{V}O_2$) can be attributed solely to differences in maximal stroke volume.

Stroke Volume: Systolic Emptying Versus Diastolic Filling

Two physiologic mechanisms regulate stroke volume and contribute in varying degrees to the increase in stroke volume noted with exercise. The first is intrinsic to the myocardium and requires enhanced cardiac filling that is followed by a more forceful contraction. The second mechanism is governed by neurohormonal influence. It involves normal ventricular filling accompanied by an increased stroke volume due to a forceful systolic ejection that brings about a greater cardiac emptying.

Greater Diastolic Filling. Greater ventricular filling during the diastolic phase of the cardiac cycle can be affected by any factor that increases venous return (referred to as *preload*) or slows the heart rate. An increase in end-diastolic volume stretches the myocardial fibers to cause a powerful ejection stroke as the heart contracts. This causes the normal stroke volume to be expelled plus additional blood that entered the ventricles to stretch the myocardium.

The relationship between the force of contraction and the resting length of muscle fibers was described by two physiologists, Frank and Starling, in their animal experiments in the early 1900s. The improved contractility is believed to result from a more optimum arrangement of myofilaments as the muscle stretches. This phenomenon applied to the

Stroke volume increase. Enhanced cardiac filling and more complete emptying are the two factors that contribute to the increase in the heart's stroke volume in exercise.

TABLE 9-4. Maximal values for oxygen uptake, heart rate, stroke volume, and cardiac output in three groups having very low, normal, and high aerobic capacities*

Group	max $\dot{V}O_2$ (l·min^{-1})	Max Heart Rate (beats·min^{-1})	Max Stroke Volume (ml)	Max Cardiac Output (l·min^{-1})
Mitral stenosis	1.6	190	50	9.5
Sedentary	3.2	200	100	20.0
Athlete	5.2	190	160	30.4

*Modified from Rowell, L. B.: Circulation. *Med. Sci. Sports,* 1:15, 1969.

TABLE 9-5. The effect of body position on cardiac output, stroke volume, and heart rate at rest and during exercise in well-trained athletes*

	Rest		Moderate Exercise		Strenuous Exercise	
	Supine	Upright	Supine	Upright	Supine	Upright
Cardiac output, l·min⁻¹	9.2	6.6	19.0	16.9	26.3	24.5
Stroke volume, ml	141	103	163	149	164	155
Heart rate, beats·min⁻¹	65	64	115	112	160	159
Oxygen uptake, ml·min⁻¹	345	384	1769	1864	3364	3387

* Data from Bevegård, S., et al.: Circulatory studies in well-trained athletes at rest and during heavy exercise, with special reference to stroke volume and the influence of body position. *Acta Physiol. Scand.*, 57:26, 1963.

myocardium has been termed *Starling's Law of the Heart.*

For many years it was taught that the Frank-Starling mechanism provided the "modus operandi" for all increases in stroke volume during exercise. Physiologists believed that the enhanced venous return in exercise caused a greater cardiac filling, so that the ventricles were stretched in diastole and subsequently responded with a more forceful ejection. In all likelihood, this is the pattern of response for stroke volume in transition from rest to exercise or as a person moves from the upright to the recumbent position. Enhanced diastolic filling probably also occurs in activities such as swimming, where the body's horizontal position optimizes blood flow into the heart.

From the data in Table 9-5, it is clear that body position has a significant effect on circulatory dynamics. Cardiac output and stroke volume are highest and most stable in the horizontal position. In this position, the stroke volume is nearly maximum at rest and increases only slightly during exercise. In contrast, the force of gravity in the upright position acts to counter the return flow of blood to the heart; this results in diminished stroke volume. This postural effect is apparent in comparing circulatory dynamics at rest in the upright and supine positions. As the intensity of upright exercise increases, however, stroke volume increases and approaches the maximum stroke volume in the supine position.

Greater Systolic Emptying. In most forms of upright exercise, the heart may not fill to an extent that would cause a significant increase in cardiac volume. Thus, the increase in stroke volume occurs mainly by means of a more complete emptying during systole, despite an increasing systolic pressure or *afterload.*

At rest in the upright position, 40 to 50% of the total end-diastolic blood volume remains in the left ventricle after a contraction; this *residual volume of the heart* amounts to approximately 50 to 70 ml of blood. Myocardial contractile force is enhanced in exercise by the sympathetic hormones epinephrine and norepinephrine that produce augmented stroke power and greater systolic emptying of the heart. In addition, endurance training enhances the contractile state of the myocardium itself and improves its capability for achieving a large stroke volume.

Heart Rate During Exercise: Training Effects

The large stroke volume of topflight endurance-trained athletes, and the increases in stroke volume of sedentary subjects following aerobic training, are usually accompanied by a proportionate heart rate reduction during submaximal exercise. The relationship between heart rate and oxygen uptake is shown in Figure 9-17. As in Figure 9-16 for stroke volume, comparisons are made between athletes and sedentary students before and after training.

The lines relating heart rate and oxygen uptake are essentially linear for both groups throughout the major portion of the exercise range. Although the untrained students' heart rates accelerated rapidly as exercise severity increased, the heart rates of the athletes accelerated to a much lesser extent; that is, the *slope* or rate of change of the lines differed considerably. Consequently, an athlete (or trained student) who has good cardiovascular response to exercise will achieve a higher level of exercise and oxygen uptake before reaching a particular submaximal heart rate than a sedentary student. At an oxygen uptake of 2.0 liters per minute, the heart rate of the athletes averaged 70 beats per minute lower than those of the sedentary students! After 55 days of training, this difference in submaximal heart rate was reduced to about 40 beats per minute. In each instance, the cardiac output was approximately the same. This means that the difference was due to the larger stroke volume.

DISTRIBUTION OF CARDIAC OUTPUT

The blood flow to specific tissues is generally proportional to their metabolic activity.

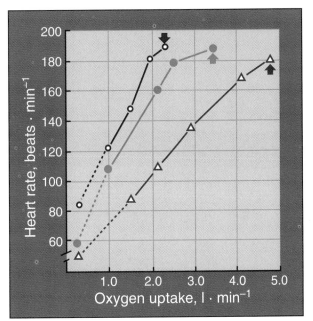

FIGURE 9-17. Heart rate in relation to oxygen uptake during upright exercise in endurance athletes (▲) and sedentary college students prior to (o) and following (●) 55 days of aerobic training; (◆= maximal values). From Saltin, B.:Physiological effects of physical conditioning. *Med. Sci. Sports,* 1: 50, 1969.)

At Rest

At rest in a comfortable environment, the 5-liter cardiac output is distributed in roughly the proportions shown in Figure 9-18. About one-fifth of the cardiac output is directed to muscle tissue whereas the major portion of blood flows to the digestive tract, liver, spleen, brain, and kidneys.

During Exercise

Table 9-6 shows the percentage distribution of the cardiac output during light, moderate, and strenuous exercise. Although regional blood flow during physical activity varies considerably depending on environmental conditions, level of fatigue, and the type of exercise, *the major portion of the exercise cardiac output is diverted to the working muscles.* At rest, about 4 to 7 ml of blood are delivered each minute to every 100 g of muscle. This output increases steadily until at maximum exertion, muscle

Training lowers heart rate. It is common for the exercise heart rate to be lowered by 12 to 15 beats per minute as a result of an aerobic conditioning program.

Blood flow to muscle. The peak blood flow to a limited amount of maximally activated muscle may reach 300 to 400 ml · min⁻¹ per 100 g.

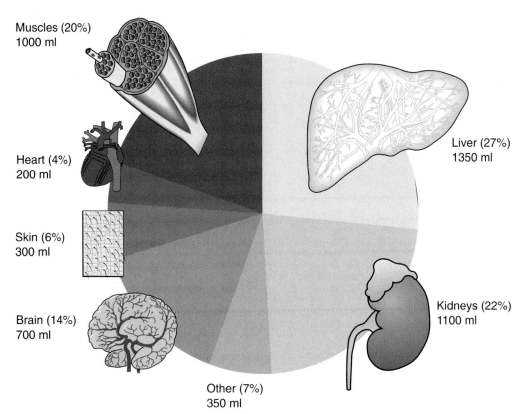

Muscles (20%)
1000 ml

Heart (4%)
200 ml

Skin (6%)
300 ml

Brain (14%)
700 ml

Liver (27%)
1350 ml

Kidneys (22%)
1100 ml

Other (7%)
350 ml

FIGURE 9-18. Relative distribution to the various organs of the five-liter cardiac output at rest. Note that despite the large mass of muscle, this tissue at rest receives approximately the same amount of blood as the much smaller kidneys.

blood flow can average about 50 to 75 ml per 100 g of tissue.

Redistribution of Blood Flow. The increase in muscle blood flow in exercise is due largely to increased cardiac output. Muscle blood flow, however, is disproportionately large in relation to blood flow in other tissues. Owing to neural and hormonal vascular regulation, including the local metabolic conditions of the muscles themselves, blood is redistributed and directed through working muscles from areas that can temporarily tolerate a reduced normal blood flow. This *shunting of blood* from specific tissues occurs primarily during maximum exercise. Blood flow to the skin increases during light and moderate exercise so metabolic heat generated in the muscles can be dissipated at the skin's surface. During intense exercise of short duration, however, this tissue temporarily restricts its

blood flow, even if exercise is performed in a hot environment.

In some instances, blood flow is reduced by as much as four-fifths of an organ's blood supply at rest! The kidneys and splanchnic tissues, for example, utilize only 10 to 25% of the oxygen available in their blood supply. Consequently, a considerable reduction in blood flow to these tissues can be tolerated before oxygen demand exceeds supply and organ function is compromised. With reduced blood flow, the energy needs of the tissues are maintained by increased extraction of oxygen from the available blood supply. A substantial reduction in blood flow to the visceral organs can be sustained for more than an hour during heavy exercise. Redistribution of blood from these tissues occurs even without an increase in cardiac output; this "frees" as much as 600 ml of oxygen per minute for use by the working muscles.

Not without a price. A prolonged reduction in liver and kidney blood flow may have its consequences; it may contribute to fatigue that eventually occurs in prolonged submaximal exercise.

TABLE 9-6. Distribution of cardiac output during light, moderate, and strenuous exercise, as well as the extraction of oxygen in these various tissues at rest[a]

Tissue	Resting a-v̄ O_2 Difference (ml O_2 per 100 ml blood)	Exercise Blood Flow, ml·min⁻¹ Light	Moderate	Maximum
Splanchnic	4.1	1100 (12%)[b]	600 (3%)	300 (1%)
Renal	1.3	900 (10%)	600 (3%)	250 (1%)
Cerebral	6.3	750 (8%)	750 (4%)	750 (3%)
Coronary	14.0	350 (4%)	750 (4%)	1000 (4%)
Muscle	8.4	4500 (47%)	12,500 (71%)	22,000 (88%)
Skin	1.0	1500 (15%)	1900 (12%)	600 (2%)
Other		400 (4%)	500 (3%)	100 (1%)
		9500	17,600	25,000

[a] Modified from Anderson, K. L.: The cardiovascular system in exercise. In *Exercise Physiology,* Edited by H. B. Falls. New York, Academic Press, 1968.
[b] Values in parentheses represent percent of total cardiac output.

Blood Flow to the Heart and Brain. Some tissues cannot compromise their blood supply (Table 9-6). The myocardium normally uses about 75% of the oxygen in the blood flowing through the coronary circulation at rest. With this limited margin of safety, the increased myocardial oxygen needs during exercise are met mainly by an increase in coronary blood flow. Thus, a four- to five-fold increase in cardiac output is accompanied by a similar increase in coronary circulation; in maximum exercise, this amounts to about 1 liter of blood per minute. Recent evidence indicates that cerebral blood flow increases by about 30% with exercise compared to rest.

CARDIAC OUTPUT AND OXYGEN TRANSPORT

At Rest

Each 100 ml of arterial blood carries about 20 ml of oxygen or 200 ml of oxygen per liter of blood (see Chapter 8). The oxygen-carrying capacity of blood normally varies only slightly because the hemoglobin content of the blood fluctuates little with one's state of training. Because about 5 liters of blood are circulated each minute at rest for trained and untrained adults, potentially 1,000 ml of oxygen are available to the body (5 liters blood x 200 ml oxygen). Because the oxygen uptake at rest averages only about 250 ml per minute, approximately 750 ml of oxygen returns "unused" to the heart. However, this is not an unnecessary waste of cardiac output. To the contrary, extra oxygen in the blood above the resting needs represents oxygen in reserve — a margin of safety that is released immediately should there be a sudden increase in a tissue's metabolic needs.

During Exercise

A person with a maximum heart rate of 200 beats per minute and a stroke volume of 80 ml per beat generates a maximum cardiac output of 16 liters (200 x 80 ml). Even during maximum exercise, the saturation of hemoglobin with oxygen is nearly complete, so each liter of arterial blood carries about 200 ml of oxygen. Consequently, 3,200 ml of oxy-

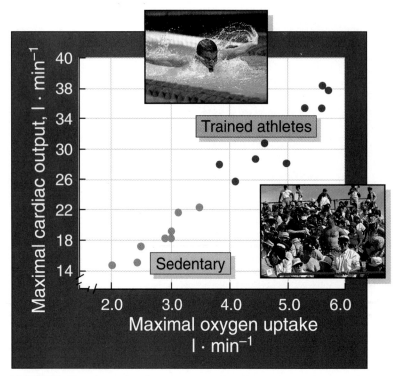

FIGURE 9-19. Relationship between maximal cardiac output and maximal oxygen uptake in trained and untrained individuals. The maximal cardiac output is related to the max $\dot{V}O_2$ in a ratio of about 6:1. Top photo courtesy of Jim Richardson, Varsity women's swim coach, University of Michigan.

Cardiac output and $\dot{V}O_2$ in children. During growth from puberty to adolescence, the oxygen cost of exercise increases as body mass increases; this in turn is closely matched by an increase in the heart's stroke volume with a proportionate increase in cardiac output.

gen are circulated each minute via a 16-liter cardiac output (16 liters x 200 ml oxygen). If all the oxygen could be extracted from this 16-liter cardiac output as it traveled through the body, the greatest possible max $\dot{V}O_2$ would be 3200 ml. However, this is only theoretical because the oxygen needs of certain tissues such as the brain do not increase greatly with exercise, yet these tissues require a rich and uninterrupted blood supply.

Any increase in the maximum cardiac output directly affects a person's capacity to circulate oxygen. Based on the preceding example, if the heart's stroke volume was increased from 80 to 200 ml per beat while the maximum heart rate remained unchanged at 200 beats per minute, maximum cardiac output would be dramatically increased to 40 liters of blood per minute. This means that the quantity of oxygen circulated in maximum exercise each minute would have increased approx-

imately 2.5 times from 3200 to 8000 ml (40 liters x 200 ml O_2). An increase in maximum cardiac output clearly results in a proportionate increase in the potential for aerobic metabolism.

Close Association Between Maximum Cardiac Output and max $\dot{V}O_2$. Figure 9-19 shows the relationship between maximum cardiac output and the capacity for achieving a high level of aerobic metabolism. Included are values for the sedentary and untrained as well as elite endurance athletes. The relationship is unmistakable. A low aerobic capacity is closely associated with a low maximum cardiac output, whereas the ability to generate a 5- or 6-liter max $\dot{V}O_2$ is always accompanied by a 30- to 40-liter cardiac output.

Figure 9-20 further amplifies the important role of cardiac output in sustaining aerobic metabolism. The cardiac output increases linearly with oxygen uptake throughout the major portion of the work range for both trained athletes and students. Each 1-liter increase in oxygen uptake above rest is generally accompanied by a 5- to 6-liter increase in blood flow. This relationship does not vary regardless of the type of exercise performed. Over a wide range of dynamic exercise, there is a tight linkage between systemic blood flow (cardiac output) and the level of oxygen uptake. The distinguishing feature for the endurance athlete is a high level of oxygen uptake and cardiac output capacity. The 35% increase in max $\dot{V}O_2$ noted in Figure 9-20 for the students after 55 days of training was accompanied by an almost proportionate increase in maximum cardiac output.

Gender Differences in Cardiac Output. The response pattern of cardiac output during exercise is similar between boys and girls and men and women. Both teenage and adult females, however, have a 5 to 10% larger cardiac output at any level of *submaximal* oxygen uptake than males. This apparent gender difference in cardiac output in submaximal exercise may be due to the roughly 10% lower hemoglobin content of the blood of women compared to values for men. Within limits, therefore, a small decrease in the blood's oxygen-carrying capacity owing to lower hemoglobin is compensated for by a proportionate increase in cardiac output in submaximal exercise.

Training and Submaximal Cardiac Output. Several reports have demonstrated that training, although improving the maximal cardiac output, also tends to reduce the minute volume of the heart during moderate exercise. In one study, the submaximal cardiac output of young men after 16 weeks of training was reduced by about 1.0 to 1.5 l·min^{-1}. As expected, maximal cardiac output increased 8% from 22.4 to 24.2 liters per minute. With the reduction in submaximal cardiac output, the exercise oxygen requirement was met by a corresponding increase in oxygen extraction (a-v̄O$_2$ difference) in the active muscles. This was presumably the result of an enhanced ability of the trained muscles to generate ATP aerobically and to function at a lower partial pressure of oxygen.

Extraction of Oxygen: The a-v̄ O$_2$ Difference

If blood flow were the only means for increasing a tissue's oxygen supply, then cardiac output would have to increase from 5 liters per minute at rest to 100 liters per minute in maximum exercise to achieve a 20-fold increase in oxygen uptake — an increase in oxygen uptake that is common among trained individuals. Fortunately, such a large cardiac output is unnecessary during exercise because hemoglobin releases its considerable "extra" oxygen from the blood that perfuses the active tissues. Consequently, two mechanisms are available to increase the capacity for oxygen uptake. The first is to speed

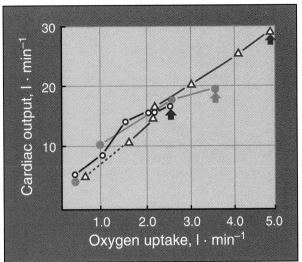

FIGURE 9-20. Cardiac output in relation to oxygen uptake during upright exercise in endurance athletes (Δ) and sedentary college students prior to (o) and following (●) 55 days of aerobic training; (▲ = maximal values). (From Saltin, B.: Physiological effects of physical conditioning. *Med. Sci. Sports,* 1: 50, 1969.)

up the rate of blood flow, that is, increase cardiac output; the second is to use the relatively large quantity of oxygen already carried by the blood, that is, expand the a-v̄ O$_2$ difference. The important relationship between cardiac output, a-v̄ O$_2$ difference, and max V̇O$_2$ is summarized in the following rearrangement of the Fick equation:

Benefit to cardiacs. A lower submaximal exercise cardiac output reduces the workload of the heart which is of real benefit to patients who suffer from exertional angina.

$$\text{Max } \dot{V}O_2 = \text{Maximal cardiac output} \times \text{Maximal a-v̄ } O_2 \text{ difference}$$

At Rest. At rest, an average of 5 ml of oxygen is used from the 20 ml of oxygen in each 100 ml of arterial blood that passes through the capillaries. Thus, 75% of the blood's original oxygen load still remains bound to hemoglobin and returns "unused" to the heart. This corresponds to an oxygen extraction (a-v̄O$_2$ difference) of 5 ml of oxygen per 100 ml of blood.

During Exercise. Figure 9-21 shows a comparison of the relationship between a-v̄ O$_2$ difference and exercise intensity for trained athletes and untrained students. The a-v̄ O$_2$ difference for the students increases steadily during light and moderate exercise and reaches a maximum value of about 15 ml of oxygen per 100 ml of blood. Following 55 days of training, the student's maximum capacity for oxygen extraction increased about 13% to 17 ml of oxygen. This means that during heavy exercise, about 85% of the oxygen was extracted from arterial blood. Actually, even more oxygen is released in the working muscles because the value for a-v̄ O_2 difference reflects an average based on calculations from *mixed* venous blood. Mixed venous blood contains blood returning from tissues whose oxygen utilization during exercise is not nearly as high as that of active muscle.

The post-training value for the maximal a-v̄ O_2 difference for the students is identical to that achieved by the endurance athletes. Obviously, the large difference in max $\dot{V}O_2$ between the athletes and students is due to the lower cardiac output capacity of the students.

In Heart Disease. The heart muscle of patients who have *advanced* coronary artery disease often shows an impaired capacity to perform work or to improve with regular exercise. As a result, training adaptations are negligible in maximal stroke volume and cardiac output. For these patients, however, improvements in exercise tolerance and aerobic capacity are still possible because regular exercise increases the skeletal muscles' ability to receive and utilize oxygen. This contributes to expanding the a-v̄ O_2 difference (and lactate threshold), and enables the patients to work at higher levels.

Factors that Affect a-v̄ O_2 Difference in Exercise

The maximal a-v̄ O_2 difference attained during exercise is influenced to some degree by one's capacity to divert a large portion of the cardiac output to working muscles. As mentioned previously, certain tissues can temporarily compromise their blood supply considerably during exercise for purposes of shunting blood and increasing the quantity of oxygen available for muscle metabolism. This redirection of the central circulation is facilitated by exercise training.

At the local level, the microcirculation of skeletal muscle is also enhanced with aerobic training. Studies with humans and animals have demonstrated a greater capillary density in specific muscles trained by endurance exercise. Muscle biopsies from the quadriceps femoris showed a significantly larger ratio of capillaries to muscle fibers in trained than in sedentary men. An increase in the capillary-to-fiber ratio would be a positive adaptation to provide a greater interface for the exchange of nutrients and metabolic gases in exercise.

Another important factor that determines the capacity for oxygen extraction is the ability of individual muscle cells to generate energy aerobically. Aerobic training improves the metabolic capacity of the specific cells trained by exercise. The mitochondria enlarge and even increase in number, as does the quantity of enzymes for aerobic energy transfer. All of the local

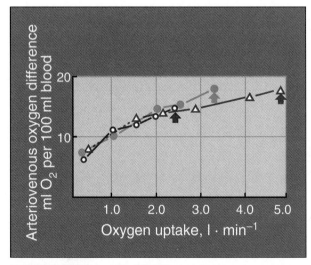

FIGURE 9-21. The a-v̄ O_2 difference in relation to oxygen uptake during upright exercise in endurance athletes (Δ) and sedentary college students prior to (o) and following (●) 55 days of training; (▲ = maximal values). (From Saltin, B.: Physiological effects of physical conditioning. *Med. Sci. Sports,* 1: 50, 1969.)

EXERCISING AFTER CARDIAC TRANSPLANTATION

The prognosis for living is not good for patients with left ventricular dysfunction who have left ventricular ejection fractions of less than 20% (referred to as end-stage heart disease). Although some minimally symptomatic or asymptomatic patients may function in a near-normal fashion and may survive for several years, the majority of symptomatic patients die within 1 year of diagnosis. Cardiac transplantation is the accepted form of treatment for these patients. The first successful human heart transplant was performed in 1967. Although long-term survival (>1 yr) was rare prior to the 1980s, survival rates have progressively increased due to improved immunosuppressive drug combinations, and utilization of the transvenous endomyocardial biopsy technique for early detection of tissue rejection.

Orthotopic transplantation involves removing the recipient's diseased heart and connecting the donor heart to the remaining great vessels and atria. For selected patients, a "piggy back" transplant is performed with the donor heart placed in the recipient's chest without removing the recipient's diseased heart. Regardless of the form of transplantation, patients generally have complicated recoveries with recurrent hospitalizations and prolonged medical care. The most common complications are

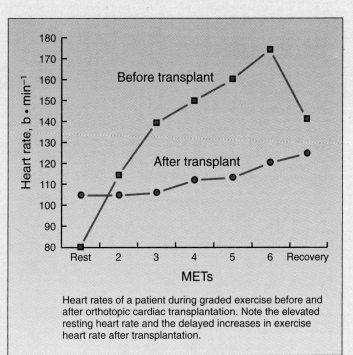

Heart rates of a patient during graded exercise before and after orthotopic cardiac transplantation. Note the elevated resting heart rate and the delayed increases in exercise heart rate after transplantation.

rejection of the donor heart and infection, and both factors are the leading causes of death.

Following successful transplantation, patients generally report a favorable quality of life, and approximately 50% of patients are able to return to work. Successful pregnancy and vaginal delivery in a cardiac transplant patient has been reported, as well as the completion of a full marathon in under 6 hours! In general, however, the cardiac transplant patient has a significantly impaired exercise capacity with diminished physiological and hemodynamic function.

The acute responses to exercise for transplant patients can be classified as abnormal. They exhibit a limited cardiac output and oxygen uptake response during exercise, and have an elevated resting heart rate and a reduced left ventricular ejection fraction. To date, the research literature includes 140 patients (136 males and 4 females) who have

undergone an exercise training program after transplant surgery. Collectively, the data show that transplant patients can respond positively to exercise training. The increase in peak $\dot{V}O_2$ is encouraging, ranging from a high of 40% to a low of 17%. This indicates that transplant patients can dramatically improve cardiorespiratory fitness, probably because the initial fitness of these men and women was so poor.

The guidelines for exercise prescription for cardiac transplant patients are essentially the same as for other post-cardiac surgery patients. The exception is that the target heart rate guidelines are not used because of the delayed heart rate response of the denervated transplanted organ. Most often, exercise intensity is prescribed using the Borg scale of perceived exertion (RPE) using ratings between "fairly light" to "somewhat hard" (RPE scale between 11 and 14). Because of the blunted heart rate response with the onset of exercise, a graded warm-up is especially important for the cardiac transplant patient. Furthermore, because the transplanted heart has no connections to the nervous system, patients who have exercise-induced ischemia do not experience the painful warnings of angina pectoris.

Reference

Squirers, R. W. Exercise training after cardiac transplantation. *Med. Sci. Sports. Exerc.* 23:686, 1991.

improvements within the muscle ultimately result in an enhanced capacity for the aerobic production of ATP.

CARDIOVASCULAR ADJUSTMENTS TO UPPER BODY EXERCISE

The highest oxygen uptake achieved by men and women during arm exercise is generally about 70 to 80% of the max $\dot{V}O_2$ during leg exercise. Similarly, the maximal values for heart rate and pulmonary ventilation are lower with arm exercise. These differences in physiologic response are probably due to the relatively small muscle mass of the upper body used in arm ergometry. The lower maximal heart rate in exercise using a smaller muscle mass such as when performed with the arms is most likely the result of: (1) a reduced output from the motor cortex (feedforward stimulation) to the cardiovascular center in the medulla or (2) a reduced feedback stimulation to the medulla from the smaller active musculature

In submaximal exercise, however, the response pattern is reversed. Figure 9-22 shows that for any level of exercise the oxygen uptake is higher when exercising the arms compared with the legs. This difference is small during light exercise but becomes larger as the intensity of effort increases. This response can be attributed to a lower economy in arm exercise owing to the static muscular contractions in this form of exercise (which does not contribute to the external work accomplished). In addition, extra musculature is required to stabilize the torso during most forms of arm exercise.

The physiologic strain is greater in upper body exercise for any level of oxygen uptake or percent of maximal oxygen uptake. Heart rate, blood pressure, ventilation, and perception of physical effort are generally higher when the arms are used as the primary means for generating power.

By understanding the differences in physiologic response between arm and leg exercise, the physician and exercise specialist can formulate prudent exercise programs using both forms of exercise. The important point is that greater metabolic and physiologic strain accompanies a standard exercise load with the arms. For this reason, exercise prescriptions based on running and bicycling cannot be applied to upper body exercise. Furthermore, because the correlation between max $\dot{V}O_2$ for arm and leg exercise is low, it is not possible to accurately predict one's capacity for arm exercise from a test using the legs, and vice versa. This further substantiates the concept of specificity for aerobic fitness.

THE "ATHLETE'S HEART"

A modest increase in size or hypertrophy is a fundamental adjustment of the healthy heart to regular exercise training. There is greater synthesis of cellular protein as the

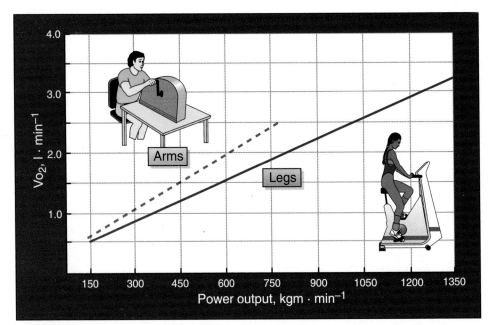

FIGURE 9-22. Arm exercise requires a greater oxygen uptake compared to leg exercise at any power output throughout the comparison range. The largest differences occurs during heavy exercise. Average data are for men and women. (From Laboratory of Applied Physiology, Queens College, NY)

individual muscle fibers thicken and the contractile elements within each fiber increase in number. This increase in size with training is transient, and heart size returns to pretraining levels when training intensity decreases.

The ultrasonic technique of *echocardiography* has evaluated the structural characteristics of the hearts of athletes, and determined if different patterns of cardiac hypertrophy and enlargement are associated with different types of physical conditioning. It is clear from the results in Table 9-7 that the structural characteristics of the hearts of apparently healthy athletes differ considerably from those of untrained individuals. Also, the pattern of these differences is related to the nature of the exercise conditioning. For example:

- The left ventricular volume was 181 ml and mass was 308 g for the swimmers, and 160 ml and 302 g for the runner. The nonathletic controls averaged 101 ml for ventricular volume and 211 g for ventricular mass. Despite their large internal ventricular dimensions, ventricular wall thickness was normal for the endurance athletes.

- The athletes involved in resistance exercise training such as weight lifters, shot putters, and wrestlers, who are regularly subjected to acute episodes of elevated arterial pressure caused by straining-type exercises, have normal ventricular volume but the ventricular wall is thickened. Undoubtedly, this represents compensation for the added workload resistance training imposes on the left ventricle.

The consequences of these apparent differences in training response on long-term cardiovascular health are unknown. However, there is no compelling scientific evidence that a normal heart can be harmed by arduous exercise training.

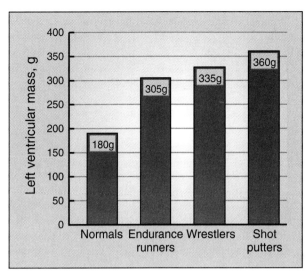

General trend in cardiac enlargement seen among the untrained and various athletic groups.

Sonar for the heart. A clearer understanding of the changes in heart size and structure with training has been provided by the ultrasonic technique of echocardiography (see Figure 9-2). With this approach, sound waves are passed through the heart to "map" the dimensions of the muscle itself as well as the volume of its cavities.

TABLE 9-7. Comparative average cardiac dimensions in college athletes, world-class athletes, and normal subjects [a]

Dimension[b]	College Runners (N = 15)	College Swimmers (N = 15)	World Class Runners (N = 10)	College Wrestlers (N = 12)	World Class Shot Putters (N = 4)	Normals (N = 16)
LVID	54	51	48–59[c]	48	43–52[c]	46
LVV, ml	160	181	154	110	122	101
SV, ml	116	—[d]	113	75	68	—[d]
LV wall, mm	11.3	10.6	10.8	13.7	13.8	10.3
Septum, mm	10.9	10.7	10.9	13.0	13.5	10.3
LV mass, g	302	308	283	330	348	211

[a] From Morganroth, J., et al.: Comparative left ventricular dimensions in trained athletes. *Ann. Intern. Med.*, 82:521, 1975.
[b] LVID, left ventricular internal dimension at end diastole; LVV, left ventricular volume; SV, stroke volume; LV wall, posterobasal left ventricular wall thickness; Septum, ventricular septal thickness; LV mass, left ventricular mass.
[c] Range.
[d] Values not reported.

OTHER TRAINING ADAPTATIONS

Endurance training may improve the vascularization of the myocardium, especially at the arteriole level, although there is considerable debate in this area. In addition, several experimenters have reported an increase in mitochondrial mass and cellular concentration of respiratory enzymes in the hearts of animals trained by endurance exercise. The significance of these vascular and cellular adaptations to the functional capacity of the heart during exercise has yet to be determined. Currently, it is believed that the healthy untrained heart does not suffer from an oxygen lack during maximum exercise. Training changes may, however, enable myocardial tissue to function at a lower percentage of its total oxidative capacity during exercise. In addition, they may provide some protection from the degenerative process of heart disease.

SUMMARY

PART 3

1. Cardiac output reflects the functional capacity of the circulatory system. Heart rate and stroke volume are the two factors that determine the heart's output capacity. The relationship is: Cardiac output = Heart rate x Stroke volume.

2. Cardiac output can be measured by invasive and noninvasive methods. Each has its specific advantages and disadvantages for use with humans, especially during exercise.

3. Cardiac output increases in proportion to the severity of exercise from about 5 liters per minute at rest to a maximum of 20 to 25 liters per minute in college-aged men and 35 to 40 liters per minute in elite male endurance athletes. These differences in maximum cardiac output are due entirely to the large stroke volumes of the athletes.

4. During upright exercise, stroke volume increases during the transition from rest to light exercise with maximum values reached at about 45% of max $\dot{V}O_2$. Thereafter, cardiac output is increased by increases in heart rate.

5. Increases in stroke volume in upright exercise are generally the result of a more complete systolic emptying rather than a greater filling of the ventricles during diastole. Systolic ejection is augmented by sympathetic hormones. Endurance training also improves myocardial strength that contributes to stroke power during systole.

6. Heart rate and oxygen uptake are linearly related in trained and untrained individuals throughout the major portion of the exercise range. With endurance training, this line shifts significantly to the right owing to improvements in the heart's stroke volume. Consequently, heart rate becomes significantly reduced at any submaximal exercise level.

7. Blood flow to specific tissues is generally regulated in proportion to their metabolic activity. This causes the major portion of exercise cardiac output to be diverted to the active muscles. In addition, a significant quantity of blood is shunted to the muscles from the kidneys and splanchnic regions because these organs can temporarily compromise their blood supply.

8. The maximal oxygen uptake is determined by the maximum cardiac output and the maximum a-v̄ O_2 difference. Large cardiac outputs clearly differentiate endurance athletes from untrained counterparts. Training also enhances the ability to generate a large a-v̄ O_2 difference.

9. Cardiac hypertrophy is a fundamental adaptation to the increased workload imposed by exercise training. The pattern of structural and dimensional changes in the left ventricle appears to vary with specific forms of exercise training. There is no scientific evidence that a normal heart is harmed by regular exercise.

American College of Sports Medicine Position Stand: Physical activity, physical fitness, and hypertension. *Med. Sci. Sports Exerc.*, 25: i-x, 1993.

Bjornstad, H., et al.: Ambulatory electro-cardiographic findings in top athletes, athletic students and control subjects. *Cardiology.* 84: 42, 1994.

Coconie, C.C., et al.: Effect of exercise training on blood pressure in 70- to 79-yr-old men and women. *Med. Sci. Sports Exerc.*, 23: 505, 1991.

Cowley, A. : Long term control of arterial blood presure. *Physiol. Revs.* 72: 231, 1992.

Coyle, E. F.: Cardiovascular function during exercise: neural control factors. Gatorade Sports Science Institute: *Sports Science Exchange*, 4 (34): 1991.

Donaldson, M. C.: Varicose veins in active people. *Phys. Sportsmed.* 18: 46, 1990.

Effron, M. B.: Effects of resistive training on left ventricular function. *Med. Sci. Sports Exerc.*, 21: 694, 1989.

Ehsani, A. A., et al.: Improvement of left ventricular contractile function by exercise training in patients with coronary artery disease. *Circulation,* 74: 350, 1986.

Fagard, R.H., and Tipton, C.M.: Physical activity, fitness, and hypertension. In *Physical Activity, Fitness, and Health.* Edited by Bouchard, C., et al., Champaign, IL, Human Kinetics, 1994.

Fagard, R.H., et al.: The effect of gender on aerobic power and exercise hemodynamics in hypertensive adults. *Med. Sci. Sports Exerc.*, 27: 29, 1995.

Fleck, S. J.: Cardiovascular adaptations to resistance training. *Med. Sci. Sports Exerc.*, 20: S146, 1988.

Fleck, S.J., et al.: Magnetic resonance imaging determination of left ventricular mass: Junior Olympic weightlifters. *Med. Sci. Sports Exerc.*, 25:522, 1993.

Gaffney, F. A., et al.: Cardiovascular and metabolic responses to static contraction in man. *Acta Physiol. Scand.*, 138: 249, 1990.

Herd, J.: Cardiovascular response to stress. *Physiol. Revs.*, 71: 305, 1991.

Hickson, R. C., et al.: Reduced training intensities and loss of aerobic power, endurance, and cardiac growth. *J. Appl. Physiol.*, 58: 492, 1985.

Holloszy, J. O., and Coyle, E. F.: Adaptations of skeletal muscle to endurance training and their metabolic consequences. *J. Appl. Physiol.*, 56: 831, 1984.

Inbar, O., et al.: Normal cardiopulmonary responses during incremental exercise in 20- to 70-yr-old men. *Med. Sci. Sports Exerc.*, 26: 538, 1994.

Keleman, M. H.: Exercise training combined with antihypertensive drug therapy: effects on lipids, blood pressure, and left ventricular mass. *JAMA,* 263: 2766, 1990.

Laughlin, M.H., et al.: Physical activity and the microcirculation in cardiac and skeletal muscle. In *Physical Activity, Fitness, and Health*, Edited by Bouchard, C., et al., Champaign, IL, Human Kinetics, 1994.

LeMarr, J. D., et al.: Cardiorespiratory responses to inversion. *Phys. Sportsmed.,* 11: 51, 1983.

Massic, B. M.: To combat hypertension, increase activity. *Phys. Sportsmed.,* 20: 89, 1992.

Miles, D. S., et al.: Cardiovascular responses to upper body exercise in normals and cardiac patients. *Med. Sci. Sports Exerc.,* 21: S126, 1989.

Mitchell, J.H., and Raven, P.B.: Cardiovascular adaptation to physical activity. In *Physical Activity, Fitness, and Health.* Edited by Bouchard, C., et al., Champaign, IL, Human Kinetics, 1994.

Nobrega, A.C.L., et al.: Cardiovascular responses to active and passive cycling movements. *Med. Sci. Sports Exerc.*, 26: 709, 1994.

Nye, P.C.G.: Identification of peripheral chemoreceptor stimuli. *Med. Sci. Sports Exerc.*, 26: 311, 1994.

Pelliccia, A., et al.: The upper limit of physiologic cardiac hypertrophy in highly trained athletes. *N. Engl. J. Med.*, 324: 295, 1991.

Rowell, L.B.: *Human Cardiovascular Control.* Cary, NC, Oxford University Press, 1994.

Saltin, B., and Strange, S.: Maximal oxygen uptake: "old" and "new" arguments for cardiovascular limitation. *Med. Sci. Sports Exerc.*, 24: 30, 1992.

Seals, D. R., and Hagberg, J. M.: The effect of exercise training on human hypertension. *Med. Sci. Sports Exerc.,* 16: 207, 1984.

Seals, D.R., and Victor, R.G.: Regulation of muscle sympathetic nerve activity during exercise in humans. *Exerc. Sport Sci. Rev.*, 19: 313, 1991.

Strange, S., et al.: Neural control of cardiovascular responses and of ventilation during dynamic exercise in man. *J. Physiol. (Lond)*: 470: 693, 1993.

Tipton, C. M.: Exercise, training, and hypertension: an update. In *Exercise and Sport Sciences Reviews.* Vol 19. Edited by J. O. Holloszy. Baltimore, Williams & Wilkins, 1991.

Toner, M. M., et al.: Cardiovascular adjustment to exercise distributed between the upper and lower body. *Med. Sci. Sports Exerc.*, 22: 773, 1990.

Wiley, R.L., et al.: Isometric exercise training lowers resting blood pressure. *Med. Sci. Sports Exerc.*, 24: 749, 1992.

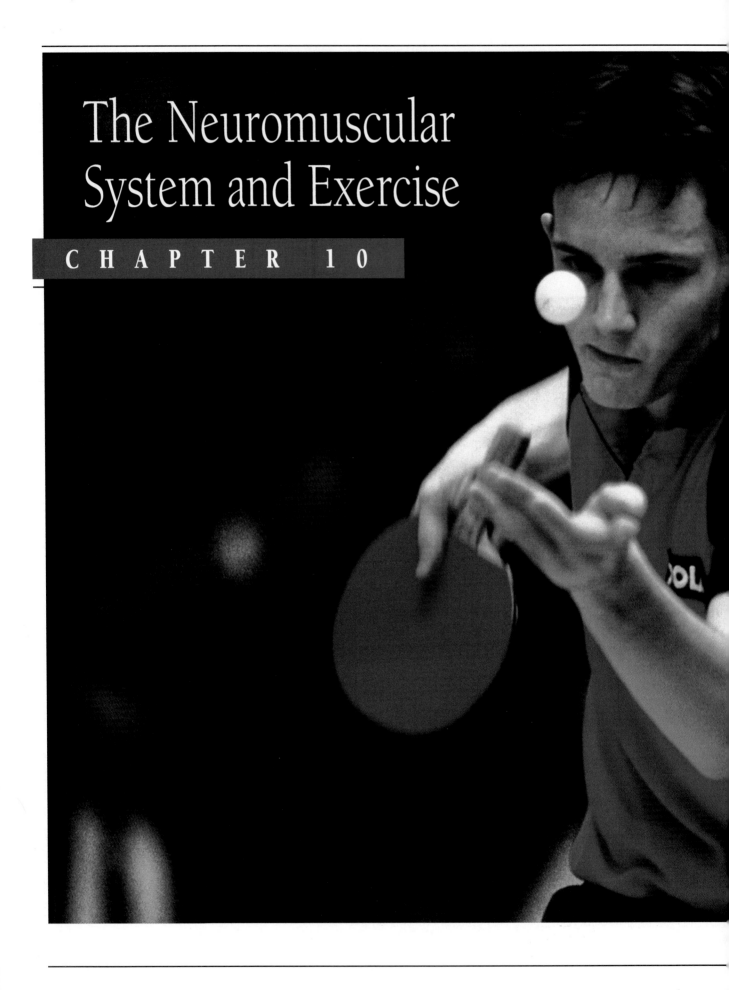

The Neuromuscular System and Exercise

CHAPTER 10

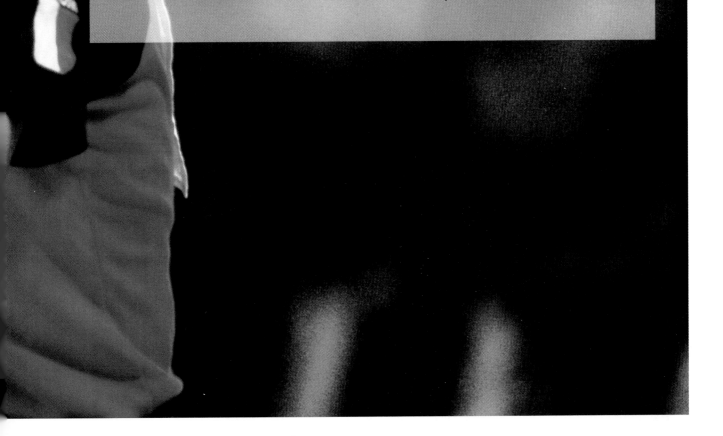

After reading this chapter, you should be able to:

- Draw the major structural components of the central nervous system involved in the control of human movement.
- Diagram the anterior motoneuron and discuss its role in human movement.
- Draw and label the basic components of a reflex arc.
- Define the following: motor unit, neuromuscular junction, autonomic nervous system, and EPSP and IPSP.
- Discuss motor units in terms of twitch characteristics, resistance to fatigue, and tension development.
- Discuss factors associated with neuromuscular fatigue.
- Define the following: muscle spindles, Golgi tendon organs, and Pacinian corpuscles.
- Draw and label the ultrastructural components of a skeletal muscle fiber.
- Outline the sequence of chemical and mechanical events during skeletal muscle contraction and relaxation.
- Contrast the characteristics of slow-twitch and fast-twitch (including subdivisions) muscle fibers. What is the distribution pattern of fiber types among elite athletes?
- Discuss whether muscle fiber type can be changed with exercise training.

All movements involve more than just the contraction of specific muscles. The correct application of the appropriate force for a given movement, such as a tennis serve, golf putt, or a slap shot in hockey, depends on a series of coordinated neural signals and the correct recruitment of specific muscle fibers. The neural circuitry in the brain and spinal cord that directs interaction between the nervous and muscular systems is somewhat analogous to a modern computer system, although the integrative and organizational structure of the human nervous system is far more advanced than any computer. In response to changing internal and external stimuli, bits of sensory input are transmitted rapidly for processing by interactive neural control mechanisms. Both simple movements that require little force and complex movements that require a large force rely on neural input that is properly organized, routed, and re-transmitted to the effector organs, the muscles.

In the sections that follow, we present a *general outline* describing the neural control of human movement. This includes the following:

- Structural organization of the neuromotor system with emphasis on the central and peripheral nervous system
- Neuromuscular transmission
- Motor unit function and activation
- Sensory input for muscular activity

ORGANIZATION OF THE NEUROMOTOR SYSTEM

The human nervous system is divided into two major parts, the *central nervous system* that includes the brain and spinal cord, and the *peripheral nervous system* that includes the nerves (cranial and spinal nerves) that exert their influence outside the brain and spinal cord. Figure 10-1 presents an overview of the human nervous system.

Central Nervous System — The Brain

Figure 10-2 illustrates that the brain is divided into six main areas: the *medulla oblongata, pons, midbrain, cerebellum, diencephalon, and telencephalon.* Each of the 12 cranial nerves has its origin in one of these anatomic areas. The bottom panel depicts the four lobes of the cerebral cortex and the sensory areas.

Brain Stem. The medulla, pons, and midbrain make up the *brain stem.* The medulla, located immediately above the spinal cord, extends into the pons and serves as a bridge between the two hemispheres of the cerebellum. The midbrain, only 1.5 cm long, is attached to the cerebellum and forms

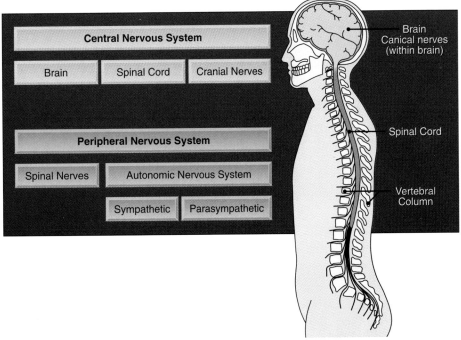

FIGURE 10-1. The human nervous system consists of two divisions. The central nervous system includes the brain and spinal cord, and the peripheral nervous system includes the spinal nerves and the nerves of the autonomic nervous system.

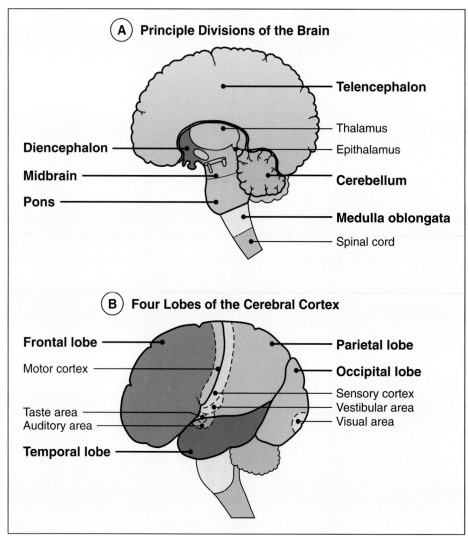

A **Principle Divisions of the Brain**

Telencephalon

Thalamus
Epithalamus

Diencephalon
Midbrain
Pons

Cerebellum

Medulla oblongata

Spinal cord

B **Four Lobes of the Cerebral Cortex**

Frontal lobe
Motor cortex

Parietal lobe
Occipital lobe

Sensory cortex
Vestibular area
Visual area

Taste area
Auditory area
Temporal lobe

FIGURE 10-2. *A.* The principal divisions of the brain. *B.* The four lobes of the cerebral cortex.

The Cerebellum. The cerebellum, made up of two lateral hemispheres and a central vermis, functions by means of intricate feedback circuits to monitor and coordinate other areas of the brain and spinal cord involved in motor control. The cerebellum receives motor output signals from the cortex and sensory information from receptors in muscles, tendons, joints, and skin as well as from visual, auditory, and vestibular end-organs. *This specialized brain tissue is the major comparing, evaluating, and integrating center for postural adjustments, locomotion, maintenance of equilibrium, perceptions of speed of body movement, and other reflex functions related to movement.*

Diencephalon. The diencephalon is found immediately above the midbrain and is a part of the cerebral hemispheres. The major structures of the diencephalon are the thalamus, hypothalamus, epithalamus, and subthalamus. The *hypothalamus,* situated below the thalamus, regulates functions ranging from metabolism to body temperature. The hypothalamus also influences activity of the autonomic nervous system (see page 286) and is affected by input from the thalamus and limbic brain system as well as various hormones (see Chapter 11). Hypothalamic activity also can be influenced by changes in arterial blood pressure and gas tension via peripheral receptors located in the aorta and carotid arteries.

Telencephalon. The telencephalon contains the two hemispheres of the cerebral cortex as well as the corpus striatum and the medulla. The cerebral cortex makes up approximately 40% of the total brain weight and is divided into four lobes: frontal, temporal, parietal, and occipital. The cortical cells have specialized sensory and motor functions. Beneath each cere-

> **Critical for skilled performance.** In essence, the cerebellum provides the "fine tuning" for muscular activity.

a connection between the pons and the cerebral hemispheres. The midbrain contains parts of the extrapyramidal motor system, specifically the red nucleus and substantia. The *reticular formation* is also located in the brain stem and provides important interconnections between the spinal cord, cerebral cortex, basal ganglia, and cerebellum. The reticular formation integrates various incoming and outgoing signals that flow through it. These signals originate from the stretching of sensors in joints and muscles, and from pain receptors in the skin, as well as visual signals from the eye and auditory impulses from the ear. Once activated, the reticular system produces either an inhibitory or facilitatory effect on other nerves.

bral hemisphere, and in close association with the thalamus is the basal ganglia, which plays an important role in the control of motor movements.

Limbic System. Various parts of the frontal and temporal lobes of the cerebral cortex, thalamus, and hypothalamus and their neural connections make up the limbic system (a group of nerves located around the brain stem). This configuration of neurons is believed to be involved with emotional behavior and learning.

Central Nervous System — The Spinal Cord

The spinal cord, illustrated in Figure 10-3, is about 45 cm long and about 1 cm in diameter and is encased by 33 vertebrae (7 cervical, 12 thoracic, 5 lumbar, 5 sacral, and 4 coccygeal). When viewed in cross section, the spinal cord has an H-shaped core of gray matter. The limbs of this core are known as the *ventral* (anterior) and *dorsal* (posterior) horns and contain principally three types of nerves: interneurons, motoneurons, and sensory neurons. The motor *efferent* neurons of the ventral horn supply extrafusal and intrafusal skeletal muscle fibers (see page 293). Sensory (*afferent*) nerves enter the spinal cord by way of the dorsal horn. Surrounding the gray core is an area of white matter that contains the ascending and descending nerve tracts within the cord itself.

Ascending Nerve Tracts. Ascending nerve tracts in the spinal cord send sensory information from peripheral sensory receptors to the brain. The sensory pathways are typically made up of three nerves. The first has its cell body in the dorsal root ganglion from which axons relay information from the peripheral receptor to the spinal cord; the cell body of the second nerve is in the cord itself, and its axon passes up the spinal cord to the

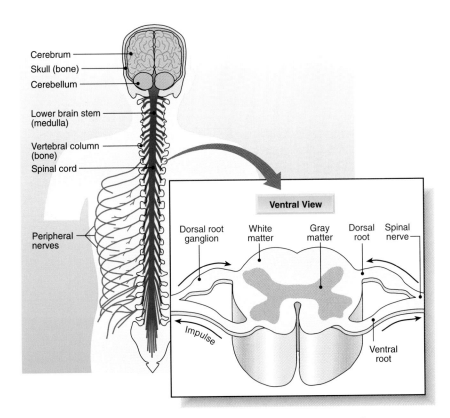

FIGURE 10-3. The human spinal cord. The insert gives a ventral view of a section of the spinal cord to illustrate both dorsal and ventral root neural pathways and the direction of the nerve impulse.

thalamus, which contains the third neuron's cell body; the axon of this third nerve passes up to the cerebral cortex.

Sensory Receptors. *Peripheral sensory nerve endings are specialized receptors to detect both conscious and subconscious sensory information.* The "conscious" receptors are sensitive to such input as body position (kinesthesia and proprioception), temperature, and pain, as well as the senses of sight, sound, smell, taste, and touch.

There are also receptors to monitor subconscious changes in the body's internal environment; these include *chemoreceptors* that respond to changes in blood gas tension (Pco_2, Po_2) and pH, and other specialized receptors called *baroreceptors* that are sensitive to changes in arterial blood pressure.

Descending Nerve Tracts. Tracts of nerve tissue descend from the brain and terminate at neurons in the spinal cord. The *pyramidal* and the *extrapyramidal tracts* are the two major pathways that serve this function.

Pyramidal Tract. Nerves in the pyramidal or corticospinal tract transmit their impulses downward through the spinal cord. By means of direct routes and interconnecting neurons in the spinal cord, these nerves eventually excite alpha motoneurons that control the various skeletal muscles.

Extrapyramidal Tract. The extrapyramidal nerves originate in the brain stem and connect at all levels of the spinal cord. The neurons of the extrapyramidal tract essentially control posture and provide a continual background level of neuromuscular tone. This is in contrast to the discrete movements stimulated by the nerves in the pyramidal tract.

The reticular formation interconnects the spinal cord, cerebral cortex, basal ganglia, and cerebellum. Once activated, the reticular system produces either an inhibitory or facilitatory effect on other neurons. The reticular inhibitory center transmits impulses that inhibit neurons to the antigravity muscles involved in postural control. Excitation of the facilitatory sensory neurons arouses the reticular nerve cells. This causes excitation in the cerebral cortex, and signals are transmitted back to the reticular system to maintain an appropriate level of cortical arousal. Superimposed on this feedback system is another feedback network that transmits impulses through the spinal cord to the muscles. For example, if the neural outflow goes to the postural muscles, the tension of these mucles becomes increased. This increased neuromuscular tone also stimulates the spindles (see page 293), the muscle's own set of sensory modulators, to redirect excitatory impulses back to the central nervous system to maintain the excitatory level of the reticular formation. This system, an example of *multiple feedback control*, is one of the most complex aspects of the nervous system.

Peripheral Nervous System

The peripheral nervous system includes afferent nerves that relay sensory information *toward* the brain and efferent nerves that transmit information *away* from the brain. The two types of efferent nerves are known as somatic and autonomic nerves.

Somatic nerves innervate skeletal muscle (called voluntary muscle), and autonomic nerves innervate smooth muscle (called involuntary muscle) like that found in the intestines, sweat and salivary glands, cardiac muscle, and some endocrine glands.

Somatic efferent nerve firing is always excitatory and results in muscle contraction, whereas autonomic nerve firing may be excitatory or inhibitory. Excitatory nerve firing is mediated by sympathetic nerve fibers, whereas inhibitory activity is mediated by parasympathetic nerve fibers

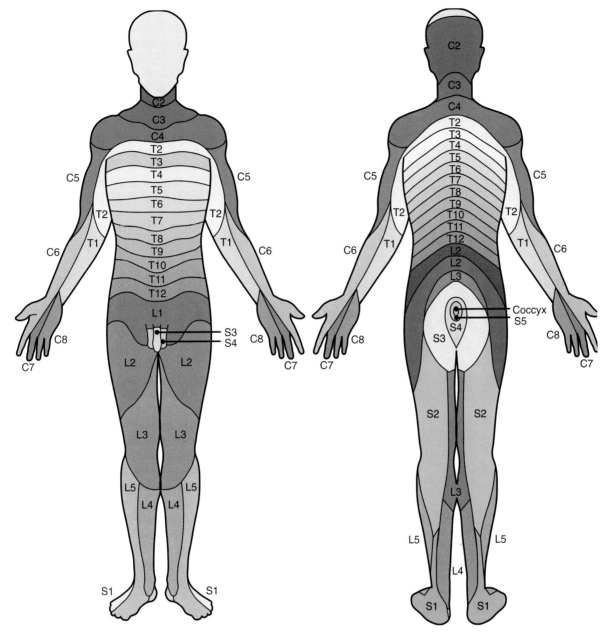

FIGURE 10-4. Location and distribution of spinal nerves (C-cervical, T-thoracic, S-sacral, L-lumbar).

(with the exception of vagal parasympathetic control of gastrointestinal motility and tone and the secretion of insulin from the pancreas, which are excitatory responses).

The peripheral nervous system consists of 31 pairs of spinal nerves and the 12 pairs of cranial nerves. Of the 31 spinal nerves, there are 8 pairs of cervical nerves, 12 thoracic, 5 lumbar, 5 sacral, and 1 coccygeal nerve. These nerves are referred to by number (e.g., C-1, first nerve from the cervical region). Careful scientific experiments have tracked their exact location, and the muscles they innervate have been mapped. Thus, when there is an injury to a specific area of the spinal cord, the result is predictable neurologic damage that results in various types of paralysis. For example, damage to the upper thoracic vertebra and the corresponding descending nerve tract almost always results in quadriplegia. Figure 10-4 shows the distribution of the different spinal nerves.

Autonomic Nerves. The autonomic nervous system is an efferent system that activates the viscera and other tissues. Tissues such as the heart and intestines, for example, display automatic excitability. It is possible, however, to exert conscious control over these tissues under some circumstances. Individuals who practice yoga or meditation can control their heart rate or even blood flow "on command." Such conscious control of the autonomic system can have some application as an alternative treatment in medicine as well as in sports. For example, when a participant is able to control heart rate or breathing cycle through relaxation techniques or by conscious control, it may be possible to affect a subsequent performance. Competitors in archery and the biathlon, for example, are able to control their cardiovascular and respiratory movements so that the normal cycle of breathing and even pulse rate become temporarily "halted" during the crucial phase of their performance.

Sympathetic and Parasympathetic Nervous System. The fibers of the sympathetic autonomic nervous system leave the spinal cord in the thoracic and upper lumbar region. The distribution of sympathetic fibers, while displaying some overlap, supply the heart, smooth muscle, sweat glands, and viscera. The parasympathetic fibers leave the brain stem and sacral segments and supply the thorax, abdomen, and pelvic regions.

Regions of the medulla, pons, and diencephalon control the autonomic nervous system. For example, blood pressure, heart rate, and respiration are controlled from fibers that originate in the lower brain stem, whereas body temperature regulation is controlled by nerve fibers of upper hypothalamic origin.

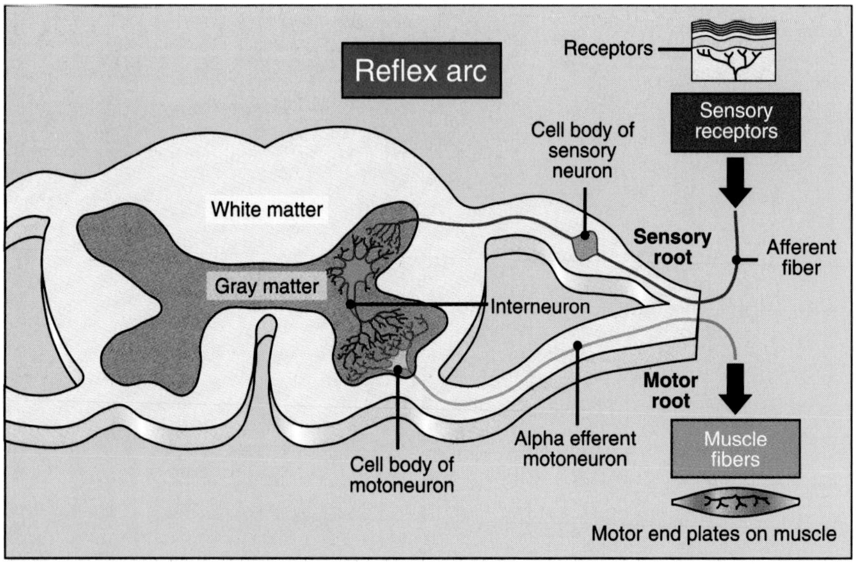

The Autonomic Reflex Arc. The diagram in Figure 10-5 shows a typical neural arrangement for an autonomic *reflex arc* in the spinal cord. Sensory input is transmitted from the receptor by sensory nerves that enter the spinal cord through the dorsal or sensory root. These nerves interconnect or *synapse* in the cord through interneurons that serve to distribute information to various levels of the cord. The impulse is then passed over the motor root pathway via anterior motoneurons to the effector organ, the muscles. The reflex arc is illustrated when one unknowingly touches a hot object. Pain receptors in the fingers are stimulated and send sensory information rapidly over afferent fibers to the spinal cord. Here the efferent or motor fibers are activated to bring about the appropriate muscular response, and the hand is rapidly pulled away. Concurrently the signal is transmitted up the cord to sensory areas in the brain, where the sensation of pain is actually "felt." The various levels of operation for sensory input, processing, and motor output, including the reflex action just described, explain how the hand is removed from the hot object before the pain is actually perceived. Many muscle functions are controlled by reflex actions in the spinal cord and

FIGURE 10-5. The reflex arc. Shown are afferent and efferent neurons plus an interneuron in a spinal cord segment. The shaded or gray matter contains the neuron cell bodies; the white matter is made up of longitudinal columns of nerve fibers. Stimulation of a single alpha motoneuron can affect as many as 3000 muscle fibers. The motoneuron and the fibers it innervates are collectively referred to as a motor unit. Only one side of the spinal nerve complex is shown.

other subconscious areas of the central nervous system.

Nerve Supply to Muscle. One nerve or its terminal branches innervates at least one of the approximately 250 million muscle fibers in the human body. Because there are only about 420,000 motor nerves, this means that a single nerve usually supplies many individual muscle fibers. *The ratio of muscle to nerve is generally related to a muscle's particular movement function.* The delicate, precise work of the eye muscles, for example, requires one neuron to control fewer than 10 muscle fibers. For less complex movements of the big muscles, a motoneuron may innervate as many as 2000 or 3000 fibers.

The next sections take a closer look at how information processed in the central nervous system is delivered to the muscles to bring about an appropriate motor response.

Motor Unit Anatomy

The functional unit of movement is the motor unit; this anatomic unit consists of the anterior motoneuron and the specific muscle fibers it innervates. Although each muscle fiber generally receives only one nerve fiber, a motor nerve may innervate many muscle fibers. This is because the terminal end of an axon forms numerous branches. Some motor units contain up to 3000 muscle fibers, whereas others contain relatively few fibers.

Anterior Motoneuron

The anterior motoneuron illustrated in Figure 10-6 consists of a *cell body, axon,* and *dendrites.* Its unique design enables it to transmit an electrochemical impulse from the spinal cord to the muscle. The cell body houses the control center — the structures involved with replication and transmission of the genetic code. This part of the

motoneuron is located within the gray matter of the spinal cord. The axon extends from the cord to deliver the impulse to the muscle; the dendrites are the short neural branches that receive impulses through numerous spinal cord connections and conduct them toward the cell body. Nerve cells conduct impulses in one direction — down the axon away from the

Innervation ratio. The finger contains 120 motor units that control 41,000 muscle fibers; the medial gastroenemius muscle (calf) has 580 motor units and 1,030,000 fibers. The ratio of muscle fibers per motor unit is therefore 340 for the finger muscle and 1,800 for the gastroenemius muscle.

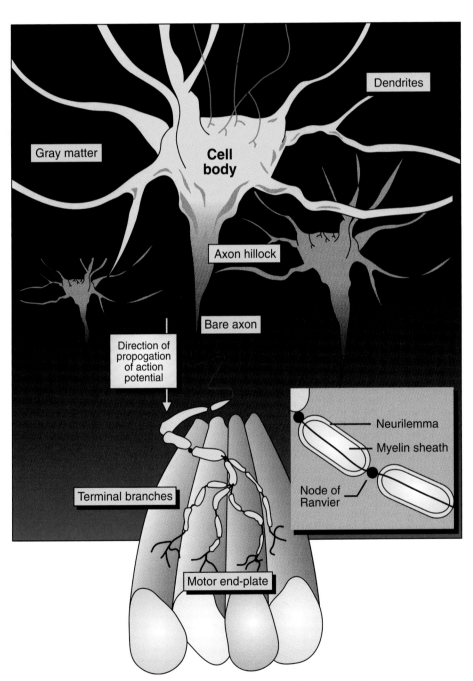

FIGURE 10-6. The anterior motoneuron consists of a cell body, axon, and dendrites. The insert illustrates a node of Ranvier that permits impulses to "jump" from one node to another as the electrical current travels toward the terminal branches at the motor end-plate.

point of stimulation. As the axon approaches the muscle, it forms hundreds of branches with each small terminal branch innervating a single muscle fiber. *Thus a whole muscle contains many motor units, each of which contains a single motoneuron and its complement of muscle fibers.* Although it may seem logical for all of the muscle fibers within a motor unit to be located in a cluster within the muscle, this is not the case. Muscle fibers of a particular motor unit are scattered over subregions of the muscle, and fibers from one motor unit are interspersed among fibers of other units. This causes the forces generated by a motor unit to be spread over a larger tissue area, thus minimizing mechanical stress.

The larger motoneurons are encased in a myelin sheath, a lipid-protein membrane that wraps around the axon over most of its length. A specialized cell known as a *Schwann cell* encases the bare axon and then spirals around it. Myelin forms a large part of this sheath and insulates the axon. A thinner membrane, the *neurilemma,* covers the myelin sheath. The Schwann cells and myelin are interrupted every 1 or 2 mm along the axon's length at the *nodes of Ranvier.* Although the myelin sheath insulates the axon to the flow of ions, the nodes of Ranvier permit depolarization of the axon to occur. This alternating sequence of myelin sheath and node of Ranvier permits impulses to "jump" from node to node as the electrical current travels toward the terminal branches at the motor end-plate. This means of conduction is responsible for the higher transmission velocity in myelinated compared with unmyelinated fibers.

Neuromuscular Junction (Motor End-Plate)

The interface between the end of a myelinated motoneuron and a muscle fiber is known as the *neuromuscular junction* or *motor end-plate.* Its function is to transmit the nerve impulse to the muscle. For each skeletal muscle fiber, there is usually only one neuromuscular junction. Figure 10-7 illustrates the details of the neuromuscular junction based on electron microscopic studies.

The terminal portion of the axon below the myelin sheath forms several smaller axon branches whose endings are the presynaptic terminals. They lie close to, but are not in contact with, the sarcolemma of the muscle fiber. The region of the postsynaptic membrane or synaptic gutter has many infoldings that increase its surface area. The region between the synaptic gutter and presynaptic terminal of the axon is

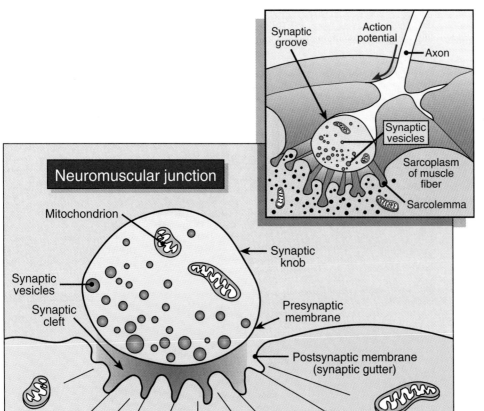

FIGURE 10-7. Microanatomy of the neuromuscular junction. Insert displays the details of the presynaptic and postsynaptic contact area between the motoneuron and the muscle fiber it innervates (From Akert, K., et al.: Freeze etching and cytochemistry of vesicles and membrane complexes in synapses of the central nervous system. In *Structures and Functions of Synapses.* Edited by G.D. Pappas and D.P. Purpa. New York, Raven Press, 1972.)

called the synaptic cleft. This is the region where the transmission of the neural impulse occurs.

Excitation. Excitation occurs only at the neuromuscular junction. The neurotransmitter responsible for changing a basically electrical neural impulse into a chemical stimulus at the motor end-plate is *acetylcholine*. This chemical is released from small, sac-like vesicles within the terminal axon to increase the postsynaptic membrane's permeability to sodium and potassium ions; this ultimately causes the impulse to spread over the entire muscle fiber as a wave of depolarization. Once this occurs, the contractile machinery of the muscle fiber is primed for its major function — contraction.

Within about 5 milliseconds after acetylcholine is released from the synaptic vesicles, it is destroyed by the enzyme *cholinesterase* that is concentrated at the borders of the synaptic cleft. This allows the postsynaptic membrane to repolarize. Acetic acid and choline, the byproducts of cholinesterase action, can be taken up by the axon and resynthesized to acetylcholine so the entire process can begin again with the arrival of another nerve impulse.

Facilitation. An action potential is generated if the change in the motoneuron's microvoltage is sufficient to reach the threshold for excitation. This change in membrane potential at the junction between two neurons (which increases the positive charges inside the cell) is referred to as the *excitatory postsynaptic potential* (EPSP). If the EPSP is subthreshold, the neuron does not discharge, but its resting membrane potential is lowered, and its tendency to "fire" is temporarily increased. The neuron fires when many subthreshold excitatory impulses arrive in rapid succession. This condition is known as *temporal summation.*

Removing inhibitory influences is important under certain exercise conditions. In all-out strength and power activities, for example, the ability to "disinhibit" and maximally activate all motoneurons required for a movement may be crucial for top-flight performance. This enhanced disinhibition could lead to full activation of muscle groups during all-out contraction and may account for the rapid, highly specific strength increases noted in the early stages of a strength development program. In fact, significant improvements in strength have been noted without increases in muscle size. Central nervous system excitation (referred to as *neuronal facilitation*) is perhaps the mechanism by which intense concentration or "psyching" enhances maximal performance. The "psychologic" influence on strength performance is discussed in Chapter 12.

Inhibition. Some presynaptic terminals set up inhibitory impulses. The inhibitory transmitter substance increases the permeability of the postsynaptic membrane to potassium and chloride ions. This produces an increase in the membrane's resting electrical potential, creating an *inhibitory postsynaptic potential* (IPSP). The IPSP hyperpolarizes the neuron, making it more difficult to fire. No action potential is generated if a motoneuron is subjected to both excitatory and inhibitory influences and if the IPSP is large. The reflex to pull one's hand away when removing a splinter, for example, can usually be overridden (inhibited) so the hand can be steadied to expedite this rather painful task. The exact neurochemical that provokes an IPSP is unknown, although gamma aminobutyric acid (GABA) and the protein glycine are thought to be involved in the inhibitory process. Neural inhibition serves protective functions and also reduces the input of "unwanted" stimuli so smooth, purposeful responses can occur.

MOTOR UNIT PHYSIOLOGY

In addition to their anatomic distinctions, motor units can be classified based on three physiologic and mechanical properties of the muscle fibers they innervate. These properties are presented in Table 10-1 and include (1) twitch characteristics (force and speed of contraction), (2) fatigability, and (3) tetanic tension characteristics.

Twitch Characteristics

Early experiments in motor unit physiology revealed that in response to a single electrical impulse, motor units developed high, low, or intermediate tension. Additionally, the motor units with low force production capacity had slow contraction times yet were fatigue resistant, whereas those with higher tensions contracted rapidly yet were prone to early fatigue. Figure 10-8 illustrates these characteristics for the three categories of motor units:

- Fast-twitch, high force, and fast fatigue (type IIb).
- Fast-twitch, moderate force, and fatigue resistant (type IIa).
- Slow-twitch, low tension, and fatigue resistant (type I).

The fast-twitch fibers are innervated by relatively large motoneurons with fast conduction velocities. This motor unit contains between 300 and 500 muscle fibers. These fast-fatiguable (FF) and fast-fatigue-resistant (FR) units reach greater peak tension and develop it nearly twice as fast as slow-twitch (S) motor units that are innervated by small motoneurons with slow conduction velocities. These units, however, are more fatigue-resistant than the fast-twitch units. As can be seen in our discussion of muscle fiber types (see page 307), the particular metabolic characteristics of all muscle fibers can be modified by specific sports training. *With prolonged aerobic training, for example, some fast-twitch units can become almost as fatigue resistant as their slow-twitch counterparts.*

All-or-None Principle. If the stimulus is strong enough to trigger an action potential in the motoneuron, all of the accompanying muscle fibers in the motor unit are stimulated to contract. There is no such thing as a strong or weak contraction from a motor unit — either the impulse is strong enough to elicit a contraction, or it is not. Once the neuron is "fired" and the impulse reaches the neuromuscular junction, the muscle cells

Force characteristics. The major reason that motor units are able to generate different tensions is that high-tension motor units have a greater number of fibers of the type that are substantially larger. These two factors, number and size of fibers, then determine the intrinsic tension differences between motor units.

TABLE 10-1. Characteristics and correspondence between motor units and muscle fiber types.

Motor Unit Designation	Force Production	Contraction Speed	Fatigue-Resistance	Sag[†]	Muscle Fiber Type in the Motor Unit
Fast Fatigable (FF)	High	Fast	Low	Yes	Fast Glycolytic (FG)
Fast Fatigue-Resistant (FR)	Moderate	Fast	High	Yes	Fast Oxidative-Glycolytic (FOG)
Slow (S)	Low	Slow	High	No	Slow Oxidative (SO)

[†]Under repetitive stimuli, some motor units respond smoothly with a systematic increase in tension, while others first increase tension and then decrease or "sag" slightly in response to the same tetanic stimulus. These sag characteristics can be used to classify the different motor units. Only the S motor units do not exhibit sag, which is probably related more to their diminished force generating capabilities than their fatigue characteristics.
Modified from Lieber, R.L.: *Skeletal Muscle Structure and Function: Implications for Rehabilitation and Sports Medicine.* Baltimore, Williams & Wilkins, 1992.

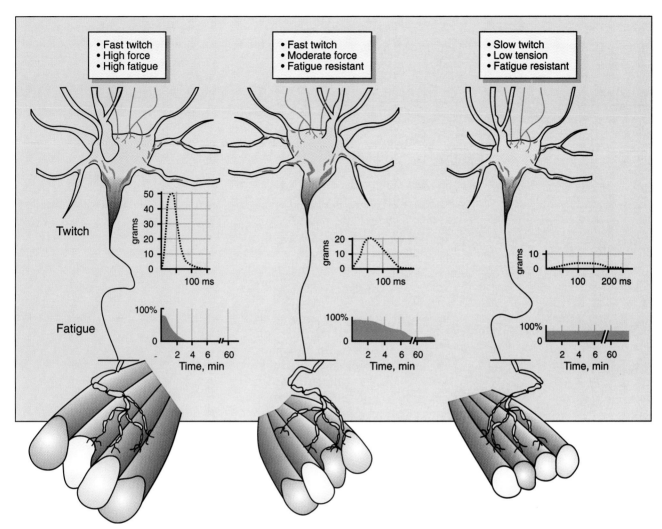

FIGURE 10-8. Speed, force, and fatigue characteristics of motor units. Motoneurons that fire rapidly with short bursts are termed phasic; those that fire slowly but continuously are tonic. (Modified from Edington, D.W., and Edgerton, V.R.: *The Biology of Physical Activity.* Boston, Houghton-Mifflin, 1976.)

always contract. This is the principle of *"all-or-none."*

Gradation of Force. The force of muscular contraction varies from slight to maximal in one of two ways: by increasing the *number* of motor units recruited for the activity and by increasing the *frequency* of discharge of the motor units. If all the motor units in a muscle are activated, the amount of force that is generated is considerable compared with that generated by the activation of only a few motor units. Also, if repetitive stimuli reach a muscle before it relaxes, there is an increase in the total tension produced. By blending these two factors, *recruitment of motor units and the rate*

of their firing, optimal patterns of neural discharge permit a wide variety of graded contractions. This is an important characteristic of skeletal muscle because it permits a variety of tensions to be produced for a selected movement. Thus, the movement can be carried out with proper timing and coordination. A good example is the golf swing, where the amount of tension in the hands, arms, and legs varies during the backswing, club-ball contact, and follow-through. There are literally thousands of examples of this phenomenon that occur daily, not just in sport activities. Although writing a letter with a pen appears to be a relatively simple task, careful analysis reveals this activity to

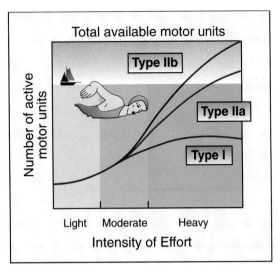

FIGURE 10-9. Recruitment of slow-twitch and fast-twitch muscle fibers (motor units) in relation to the intensity of exercise. As the effort becomes more intense, progressively more fast-twitch fibers are recruited. (From data of Edgerton, V. R.: Mammalian muscle fiber types and their adaptability. *Am. Zoology, 18*:113, 1978.)

be quite complex involving a myriad of coordinated neuromuscular forces and actions.

Motor Unit Recruitment. For low force contractions, few motor units are activated and for higher force contractions, more units are enlisted. This process of adding more motor units to increase muscle force is known as *motor unit recruitment.* Several factors determine motor unit recruitment and hence modulation of muscle force production. As muscle force increases, motoneurons with progressively larger axons are recruited. This is known as the *size principle* that provides an anatomic basis for the orderly recruitment of motor units to produce a smooth contraction.

Figure 10-9 illustrates that not all of the motor units in a muscle fire at the same time. If they did, it would be virtually impossible to control the force of a contraction. This is easy to demonstrate if one considers the tremendous gradation of forces and speeds that muscles generate. For example, when lifting a barbell, specific muscles contract to move the limb and weight at some particular speed of movement under a given rate of tension development. If the weight is not too heavy, it can be lifted at numerous speeds. If a heavier weight is used, the speed options decrease accordingly. *From the standpoint of neural control, the fast-twitch and slow-twitch motor units are selectively recruited and modulated in their firing pattern to produce the desired response.* In muscular activity requiring contractions of increasing force, the slow-twitch fibers (motor units) with the lowest functional threshold are selectively recruited predominantly during lighter effort. This is followed by activation of the more powerful, higher threshold, fast-twitch units

when peak force is required. During sustained activities such as jogging or cycling on a level grade or lifting a light weight at a slow speed, motor units of slow-twitch fibers are selectively recruited; in rapid, powerful movements such as taking a slap shot in ice hockey or throwing the javelin, the fast-twitch fibers, especially the type IIb fibers, come into play. As a runner or bicyclist reaches a hill during a distance race some fast-twitch units are also activated so a constant pace is maintained over varying terrain.

The differential control of the motor unit firing pattern is probably the major factor that distinguishes not only skilled from unskilled performances, but also specific athletic groups. Weightlifters, for example, generally demonstrate a *synchronous* pattern of motor-unit firing (i.e., many motor units recruited simultaneously during lifting), whereas the firing pattern of endurance athletes is mainly *asynchronous* (i.e., some motor units fire while others recover). As discussed previously, the compositional characteristics of a muscle in terms of its specific motor units (muscle fibers) contribute to the performance characteristics of various athletes. The synchronous firing of a muscle's fast-twitch fibers certainly aids the weight lifter to generate force quickly for the desired lift. For the endurance athlete, the asynchronous firing of predominantly slow-twitch, fatigue-resistant units provides a built-in recuperative period to permit performance to continue for relatively uninterrupted time periods with minimal fatigue.

· · · · · · · · · · · · · · ·

NEUROMUSCULAR FATIGUE

A second property distinguishing differences in motor units is their resistance to fatigue, defined as the decline in muscle tension with repeated stimulation. Muscular fatigue is the result of many factors, each related to the specific exercise demand that produces it. There are four main components involved in voluntary muscle contractions. These are in order of hierarchy:

- Central nervous system
- Peripheral nerves
- Neuromuscular junction
- Muscle fiber

Fatigue results if the chain of events is interrupted between the central nervous system and the muscle fiber, independent of the reason.

- A significant reduction in muscle glycogen is related to fatigue during prolonged, submaximal exercise. This "nutrient fatigue" within muscle occurs even though sufficient oxygen is available to generate energy through aerobic metabolic pathways.
- Muscle fatigue in short-term maximal exercise is associated with oxygen lack, an increased level of lactic acid accumulation, and a dramatic increase in H^+ concentration in the active muscle. Such drastic intracellular changes could lead to an interference in the contractile mechanism, a depletion of stored high-energy phosphates, an impaired energy transfer via glycolysis owing to reduced activity of key enzymes, a disturbance in the tubular system for transmitting the impulse throughout the cell, and ionic imbalances. Certainly a change in Ca^{++} distribution could alter the activity of the myofilaments and impair muscular performance.
- Fatigue also can be demonstrated at the neuromuscular junction when an action potential fails to cross from the motoneuron to the muscle fiber. The precise mechanism is unknown for this aspect of "neural fatigue."

As muscle function becomes impaired during prolonged submaximal exercise, additional motor-unit recruitment takes place to maintain the required force output for the particular activity. In all-out exercise, when all motor units are presumably maximally activated, fatigue is accompanied by a decrease in neural activity (as measured by the electromyogram [EMG]). The fact that neural activity decreases supports the argument that this form of fatigue is partially caused by a failure in neural or myoneural transmission.

RECEPTORS IN MUSCLES, JOINTS, AND TENDONS: THE PROPRIOCEPTORS

Specialized sensory receptors in the muscles, joints, and ligaments are sensitive to stretch, tension, and pressure. These end-organs, known as *proprioceptors,* rapidly relay information concerning muscular dynamics and limb movement to conscious and unconscious portions of the central nervous system for processing. Thus the progress of any movement or sequence of movements is continually monitored within the neuromuscular network to provide the basis for modifying subsequent motor patterns.

Muscle Spindles

The muscle spindles provide sensory information concerning changes in the length and tension of muscle fibers. Their main function is to respond to stretch on a muscle and, through reflex action, to initiate a stronger contraction to reduce this stretch.

Structural Organization. Figure 10-10 illustrates that the spindle is fusiform in shape and is attached in parallel to the regular or extrafusal fibers of the muscle. Consequently when the muscle is stretched, so is the spindle. The number of spindles contained per gram of muscle varies widely depending on the muscle group. On a relative basis, there are more spindles in muscles that perform complex movements. Within the spindle, there are two types of specialized muscle fibers called *intrafusal fibers.* A unique property of the intrafusal fibers is that their ends are capable of contracting.

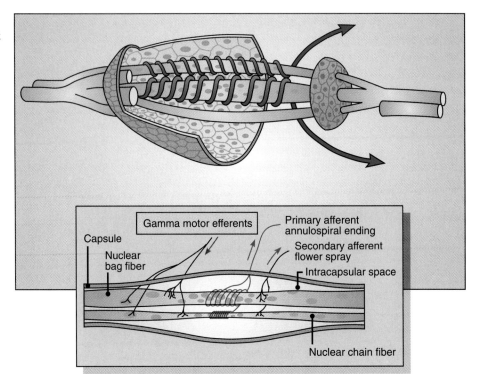

FIGURE 10-10. Structural organization of the muscle spindle. The insert shows an enlarged view of the equatorial region of the spindle. (Modified from Schade, J.P., and Ford, D.H.: *Basic Neurology,* 2nd ed. Amsterdam, Elsevier/North-Holland Biomedical Press, 1973.)

Three different nerve fibers service the spindles; two are afferent or sensory, and one is efferent or motor.

The third type of spindle nerve fiber has a motor function. These are the thin *gamma efferent fibers* that innervate the contractile, striated ends of the intrafusal fibers. These fibers, activated by higher centers in the brain, provide the mechanism for maintaining the spindle at peak operation at all muscle lengths.

Stretch Reflex. The functional significance of the muscle spindle is its ability to detect, respond to, and control changes in the length of extrafusal muscle fibers. This is important in the regulation of movement and maintenance of posture. Postural muscles are continuously bombarded by neural input; they must maintain their readiness to respond to voluntary movements or to maintain some degree of constant activity to counter the pull of gravity for upright posture. The stretch reflex is fundamental to achieving this end.

The stretch reflex has three main components:

- Muscle spindle, the sensory receptor within the muscle that responds to stretch
- Afferent nerve fiber that carries the sensory impulse from the spindle to the spinal cord
- Efferent motor neuron in the spinal cord that signals the muscle to contract

Figure 10-11 illustrates schematically the neural pathways involved in this basic reflex. In part A, the biceps muscle is contracted to maintain the bony lever at a 90 degree angle while holding a 1.0-kg book. If the book is suddenly increased twofold in weight (part B), the muscle is stretched. This causes the spindles' sensory endings to direct impulses through the dorsal root into the spinal cord, where they directly activate the motoneuron. The returning motor impulses (part C) cause the muscle to contract more forcefully to return the limb to its original position. During this reflex process, interneurons in the cord are also activated to facilitate the appropriate movement response. Excitatory impulses are conveyed to synergistic muscles that support the desired movement, whereas inhibitory impulses flow to the neurons of muscles that are antagonists of the movement. In this way, the stretch reflex acts as a self-regulating or compensating mechanism; it enables the muscle to adjust automatically to differences in load (and length) without immediately processing information through higher neural centers.

Golgi Tendon Organs

In contrast to muscle spindles that lay parallel to the extrafusal muscle fibers, the Golgi tendon organs are connected in series to as many as 25 extrafusal fibers. *These sensory receptors are also located in the ligaments of joints and are mainly responsible for detecting differences in muscle tension rather than length.* As shown in Figure 10-12, the Golgi tendon organs respond as a feedback monitor to discharge impulses under one of two conditions: (1) in response to tension created in the muscle when it shortens and (2) in response to tension when the muscle is passively stretched.

When stimulated by excessive tension or stretch, the Golgi receptors conduct their signals rapidly to bring about a *reflex inhibition* of the muscles they supply. This occurs because of the overriding influence of the inhibitory spinal interneuron on the motoneurons supplying the muscle. If the change in tension or stretch is too great, the sensor's discharge increases; this further depresses the activity of the motoneurons and reduces the tension generated in the muscle fibers. If the muscle contraction produces little tension, Golgi receptors are only weakly activated and exert little influence. *The ultimate function of the Golgi tendon organs is to protect the muscle and its connective tissue harness from injury due to an excessive load.*

Pacinian Corpuscles

Pacinian corpuscles are small, ellipsoidal bodies located close to the Golgi tendon organs. These small, onion-like sensory receptors are sensitive to quick movement and deep pressure. Deformation or compression of the capsule by a mechanical stimulus transmits pressure to the sensory nerve endings within its core. This produces a change in the electric potential of the nerve ending.

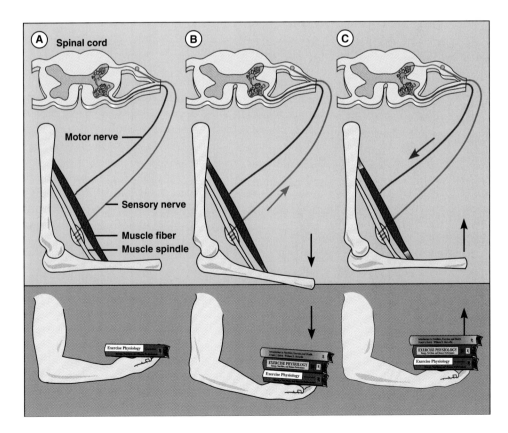

FIGURE 10-11. Schematic representation of the stretch reflex. Because the spindles are arranged parallel with the extrafusal fibers, they become stretched when these fibers are elongated. The spindle's sensory receptors fire when the intrafusal fibers are stretched. This activation of the spindle's sensory receptors reflexly stimulates the alpha motoneurons and causes contraction of the extrafusal fibers. This takes the stretch off of the intrafusal fibers and silences the spindle afferents. In the diagram, the stretch reflex acts as a self-regulating mechanism to maintain the relative constancy of limb position.

FIGURE 10-12. The Golgi tendon organ. Excessive tension or stretch on a muscle activates the tendon's Golgi receptors. This brings about a reflex inhibition of the muscles they supply. In this way, the Golgi tendon organ functions as a protective sensory mechanism to detect and subsequently inhibit undue strain within the muscle-tendon structure.

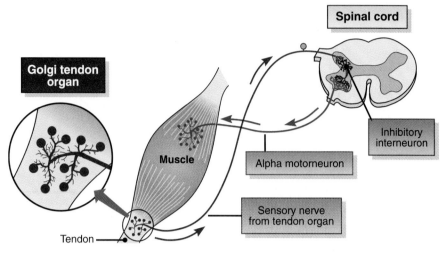

If this generator potential is of sufficient magnitude, a sensory signal is established and propagated down the myelinated axon leaving the corpuscle.

Pacinian corpuscles are "fast-adapting" mechanical sensors because they discharge a few impulses at the onset of a steady stimulus and then remain electrically silent or may discharge a second volley of impulses when the stimulus is removed. Consequently, they detect *changes* in movement or pressure, rather than how much movement occurred or how much pressure was applied.

S·U·M·M·A·R·Y

PART 1

1. Human movement is finely regulated by neural control mechanisms located in the central nervous system. In response to internal and external stimuli, bits of sensory input are automatically and rapidly routed, organized, and transmitted to the effector organs, the muscles.

2. Tracts of nerve tissue descend from the brain to influence neurons in the spinal cord. Neurons in the extrapyramidal tract control posture and provide a continual background level of neuromuscular tone; the pyramidal tract neurons provide for discrete muscular movement.

3. The cerebellum is the major comparing, evaluating, and integrating center that provides the "fine-tuning" for muscular activity.

4. Many muscular functions are controlled in the spinal cord and other subconscious areas of the central nervous system. The reflex arc is the basic mechanism for processing these automatic muscular movements.

5. The number of muscle fibers in a motor unit depends on the muscle's movement function. Intricate movement patterns require a small fiber-to-neuron ratio, whereas for gross movements, a single neuron may innervate several thousand muscle fibers.

6. The anterior motoneuron (cell body, axon, and dendrites) transmits the electrochemical nerve impulse from the spinal cord to the muscle. The dendrites receive impulses and conduct them toward the cell body, whereas the axon transmits the impulse in one direction only — down the axon to the muscle.

7. The neuromuscular junction is the interface between the motoneuron and the muscle fiber. Acetylcholine is released at this junction to provide the chemical stimulus that activates muscles.

8. Excitatory and inhibitory impulses continually bombard the synaptic junctions between neurons. These alter a neuron's threshold for excitation by either increasing or decreasing its tendency to "fire." In all-out power exercise, a high degree of disinhibition is beneficial because it enables maximal activation of a muscle's motor units.

9. There are three types of motor units depending on speed of contraction, force generated, and fatigability: (1) fast-twitch, high force, and high fatigue; (2) fast-twitch, moderate force, and fatigue resistant, and (3) slow-twitch, low tension, and fatigue resistant.

10. Gradation of muscle force is accomplished through an interaction of factors that regulate the number and type of motor units recruited as well as their frequency of discharge. Light exercise is accomplished through predominant recruitment of slow-twitch units followed by activation of the fast-twitch units when a more powerful force is required.

11. Alterations in motor unit recruitment and firing pattern probably explain a large portion of the strength improvement with resistance training, especially during the early stages of training.

12. Special sensory receptors in muscles, tendons, and joints relay information concerning muscular dynamics and limb movement to specific portions of the central nervous system. This provides important sensory feedback during physical activity.

Human movement depends on transforming the chemical energy bound in ATP into mechanical energy of motion. This specific energy transformation is achieved through the action of skeletal muscles. Muscular forces acting on the body's bony lever system cause one or more bones to move about their joint axis.

In the sections that follow, we present the architectural organization of skeletal muscle and focus on its gross and microscopic structure. The discussion includes the sequence of chemical and mechanical events in muscular contraction and relaxation, as well as the differences in muscle fiber characteristics and their contribution to exercise performance.

GROSS STRUCTURE OF SKELETAL MUSCLE

Each of the more than 430 voluntary muscles in the body contains various wrappings of fibrous connective tissue. Figure 10-13 shows the cross section of a muscle that consists of thousands of cylindric muscle cells called fibers. These long, slender multinucleated fibers (whose number is probably fixed by the second trimester of fetal development) lie parallel to each other, and the force of contraction is along the long axis of the fiber.

Each fiber is wrapped and separated from its neighboring fibers by a fine layer of connective tissue called the *endomysium*. Another layer of connective tissue, the *perimysium,* surrounds a bundle of up to 150 fibers called a *fasciculus.* Surrounding the entire muscle is a fascia of fibrous connective tissue known as the *epimysium.* This protective sheath is tapered at its distal end as it blends into and joins the intramuscular tissue sheaths to form the dense, strong connective tissue of the *tendons.* The tendons connect both ends of the muscle to the outermost covering of the skeleton, the *periosteum.* Thus, the force of muscular contraction is transmitted directly from the muscle's connective tissue harness to the tendons,

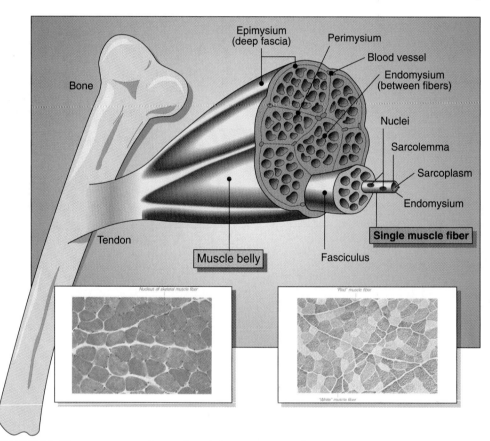

FIGURE 10-13. Cross section of a muscle and the arrangement of its connective tissue wrappings. The individual fibers are covered by the endomysium. Groups of fibers called fasciculi are surrounded by the perimysium, and the entire muscle is wrapped in a sheath of connective tissue, the epimysium. The sarcolemma is a thin, elastic membrane that covers the surface of each muscle fiber. The insert photos display transverse sections of striated muscle with different staining procedures to display various types of muscle fibers. (From Sobotta, J., and Hammersen, F.: *Histology. Color Atlas of Microscopic Anatomy.* 3rd ed. Baltimore, Urban & Schwarzenberg, 1992.)

which in turn pull on the bone at their points of attachment.

Beneath the endomysium and surrounding each muscle fiber is the *sarcolemma*. This thin, elastic membrane encloses the fiber's cellular contents. The aqueous protoplasm or *sarcoplasm* of the cell contains the contractile proteins, enzymes, lipid and glycogen particles, nuclei, and various specialized cellular organelles. Embedded within the sarcoplasm is an extensive interconnecting network of tubular channels and vesicles known as the *sarcoplasmic reticulum*. This highly specialized system provides the cell with structural integrity and also serves important functions in muscular contraction.

Chemical Composition

Approximately 75% of skeletal muscle is water, 20% is protein, and the remaining 5% is made up of inorganic salts and other substances that include high-energy phosphates, urea, lactic acid, the minerals calcium, magnesium, and phosphorus, various enzymes and pigments; ions of sodium, potassium, and chloride; and amino acids, lipids, and carbohydrates.

Blood Supply

During exercise that requires an oxygen uptake of 4,000 ml per minute, the muscle's oxygen uptake increases nearly 70 times to about 3,400 ml per minute. To accommodate the large oxygen requirement of exercising muscles, the local vascular bed must channel large quantities of blood through the active tissues. In rhythmic exercise such as running, swimming, or cycling, the blood flow fluctuates; it decreases during the muscle's contraction phase and increases during the relaxation period. This provides a "milking action" that facilitates blood flow through the muscles and back to the heart. Complementing this pulsatile flow is the rapid dilatation of previously dormant capillaries to increase the effective surface for nutrient and gaseous exchange.

Straining-type activities present a somewhat different picture. When a muscle contracts to about 60% of its force-generating capacity, blood flow to the muscle is occluded as a result of elevated intramuscular pressure. With a sustained static or isometric contraction, the compressive force of the contraction can actually stop the flow of blood. Under such conditions, energy for continued muscular effort is generated mainly from the stored phosphagens and through the anaerobic reactions of glycolysis.

Capillarization of Muscle. One factor often proposed for the improved exercise capacity with training is an increase in capillary density of the trained muscles. Aside from its role in delivering oxygen, nutrients, and hormones, the capillary circulation also provides the means for removing heat and metabolic byproducts from the active tissues. All of these functions would be enhanced by a higher capillary density in muscle tissue.

Several investigations show favorable effects of endurance training on the capillarization of skeletal muscle. In one study using the electron microscope, the number of capillaries per muscle (as well as the capillaries per square millimeter of muscle tissue) averaged about 40% greater in endurance athletes than in untrained counterparts. The functional significance of this training response is that increased capillarization enhances the oxygenation of the entire muscle cell. This would be beneficial during strenuous exercise that requires a high level of steady-rate aerobic metabolism.

ULTRASTRUCTURE OF SKELETAL MUSCLE

The ultrastructure or microscopic anatomy of skeletal muscle has been

The microcirculation. Skeletal muscle is served by between 200 and 500 capillaries for each mm^2 of tissue. There are often as many as four capillaries in direct contact with each muscle fiber, and this number can be significantly increased with aerobic training.

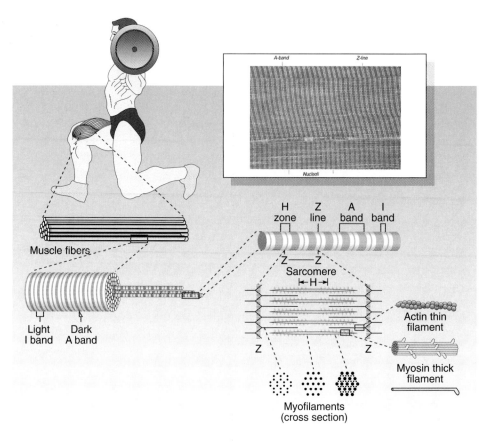

FIGURE 10-14. Microscopic organization of skeletal muscle. The whole muscle is composed of fibers; these in turn are made up of myofibrils, of which the actin and myosin protein filaments are a part. If viewed under a microscope, magnification would be approximately x 205,000. The insert figure displays a microscopic view of skeletal muscle fibers with prominent cross-striations. (From Vander, A.J., et al.: *Human Physiology*. 3rd ed. New York, McGraw Hill, 1985. Insert graph from Sobotta, J., and Hammersen, F. : *Histology. Color Atlas of Microscopic Anatomy*. 3rd ed. Urban & Schwarzenberg. Baltimore, 1992.)

Muscle proteins. The most abundant muscle proteins, in relation to the muscle's total protein content, are myosin, actin, and tropomyosin. Also, about 700 mg of the conjugated protein myoglobin are incorporated into each 100 g of muscle tissue.

revealed with the aid of electron microscopy, x-ray diffraction, and histochemical staining techniques. Figure 10-14 shows the different levels of subcellular organization within skeletal muscle fibers.

Each muscle fiber is composed of smaller functional units that lie parallel to the long axis of the fiber. These *fibrils* or *myofibrils* are approximately 1 μ in diameter and are composed of even smaller subunits, the *filaments* or *myofilaments,* that also lay parallel to the long axis of the myofibril. The myofilaments consist mainly of two proteins, actin and myosin, that account for about 84% of the myofibrillar complex.

The Sarcomere

At low magnification, the alternating light and dark bands along the length of the muscle fiber give it its characteristic striated appearance. Figure 10-15 illustrates the structural

details of this cross-striation pattern within a myofibril.

The lighter area is known as the *I band,* and the darker zone the *A band.* The *Z line* bisects the I band and adheres to the sarcolemma to give stability to the entire structure. The repeating unit between two Z lines is called the *sarcomere,* which is the functional unit of the muscle cell. The actin and myosin filaments within the sarcomere are primarily involved in the mechanical process of muscular contraction.

The position of the thin actin and thicker myosin proteins in the sarcomere results in an overlap of the two filaments. The center of the A band contains the *H zone,* a region of lower optical density owing to the absence of actin filaments in this area. The central portion of the H zone is bisected by the *M line,* which delineates the sarcomere's center. The M line consists of the protein structures that support the arrangement of the myosin filaments.

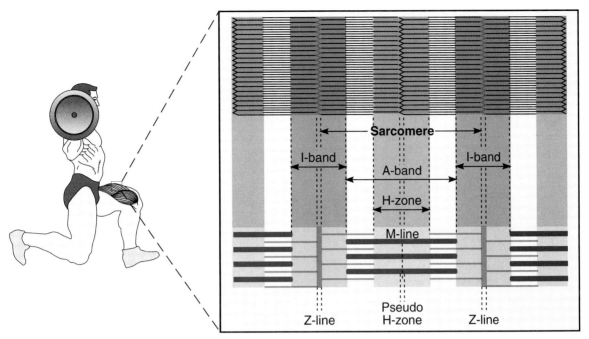

FIGURE 10-15. Structural position of the myofilaments in a sarcomere. A sarcomere is bounded at both ends by the Z line.

Actin-Myosin Orientation

Part A of Figure 10-16 illustrates the actin-myosin orientation within a sarcomere at resting length.Part B shows the hexagonal arrangement of actin and myosin filaments. A thick filament (150 Å in diameter and 1.5 m long) is bordered by six thinner filaments, each about 50 Å in diameter and 1 μ long. Three thick filaments surround each thin filament. This muscular substructure is extremely impressive. For example, a myofibril 1 μ in diameter contains about 450 thick filaments in the center of the sarcomere and 900 thin filaments at each end of the sarcomere. A single muscle fiber 100 μ in diameter and 1 cm long contains about 8000 myofibrils, each myofibril consisting of 4500 sarcomeres. This results in a total of 16 billion thick and 64 billion thin filaments in a single fiber.

Figure 10-17 is a detailed illustration of the spatial orientation of the various proteins that comprise the contractile filaments. Projections or "cross-bridges" spiral about the myosin filament at the region where the filaments of actin and myosin overlap. These cross-bridges are

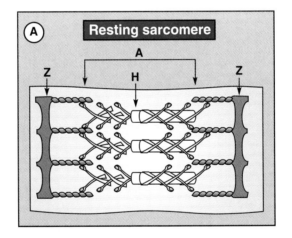

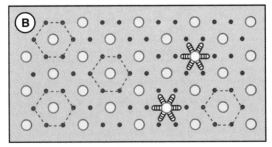

FIGURE 10-16. *A.* Ultrastructure of actin-myosin orientation within a resting sarcomere. *B.* Representation of electron micrograph through a cross section of myofibrils in a single muscle fiber. Note the hexagonal orientation of the smaller actin and larger myosin filaments, as well as cross-bridges that extend from a thick to thin filament.

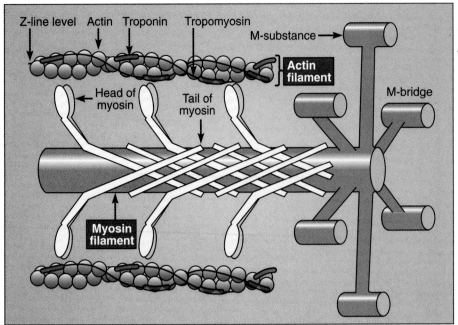

FIGURE 10-17. Details of the thick and thin protein filaments, including tropomyosin, troponin, and the M line. The myosin ATPase is located on the globular heads of the myosin; this "active" head frees the energy from ATP to be used in muscle contraction. (Modified from Edington, D.W., and Edgerton, V.R.: *The Biology of Physical Activity.* Boston, Houghton-Mifflin, 1976.)

repeated at intervals of about 450 Å along the filament. Their globular "lollipop-like" heads extend perpendicularly to interact with the thinner strands of actin; this is the structural and functional link between the myofilaments.

Tropomyosin and troponin are two other important constituents of the actin helix structure. These proteins appear to regulate the make-and-break contacts between the myofilaments during contraction. Tropomyosin is distributed along the length of the actin filament in a groove formed by the double helix. It is believed to inhibit actin and myosin interaction or coupling and prevent a permanent bonding of these filaments. Troponin, which is embedded at fairly regular intervals along the actin strands, has a high affinity for calcium ions (Ca^{++}). This mineral plays a crucial role in muscle function. It is the action of Ca^{++} and troponin that triggers the myofibrils to interact and slide past each other. When the fiber is stimulated, the tro-

ponin molecules appear to undergo a conformational change that in some way "tugs" on the tropomyosin protein strand. This moves the tropomyosin deeper into the groove between the two actin strands and "uncovers" the active sites of the actin allowing contraction to proceed.

The M line consists of transversely and longitudinally oriented proteins that serve to maintain the proper orientation of the thick filament within a sarcomere. As can be observed in Figure 10-16B, the perpendicularly oriented M bridges connect with six adjacent thick (myosin) filaments in a hexagonal pattern.

Intracellular Tubule Systems

Figure 10-18 illustrates the tubule system within a muscle fiber. An extensive network of interconnecting tubular channels, the sarcoplasmic reticulum, lies parallel to the myofibrils. The lateral end of each tubule terminates in a sac-like vesicle that stores Ca^{++}. Another network of tubules known as the *transverse tubule system,* or *T system,* runs perpendicular to the myofibril. The T tubules are situated between the lateral-most portion of two sarcoplasmic channels with the vesicles of these structures abutting the T tubule. This repeating pattern of two vesicles and T tubules in the region of each Z line is known as a *triad.* There are two triads in each sarcomere, and the pattern is repeated regularly throughout the length of the myofibril.

The T tubules pass through the fiber and open externally from the inside of the muscle cell. The triad and T tubule system appear to function as a microtransportation or plumbing network for spreading the action potential (wave of depolarization) from the fiber's outer membrane inward to the deep regions of the cell. During this depolarization process, Ca^{++} are released from the triad sacs

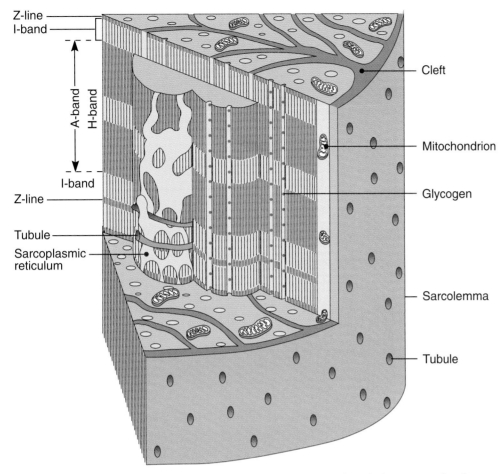

Z-line
I-band
A-band
H-band
I-band
Z-line
Tubule
Sarcoplasmic reticulum

Cleft

Mitochondrion

Glycogen

Sarcolemma

Tubule

FIGURE 10-18. Three-dimensional view of sarcoplasmic reticulum and T tubule system within the muscle fiber. (From Graham, H.: How is muscle turned on and off? *Sci. Am.;* 222:84, 1970.)

and diffuse a short distance to the filaments, presumably to "activate" the actin filaments. Contraction is initiated when the cross-bridges of the myosin filaments are attracted to the active sites on the actin filaments. When electrical excitation ceases, there is a decrease in free calcium concentration in the cytoplasm; this is associated with the relaxation of the muscle.

. . . .

CHEMICAL AND MECHANICAL EVENTS DURING CONTRACTION AND RELAXATION

The electron microscope has unraveled many secrets of cellular structure that have led to the formulation of reasonable hypotheses concerning the chemical and mechanical events during muscular contraction and relaxation. Although many gaps remain, there is considerable evidence to support a *"sliding-filament theory"* of muscle contraction that fits nicely with the detailed ultrastructure of muscle discussed previously.

Sliding-Filament Theory

The sliding-filament theory proposes that a muscle shortens or lengthens because the thick and thin myofilaments slide past each other without the filaments themselves changing length. This causes a major change in the relative size of the various zones and bands within a

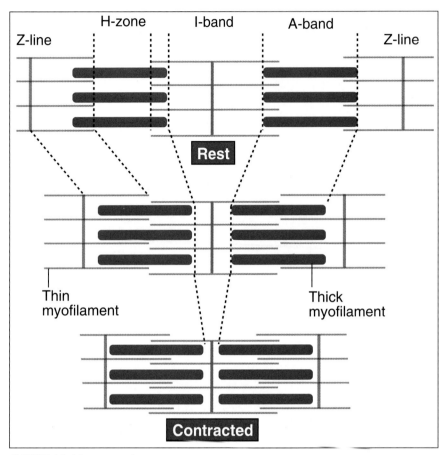

FIGURE 10-19. Structural rearrangement of actin and myosin filaments at rest and during muscle shortening.

sarcomere. Figure 10-19 illustrates that the thin actin myofilaments slide past the myosin myofilaments and move into the region of the A band during contraction (and move out in relaxation).

The major structural rearrangement during contraction occurs in the region of the I band which decreases markedly. The Z bands are essentially pulled toward the center of each sarcomere. There is no change in the width of the A band, although the H zone can disappear when the actin filaments are in contact at the center of the sarcomere. In an isometric muscular action, force is generated while the fiber's length remains relatively unchanged and the relative spacing of I and A bands stays constant; in this situation, the same molecular groups react with one another repeatedly. In an eccentric action in which force is generated while the muscle lengthens, the A band becomes broader.

Mechanical Action of the Cross-Bridges. The globular head of the myosin cross-bridge provides the mechanical means for the actin and myosin filaments to slide past each other. Figure 10-20 shows schematically the oscillating to-and-fro nature of the cross-bridges, which move in a way somewhat similar to the action of oars in water. Unlike oars, however, the cross-bridges do not all move in a synchronous manner. During contraction, each cross-bridge undergoes many repeated but independent cycles of movement. Thus, at any one time, only about 50% of the bridges are in contact with the thin actin filaments to form the protein complex actomyosin, which has contractile properties; the others are at some other position in their vibrating cycle.

As illustrated in the right side of Figure 10-20, each action of a cross-bridge contributes only a small longitudinal displacement in terms of the total sliding action of the filaments. This process has been likened to the action of a person climbing a rope. The arms and legs represent the cross-bridges. Climbing is accomplished by first reaching with the arms; then grabbing, pulling, and breaking contact; and then repeating this process over and over throughout the climb.

Link Between Actin, Myosin, and ATP. The interaction and movement of the protein filaments during muscular action necessitate that the myosin cross-bridges continually undergo oscillatory movements by combining, detaching, and recombining to new sites along the actin strands.

The detachment of the myosin cross-bridges from the actin filament is brought about when the ATP molecule is joined to the actomyosin complex. This reaction enables the myosin cross-bridge to return to its original state so it is available to bind a new active site on the actin. The dissocia-

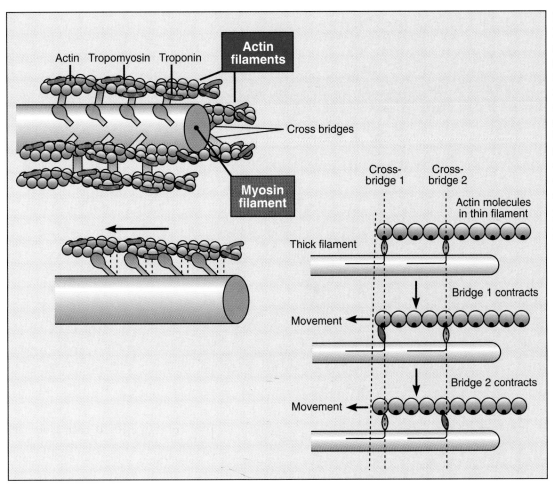

FIGURE 10-20.
Relative positioning of actin and myosin filaments during the oscillating movement of the cross-bridges. The action of each bridge contributes a small displacement of movement. For clarity, one of the actin strands is omitted from the left-hand portion of the figure.

tion of actomyosin occurs in the following way:

$$Actomyosin + ATP \longrightarrow Actin + Myosin\text{-}ATP$$

ATP also serves an important function in the contraction process. Energy is provided for cross-bridge movement when the terminal phosphate is split from ATP. One of the reacting sites on the globular head of the myosin cross-bridge binds to the reactive site on actin. The other myosin active site acts as the enzyme myofibrillar adenosine triphosphatase, or more commonly *myosin ATPase*. This enzyme splits ATP so its energy can be used for muscle contraction. The rate of ATP splitting is relatively slow if myosin and actin remain apart; when they join, however, the reactive rate of myosin ATPase increases considerably. It is believed that energy released from ATP splitting somehow activates the cross-bridges, causing them to oscillate. It is possible that this energy transfer process causes a conformational change in the shape of the globular head of the myosin cross-bridge so it interacts with the appropriate actin molecule.

It is tempting to speculate that specific forms of speed and power training modify enzymatic activity in a manner that facilitates the sequence of events in muscular contraction. More will be said shortly concerning fiber types and training effects.

Excitation-Contraction Coupling

Excitation-contraction is the physiologic mechanism whereby an electric discharge at the muscle initiates the chemical events that lead to contraction.

Like a cocked spring. Recent research indicates that the elongated, pear-shaped myosin is not rigid. In fact, prior to the muscle action the myosin head literally bends around the ATP molecule and becomes cocked, almost like a spring. The myosin then interacts with the adjacent action filaments, splits a phosphate from ATP, and straightens. This forces the sliding motion that makes the muscle contract.

Actin + Myosin ATPase ⟶ Actomyosin ATPase

Actomyosin ATPase ⟶ Actomyosin + ADP + P + Energy

In the resting state, a muscle's Ca^{++} concentration is low. When a muscle fiber is stimulated to contract, there is an immediate increase in intracellular Ca^{++}. This is initiated by the arrival of the action potential at the transverse tubules that causes Ca^{++} to be released from the lateral sacs of the sarcoplasmic reticulum. The inhibitory action of troponin that prevents actin-myosin interaction is released when Ca^{++} ions bind rapidly with troponin in the actin filaments. In a sense, the muscle is now "turned on."

When the active sites on the actin and myosin are joined, myosin ATPase is activated, which in turn splits ATP. During this process, the transfer of energy causes movement of the myosin cross-bridges, and the muscle generates tension.

The cross-bridges uncouple from actin when ATP binds to the myosin bridge. Coupling and uncoupling continue as long as the Ca^{++} concentration remains at a sufficient level to inhibit the troponin-tropomyosin system. When the nerve stimulus to the muscle is removed, Ca^{++} moves back into the lateral sacs of the sarcoplasmic reticulum. This restores the inhibitory action of the troponin-tropomyosin, and actin and myosin remain separated as long as ATP is present. Figure 10-21 illustrates the interaction between the actin and myosin filaments, Ca^{++}, and ATP in a relaxed and contracted muscle.

Relaxation

When a muscle is no longer stimulated, the flow of Ca^{++} ceases, and troponin is free once again to inhibit actin-myosin interaction. During recovery, Ca^{++} is actively pumped into the sarcoplasmic reticulum where it concentrates in the lateral vesicles. The retrieval of Ca^{++} from the troponin-tropomyosin proteins "turns off" the active sites on the actin filament. This deactivation accomplishes two things: (1) It prevents any mechanical link between the myosin cross-bridges and the actin filaments; (2) it reduces the activity of myosin ATPase so there is no more ATP splitting. The muscle's relaxation is brought about by the return of the actin and myosin filaments to their original state.

Sequence of Events in Muscular Contraction

The following is a list of the main events in muscular contraction and relaxation. The sequence begins with the initiation of an action potential by the motor nerve. This impulse is then propagated over the entire surface of the muscle fiber as the cell membrane becomes depolarized:

- The muscle action potential depolarizes the transverse tubules at the A-I junction of the sarcomere.
- The depolarization of the transverse or T tubules causes Ca^{++} to be released from the lateral sacs of the sarcoplasmic reticulum.

FIGURE 10-21. Interaction between the actin-myosin filaments, Ca^{++}, and ATP in relaxed and contracted muscle. In the relaxed state, troponin and tropomyosin interact with actin preventing the coupling of the myosin cross-bridge to actin. During contraction, the cross-bridge couples with actin as a result of the binding of Ca^{++} with troponin-tropomyosin. (From Vander, A.J., et al.: *Human Physiology.* 3rd ed. New York, McGraw-Hill, 1985.)

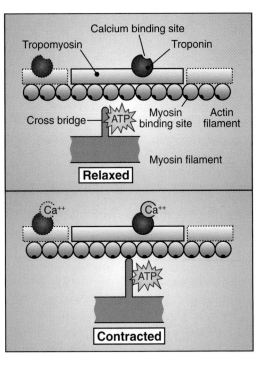

- Ca⁺⁺ ions bind to troponin-tropomyosin in the actin filaments. This releases the inhibition that prevented actin from combining with myosin.
- Actin combines with myosin-ATP. Actin also activates myosin ATPase, which then splits ATP. Tension is created because the energy from this reaction is used to produce movement of the myosin cross-bridge.
- ATP binds to the myosin bridge. This breaks the actin-myosin bond and allows the cross-bridge to dissociate from actin. This leads to a relative movement or sliding of the thick and thin filaments past each other, and the muscle shortens.
- Cross-bridge activation continues as long as the concentration of Ca⁺⁺ remains high enough (owing to membrane depolarization) to inhibit the action of the troponin-tropomyosin system.
- When the muscle is no longer stimulated, the concentration of Ca⁺⁺ ions rapidly decreases as they move back into the lateral sacs of the sarcoplasmic reticulum by an energy process that splits ATP.
- The removal of Ca⁺⁺ ions restores the inhibitory action of troponin-tropomyosin. In the presence of ATP, actin and myosin remain in the dissociated, relaxed state.

MUSCLE FIBER TYPE

Skeletal muscle is not simply a homogeneous group of fibers with similar metabolic and functional properties. Although considerable confusion has existed concerning the method and terminology for classifying human skeletal muscle, two distinct fiber types have been identified and classified by their contractile and metabolic characteristics.

Fast-Twitch Fibers

Fast-twitch muscle fibers have a high capability for the electrochemical transmission of action potentials, a high activity level of myosin ATPase, a rapid level of calcium release and uptake by the sarcoplasmic reticulum, and a high rate of cross-bridge turnover, all of which relate to their ability to transfer energy rapidly for quick, forceful contractions. Recall that it is myosin ATPase that splits ATP to provide energy for muscle action. In fact, the fast-twitch fiber's intrinsic speed of contraction and tension development is two to three times as fast as that of fibers classified as slow-twitch fibers (see next section). The fast-twitch fibers rely largely on a well-developed, short-term glycolytic system for energy transfer. They have been labeled *FG fibers* to signify their fast-glycogenolytic capabilities. Fast-twitch fibers are generally activated in short-term, high-power output activities as well as other forceful muscular contractions that depend almost entirely on anaerobic metabolism for energy. The metabolic and contractile capacities of these fibers are also important in the stop-and-go or change-of-pace sports such as basketball or field hockey, which at times require rapid energy that only the anaerobic metabolic pathways supply.

Fast-Twitch Subdivisions. Subdivisions of the fast-twitch fiber are present in humans. The *type IIa fiber* is considered intermediate because its fast contraction speed is combined with a moderately well-developed capacity for both aerobic (possesses a high level of the aerobic enzyme *succinic dehydrogenase* [SDH]) and anaerobic (possesses a high level of the anaerobic enzyme *phosphofructokinase* [PFK]) energy transfer. These are called the *fast-oxidative-glycolytic (FOG) fibers.* Another subdivision, the *type IIb fiber,* possesses the greatest anaerobic potential and is the "true" *FG fiber.*

High levels of myosin ATPase. Fast-twitch muscle fibers, with the ability for rapid and powerful contraction, possess a relatively high activity level of the enzyme myosin ATPase.

Individuals who engage in weightlifting often exhibit remarkable muscular hypertrophy. It is not unusual to observe these relatively large individuals with a lean body mass of 90% or more of their total body mass. This compares to the average lean body mass of 80 to 85% for normal nonweightlifting men.

Although many athletes use weight training to increase strength to enhance performance of a specific sport, bodybuilders lift weights solely to improve body configuration and form. Although it is obvious that bodybuilders have enormous muscular hypertrophy, the quantification of the differences in muscle accumulation is poorly documented between groups of athletes and nonathletes.

It is difficult to quantify the amount of excess muscle, i.e., the amount of muscle in excess of that to be expected based on body mass. Newer x-ray techniques have not yet been applied to the study of excess muscle. However, by measuring the body's potassium content (a mineral found mainly in muscle that closely predicts muscle mass), it is possible to make a rea-

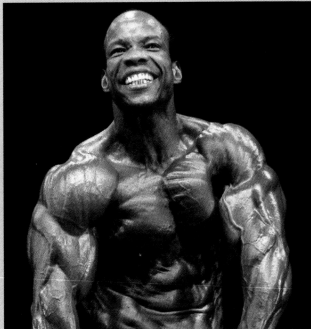

sonable estimate of the muscle content of the body. It is also possible to calculate excess muscle using an anthropometric technique devised by the noted scientist Dr. A.R. Behnke. It was Behnke's assertion that because the lower trunk region (hips) with weight training does not hypertrophy to the degree of other body areas, it is possible to make a presumptive estimate of body mass before weight training by calculating the weight equivalent of the hips (designated as $W_{[hips]}$). Scale weight minus $W_{[hips]}$ would then provide an estimate of excess muscle.

Research has presented data about estimates of excess muscle in bodybuilders, weightlifters, and pro-

fessional football players (interior linemen). For the bodybuilders, their excess muscle of 34.6 lbs accounts for approximately 21% of their lean body mass; for the weightlifters, excess muscle of 30.6 lbs accounts for 19% of lean body mass. For the football players, even though they can weigh 60 to 70 lbs more than the weightlifters and bodybuilders, respectively, their excess muscle (in relation to that expected for body mass) was only 16.8 lbs and accounted for merely 8% of their lean body mass. The amount of excess muscle for bodybuilders is truly remarkable and attests to these athletes' extreme degree of muscular development. Such muscularity takes incredible dedication to training and proper nutrition. The average national or international competitive body builder has trained for a minimum of 10 years, 2 hours a day, 5 days a week.

Reference

Katch, V. L,. et al.: Extreme muscular development in man: Body composition of competitive Olympic lifters, power lifters, and body builders. *Med. Sci. Sports* 12:340, 1980.

Slow-Twitch Fibers

Slow-twitch fibers generate energy for ATP resynthesis predominantly by means of the relatively long-term system of aerobic energy transfer. They are distinguished by a low activity level of myosin ATPase, a slow speed of contraction, and a glycolytic capacity less well developed than their fast-twitch counterparts. The slow-twitch fibers, however, contain relatively large and numerous mitochondria and accompanying iron-containing cytochromes. Accompanying this enhanced metabolic machinery is a high concentration of mitochondrial enzymes required to sustain aerobic metabolism. Thus, slow-twitch fibers are fatigue resistant and well suited for prolonged aerobic exercise. These fibers have been labeled *SO fibers* to describe their slow contraction speed and great reliance on oxidative metabolism.

In contrast to the FG fibers that fatigue readily, the SO fibers (more precisely, motor units) are adapted for prolonged work and are recruited for aerobic activities. In fact, studies of muscle glycogen depletion indicate that in prolonged, moderate exercise there is almost exclusive reliance on the slow-twitch muscle fibers. Even after 9 to 12 hours of moderate aerobic exercise the limited glycogen that is available is found mostly in the "unused" fast-twitch fibers. It also appears that the capacity for blood flow through muscle is determined by differences in the oxidative capacity of the two fiber types, with the slow-twitch fibers receiving proportionately more blood during exercise than their fast-twitch counterparts.

Many researchers classify slow-twitch fibers as *type I,* and the fast-twitch fibers (and proposed subdivisions) are categorized as *type II.* When a person exercises at near maximum aerobic and anaerobic levels, as in middle-distance running or swimming, or in multiple sprint sports such as basketball, field hockey, or soccer, both types of muscle fibers are activated because these activities require a blend of aerobic and anaerobic energy.

Differences Between Athletic Groups

Several interesting observations can be made concerning muscle fiber types and the possible influence of specific training on fiber composition and metabolic capacity. For one thing, sedentary men and women as well as young children possess 45 to 55% slow-twitch fibers. For fast-twitch fibers, the percentage is probably equally distributed between subdivisions. Although there are no gender differences in fiber distribution, the individual variation is large. Generally the trend in one's muscle fiber type distribution is consistent throughout the body's major muscle groups.

Certain patterns of fiber distribution are readily apparent among highly proficient athletes. Successful endurance athletes, for example, generally demonstrate a predominance of slow-twitch fibers in the muscles activated in their sport. For successful sprint athletes, the fast-twitch muscle fiber predominates. This is shown in Figure 10-22 for top Scandinavian competitors who represent different sports. Athletic groups with the highest aerobic and endurance capacities, such as distance runners and cross-country skiers, also have the highest relative number of slow-twitch fibers, often as high as 90%! Weightlifters, ice-hockey players, and sprinters, on the other hand, tend to have more fast-twitch fibers and a relatively lower max $\dot{V}O_2$. As might be expected, men and women who perform in middle-distance events have an approximately equal percentage of the two types of muscle fibers. This distribution also occurs for power athletes, such as throwers, jumpers, and high jumpers. These relatively clear-cut distinctions between performance and muscle fiber composition are for elite athletes who have achieved prominence in a specific sport category. Figure 10-23 presents additional data for the per-

A reddish looking muscle fiber. It is the concentration of mitochondria combined with high levels of myoglobin that give the slow-twitch fibers their characteristic red pigmentation.

Both fibers are important. It should be noted that both fiber types are involved in most activities; it is just that certain activities require activation of a much greater proportion of one fiber type over another.

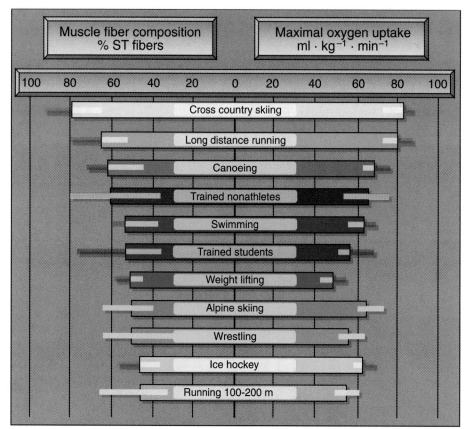

| Muscle fiber composition % ST fibers | | | | | | Maximal oxygen uptake ml · kg⁻¹ · min⁻¹ | | | | |

| 100 | 80 | 60 | 40 | 20 | 0 | 20 | 40 | 60 | 80 | 100 |

Cross country skiing

Long distance running

Canoeing

Trained nonathletes

Swimming

Trained students

Weight lifting

Alpine skiing

Wrestling

Ice hockey

Running 100-200 m

FIGURE 10-22. Muscle fiber composition (percent slow-twitch fibers, left side) and maximal oxygen uptake (right side) in athletes representing different sports. The outer, lightly shaded bars denote the range. (From Bergh, U., et al.: Maximal oxygen uptake and muscle fiber types in trained and untrained humans. *Med. Sci. Sports, 10*:151, 1978.)

Muscle fiber training specificity. Why do some highly trained athletes who switch to a sport requiring different muscle groups feel essentially untrained for the new activity? The answer is that only the specific muscles (more precisely, muscle fibers) used in training show adaptation to exercise. Within this framework, swimmers or canoeists will not necessarily transfer their upper body "fitness" to a running sport (unless they now train for that sport).

centage of slow-twitch and fast-twitch fiber type in three muscle groups in US male and female top athletes.

A person's fiber composition, however, is clearly not the sole determinant of performance. Several researchers have shown that for a particular group, either trained or untrained, knowledge of a person's predominant fiber type is of limited value in predicting the outcome of specific exercise performances. *This is not surprising because performance capacity is the end result of the blending of many physiologic, biochemical, neurologic, and biomechanical "support systems" — and is not simply determined by a single factor such as muscle fiber type.*

In terms of muscle size, endurance athletes exhibit slow-twitch fibers that are slightly enlarged in relation to normal. Weightlifters and other power athletes show a definite enlargement, especially in the fast-twitch fibers. These fibers may be 45% larger than those of endurance athletes or of sedentary individuals of the same age. This is because power and strength training induce a definite enlargement of the fiber's contractile apparatus — specifically the actin and myosin filaments as well as its total glycogen content.

Can Fiber Type be Changed?

To determine whether the fiber composition characteristics of specific athletic groups are due to training or natural endowment (that is, can fiber composition be changed?), six men participated in a 5-month program of aerobic bicycle training. Muscle biopsy specimens from the lateral portion of the quadriceps before and after training indicated no change in fiber composition, although all men improved considerably in work capacity and aerobic power. Similar observations have been reported for the fiber composition of subjects after endurance or sprint training program, or after a period of weight training. These data are often used to support the argument that a fast-contracting fiber before training will still be a fast-contracting fiber after training, with the same holding true for the slow-twitch fibers.

Additional studies with both humans and animals, however, suggest the possibility of changes in biochemical-physiologic properties of muscle fibers with a progressive transformation in fiber type with specific and chronic training. In one study of 18 weeks of "aerobic" and 11 weeks of "anaerobic" training in four athletes, the anaerobic training caused an increase in the percentage of type II fibers and a decrease in the percentage of type I fibers; the opposite was observed in the aerobic phase of the training sequence. Similarly, research has shown a 23% increase in the per-

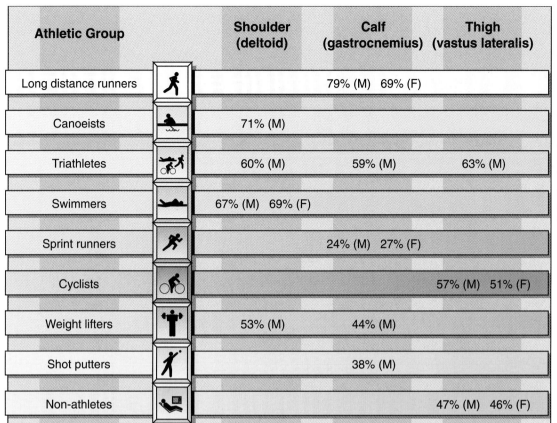

Athletic Group		Shoulder (deltoid)	Calf (gastrocnemius)	Thigh (vastus lateralis)
Long distance runners			79% (M) 69% (F)	
Canoeists		71% (M)		
Triathletes		60% (M)	59% (M)	63% (M)
Swimmers		67% (M) 69% (F)		
Sprint runners			24% (M) 27% (F)	
Cyclists				57% (M) 51% (F)
Weight lifters		53% (M)	44% (M)	
Shot putters			38% (M)	
Non-athletes				47% (M) 46% (F)

FIGURE 10-23. Percentage of slow-twitch fibers in three muscle groups of male (M) and female (F) athletes. The percentage of fast-twitch fibers is calculated as the difference between 100% and the percentage of slow-twitch fibers.

centage of fast-twitch fibers and a commensurate decrease in slow-twitch fiber percentage after only 6 weeks of sprint training. These findings suggest that specific training (and perhaps inactivity) may induce an actual conversion of type I to type II fibers or vice versa (It is likely that some type IIa fibers are "transitional" fibers able to take on type I characteristics and functions under an aerobic training stimuli.) It is clear that more research needs to be done in this intriguing area before definitive statements can be made concerning the fixed nature of a muscle's fiber composition. At present, it appears that some transformation in muscle fiber type with chronic activity is in fact possible.

Metabolic Adaptations are Real and Significant

The muscle fiber type distribution appears to be determined largely by genetic code, with the major direction of a muscle's fiber composition

and perhaps fiber number being fixed before birth or early puberty. Whether this status can be significantly modified with prolonged training is still open to question. It also seems likely that, at elite levels of certain sports performances, a particular fiber distribution is "required" for success. Although this suggests an obvious genetic predetermination for sports success, it is a well-documented fact that specific training significantly enhances aerobic and possibly anaerobic power of both fiber types regardless of age. In fact, enhancement of the oxidative capacity of fast-twitch fibers with high-intensity endurance training brings them to a level at which they are almost as well equipped for oxidative metabolism as are the slow-twitch fibers of untrained subjects. This training adaptation in both young and mature adults is brought about by the well-documented increase in mitochondrial size and number and the accompanying enhancement in the quantity of enzymes relevant to Krebs cycle and electron transport function.

Age is no barrier to skeletal muscle fiber adaptation. If the training stimulus is adequate, the skeletal muscles of older men and women adapt (fiber size, capillarization, glycolytic and respiratory enzymes) to both endurance and resistance training exercise in a manner similar to younger people.

TABLE 10-2. Effects of specific forms of training on skeletal muscle*

Muscle Factor	Slow-Twitch Fibers		Fast-Twitch Fibers	
	Type of Training			
	Strength	Endurance	Strength	Endurance
Percent composition	0 or ?	0 or ?	0 or ?	0 or ?
Size	+	0 or +	+ +	0
Contractile property	0	0	0	0
Oxidative capacity	0	+ +	0	+
Anaerobic capacity	? or +	0	? or +	0
Glycogen content	0	+ +	0	+ +
Fat oxidation	0	+ +	0	+
Capillary density	?	+	?	? or +
Blood flow during work	?	? or +	?	?

0 = no change; ? = unknown; + = moderate increase; + + = large increase.
*Modified from Gollnick, P.D., and Sembrowich, W.L.: Adaptations in human skeletal muscle as a result of training. *In Exercise in Cardiovascular Health and Disease.* Edited by E.A. Amsterdam, et al., New York, Yorke Medical Books, 1977.

Individuals who have adapted to endurance training may show some conversion in the type IIb fiber to the more aerobic type IIa fiber. This is accompanied by a large increase in mitochondrial content and aerobic enzyme levels in these specific fibers.

The changes that occur in skeletal muscle from specific training are summarized in Table 10-2.

SUMMARY

PART 2

1. Skeletal muscle is encased in various wrappings of connective tissue. These eventually blend into and join the tendinous attachment to bone. This harness enables muscles to act on the bony levers to transform the chemical energy of ATP into mechanical energy and motion.

2. Seventy-five percent of skeletal muscle is water, 20% is protein; and the remainder consists of inorganic salts, enzymes, pigments, lipids, and carbohydrates.

3. In vigorous exercise, the muscle's oxygen uptake increases nearly 70 times above the resting level. Supporting this metabolic requirement are immediate adjustments and longer term training adaptations in the local vascular bed.

4. The sarcomere is the functional unit of the muscle cell. It contains the contractile proteins actin and myosin. There are 4500 sarcomeres and a total of 16 billion thick (myosin) and 64 billion thin (actin) filaments in an average-sized fiber.

5. Projections or cross-bridges provide the structural link between the thin and thick contractile filaments. Tropomyosin and troponin, two proteins of the myofibrillar complex, regulate the make-and-break contacts between the filaments during contraction. Tropomyosin inhibits actin and myosin interaction; troponin with calcium triggers the myofibrils to interact and slide past each other.

6. The triad and T tubule system serve as a microtransportation network for spreading the action potential from the fiber's outer membrane inward to deep regions of the cell. Contraction occurs when calcium activates actin, causing the myosin cross-bridges to attach to active sites on the actin filaments. Relaxation occurs when calcium concentration decreases.

7. The sliding filament theory proposes that a muscle shortens or lengthens because the protein filaments slide past each other without changing their length. The mechanisms for excitation-contraction coupling are the electro-chemical and mechanical events linked to achieve muscular contraction.

8. Two types of muscle fibers can be classified by their contractile and metabolic characteristics: (1) fast-twitch fibers, in which energy is predominantly generated anaerobically and rapidly for a quick, powerful contraction, and (2) slow-twitch fibers that contract relatively slowly and generate energy for ATP resynthesis predominantly via aerobic metabolism.

9. The percentage distribution of fiber type differs significantly among individuals. This distribution is probably largely determined by genetic code, although some modification may take place with physical training.

10. Both fiber types can be markedly improved in metabolic capacity by specific training.

SELECTED REFERENCES

Antonio, J., and Gonyea, W.J.: Skeletal muscle fiber hyperplasia. *Med. Sci. Sports Exerc.*, 25: 1333, 1993.

Asmussen, E.: Muscle fatigue. *Med. Sci. Sports Exerc.*, 25:412, 1993.

Armstrong, R.B.: Muscle fiber recruitment patterns and their metabolic correlates. *In Exercise, Nutrition, and Energy Metabolism.* Edited by E.S. Horton and R.L. Terjung, New York, Macmillan, 1988.

Basmajian, J.V., and Deluca, C.J.: *Muscles Alive. Their Functions Revealed by Electromyography.* 5th Ed., Baltimore, Williams & Wilkins, 1985.

Bigland-Richie, B., et al.: Changes in motoneurone firing rates during sustained maximal voluntary contractions. *J. Physiol.* (London), 340:335, 1983.

Criswell, D., et al.: High intensity training-induced changes in skeletal muscle antioxidant enzyme activity. *Med. Sci. Sports Exerc.*, 25: 1135, 1993.

Freund, H.J.: Motor unit and muscle activity in voluntary motor control. *Physiol. Rev.*, 63:387, 1983.

Gaffney, F.A.: Cardiovascular and metabolic responses to static contraction in man. *Acta Physiol. Scand.*, 138:249, 1990.

Hakkinen, K., and Komi, P.V.: Electromyographic changes during strength-training and detraining, *Med. Sci. Sports Exerc.*, 15:455, 1983.

Hakkinen, K., et al.: Effect of combined concentric and eccentric strength training and detraining on force-time, muscle fiber, and metabolic characteristics of leg extensor muscles. *Scand. J. Sports Sci.*, 3:50, 1981.

Hogan, N., et al.: Controlling multijoint motor behavior. In *Exercise and Sport Sciences Reviews.* Vol. 15. Edited by K.B. Pandolf. New York, Macmillan, 1987.

Holloszy, J.O., and Coyle, E.F.: Adaptations of skeletal muscle to endurance training and their metabolic consequences. *J. Appl. Physiol.*, 56:831, 1984.

Klug, G.A., and Tibbits, G.F.: The effects of activity on calcium-mediated events in striated muscle. In *Exercise and Sport Sciences Reviews.* Vol. 16. Edited by K.B. Pandolf. New York, Macmillan, 1988.

Kraus, W.E., et al.: Skeletal muscle adaptation to chronic low-frequency motor nerve stimulation. *Exerc. Sport Sci. Rev.*, 22: 313, 1994.

Lieber, R.L.: *Skeletal muscle Structure and Function: Implications for Rehabilitation and Sports Medicine.* Baltimore, Williams & Wilkins, 1992.

MacLaren, C.P., et al: A review of metabolic and physiological factors in fatigue. In *Exercise and Sport Sciences Reviews.* Vol. 17. Edited by K.B. Pandolf. Baltimore, Williams & Wilkins, 1989.

Moratini, T., and DeVries, H.: Neural factors versus hypertrophy in the time course of muscle strength gain. *Am. J. Phys. Med.*, 58:115, 1979.

Nemete, P., et al.: Comparison of enzyme activities among single muscle fibers within defined motor units. *J. Physiol.* (London), 311:489, 1985.

Otten, E.: Concepts and models of functional architecture in skeletal muscle. In *Exercise and Sport Sciences Reviews.* Vol. 16. Edited by K.B. Pandolf. New York, Macmillan, 1988.

Ottoson, D.: *Physiology of the Nervous System.* London, Macmillan, 1983.

Ozmun, J.C., et al.: Neuromuscular adaptations following prepubescent strength training. *Med. Sci. Sports Exerc.*, 26: 510, 1994.

Pette, D., and Vrbova, G.: Neural control of phenotypic expression in mammalian muscle fibers. *Muscle Nerve*, 8:676, 1985.

Roman, W.J., et al.: Adaptations in the elbow flexors of elderly males after heavy-resistance training. *J. Appl. Physiol.*, 74: 750, 1993.

Sale, D. G., et al.: Neural adaptation to resistance training. *Med. Sci. Sports Exerc.*, 20:S135, 1988.

Saltin, B., et al.: Fiber types and metabolic potentials of skeletal muscles in sedentary man and endurance runners. *Ann. N.Y. Acad. Sci.*, 301:3, 1977.

Seals, D.R., and Victor, R.G.: Regulation of muscle sympathetic nerve activity during exercise in humans. In *Exercise and Sport Sciences Reviews.* Vol. 19. Edited by J.O. Holloszy. Baltimore, Williams & Wilkins, 1991.

Spectar, S.A., et al.: Muscle architecture and force-velocity characteristics of cat soleus and medial gastrocnemius: Implications for motor control. *J. Neurobiol.*, 44:951, 1980.

Hormones, Exercise, and Training

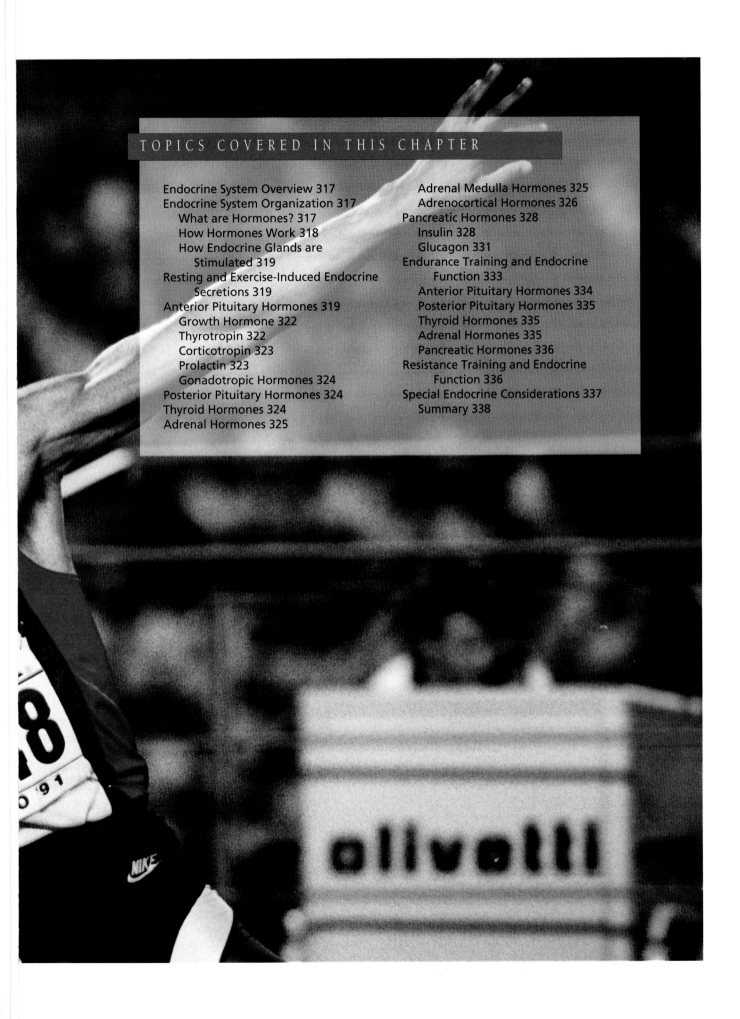

TABLE 11-1. Endocrine glands, their secretions, functions, control factors, effects of hypo- and hypersecretion, and the effects of exercise on hormone output

Host Gland	Hormone	Hormone Effects	Control of Hormone Secretion	Effects of Hyposecretion and Hypersecretion	Exercise Effects on Hormone Secretion
Anterior pituitary	Growth hormone (GH; somato-tropin)	Stimulates tissue growth; mobilizes fatty acids for energy; inhibits CHO metabolism	Hypothalamic releasing factor (GHRF)	*Hypo-* dwarfism in children; *Hyper-* gigantism in children; acromegly in adults	↑ with increasing exercise
	Thyrotropin (TSH)	Stimulates production and release of thyroxine from thyroid gland	Hypothalamic TSH-releasing factor; thyroxine	*Hypo-* cretinism in children (stunted growth, mental retardation); myxedema in adults (low BMR, constipa-tion, dry skin, puffy eyes, edema, lethargy); *Hyper-* Graves' disease (autoimmune disease — elevated BMR, weight loss, irregular heartbeat), heart disease	↑ with increasing exercise
	Corticotropin (ACTH)	Stimulates produc-tion and release of cortisol, aldoster-one, and adrenal hormones	Hypothalamic ACTH-releasing factor; cortisol	*Hypo-* rarely seen; *Hyper-* Cushing's disease	unknown
	Gonadotropic (FSH and LH)	FSH works with LH to stimulate pro-duction of estro-gen by ovaries, LH works with FSH to stimulate produc-tion of estrogen and progesterone by ovaries and testosterone by male testes	Hypothalamic FSH and LH releasing factor; female — estrogen and progesterone; male — testosterone	*Hypo-* failure of sexual maturation; *Hyper-* none	No change
	Prolactin (PRL)	Inhibits testoster-one; mobilizes fatty acids	Hypothalamic PRL-inhibiting factor	*Hypo-* poor milk production in nursing women, *Hyper-* galactorrhea, cessation of menses in females, impotence in males	↑ with increasing exercise
	Endorphins	Blocks pain; pro-motes euphoria; affects feeding and female men-strual cycle	Stress — physi-cal/emotional (may be inten-sity related)	Unknown	↑ with long dura-tion exercise
Posterior pituitary	Vasopressin (ADH)	Controls water ex-cretion by kidneys	Hypothalamic secretory neurons	*Hypo-* diabetes; *Hyper-* unknown	↑ with increasing exercise
	Oxytocin	Stimulates muscles in uterus and breasts; important in birthing and lactation	Hypothalamic secretory neurons	Unknown	unknown
Adrenal cortex	Cortisol Corticosterone	Promotes use of fatty acids and protein catabolism; conserves blood sugar/insulin antagonist; has anti-inflammatory effects with epinephrine	ACTH; stress	*Hypo-* Addison's disease (weight loss; glucose and sodium levels drop and potassium levels rise, result-ing in hypotension and dehy-dration); *Hyper-* Cushing's disease (persistent hyperglycemia, dramatic losses in muscle and bone protein, and water and salt retention leading to hypertension)	↑ in heavy exercise only

TABLE 11-1. (cont'd)

Host Gland	Hormone	Hormone Effects	Control of Hormone Secretion	Effects of Hyposecretion and Hypersecretion	Exercise Effects on Hormone Secretion
	Aldosterone	Promotes retention of sodium, potassium, and water by the kidneys	Angiotensin and plasma potassium concentration; renin	*Hypo-* Addison's disease; *Hyper-* aldosteronism (excessive sodium and water retention and accelerated excretion of potassium)	↑ with increasing exercise
Adrenal medulla	Epinephrine Norepinephrine	Facilitates sympathetic activity, increases cardiac output, regulates blood vessels, increases glycogen catabolism and fatty acid release	Stress stimulated hypothalamic sympathetic nerves	*Hypo-* unimportant; *Hyper-* hypertension, increased metabolism	Epinephrine, ↑ in heavy exercise Norepinephrine, ↑ with increasing exercise
Thyroid	Thyroxine (T_4) Triiodothyronine (T_3)	Stimulates metabolic rate; regulates cell growth and activity	TSH; whole body metabolism	*Hypo-* decreased BMR and body temperature, cold intolerance, decreased appetite, weight gain, decreased glucose metabolism, elevated cholesterol, decreased protein synthesis, hypotension, muscle cramps, growth retardation, depressed ovarian function; *Hyper-* increased BMR, temperature, heat intolerance, increased appetite, weight loss, hypertension, enhanced catabolism of glucose, fat, and protein, loss of muscle, muscle atrophy, depressed ovarian function	↑ with increasing exercise
Pancreas	Insulin	Promotes CHO transport into cells; increases CHO catabolism and decreases blood glucose; promotes fatty acid and amino acid transport into cells	Plasma glucose levels	*Hypo-* diabetes; *Hyper-* hypoglycemia, anxiety, nervousness, weakness	↓ with increasing exercise
	Glucagon	Promotes release of glucose from liver to blood; increases fat metabolism, reduces amino acid levels	Plasma glucose levels	*Hypo-* chronic hypoglycemia, low circulating amino acids; *Hyper-* hyperglycemia	↑ with increasing exercise
Parathyroid	Parathormone	Raises blood calcium; lowers blood phosphate	Plasma calcium concentration	*Hypo-* hypocalcemia, respiraory paralysis, uncontrolled spasms and convulsions; *Hyper-* hypercalcemia, extreme leaching of calcium from bones, depression of nervous system activity, muscle weakness, formation of kidney stones	↑ with long-term exercise
Ovaries	Estrogen Progesterone	Controls menstrual cycle; increases fat deposition; promotes female sex characteristics	FSH, LH	*Hypo-* (estrogen); *Hyper-* (progesterone) masculinization or virilization	↑ with exercise; depends on menstrual phase
Testes	Testosterone	Controls muscle size; increases RBC; decreases body fat; promotes male sex characteristics		*Hypo-* feminization; *Hyper-* masculinization or virilization	↑ with exercise
Kidney	Renin	Stimulates aldosterone secretion	Plasma sodium	*Hypo-* hypertension; *Hyper-* hypotension	↑ with increasing exercise

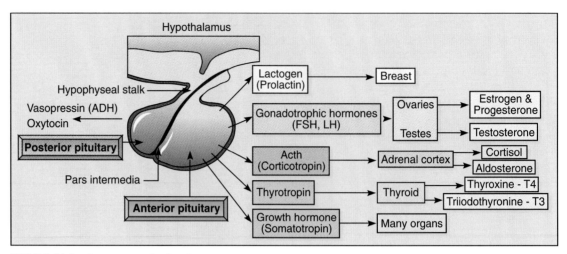

FIGURE 11-2. The pituitary gland and its secretions.

Growth Hormone

Growth hormone (GH or *somatotropin*) has widespread physiologic activity because it promotes cell division and cellular proliferation throughout the body. GH facilitates protein synthesis by increasing amino acid transport through cell membranes, stimulating RNA formation, or activating cellular ribosomes that increase protein synthesis. The release of GH also results in decreased carbohydrate utilization with a subsequent increased use of lipids for energy.

GH secretion during rest is influenced by a GH-releasing factor that acts directly on the anterior pituitary gland. In fact, each of the primary pituitary hormones has its own hypothalamic releasing hormone, sometimes called a *releasing factor*. These releasing hormones are controlled by neural input to the hypothalamus by factors such as anxiety, stress, and exercise.

GH, Exercise, and Tissue Synthesis. Studies of exercise-induced production of GH have revealed an increased secretion a few minutes after exercise begins. With increasing exercise intensity, there is a sharp rise in GH production and total secretion. In fact, GH secretion is more related to the peak intensity of exercise than to duration or total work output. The exact stimulus for increased GH production with exercise has not been identified. Most probably, neural factors provide for primary control.

The mechanism by which GH and exercise interact to bring about increases in protein synthesis (and subsequent muscle hypertrophy), cartilage formation, skeletal growth, and cell proliferation is not entirely clear. One hypothesis suggests that exercise directly stimulates GH production that in turn stimulates anabolic processes. It has been shown that exercise is directly associated with the doubling of both GH pulse frequency and amplitude. Furthermore, exercise stimulates the production of endogenous opiates that facilitate GH release by inhibiting the liver's production of *somatostatin,* a hormone that blunts the release of GH.

Figure 11-3 shows a proposed plan for classifying the overall metabolic actions of GH. In terms of exercise modulation, GH stimulates lipid release from adipose tissue while inhibiting glucose uptake by the cells, thus maintaining blood sugar at fairly high levels. This sparing of glucose would certainly contribute to one's ability to perform endurance exercise.

Thyrotropin

Thyrotropin, sometimes called *thyroid-stimulating hormone* (TSH), controls the amount of hormone secreted by the thyroid gland. This hormone acts to maintain growth and develop-

ions that
reabsorbe
with inc
little sodi
contrast.
into the u
terone se
exchange
gen ion f
ion, aldc
the main
and pH.
for nerv
function
would be
ulation o

An in
tion proc
extracell
sorbed fr
es blood
by a con
output ar

Durin
the symp
stricts bl
This red
stimulate
hormone
Increase
duction
mone, ai
adrenal c
Aldoster
sively du
ma aldos
as six tir
rest, the
stimulate
sure in t
kidneys,
tion.

Glucoco
hydroco
corticoid
tex. The
cortisol r
metaboli
  • Stin
    ami
    boc
    "lib
    to t

is t
in
wh
lisr
tha
thy
ing
Co
me
prc
dec
ite
Fig

"fre
inc
the
cise
era
imr
atic

AD

cap
eac
two
the
cor
sec
and
erec

Adr

syn
to p
effe
epir
tive
mec
forr
dire
The
bloc
ly tl
by t

C
adre
cise
incr

ment of the thyroid gland as well as to increase activity of the thyroid cells. In light of the important role of thyroid hormone in regulating cellular metabolism, it is not surprising that TSH output from the pituitary increases during exercise, although this effect may not be consistent.

Corticotropin

Corticotropin, or *adrenocorticotropic hormone* (ACTH), regulates the output of the hormones secreted by the adrenal cortex in a manner similar to the way TSH controls thyroid hormone secretion. ACTH acts to directly enhance lipid mobilization from adipose tissue, increase the rate of gluconeogenesis, and stimulate protein catabolism. Evidence suggests that

ACTH concentrations increase with exercise duration if intensity is higher than 25% of aerobic capacity.

Prolactin

The hormone prolactin (PRL) initiates and supports milk secretion from mammary glands. PRL levels increase with higher intensities of exercise and return toward baseline within 45 minutes of recovery. Owing to its important role in female sexual function, it is possible that repeated exercise-induced PRL release may inhibit the ovaries and contribute to the alterations in menstrual cycle often observed among athletic women. Evidence also shows that PRL increases in males following acute maximal exercise.

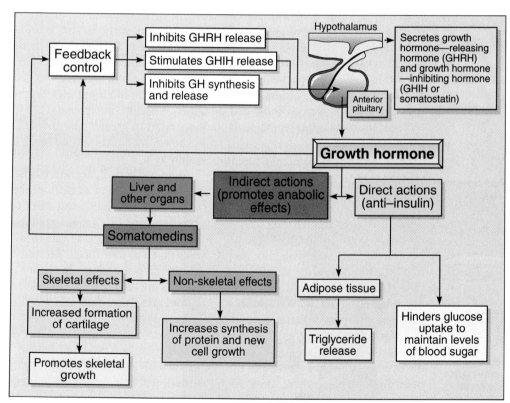

FIGURE 11-3. Overview plan for classifying the actions of growth hormone (GH). GH stimulates the breakdown and release of triglycerides from adipose tissue and hinders glucose uptake by the cells to maintain relatively high levels of blood sugar. GH exerts an anti-insulin effect because its action is opposite to insulin. The indirect anabolic effects of GH are mediated through somatomedins. Elevated levels of GH and somatomedins feed back to promote growth-hormone-inhibiting hormone release and depress the release of growth-hormone-releasing hormone by the hypothalamus; this further inhibits GH release by the anterior pituitary.

tion." It also appears that the opiates produced in the body during exercise are degraded more slowly in the blood of trained individuals compared with the untrained. Certainly, this slower rate of disposal would facilitate a given opiate response and might augment one's tolerance for extended exercise.

SUMMARY

1. The endocrine system consists of a host organ, a hormone, and a target or receptor organ. Hormones are either steroids or amino acid (polypeptide) derivatives.

2. The major function of hormones is to alter the rates of cellular reactions. Hormones act at specific receptor sites by either enhancing or inhibiting enzyme function.

3. Hormone concentration in the blood is determined by the amount of hormone synthesized, the amount released, the amount taken up by the target organ, and the rate of hormone removal from the blood.

4. The anterior pituitary is responsible for the secretion of at least six hormones: PRL, the gonadotropic hormones FSH and LH, corticotropin, thyrotropin, and GH.

5. GH promotes cell division and cellular proliferation; thyrotropin controls the amount of hormone secreted by the thyroid gland; ACTH regulates the output of the hormones secreted by the adrenal cortex; PRL is important in reproduction and in the development of secondary sex characteristics of females; and FSH and LH stimulate the ovaries to secrete estrogen in women and sperm in men.

6. The posterior pituitary secretes antidiuretic hormone that controls water excretion by the kidneys. It also secretes oxytocin, which is an important hormone in birthing and milk secretion.

7. Thyroxine increases the metabolic rate of all cells and increases the breakdown of carbohydrate and lipid in energy metabolism.

8. The inner (medulla) and the outer (cortex) portions of the adrenal gland secrete two different types of hormones. The medulla secretes the catecholamines, epinephrine and norepinephrine. The adrenal cortex secretes mineralocorticoids, which regulate extracellular sodium and potassium, glucocorticoids, which stimulate gluconeogenesis and serve as an insulin antagonist, and androgens, which control male secondary sex characteristics.

9. The main function of insulin, secreted from the pancreas, is to increase the rate of glucose transport into cells and thereby control the body's rate of carbohydrate metabolism. Diminished insulin production results in the condition of diabetes. The pancreas also secretes glucagon, an insulin antagonist that acts to raise the level of blood sugar.

10. Exercise training has differential effects on resting and exercise-induced hormone production and release. Trained persons exhibit elevated hormone response during exercise for ACTH and cortisol, depressed values for GH, PRL, FSH, LH, testosterone, ADH, T_4, and insulin, and no training response for aldosterone, renin, and angiotensin.

11. Exercise-induced elevation of beta-endorphins has been associated with euphoria, increased pain tolerance, the "exercise high," and altered menstrual function.

Borer, K.T.: Exercise-induced facilitation of pulsatile growth hormone (GH) secretion and somatic growth. In *Hormones and Sport*. Vol. 55. Edited by Z. Laron and A. D. Rogol. Serono Symposia Publications. New York, Raven Press, 1989.

Carrol, J.F., et al.: Effect of training on blood volume and plasma hormone concentrations in the elderly. *Med. Sci. Sports Exerc.*, 27: 79, 1995.

Craig, B.W., and Kang, H-O.: Growth hormone release following single versus multiple sets of back squats: total work versus power. *J. Strength Cond. Res.*, 8(4):270, 1994.

Criswell, D., et al.: Fluid replacement beverages and maintenance of plasma volume during exercise: Role of aldosterone and vasopressin. *Eur. J. Appl. Physiol.*, 65:445, 1992.

Deschenes, M., et al.: Exercise-induced hormonal changes and their effects upon skeletal muscle tissue. *Sports Med.*, 12:80, 1991.

DeSousa, M.J., et al.: Menstrual status and plasma vasopressin, renin activity, aldosterone, and exercise response. *J. Appl. Physiol.*, 67:736, 1989.

Deyssig, R., et al.: Effect of growth hormone treatment on hormonal parameters, body composition and strength in athletes. *Acta Endocrinol*, 128: 313, 1993.

Dolkas, C.B., et al.: Effect of body weight gain on insulin sensitivity after retirement from exercise training. *J. Appl. Physiol.*, 68:520, 1990.

Farrell, P.A.: Decreased insulin response to sustained hyperglycemia in exercise trained rats. *Med. Sci. Sports Exerc.*, 22:469, 1988.

Farrell, P.A., et al.: Enkephalins, catecholamines, and psychological mood alterations: effects of prolonged exercise. *Med. Sci. Sports Exerc.*, 19:347, 1987.

Fogelholm, G.M., et al.: Low-dose amino acid supplementation: no effects on serum human growth hormone and insulin in male weight lifters. *Int. J. Sports Nutr.*, 3: 290, 1993.

Francesconi, R.P.: Endocrinological responses to exercise in stressful environments. In *Exercise and Sport Sciences Reviews*. Vol. 16. Edited by K.B. Pandolf. New York, Macmillan, 1988.

Fry, A., et al.: Endocrine and performance responses to high volume training and amino acid supplementation in elite junior weightlifters. *Int. J. Sports Nutr.*, 3: 306, 1993.

Galbo, H.: *Hormonal and Metabolic Adaptation to Exercise*. New York, G. T. Verlag, 1983.

Gerra, G., et al.: ACTH and beta-endorphic responses to physical exercise in adolescent women tested for anxiety and frustration. *Psychiatry Res.*, 41:179, 1992.

Helmrich, S.P. et al.: Prevention of non-insulin-dependent diabetes mellitus with physical activity. *Med. Sci. Sports Exerc.*, 26: 824, 1994.

Houmard, J.A., et al.: Testosterone, cortisol, and creatine kinase levels in male distance runners during reduced training. *Int. J. Sports Med.*, 11:41, 1990.

Kjaer, M.: Regulation of hormonal and metabolic responses during exercise in humans. In *Exercise and Sport Sciences Reviews*. Vol. 20. Edited by J.O. Holloszy. Baltimore, Williams & Wilkins, 1992.

Kraemer, W.J., et al.: Changes in hormonal concentrations after different heavy-resistance exercise protocols in women. *J. Appl. Physiol.*, 75: 594, 1993.

Kraemer, W.J., et al.: Effects of different heavy-resistance exercise protocols on plasma β-endorphin concentrations. *J. Appl. Physiol.*, 74, 450, 1993.

Kraemer, W.J., et al.: Influence of the endocrine system on resistance training adaptations. *National Strength Cond. Assoc. J.*, 14:47, 1992.

Kraemer, W.J.: Endocrine responses and adaptations to strength training. In *Encyclopedia of Sports Medicine: Strength and Power*. Edited by P.V. Komi. London, Blackwell Scientific, 1992.

Kraemer, W.J., et al.: Endogenous anabolic hormonal and growth factor responses to heavy resistance exercise in males and females. *Int. J. Sports Med.*, 12:228, 1991.

Kriska, A.M., et al.: The potential role of physical activity in the prevention of non-insulin-dependent diabetes mellitus: the epidemiological evidence. *Exerc. Sport Sci. Rev.* 22: 121, 1994.

Loucks, A.B., and Callister, R.: Induction and prevention of low-T_3 syndrome in exercising women. *Am. J. Physiol.*, 264: R924, 1993.

MacKinnon, L.T.: Current challenges and future expectations in exercise immunology: back to the future. *Med. Sci. Sports Exerc.*, 26: 191, 1994.

MacNeil, B., and Hoffman-Goetz, L.: Chronic exercise enhances in vivo and in vitro cytotoxic mechanisms of natural immunity in mice. *J. Appl. Physiol.*, 74: 388, 1993.

Morgan, W.P.: Affective beneficence of vigorous physical activity. *Med. Sci. Sports Exerc.*, 17:94, 1985.

Nieman, D.C., et al.: Physical activity and immune function in elderly women. *Med. Sci. Sports Exerc.*, 25: 823, 1993.

Nieman, D.C.: Exercise, upper respiratory tract infection, and the immune system. *Med. Sci. Sports Exerc.*, 26: 128, 1994.

Nieman, D.C.: Physical activity, fitness, and infection. In *Physical Activity, Fitness, and Health*. Edited by Bouchard, C., et al., Champaign, IL, Human Kinetics, 1994.

Peters, E.M., et al.: Vitamin C supplementation reduces the incidence of post-race symptoms of upper-respiratory-tract infection in ultramarathon runners. *Am. J. Clin. Nutr.*, 57: 170, 1993.

Pratley, R., et al.: Strength training increases resting metabolic rate and norepinephrine levels in healthy 50- to 65-yr-old men. *J. Appl. Physiol.*, 73: 133, 1994.

Richter, E.A., and Sutton, J.R.: Hormonal adaptation to physical activity. In *Physical Activity, Fitness, and Health*. Edited by Bouchard, C., et al., Champaign, IL, Human Kinetics, 1994.

Rocchini, A. P., et al.: The effects of weight loss on the sensitivity of blood pressure to sodium in obese adolescents. *N. Engl. J. Med.*, 321:580, 1989.

Saltin, B.: Physiological effects of physical conditioning. *Med. Sci. Sports Exerc.*, 1:50, 1969.

Schneider, S.H., et al.: Exercise and

NIDDM. Technical Report. *Diabetes Care,* 15(Suppl. 2):50, 1992.

Sutton, J.R., and Farrell, P.: Endocrine responses to prolonged exercise. *In Exercise Science and Sports Medicine.* Vol. 1. Edited by D.R. Lamb, and R. Murray. Indianapolis, Benchmark Press, 1988.

Tarnopolsky, L., et al.: Gender differences in hormonal and metabolic responses to prolonged exercise in males and females. *J. Appl. Physiol.,* 68:650, 1990.

Vitug, A., et al.: Exercise and Type I diabetes mellitus. In *Exercise and Sport Sciences Reviews.* Vol. 16. Edited by K.B. Pandolf. New York, Macmillan, 1988.

Wallberg-Henriksson, H.: Exercise and diabetes mellitus. In *Exercise and Sport Sciences Reviews.* Vol. 20. Edited by J.O. Holloszy. Baltimore, Williams & Wilkins, 1992.

Wasserman, D.H., et al.: Interaction of exercise and insulin action in humans. 260:E37, 1991.

EXERCISE TRAINING AND ADAPTATIONS IN FUNCTIONAL CAPACITY

Exercise training for sports is often more art than science. The success of different conditioning programs is usually evaluated by individual achievements or won-loss records rather than by scientific inquiry and discovery. Many coaches in sports such as basketball and soccer often place considerable importance on the development of cardiovascular or aerobic capacity, yet devote little time to various phases of vigorous anaerobic conditioning. While such sports do require a relatively steady release of aerobic energy, there are crucial situations that demand all-out effort. If the relative capacity of the athlete's anaerobic energy transfer system is poor, the player may be unable to perform at full potential. Training the anaerobic capacity of endurance athletes, on the other hand, would be wasteful because the contribution of anaerobic energy transfer to successful performance is minimal. Rather, these activities demand a well-conditioned heart and vascular system capable of circulating large quantities of blood as well as a high capacity of muscle cells to generate ATP aerobically. At the other extreme, one's capacity for aerobic metabolism contributes little to overall success in sprint activities and sports such as football. Here, performance largely depends on muscular strength and power where energy is generated primarily from reactions that do not use oxygen.

With a clear understanding of energy transfer and the effects of specific training on the systems of energy delivery and utilization, it is possible to construct a sound training program to achieve optimum performance. The focus of Chapters 12 and 13 is the basis of training for aerobic and anaerobic power and muscular strength, the physiologic consequences of such training, and the important factors that affect training success.

Training the Anaerobic and Aerobic Energy Systems

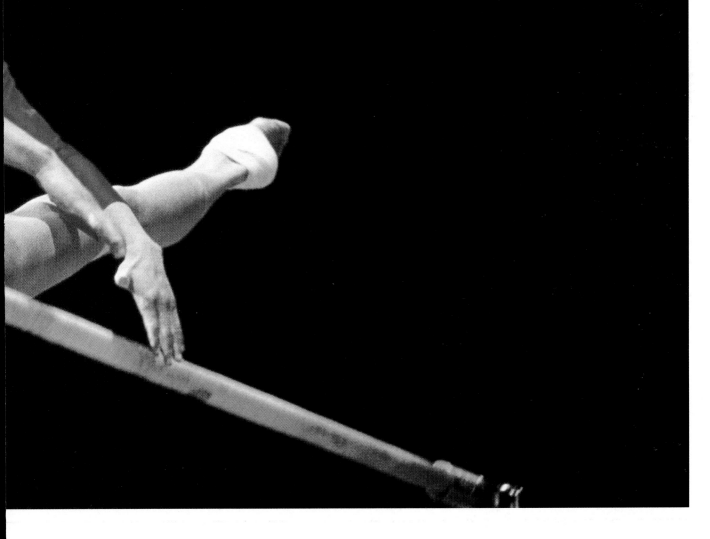

After reading this chapter, you should be able to:

- Discuss the following principles as they apply to exercise training: (1) Overload, (2) Specificity, (3) Individual Differences, and (4) Reversibility.

- Explain how the overload principle is applied in training the (1) high-energy phosphates, and (2) the glycolytic system. What specific adaptations take place in each system as a result of such training?

- Graph the heart rate response during and in recovery from a 3-minute step test for an aerobically trained and sedentary student.

- Administer the Queens College Step Test and the Tecumseh Step Test to a young adult.

- Describe how the following factors affect the results of an aerobic training program: (1) initial fitness level, (2) genetics, (3) training frequency, (4) training duration, and (5) training intensity.

- Indicate how to use exercise heart rate to establish the appropriate exercise intensity for an aerobic training program.

- Discuss what is meant by the "training sensitive zone".

- Explain why you should adjust the "training sensitive zone" for swimming and other forms of upper body exercise compared to bicycling and running.

- Discuss the influence of age on maximum heart rate and the "training sensitive zone".

- Contrast continuous versus intermittent aerobic exercise training.

- Discuss potential benefits and risks of exercising during pregnancy.

Many forms of physical activity require a rapid generation of energy. Because energy release is required almost instantaneously, sufficient oxygen cannot be delivered to the muscles quickly enough to match energy requirements. Even if oxygen was immediately available, sufficient aerobic energy could not be provided fast enough to be of much use. Consequently anaerobic energy capacity determines success in plowing through the line in football, spiking in volleyball, or running out an infield hit in softball. The apparent steady-rate sports, such as basketball, tennis, field hockey, lacrosse, and soccer also involve sprinting, dashing, darting, and stop-and-go, where the capacity to generate short bursts of anaerobic power plays an important role. At the other extreme, success in the true endurance activities necessitates a highly trained aerobic energy system that depends upon a well-conditioned heart and vascular system capable of delivering a large quantity of oxygen to the active tissues for an extended time.

· · · · · · · · · · · · · · ·

ENERGY FOR EXERCISE: IT'S THE BLEND THAT'S IMPORTANT

Figure 12-1 summarizes the relative involvement of the systems of anaerobic and aerobic energy transfer during "all-out" exercise of varying durations. Keep in mind that the three energy systems — the adenosine triphosphate-creatine phosphate (ATP-CP) system, the lactic acid system, and the aerobic system — are often operating simultaneously during physical activity. However, their *relative contribution* to the total energy requirement can differ markedly depending on the duration and intensity of the activity.

With an immediate, maximum burst of effort as in the tennis serve, golf swing, front flip in gymnastics, and even the 60- or 100-yard dash, energy is provided anaerobically almost exclusively by the stored high-energy phosphates ATP and CP. In a performance that lasts between 10 and 90 seconds, as in a 100-yard swim or 220-yard run, energy is still supplied predominantly by anaerobic reactions. In these cases, however, the primary role is played by energy from the initial glycolytic phase of carbohydrate breakdown with subsequent lactic acid formation. Training for such activities must be of sufficient intensity and duration to overload this specific anaerobic energy system. In wrestling, boxing, ice hockey, a 400- or 1500 meter run, or a full court press in basketball, the magnitude of energy generated from anaerobic sources depends on the person's capacity and tolerance for lactic acid accumulation. In these activities, aerobic energy metabolism also plays an important role. As exercise intensity diminishes somewhat and the duration extends between 2 and 4 minutes, dependence on energy from the anaerobic pathways decreases, while energy release from oxygen-consum-

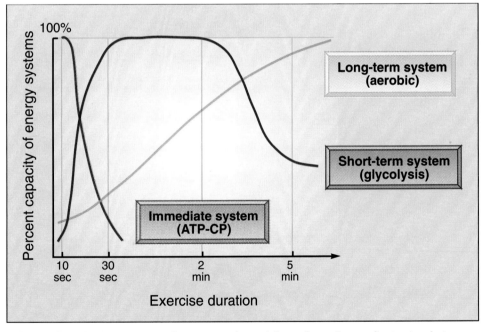

FIGURE 12-1. The three systems of energy transfer, and their relative degree of activation during all-out exercise of different durations.

ing reactions predominates. With exercise that continues beyond 4 minutes, the activity becomes progressively more dependent on aerobic energy; in a marathon run or long-distance swim, the body is powered almost exclusively by the energy from aerobic reactions.

In training for a particular sport or performance goal, the activity must be carefully evaluated in terms of its energy components. Based on such an analysis, an appropriate amount of time and "energy" can then be devoted to the specific training of each energy system.

PRINCIPLES OF TRAINING

The major objective in exercise training is to cause biologic adaptations to improve performance in specific tasks. This requires adherence to carefully planned and executed activities. Attention is focused on factors such as frequency and length of workouts, type of training, speed, intensity, duration, and repetition of the activity, and appropriate competition. Although these factors vary depending on the performance goal, it is possible to identify several principles of physiologic conditioning common to the performance classifications shown in Figure 12-2.

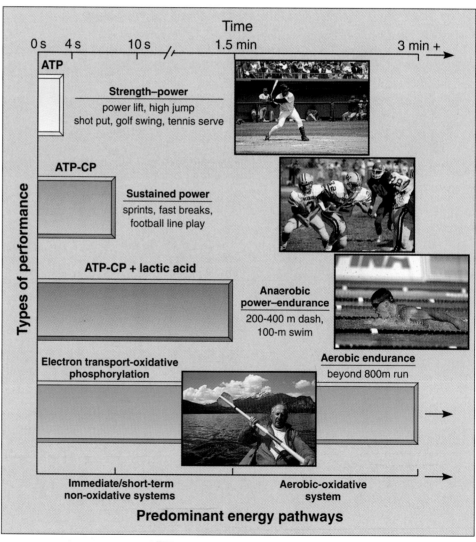

FIGURE 12-2. Classification of physical activity based on the duration of all-out exercise and the corresponding, predominant intracellular energy pathways.

TABLE 12-1. Effects of 10 weeks of interval swim training on changes in max $\dot{V}O_2$ and endurance performance as measured during running and swimming*

Subjects	Measure	Running Test			Swimming Test		
		Pre-Training	Post-Training	% Change	Pre-Training	Post-Training	% Change
Swim Training							
Max $\dot{V}O_2$							
	$L\cdot min^{-1}$	4.05	4.11	+1.5	3.44	3.82	+11.0
	$ml\cdot kg^{-1}\cdot min^{-1}$	54.9	55.7	+1.5	46.6	51.8	+11.0
Max work time, min		19.6	20.5	+4.6	11.9	15.9	+34.0
Nontraining Controls							
Max $\dot{V}O_2$							
	$L\cdot min^{-1}$	4.12	4.18	+1.5	3.51	3.40	3.1
	$ml\cdot kg^{-1}\cdot min^{-1}$	55.1	55.5	+0.7	46.8	45.0	–3.8
Max work time, min		20.7	19.7	–4.8	11.5	11.5	0

*From Magel, J. R., et al.: Specificity of swim training on maximum oxygen uptake. *J. Appl. Physiol.,* 38:151, 1975.

Overload Principle

A specific exercise *overload* must be applied to enhance physiologic improvement effectively and to bring about a training change. By exercising at a level above normal, a variety of adaptations take place that enable the body to function more efficiently. The appropriate overload for each person can be achieved by manipulating combinations of training *frequency, intensity, mode, and duration.* This concept of individualized and progressive overload applies to the athlete, the sedentary person, the disabled, and even the cardiac patient.

Specificity Principle

A common inquiry concerning exercise participation deals with whether swimming, cycling, or running is the most effective in developing aerobic capacity. The proper answer concerning specificity of training is that each is equally effective because all three are "big muscle" activities that can provide sufficient cardiovascular overload. In fact, champion athletes in the distance events in each activity are noted for their high level of aerobic fitness in their particular activity.

When applied to training, specificity refers to adaptations in the metabolic and physiologic systems depending on the type of overload imposed. It is known that a specific exercise stress such as strength-power training induces specific strength-power adaptations, and that specific aerobic or cardiovascular exercise elicits specific endurance-training adaptations with essentially little interchange between strength and aerobic training. The specificity principle, however, is really more encompassing because development of aerobic fitness for swimming, bicycling, running or arm exercise is most effectively achieved when the exerciser trains the specific muscles involved in the desired performance. *In essence, specific exercise elicits specific adaptations creating specific training effects.* This is often referred to as the SAID principle (Specific Adaptations to Imposed Demands).

The fundamental training principle. The concept of individualized and progressive overload applies to the athlete, the sedentary person, the disabled, and even the cardiac patient.

World's fittest man — specificity in action. Steve Sokol, a specialist in fitness training and education from San Jose, California, holds the following world records for a variety of fitness activities:

- 52,003 situps in 32 hours, 17 minutes
- 3,336 situps in 1 hour
- 13,013 leg lifts in 5 hours, 45 minutes
- 3,522 leg lifts in 1 hour
- 30,000 jumping jacks in 7 hours, 30 minutes
- 4,412 jumping jacks in 1 hour
- 3,333 squat thrusts in 4 hours
- Rode 500 miles from San Francisco to Los Angeles in 43 hours without sitting down on the seat of the bicycle!

Aerobic Power. In an experiment in one of our laboratories to study the specificity of training (Table 12-1), 15 men trained 1 hour a day, 3 days a week, for 10 weeks.

Training heart rates averaged between 85 and 95% of each subject's maximum. All subjects were measured during treadmill running, an exercise involving predominantly the leg muscles, and swimming that mainly uses the muscles of the arms and upper body. The results showed there was essentially complete specificity for improvements in aerobic capacity with swim training. Although improvements in max $\dot{V}O_2$ averaged 11% when the subjects were measured while swimming, they showed no change while running on the treadmill. This was surprising, because the expectation was at least a minimal improvement on the running test from the intense nature of the "general" cardiovascular overload during swim training. Apparently, there was no "transfer" in the improved aerobic capacity from swim training to running.

Based on available research, it is reasonable to advise that in training for specific aerobic activities such as cycling, swimming, rowing, or running, the overload must engage the appropriate muscles required by the activity, as well as provide an exercise stress for the central cardiovascular system. Little improvement is noted when aerobic capacity is measured by a dissimilar exercise, yet improvements are significant when the test exercise is the same exercise used in training. Thus, one can appreciate how difficult it is to be in "good shape" for diverse forms of aerobic exercise such as performed by a triathlete.

Local Adaptations. In endurance training, the overload of specific muscle groups improves exercise performance and aerobic power by enhancing both oxygen transport and utilization in the trained muscles. The oxidative capacity of the vastus lateralis muscle, for example, is greater in well-trained cyclists than in endurance runners and is improved significantly following training on a bicycle ergometer. Such adaptations would certainly increase the capacity of the trained muscles to generate ATP aerobically. The specificity of aerobic improvement also may result from greater regional blood flow in trained tissues, owing to increased microcirculation or to more effective distribution of cardiac output, or both. Regardless of the mechanism involved, these training adaptations will usually occur *only* in the specifically trained muscles and would *only* be seen when these muscles were activated.

Individual Differences Principle

Many factors contribute to individual variation in training response. The person's relative fitness level at the start of training is important. It is unrealistic to expect different people to be in the same "state" of training at the same time. Consequently, it is counter-productive to insist that all performers on a team (or even the same event) train the same way or at the same relative or absolute exercise rate. It is also unrealistic to expect all individuals to respond to a given training dosage in precisely the same manner. Benefits are optimized when training programs are planned to meet individual needs and capacities. Coaches and trainers must recognize how each of their athletes or trainees responds to a given exercise stimulus and adjust the exercise prescription in relation to that response.

Reversibility Principle

Detraining occurs rapidly when a person stops exercising. After only a week or two of detraining, significant reductions in both physiologic and exercise capacity can be measured, and many of the training improvements are lost within several months.

TABLE 12-2. Changes in physiologic and metabolic values resulting from various durations of detraining
*Number in parentheses refers to study in footnote.

Study*	N	Gender	Duration (Days)	Variable	Pre-Detraining Average	Post-Detraining Average	Percent Change
(1)	5	M	20 (bedrest)	Max $\dot{V}O_2$, L·min^{-1}	3.3	2.4	−27
				Stroke volume, ml·beat^{-1}	116	88	−24
				Cardiac output, L·min^{-1}	20.0	14.8	−26
(2)	7	F	84	Max $\dot{V}O_2$, ml·kg^{-1}·min^{-1}	47.8	40.4	−15.5
				V_E max, L·min^{-1}	77.5	69.5	−10.3
				O_2 pulse, ml·beat^{-1}	12.7	10.9	−14.2
(3)	17	M	70	Sum of 3-min recovery heart rate	190	237	−24.7
(4)	9	M	35	CP, mmols·g wet wt^{-1}	17.9	13.0	−27.4
				ATP, mmols·g wet wt^{-1}	5.97	5.08	−14.9
				Glycogen, mmols·g wet wt^{-1}	113.9	57.4	−49.6
				Elbow extension strength, ft-lb	39.0	25.5	−34.6
(5)	6	M	56	Max $\dot{V}O_2$, L·min^{-1}	4.22	3.67	−14
	1	F		Max $\dot{V}O_2$, ml·kg^{-1}·min^{-1}	62.1	53.2	−14
				HR max, b·min^{-1}	187	199	+6
				Stroke volume, ml·beat^{-1}	148	127	−14
				Cardiac output, L·min^{-1}	27.8	25.2	−9
				Max a-$\bar{v}O_2$ diff, ml·100 ml^{-1}	15.1	14.5	−19
				Citrate synthase, mol·kg protein^{-1}·h^{-1}	10.0	6.0	−40.6
				SDH, mol·kg protein^{-1}·h^{-1}	4.43	2.73	−38.4

[1] Saltin, B., et al.: Response to exercise after bed rest and after training. *Circulation,* 38(Suppl. 7), 1968.
[2] Drinkwater, B., and Horvath, S.: Detraining effects on young women. *Med. Sci. Sports,* 4:91, 1972.
[3] Michael, E., et al.: Physiological changes of teenage girls during five months of detraining. *Med. Sci. Sports,* 4:214, 1972.
[4] MacDougall, J.D., et al.: Biochemical adaptation of human skeletal muscle to heavy resistance training and immobilization. *J. Appl. Physiol.,* 43:70, 1977.
[5] Coyle, E.F., et al.: Time course of loss of adaptations after stopping prolonged intense endurance training. *J. Appl. Physiol.,* 57:1857, 1984.

Table 12-2 lists the physiologic and metabolic consequences of various durations of detraining as evaluated in several studies.

In one experiment the max $\dot{V}O_2$ decreased 25% in five subjects confined to bed for 20 consecutive days; this was accompanied by a similar decrement in maximal stroke volume and cardiac output. These findings showed that an approximately 1% decrease occurred in aerobic capacity each day. Additionally, the number of capillaries within trained muscle decreased between 14 and 25% within only 3 weeks of detraining.

The important point is that even among highly trained athletes *the beneficial effects of exercise training are transient and reversible.* For this reason, most athletes begin a reconditioning program several months before the start of the competitive season, or maintain some moderate level of sport-specific exercise to slow down the rate of deconditioning. Many ex-athletes are in poorer physiologic condition several years after they retire from active participation than the business executive who exercises on a regular basis.

ANAEROBIC CONDITIONING

The capacity to perform all-out exercise of up to 90 seconds duration depends mainly on anaerobic energy metabolism.

Prolonged recovery. Recovery time can be considerable with exercises that produce large amounts of lactic acid. For this reason, intervals of anaerobic training should occur at the end of the workout. Otherwise, fatigue from this high intensity training would carry over and perhaps hinder the ability to perform subsequent aerobic training.

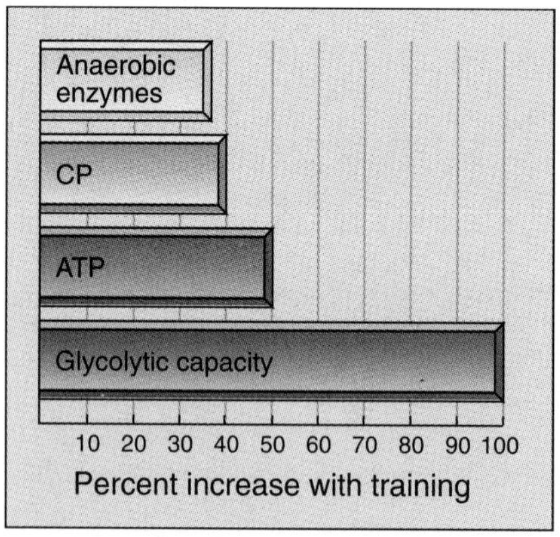

FIGURE 12-3. Potential for increases in the anaerobic energy metabolism of skeletal muscle with heavy physical training.

The overload principle must be applied to improve this energy-generating capacity.

The Anaerobic Energy System

Recall that energy is generated anaerobically from the breakdown of the high-energy phosphates ATP and CP and in the reactions of glycolysis, in which glucose is transformed into lactic acid.

High Energy Phosphates. During the first 6 seconds of all-out exercise, energy is made available almost immediately from the anaerobic breakdown of the energy currency ATP and the energy reservoir CP. *Maximum overload of this phosphate pool in specific muscles can be achieved with all-out bursts of effort for 5 to 10 seconds.* During swim training, a sprinter might swim intervals of 20 to 25 yards to overload the arms and upper body, whereas the sprint runner could similarly overload the phosphate pool of the leg muscles by running 60- to 100-yard sprints. A football lineman may sprint for only 2 to 3 seconds on any one play. To increase the intensity of overload during this relatively short but intense exercise period, the player could practice running with a weighted belt or vest, or sprint up hills or stairs. Because high-energy phosphates supply the energy for such brief, intermittent exercise, only a small amount of lactic acid is produced and recovery is rapid. Thus, a subsequent exercise bout can begin after only a 30- to 60-second recovery.

As a general rule, in training to enhance a muscle's ATP-CP energy capacity, the individual should undertake repetitive bouts of intense, short duration exercise. *The training activities selected must engage the muscles in the movement patterns for which the person desires improved anaerobic power.* This enhances the metabolic capacity of the specifically trained muscle fibers and facilitates neuromuscular adaptations to the specific rate and pattern of movement.

Glycolytic Capacity. As the duration of all-out effort extends beyond 10 seconds, the contribution of total energy from the phosphates decreases, while the quantity of anaerobic energy generated from the formation of lactic acid increases. To improve capacity for energy release by the lactic acid system, training must overload this specific form of energy metabolism.

Anaerobic training of the lactic acid system is physiologically and psychologically taxing and requires considerable motivation. Bouts of up to 1 minute of intense running, swimming, or cycling, stopped 30 to 40 seconds before exhaustion, cause large increases in lactic acid. To ensure that maximum levels of lactic acid are produced during each training session, the exercise bout should be repeated several times, interspersed with 3 to 5 minutes' recovery. Each successive exercise interval causes a "lactate stacking" that results in higher levels of lactic acid than would occur with just one bout of all-out effort to the point of voluntary exhaustion. Of course, it is critical to engage the specific muscle groups that require enhanced anaerobic capacity.

Adaptations in the Anaerobic System

Figure 12-3 summarizes the metabolic adaptations in anaerobic function that accompany strenuous anaerobic physical training. In keeping with the concept of specificity of training, activities that demand a high level of anaerobic metabolism bring about specific changes in the immediate and short-term energy systems, without a concomitant increase in aerobic functions. Specifically the metabolic changes that occur with sprint and power-type training include:

- Increases in resting levels of anaerobic substrates (ATP, CP, and glycogen)

- Increases in the quantity and activity of key enzymes (especially in fast-twitch muscle fibers) that control the anaerobic phase of glucose breakdown
- Increases in the capacity to generate high levels of blood lactate during all-out exercise. This is probably due to enhanced levels of glycogen and glycolytic enzymes as well as to an improved motivation and "pain" tolerance for fatiguing exercise

AEROBIC TRAINING

The current interest in exercise training results largely from the desire of many people to improve their ability to sustain physical activity without undue fatigue. Often this desire is directed toward sports participation, although a variety of recreational, leisure, household, and occupational activities require a continuous, fairly high level of aerobic energy expenditure. In the following discussion, we present a relatively simple method to evaluate one's present status for aerobic exercise. We also outline the principles that govern effective overload of the aerobic energy system.

The Aerobic Energy System

Under conditions of aerobic metabolism, pyruvic acid from carbohydrate metabolism as well as the carbon compounds from lipid and protein breakdown enter the Krebs cycle for oxidation and ATP resynthesis. If the supply and utilization of oxygen are adequate to meet energy requirements, exercise continues in a steady rate and feelings of fatigue are minimal. If aerobic metabolism is inadequate, anaerobic energy transfer increases and fatigue sets in. *The intensity at which exercise can be sustained beyond several minutes depends on the body's capability for aerobic metabolism.* This, in turn, depends

on the functional capacity of the support systems for oxygen transport—the lungs, heart, and vascular system—as well as the muscles' ability to process oxygen as it is delivered.

Heart Rate Response: A Useful Method to Evaluate Cardiovascular Fitness. A low heart rate due to a large stroke volume during submaximal exercise generally reflects a high level of cardiovascular fitness (see Chapter 9). If a large quantity of blood is pumped with each heartbeat, only a small increase in heart rate is required to deliver blood with its complement of oxygen to the exercising muscles. *A step test provides a convenient means to use heart rate to evaluate the efficiency of the cardiovascular response to aerobic exercise.*

Suppose three people perform 3 minutes of step-up exercise on a bench to the cadence of a metronome. Figure 12-4 illustrates the heart rate response of each person during the 3 minutes of stepping. Heart rate increases rapidly during the first minute and then starts to level off. Subject A, a varsity lacrosse player, attains a heart rate of 120 beats per

Step training — the new kid on the bench. Choreographed bench stepping exercise or "stairaerobics" has become the current craze in the fitness marketplace. Nearly a dozen step benches have been designed and a variety of videos are on the market or in preparation. This form of training involves stepping to music on and off a bench platform between 4 and 12 inches high using a variety of foot, arm, and leg movements. Intensity of effort is generally regulated by bench height and body movements, although speeding up the beat of the music can also contribute to the cardiovascular demands of this low-impact exercise.

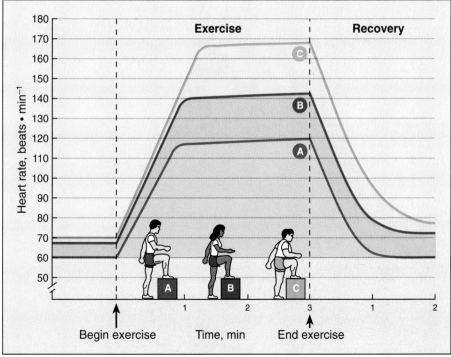

FIGURE 12-4. Heart rate response during stepping exercise and in recovery for three students with different levels of cardiovascular fitness.

minute at the end of 3 minutes, while the heart rate of subject B, a kinesiology major, is 142 beats per minute. For subject C, a sedentary college student, the heart rate response to this exercise is 170 beats per minute. Clearly, the cardiovascular stress of bench stepping for student C is considerably greater than for the other two students, especially student A, whose heart rate increase is minimal. It is reasonable to conclude that cardiovascular capacity is greatest for the athlete, less for the kinesiology major, and relatively poor for the sedentary student. Figure 12-4 also illustrates the pattern of heart rate recovery for the three students in the 2 minutes immediately following bench stepping. Notice that on completion of exercise, heart rate decreases rapidly during the first 30 seconds; it then continues to decline but at a much slower rate. After 2 minutes, the heart rate has essentially returned to resting values. The most noticeable differences between students A, B, and C are observed in the period immediately following exercise. Thus, if recovery heart rate is measured as soon as exercise stops, it is still possible to discriminate between subjects in terms of their heart rate response to the stress of exercise.

The Queens College Step Test. Heart rate response to the Queens College Step Test has been measured in thousands of male and female students to evaluate their cardiovascular response to exercise. To measure large numbers at the same time, stepping was done using the bottom step of the gymnasium bleachers which was 41.3 cm (16 1/4 inches) high. For women, the stepping cadence was set by a metronome at 88 beats per minute (22 complete step-ups per minute); for men, it was set at 96 beats (24 step-ups per minute). One complete stepping cycle on the bench represented 4 beats on the metronome, "up-up, down-down." After a demonstration, students were given 15 seconds of practice stepping to adjust to the cadence of the

metronome. The test was then begun and continued for 3 minutes. On completion of stepping, the students remained standing while the pulse (which is easily located by pressing *softly* at the carotid artery along the trachea in the neck) was counted for a 15-second interval beginning 5 seconds after the end of stepping (5 seconds to 20 seconds postexercise). This 15-second pulse rate value was then multiplied by 4 to express the heart rate in beats per minute. Table 12-3 presents percentile rankings for the various heart rate scores for men and women. Accompanying these scores are the corresponding values for maximal oxygen uptake that were predicted from the heart rate values (see the following section).

In comparing heart rate response on the stepping exercise with the standards of these students, one must follow the exact procedures for administering the test. The stepping cadence *must* be 22 steps per minute for women and 24 steps per minute for men. The bench height *must* be 41.3 cm, and recovery heart rate *must* be measured during the 5- to 20-second interval at the end of exercise.

Prediction of Maximal Oxygen Uptake. The limitations in predicting maximal oxygen uptake from submaximal measures of heart rate have been discussed in Chapter 5. It is reasonable, however, to expect that a person having a low heart rate during stepping exercise and in recovery is in better aerobic condition than someone whose heart rate on the same test is relatively higher. To evaluate the validity of this expectation, laboratory studies were conducted on a sample of men and women who were part of the larger study of the Queens College Step Test. Maximal oxygen uptake was measured using treadmill test procedures. Each subject's max $\dot{V}O_2$ score was then plotted in relation to the corresponding recovery heart rate score obtained on the step test. Figure 12-5 illustrates these results for the sample of women.

A useful fitness test. The heart rate response to a step test can serve as the frame of reference for evaluating cardiovascular adaptation to a particular program of aerobic conditioning. The important consideration is that the procedures for administering a step test must be identical each time the test is taken.

The step test is a practical test. While the step test prediction method certainly does not possess the accuracy required for use in research, it does provide a valid method for classification purposes.

TABLE 12-3. Percentile rankings for recovery heart rate and predicted maximal oxygen uptake for male and female college students*

Percentile Ranking	Recovery HR, Female	Predicted max $\dot{V}O_2$ (ml · kg^{-1} · min^{-1})	Recovery HR, Male	Predicted max $\dot{V}O_2$ (ml · kg^{-1} · min^{-1})
100	128	42.2	120	60.9
95	140	40.0	124	59.3
90	148	38.5	128	57.6
85	152	37.7	136	54.2
80	156	37.0	140	52.5
75	158	36.6	144	50.9
70	160	36.3	148	49.2
65	162	35.9	149	48.8
60	163	35.7	152	47.5
55	164	35.5	154	46.7
50	166	35.1	156	45.8
45	168	34.8	160	44.1
40	170	34.4	162	43.3
35	171	34.2	164	42.5
30	172	34.0	166	41.6
25	176	33.3	168	40.8
20	180	32.6	172	39.1
15	182	32.2	176	37.4
10	184	31.8	178	36.6
5	196	29.6	184	34.1

*From McArdle, W. D., et al.: Percentile norms for a valid step test in college women. *Res. Q.*, 44:498, 1973.

It was clear that a definite relationship existed. Subjects with a higher max $\dot{V}O_2$ tended to have lower heart rate recovery scores on the step test. Although the relationship was not a perfect one, significant information about aerobic capacity was obtained by knowing an individual's heart rate score. A mathematical equation was developed to describe the line of "best fit" that passed through the scores for recovery heart rate and max $\dot{V}O_2$. Based on this equation, a max $\dot{V}O_2$ value was predicted from heart rate with the value expressed in relation to body mass as milliliters of oxygen per kilogram of body mass per minute (ml·kg^{-1}·min^{-1}). Table 12-3 also presents the predicted max $\dot{V}O_2$ scores for college-aged men and women. For example, if the step test recovery heart rate for a woman was 156 beats per minute, the predicted max $\dot{V}O_2$ would be 37.0 ml·kg^{-1}·min^{-1}; a heart rate of 172 beats per minute for a man results in a predicted max $\dot{V}O_2$ value of 39.1

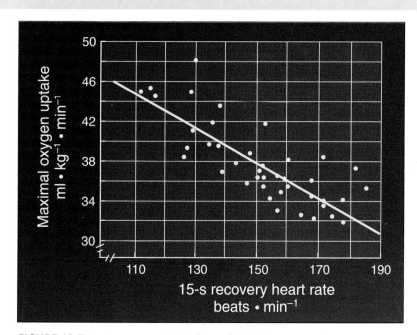

FIGURE 12-5. Scattergram and line of "best fit" relating step-test heart rate scores and maximal oxygen uptakes in college women. (From McArdle, W. D., et al.: Reliability and interrelationships between maximal oxygen uptake, physical work capacity, and step test scores in college women. *Med. Sci. Sports*, 4: 182, 1972.)

TABLE 12-4. Aerobic capacity classification based on gender and age.

| AGE | Maximal Oxygen Uptake (ml $\cdot$ kg^{-1} $\cdot$ min^{-1}) | | | | |
	LOW	FAIR	AVERAGE	GOOD	HIGH
Woman					
20–29	28	29–34	35–40	41–46	>47
30–39	27	38–41	34–38	39–45	>46
40–49	25	26–31	30–37	38–43	>44
50–65	21	22–28	27–34	35–40	>41
Men					
20–29	37	38–41	42–50	51–55	>56
30–39	33	34–37	38–42	43–50	>51
40–49	29	30–35	36–40	41–46	>47
50–59	25	26–30	31–38	39–42	>43
60–69	21	22–25	26–33	34–37	>38

The Tecumseh Step Test: A Valid Alternative. The Tecumseh Step Test can be used with adult men and women of all ages. Although a heart rate score on this test cannot be transposed into a max $\dot{V}O_2$ value, the recovery heart rates are valid for showing relative fitness for aerobic exercise. The fitness classifications were constructed from average values based on a large sample from Tecumseh, Michigan, a representative midwestern community. The test is attractive from a practical standpoint because the exercise level is relatively moderate and the stepping surface is the approximate height of most stairs found in the home.

The test can be performed alone, but it is much easier with a partner. Find a stair or stool 8 *inches high* (20.3 cm). The correct stepping height is important and easily can be achieved by adjusting the stepping or floor surface with a board or similar hard, flat object. As with all standardized step tests, the correct stepping cadence is crucial, so a brief practice is required to insure that the person steps up and down *twice* within a 5-second span, or 24 *complete step-ups each minute for 3 minutes*. A partner can chant "Up-up, down-down, up-up, down-down" within a 5-second span to establish the proper cadence. Each new sequence starts at 5, 10, 15, 20, and so on. For more precision, set a metronome at 96 beats per minute; this gives one foot-step per beat.

At the completion of 3 minutes of stepping, the person remains standing and the pulse rate is located. Exactly 30 seconds after stopping, pulse rate is measured for 30 seconds. The number of pulse beats from 30 seconds after stepping to 1 minute postexercise is the heart rate score.

Refer to Table 12-5 to obtain the cardiovascular fitness classification for age and gender.

ml $\cdot$ kg^{-1} $\cdot$ min^{-1}. In terms of accuracy of prediction, one can be 95% confident that the predicted max $\dot{V}O_2$ will be within ± 16% of the person's actual value.

Ideally, the most accurate measurement of max $\dot{V}O_2$ takes place in the laboratory with sophisticated equipment. This type of test also requires near-maximal effort from the subject. Although not possessing the accuracy required for research, the step test provides as good an estimate of max $\dot{V}O_2$ as obtained with other submaximal prediction tests that require a bicycle ergometer or treadmill (e.g., Åstrand test) or performance in a running test on a track (e.g., Cooper 12-min run). Such prediction tests are useful for placing individuals into different categories of cardiovascular fitness (e.g., low, medium, high).

Max $\dot{V}O_2$ Rating. A person's maximal oxygen uptake score can be evaluated against the aerobic capacity classifications in Table 12-4. Although such classifications are subjective, they have been constructed from average max $\dot{V}O_2$ values of physically active (but not college varsity caliber athletic competitors) and sedentary men and women measured in the United States and abroad.

TABLE 12-5. Step test classifications for Tecumseh Step Test based on 30-second recovery heart rate for men and women

CLASSIFICATION AGE	NUMBER OF BEATS*			
	20–29	30–39	40–49	50 & OLDER
Men				
Outstanding	34–36	35–38	37–39	37–40
Very good	37–40	39–41	40–42	41–43
Good	41–42	42–43	43–44	44–45
Fair	43–47	44–47	45–49	46–49
Low	48–51	48–51	50–53	50–53
Poor	52–59	52–59	54–60	54–62
Women				
Outstanding	39–42	39–42	41–43	41–44
Very good	43–44	43–45	44–45	45–47
Good	45–46	46–47	46–47	48–49
Fair	47–52	48–53	48–54	50–55
Low	53–56	54–56	55–57	56–58
Poor	57–66	57–66	58–67	59–66

*Thirty-second heart rate is counted beginning 30 seconds after exercise stops.
Based on information in Montoye, H. J.: *Physical Activity and Health: An Epidemiologic Study of an Entire Community.* Englewood Cliffs, N.J., Prentice-Hall, 1975.

Factors that Affect Aerobic Conditioning

Figure 12-6 illustrates the two major goals of aerobic conditioning:
- To enhance the capacity of the central circulation to deliver blood.
- To develop the "metabolic machinery" to consume oxygen within the active muscles.

Four Factors Influence Aerobic Conditioning
- Initial level of cardiovascular fitness
- Frequency of training
- Duration of training
- Intensity of training

Initial Level of Cardiovascular Fitness. As a general rule, the amount of improvement through training depends on a person's initial fitness level. In simple terms, if you rate low at the start, there is room for considerable improvement. If aerobic capacity is already high, naturally there will be relatively less improvement. Of course, a 5% improvement in physio-

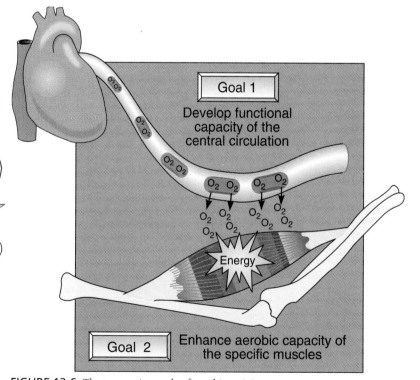

Goal 1

Develop functional capacity of the central circulation

Energy

Goal 2 Enhance aerobic capacity of the specific muscles

FIGURE 12-6. The two major goals of aerobic training.

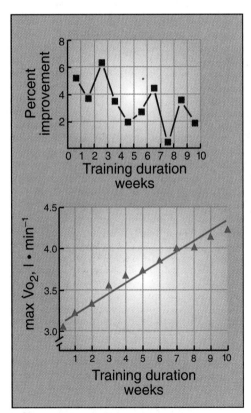

FIGURE 12-7. Continuous improvements in max $\dot{V}O_2$ over 8 weeks of high-intensity, aerobic training. (From Hickson, R. C., et al.: Linear increases in aerobic power induced by a program of endurance exercise. *J. Appl. Physiol.*, 42: 373, 1977.)

logic function for an elite athlete is just as important to that person as a 40% increase is for a sedentary person.

How Long Before Improvement Occurs? Positive adaptations in cardiovascular fitness and aerobic capacity occur rapidly, often being noted within several weeks. Figure 12-7 shows absolute and percentage improvements in max $\dot{V}O_2$ for men who trained 6 days a week for 10 weeks. Training consisted of 30- minutes of bicycling 3 days a week combined with running up to 40 minutes on alternate days. There was a continuous week-by-week improvement in aerobic capacity. Of course, these adaptive responses eventually begin to level off as a person reaches the "genetically determined" maximum.

Although fewer studies have been conducted with women, the amount and rate of improvement in aerobic capacity with training is similar to that for men.

Genetics Play a Role. Genetic factors play an important role in influencing the amount of improvement with training. This makes it difficult to predict exactly how much improvement can be expected based on a subject's pre-training test results. Because of inherited traits, some people possess a relatively high aerobic capacity without having had any previous training experience. In addition, some individuals are more "training responsive" or "trainable" than others. Dr. Åstrand, a renowned Swedish physiologist, contends that a high level of aerobic capacity is as much determined by who one's parents are as by participation in vigorous conditioning programs.

Frequency of Training. Exercising at least 3 days a week generally is necessary to bring about adaptive changes in the aerobic system. Of course, it is possible to locate one or two research

studies that report a significant improvement with training only 1 day a week. The subjects in those studies had been quite sedentary, however, and for them, any form of overload even though infrequent would stimulate cardiovascular improvement. The majority of experiments dealing with training frequency, however, indicate that a training response occurs if exercise is performed at least 3 times weekly for at least 6 weeks. Interestingly, several studies have shown that the improvements from training 4 or 5 times a week were either no greater or only slightly greater compared with exercising only 3 times a week. For the average person, an extra investment of time may not be that profitable for improving physiologic function, at least as measured by max $\dot{V}O_2$. If exercise is used primarily for weight control, daily exercise can represent a considerable caloric expenditure.

Duration of Training. One of the most common inquiries concerning exercise participation deals with the duration of the daily workout. For example, are 10 minutes twice as beneficial as 5 minutes of jogging? Would a run of 2 or 3 minutes that is repeated 8 to 10 times be recommended over a run at similar intensity performed continuously for 20 to 30 minutes? Precise answers to these questions are difficult because the mechanisms underlying the improvement in aerobic capacity are not fully understood. What is known, however, is that both continuous and more intense intermittent overload are effective in improving aerobic capacity. In general, performing less exhaustive, moderate-paced exercise for 20 to 30 minutes per session is a realistic recommendation for exercising in terms of intensity of effort and time commitment. This may be far from optimal, however, because most competitive endurance athletes spend from 2 to 3 hours or more per training session in activities geared to enhance the functional capacity of their physiologic systems.

Intensity of Training. *Intensity of training is the most critical factor related to successful aerobic conditioning.* Intensity of exercise reflects both the energy requirements of the activity and the specific energy systems activated. Intensity can be expressed in several ways:

- As calories expended per unit time
- As a particular exercise level or power output
- As a level of exercise below, at, or above the lactate threshold
- As a percentage of max $\dot{V}O_2$
- As a particular heart rate or some percentage of maximum heart rate
- As multiples of the resting metabolic rate (MET) required to perform the exercise

By far, the most practical means to assess the strenuousness of exercise is the exercise heart rate. Researchers frequently use exercise heart rate to structure a training program and evaluate the effectiveness of various training intensities. In general, for college-age men and women, the exercise must be of sufficient intensity to increase heart rate to at least 130 to 140 beats per minute. *This is equivalent to about 50 to 55% of max $\dot{V}O_2$, or 70% of the maximum exercise heart rate. As a general rule, this exercise intensity represents the minimal stimulus to cardiovascular improvement.* Although this level of cardiovascular stress is the threshold for aerobic improvement, more intense exercise is even more effective. Conversely, intensity of effort below the threshold level can also induce fitness improvements if the duration of the exercise session is extended.

An alternate, equally effective method to establish the training threshold is to exercise at a heart rate that is about 60% of the difference between resting and maximum. This use of the "heart rate reserve" in determining the threshold training heart rate (called the *Karvonen method* after the Finnish physiologist who first introduced this concept), gives a somewhat higher value compared with the heart rate computed simply as 70% of HRmax. The Karvonen method is calculated as follows:

$$HR_{threshold} = HR_{rest} + 0.60 \, (HR_{max} - HR_{rest})$$

Exercise Need Not Be Overly Strenuous. An exercise heart rate of 70% maximum (140 beats per minute for young adults) represents only moderate exercise that can be continued for long duration with little or no physiologic discomfort. This training level is frequently referred to as "conversational exercise"; it is sufficiently intense to stimulate a training effect yet not so strenuous that it limits a person from talking during the workout.

Figure 12-8 shows that as aerobic fitness improves, heart rate at a given submaximal level of exercise or oxygen uptake gradually becomes reduced. Consequently, to keep pace with improving fitness, the exercise level must increase periodically to achieve the same threshold heart rate

To help combat obesity, increase exercise duration. The ideal aerobic prescription for the individual who needs to reduce excess fat is approximately 60 minutes of moderate exercise daily, seven days a week! Walking is a preferred mode of exercise. The daily exercise can be split into 10-, 20-, or 30-minute sessions, as long as the daily total is 60 minutes or more. For an individual who weighs 216 pounds, the caloric expenditure during slow walking on the level would be approximately 7.8 calories a minute or 470 calories an hour. In one month, this would equal 14,400 calories (480 kcal x 30 days), or the equivalent of 4.1 pounds of body fat (14,400 kcal÷3500 kcal a pound). In one year, as long as caloric intake remains constant, fat loss without dieting would translate to a loss of about 50 pounds!

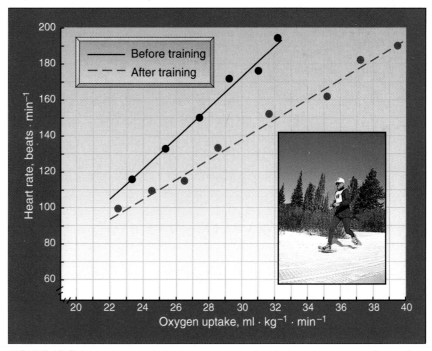

FIGURE 12-8. Improvements in heart rate response in relation to oxygen uptake resulting from training. A significant reduction in exercise heart rate with training is assumed to reflect an enhanced stroke volume of the heart.

The first Ironman triathlon was conducted in Hawaii in 1978 with 14 competitors. The Ironman triathlon competition consists of a marathon run (26.2 miles), a 112 mile bicycle ride, and a 2 mile endurance swim. Since this initial triathlon, the competition has flourished. In 1993 there were 2500 competitors, and by the mid 1990's, more than 2 million individuals will participate in triathlons of various distance throughout the United States.

While ample data describe the physical and physiological characteristics of elite athletes training for single sports, there are only a few reports on triathletes. Such studies may yield insight concerning the specificity of training. For example, research with untrained subjects indicates that the max $\dot{V}O_2$ is highly dependent on the mode of testing, with the highest values attained during treadmill running. When the aerobic capacity of these individuals is tested during cycling, the max $\dot{V}O_2$ is generally 8 to 12% below that running, and the aerobic capacity falls 18 to 22% below the value achieved during running when max $\dot{V}O_2$ is measured during a graded swimming test. With single sport-spe-

cific training, cyclists often equal or exceed their treadmill values for max $\dot{V}O_2$ when tested on a cycle ergometer, and highly trained swimmers may equal their running max $\dot{V}O_2$ during a tethered or free swimming test. Because triathletes train specifically for three

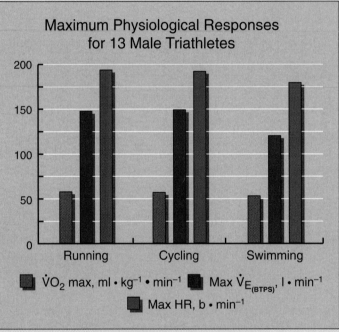

events, it is interesting to speculate whether they can (a) attain equivalent values for aerobic capacity in each of the three triathlon modes of exercise, or (b) maintain the running-cycling-swimming differential in aerobic capacity observed for untrained persons.

The insert table shows the results for aerobic capacity of 13 triathletes with an average of 2 years competition. The weekly training mileage for

these athletes was 32 miles of running, 155.8 miles of cycling, and 5.3 miles of swimming.

The cycling max $\dot{V}O_2$ averaged 95.7% of the running value, while the aerobic capacity during swimming was 86.8% of that achieved running. These differences are essentially the same as those noted for trained single sport athletes, and suggest that triathletes undergo highly specific adaptations that are linked to the mode of training. Perhaps triathletes do not attain as high a cycling or swimming max $\dot{V}O_2$ compared to the value running because of differences in training volume. While a triathlete spends considerable time training for each activity, the total training volume per sport is necessarily less than if training was solely focused on only one sport. These data argue against a generalized cross-training effect and suggest that triathletes are truly a superb class of aerobic athletes who attain world class physiology and performance in more than one sport.

Reference

Kohrt, W. M., et al.: Physiological responses of triathletes to maximal swimming, cycling and running. *Med. Sci. Sports Exerc.*, 19:51, 1987.

or whatever target rate has been selected. A person who began training by walking would have to walk more briskly; this would be gradually replaced by jogging for selected periods of the workout. Eventually, continuous running would be required to achieve the same relative strenuousness at the desired training heart rate.

Although there may be a minimal threshold intensity below which a training effect does not occur, there may also be a ceiling "threshold" above which there are no further gains. The lower and upper limits may depend on the participant's initial capacity and state of training. For people in relatively poor condition and for older men and women, the training threshold may be closer to 60% of HR max that corresponds to about 45% max $\dot{V}O_2$; individuals at higher fitness levels generally have a higher threshold level. The ceiling for training intensity is unknown, although 85% max $\dot{V}O_2$ (corresponding to 90% HR max) is thought to be the upper limit. At present, no definitive research is available to either prove or disprove this notion.

DEVELOPING AN AEROBIC TRAINING PROGRAM

In this section, we present guidelines for initiating aerobic training and describe a method for gauging the intensity of that training. We also discuss the advantages and possible limitations of aerobic conditioning through intermittent or continuous training procedures. (See Chapter 18 for guidelines on the medical screening of adults for exercise.)

Guidelines

Regardless of one's present physical condition, there are some basic guidelines to follow when beginning an aerobic exercise program. These are based on both research and common sense, and are designed to help improve fitness effectively and enjoyably.

- **Start slowly.** Injury may occur after any sudden burst of vigorous activity following a few years of sedentary living. Although it is normal to feel minor muscle aches and twinges of joint pain when starting an exercise program, it is not normal to experience severe muscular discomfort or excessive cardiovascular strain. Anyone who has felt such discomfort knows that there is no greater discouragement to continuing a program of regular exercise.
- **Warm up.** Before beginning to exercise, it is prudent to stretch gently and limber up. There are numerous warm-up and calisthenic exercises to limber joints and stretch muscles. Mild aerobic exercise such as running in place, jogging on a treadmill, skipping rope, or cycling on a stationary bicycle for several minutes, provides an adequate cardiovascular warmup *immediately before* the aerobic phase of the workout. The important point is to perform a variety of big muscle exercises in a rhythmic, moderate, and continuous manner so the pulse attains between 50 and 60% of its maximum.
- **Allow a cool-down period.** After exercising, allow 5 to 10 minutes to slow down gradually before stopping. This allows metabolism to progress to resting levels. More importantly, a gradual cool down prevents blood from pooling in the large veins of the previously exercised muscles. Venous pooling could bring about a drop in blood pressure and cause less blood to circulate to the heart and brain. This can cause dizziness, nausea, and even fainting, whereas a reduction in blood to the heart muscle itself may precipitate a series of irregular heart beats

Guidelines for children. Physical activity programs for children should be more general in nature compared to the rather specific formulations put forth for the "training" of adults. The following are general recommendations for physical activity and fitness activities for children summarized from various professional organizations and individual researchers in the area:

Exercise Type	Frequency	Intensity	Duration
Large muscle, rhythmic, aerobic	3–5 days/wk	50–80% maximal functional capacity	30–60 min

Swimming tops the list of sports participation. In 1989, 70.4 million people went swimming at least once during the year. This was followed closely by exercise walking (66.6 million); aerobic dancing and volleyball were last with 25.1 million participants.

TABLE 12-6. Relationship between percent max heart rate and percent max $\dot{V}O_2$

Percent max HR	Percent max $\dot{V}O_2$
50	28
60	42
70	56
80	70
90	83
100	100

that could trigger a dangerous cardiac episode.

Determining the Training Intensity

The term "intensity" is quite relative in terms of establishing an appropriate level of exercise for a specific individual. What could pose a considerable exercise stress for one person might well be below the threshold intensity of 70% maxHR for an elite athlete. Thus, it is necessary to evaluate exercise in terms of the stress it places on each person's aerobic system. Several methods have been proposed to individualize aerobic exercise training.

Train at a Percentage of max $\dot{V}O_2$. With this method, the oxygen uptake during exercise is either actually determined or estimated so that an individual can train at a percentage of the max $\dot{V}O_2$. For example, if jogging at 5.5 miles per hour requires an oxygen uptake of 33 ml $O_2 \cdot kg^{-1} \cdot min^{-1}$ and the jogger's max $\dot{V}O_2$ is 60 ml $O_2 \cdot kg^{-1} \cdot min^{-1}$, this exercise would represent an aerobic stress of 55% of aerobic capacity. For another individual with a lower aerobic capacity of 40 ml $O_2 \cdot kg^{-1} \cdot min^{-1}$, the oxygen cost of jogging at 5.5 miles per hour would still be approximately 33 ml $O_2 \cdot kg^{-1} \cdot min^{-1}$, yet this person would be exercising at 83% of maximum. To provide a similar overload of 83% of max $\dot{V}O_2$ for the first jogger, the pace would have to be increased to a run requiring about 48 ml $O_2 \cdot kg^{-1} \cdot min^{-1}$ or an increase in pace to about 8.6 miles per hour.

Although the assessment of exercise intensity by direct measurement of oxygen uptake is accurate, it is impractical without a fairly extensive laboratory. An alternative is to use heart rate to classify exercise in terms of intensity or strenuousness for a specific individual. This makes it possible to personalize an exercise program and regulate the intensity

of exercise to keep pace with improving fitness.

Train at a Percentage of Maximum Heart Rate. An effective alternative to the measurement of oxygen uptake is to use heart rate to classify exercise in terms of relative intensity and to establish a training protocol. This practice is based on the fact that percent max $\dot{V}O_2$ and percent maxHR are related in a predictable way. Selected values for percent max $\dot{V}O_2$ and corresponding percentages of maxHR are presented in Table 12-6.

The error in estimating percent max $\dot{V}O_2$ from percent maxHR, or vice versa, is about ± 8%. Because of this intrinsic relationship, it is only necessary to monitor heart rate to estimate percent max $\dot{V}O_2$. *The relationship between percent max $\dot{V}O_2$ and percent maxHR is essentially the same regardless of gender, fitness level, or age.* This also holds true for either arm or leg exercise for both healthy people and cardiac patients. The important point is that maximum heart rate is significantly lower in arm exercise, and this difference must be considered in formulating the exercise prescription for different exercise modes.

To train at a percentage of maximum heart rate requires knowledge of what the heart rate would be during near-exhausting exercise. A person's actual maximum heart rate can be determined immediately after 3 or 4 minutes of all-out running or swimming. This procedure is inadvisable, however, because such intense exercise requires considerable motivation and could be dangerous for people predisposed to coronary heart disease. *For this reason, people should consider themselves "average" and use the age-predicted maximum heart rates shown in Figure 12-9.* In addition to the average maximum heart rates by age, Figure 12-9 illustrates the "training-sensitive zone" that represents the lower threshold level of 70% and the upper level of 90% of maximum heart rate for each age group. *Conditioning of the aerobic systems occurs as long as the exercise heart rate is within this zone.*

Example: If a 30-year-old man wishes to train at moderate intensity, yet still be at the threshold level, the training heart rate selected would be equal to 70% of his age-predicted maximum (190 beats per minute), or a target exercise heart rate of 133 beats per minute (0.70 x 190). For a 40-year-old woman, on the other hand, the target heart rate would be 126 beats per minute (0.70 x 180). By trial and error using progressive increments of exercise, each person can arrive at a walking, jogging, or cycling speed to produce the desired target heart rate.

In carrying out this procedure, the person should exercise moderately for 3 to 5 minutes and count the pulse rate for 10 seconds immediately afterward. If the exercise is not intense enough to produce the desired target heart rate, the same exercise is repeated but at a faster pace— jogging instead of walking, pedaling faster or switching to a lower gear while cycling, or cycling faster to cover a greater distance within a specified time. If the 30-year-old man wishes to train at 85% of maximum heart rate, exercise intensity would be increased to produce a heart rate of 161 beats per minute (0.85 x 190).

Adjust for Swimming and Other Upper Body Exercise. The maximum heart rate for swimming averages about *13 beats per minute lower* than for running. This occurs in both trained and untrained subjects, and is probably the result of using the arms primarily during swimming exercise. Therefore, if swimming or other forms of upper body exercise such as arm cranking is selected as the training exercise, consider the decrease in maximum heart rate in this form of work when establishing the exercise intensity. We recommend that 13 beats per minute be subtracted from the age-predicted maximum heart rate values in Figure 12-9. Consequently, a 25-year-old person wishing to swim at 80% of maximum heart rate would select a swimming speed that produces a heart rate of about 146 beats per minute (0.80 x [195–13]). This represents more accurately the appropriate training heart rate for swimming.

Is Less Intense Exercise Effective? The recommendation for training at 70% of maximum heart rate as the threshold for aerobic improvement should be viewed as a *general guideline* for establishing an effective, yet comfortable exercise level. Although 20 to 30 minutes of continuous exercise at the 70% level will stimulate a training effect, exercise at a lower intensity of 60% for 45 minutes will also prove beneficial. *In general, lower exercise intensity often can be offset by longer exercise duration.* The important point is that regardless of the exercise level selected, more is not necessarily better. Excessive exercise increases the chance for bone, joint,

A low impact training alternative. Running in shallow water is an effective low impact way to elicit cardiovascular and metabolic responses that are comparable to treadmill running. In fact, the shallow water exercise produces higher responses than running in deeper water.

The ideal aerobic workout. The ideal workout to improve cardiovascular fitness consists of a 5-minute warm-up, a minimum of 30 minutes of large muscle activity at an intensity between 70 and 85% of maximum heart rate, and a recovery period of less intensive exercise. Exercise during the 30-minute workout is known as the conditioning phase of the regimen.

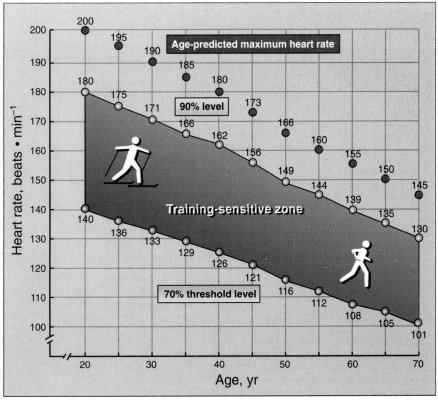

FIGURE 12-9. Maximal heart rates and the training-sensitive zone for use in aerobic training programs for men and women of different ages.

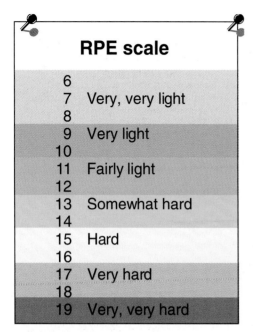

RPE scale

6	
7	Very, very light
8	
9	Very light
10	
11	Fairly light
12	
13	Somewhat hard
14	
15	Hard
16	
17	Very hard
18	
19	Very, very hard

FIGURE 12-10. The Borg scale used for rating perceived exertion (RPE) during exercise. (From Borg, G. A.: Psychological basis of physical exertion. *Med. Sci. Sports Exerc.,* 14: 377, 1982.)

and muscle injury. In Chapter 18 we point out that the health benefits from regular exercise do not require heroic levels of physical activity. Unfortunately, far too many people push themselves, adhering to the slogan, "no pain, no gain."

Train at a Perception of Effort. In addition to oxygen uptake and heart rate as indicators of exercise intensity, one can also use the *rating of perceived exertion* (RPE). With this approach, the exerciser rates on a numerical scale (Borg scale) how they feel in relation to the level of exertion. The levels of exercise that correspond to higher levels of energy expenditure and physiologic strain result in higher ratings. For example, an RPE of 13 or 14 ("somewhat hard"), illustrated in Figure 12-10, coincides with an exercise heart rate of about 70% maximum which is the generally accepted threshold for the training-sensitive zone. Individuals can quickly learn to exercise at a specific RPE based on

their subjective feeling of exertion. These subjective measures coincide nicely with objective measures of exercise intensity. In this sense, it is appropriate to consider the axiom, "listen to your body."

Train At The Lactate Threshold. Research indicates that it is also desirable to set exercise training at or slightly above the level of exercise that represents an individual's lactate threshold. This exercise level can be determined by plotting exercise intensity, such as running speed, in relation to the level of blood lactate as illustrated in Figure 12-11. In this example, the running speed at which 4 mmol of lactate accumulated per liter of blood was the recommended training intensity. This represents a level of exercise just above the lactate threshold. Periodic re-evaluation of the lactate threshold-exercise intensity relationship is required as aerobic fitness improves.

One difference between the heart rate and lactate threshold methods for setting the training intensity lies in the physiologic system being overloaded. More than likely, the heart rate method establishes an exercise stress for the central circulation (e.g., stroke volume, cardiac output), whereas adjusting training to the lactate threshold considers the response and capability of the periphery (local vasculature and active muscles) for aerobic metabolism.

Continuous Versus Intermittent Aerobic Training

Continuous Training. Continuous or long slow distance training (LSD training) involves steady-rate aerobic exercise performed at either moderate or high intensity for a sustained period. By its nature, continuous exercise training is submaximal and can be performed for considerable time in relative comfort. Such training is suitable for people just beginning an exercise program or desiring to expend considerable calories for purposes of weight control. It is certainly a more

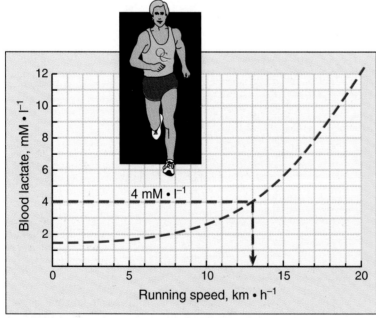

FIGURE 12-11. Blood lactate level in relation to running speed for one subject. At a lactate level of 4 mmol $\cdot$ l^{-1}, the corresponding running speed was approximately 13 km $\cdot$ hr^{-1}. This running speed then became the subject's initial training intensity.

pleasant method of training the aerobic system than the more intense method of interval training discussed in the next section. LSD training can be maintained at the threshold intensity of 70% maxHR or increased to the 85% or even 90% level.

Continuous exercise training is desirable for endurance athletes because it allows them to train at nearly the same intensity as in actual competition. A champion middle-distance runner may run 5 miles continuously in 25 minutes during workouts at a heart rate of 180 beats per minute; this pace would not be exhausting but would still nearly duplicate race conditions. By finishing each exercise session with several all-out sprints stopped 30 to 40 seconds before exhaustion, the athlete can also train the anaerobic system that does play a small role in such middle-distance events, especially at the race's finish. The marathon runner will train at a slightly slower pace than the middle-distance athlete because a much longer distance must be run in both practice and competition.

Interval Training. Many daily activities and sports are intermittent, characterized by periods of intense activity interspersed with periods requiring only a moderate to low level of energy expenditure. Interval exercise training requires correct spacing of exercise and rest periods so a person can accomplish a tremendous amount of exercise with minimal fatigue. The rest-to-exercise intervals can vary from a few seconds to several minutes. A training prescription should be based on the following:

  • Intensity of exercise
  • Duration of the exercise interval
  • Length of recovery
  • Number of repetitions of the exercise-recovery interval

For example, running continuously at a "4-minute mile" pace would exhaust most people within a minute. However, running at this speed for only 15 seconds followed by a 30-second rest period would enable many

people to run 4 minutes at this near-record pace. Of course, this is not equivalent to a 4-minute mile; but during 4 minutes of actual running, 1 mile would have been run even though the combined work and rest intervals would have taken 11 minutes 30 seconds.

Rationale for interval training. The rationale for interval training has a sound basis in physiology. In the example of the continuous run at a 4-minute mile pace, a major portion of energy would be supplied through the anaerobic production of lactic acid. Exhaustion occurs as the level of this acid metabolite rises. On the other hand, intermittent exercise performed for repeated intervals of 15 seconds or less would allow a severe load to be imposed on the muscles before appreciable accumulation of lactic acid. Recovery from these brief, yet intense exercise intervals would be predominantly "alactic" in nature and would take place quickly. The subsequent exercise interval could then begin again after only a brief rest period. These repetitive exercise intervals eventually place considerable demand on the aerobic system.

In interval training, as in other forms of physiologic conditioning, the intensity of exercise should be geared to the particular energy systems the person desires to train. A practical system for determining interval training exercise rates is presented in Table 12-7. The following illustrates how to establish the exercise interval and the relief interval.

  • **Exercise interval.** To determine the exercise interval, 1.5 to 5.0 seconds is added to the exerciser's "best time" for training distances between 60 and 220 yards for running and 15 and 55 yards for swimming. If a person can run 60 yards from a running start in 8 seconds, the training time for each repeat would therefore be 8 + 1.5 or 9.5 seconds. For interval training distances of 110 and 220 yards, 3 and 5 seconds are added,

TABLE 12-7. Guidelines for determining interval-training exercise rate for running and swimming different distances*

Interval Training Distances (Yards)		Work Rate for Each Exercise Interval or Repeat	
Run	Swim		
55	15	1.5	seconds *slower* than best times from a running (or swimming) start for each distance
110	25	3.0	
220	55	5.0	
440	110		1 to 4 seconds *faster* than the average run or 110-yard swim times recorded during a mile run or 440-yard swim
660–1320	165–320		3 to 4 seconds *slower* than the average run or 100-yard swim times recorded during a mile run or 440-yard swim

*From Fox, E. L., and Mathers, D. K.: *Interval Training*. Philadelphia, W. B. Saunders, 1974.

A healthful tip from the experts. The U.S. Centers for Disease Control and Prevention and the American College of Sports Medicine recommend a healthy lifestyle in which "every American adult should accumulate 30 minutes or more of moderate intensity physical activity over the course of most days of the week". This amount of exercise can be in recreational and household activities, or planned exercise such as jogging, swimming, and cycling.

Exercise in moderation during pregnancy. For a previously active, healthy woman during an uncomplicated pregnancy, moderate aerobic exercise does not produce circulatory alterations that compromise fetal oxygen supply.

to the best running times. This particular application of interval training is suited for training the high-energy-phosphate component of the anaerobic energy system. For training distances of 440 yards running or 110 yards swimming, the exercise rate is determined by subtracting 1 to 4 seconds from the average 440-yard portion of a mile run or 110-yard portion of a 440-yard swim. If a person runs a 7-minute mile (averaging 105 seconds per 440 yards), 3 to 5 seconds are added for each 440-yard portion of the interval distance. In running an interval of 880 yards, the 7-minute miler would thus run each interval at about 216 seconds ([105 + 3] x 2 = 216).

- **Relief Interval.** The relief interval can be either passive (rest-relief) or active (exercise-relief). The recommended duration of relief is usually expressed as a ratio of exercise duration to recovery duration. The ratio of 1:3 is generally recommended for training the immediate energy system. Thus, for a sprinter who runs 10-second intervals,

the relief interval is usually about 30 seconds. For training the short-term glycolytic energy system, the relief interval is twice as long as the exercise interval for an exercise to relief ratio of 1:2. These specified ratios of exercise to relief for anaerobic training provide for sufficient restoration of the high-energy-phosphate pools or lactic acid removal so the next exercise bout can proceed without undue fatigue.

At present, there is insufficient evidence to claim superiority for either continuous or interval training for aerobic fitness. Both methods provide results, and they probably can be used interchangeably.

Maintaining Aerobic Fitness

An interesting question concerning fitness maintenance is the optimal frequency, duration, and intensity of exercise required to retain the improved aerobic fitness attained through training. Studies reveal that if exercise *intensity* is maintained, the frequency and duration of training can be reduced considerably without decrements in aerobic performance (e.g., 6 days a week training reduced to 2 days; 40 minutes a day training reduced to 13 minutes). However, a small reduction in exercise intensity, keeping training frequency and duration constant, would cause a significant decline in aerobic fitness.

EXERCISING DURING PREGNANCY

With a considerable number of women involved in physically demanding occupations and active lifestyles, there is growing interest in topics related to exercise and pregnancy. Questions include:

- To what degree does pregnancy affect the energy cost and physiologic demands of exercise?
- What are the effects of exercise intensity on fetal blood supply?

- What are the effects of regular exercise on the course and outcome of pregnancy?

Energy Cost and Physiologic Demands of Exercise

The cardiovascular responses during exercise in pregnancy follow normal patterns. In addition, other than the strain provided by the additional weight gain and possible encumbrance of fetal tissue, an uncomplicated pregnancy offers no greater physiologic strain to the mother during moderate exercise. This means that as pregnancy progresses, the increase in maternal body mass adds significantly to the exercise effort in weight-bearing activities such as walking, jogging, and stair climbing. If body mass is supported during exercise as it is in stationary bicycling and to some extent swimming, the exercise response for heart rate and oxygen uptake during pregnancy is essentially identical to that observed in the non-pregnant state.

Fetal Blood Supply

Studies of uterine blood flow during exercise in various species of mammals indicate that for healthy animals, oxygen supply to the developing fetus is maintained during moderate to heavy levels of maternal exercise. However, in animals with one umbilical artery tied off to restrict circulation to the placenta, oxygen supply to the fetus was considerably reduced with maternal exercise. The researchers concluded that vigorous maternal exercise is well tolerated by the fetus during a normal pregnancy, but could be potentially harmful to a fetus with some limitation of the umbilical circulation.

Because vigorous exercise probably diverts some blood from the uterus, and this could pose a hazard to a fetus with restricted placental blood flow, it is prudent for a pregnant woman to exercise in moderation, especially if the pregnancy is compromised to any degree. In addition, an elevation in maternal core temperature could

hinder heat dissipation from the fetus through the placenta. During warm weather, it is therefore prudent for pregnant women to exercise in the cool part of the day and for shorter intervals while maintaining regular fluid intake before, during, and after exercising to prevent dehydration.

Outcome

Although regular aerobic exercise can serve an important role in maintaining the physical fitness, optimal body weight, and general well-being of a pregnant woman, it remains unclear whether extremes of maternal exercise are beneficial to the developing fetus and whether exercise enhances the course of pregnancy, including labor, delivery, and outcome.

ADAPTATIONS IN THE AEROBIC SYSTEM

Aerobic overload training is associated with adaptations in a variety of functional capacities related to oxygen transport and utilization. The most notable adaptations accompanying aerobic training are discussed here.

Metabolic Adaptations

- *Metabolic Machinery*. Mitochondria from trained skeletal muscle have a greatly increased capacity to generate ATP aerobically by oxidative phosphorylation.
- *Enzymes*. Associated with the increased capacity for mitochondrial oxygen uptake is an

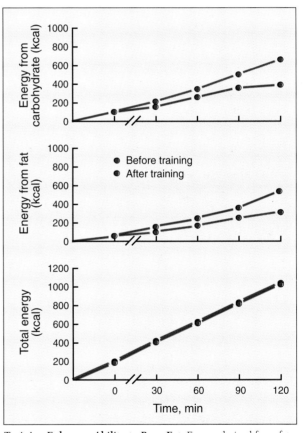

Training Enhances Ability to Burn Fat. Energy derived from fat oxidation in prolonged exercise is significantly increased following aerobic training with a corresponding decrease in carbohydrate breakdown. This carbohydrate-sparing adaptation may be due to a facilitated release of fatty acids from adipose tissue depots, as well as increased imtramuscular fat in the endurance trained individual. (Data from Hurley. B.F., et al.: Muscle triglyceride utilization during exercise: effect of training. *J. Appl. Physiol.,* 5: 62,1986)

increase in both the size and number of mitochondria, and a potential twofold increase in the level of aerobic system enzymes. These changes may be important for sustaining a high percentage of aerobic capacity during prolonged exercise.

- *Lipid Metabolism.* There is an increase in the trained muscle's reliance on lipid metabolism. This occurs by an increase in blood flow within muscle and an increase in the activity of fat-mobilizing and fat-metabolizing enzymes. Thus at any submaximal exercise level, a trained person uses more free fatty acids for energy than an untrained counterpart.
- *Carbohydrate Metabolism.* The trained muscle exhibits a greater capacity to oxidize carbohydrate. Consequently, large quantities of pyruvic acid move through the aerobic energy pathways during high intensity aerobic effort. This is consistent with the increased oxidative capacity of the mitochondria and increased glycogen storage within the trained muscles.
- *Fiber Type.* Training produces aerobic metabolic adaptations in both types of muscle fibers, causing each to develop their already existing aerobic potential. The possibility is probably small for producing actual changes in muscle fiber type.

Cardiovascular and Pulmonary Adaptations

Because the cardiovascular and pulmonary systems are intimately linked with aerobic processes, related changes occur that are both functional and dimensional. These include:

- *Heart Size.* A mild cardiac hypertrophy is a normal training adaptation characterized by an increase in the size of the left ventricular cavity, as well as by a slight thickening of its walls.

Cardiac enlargement returns to control levels with reduced training intensity.

- *Plasma Volume.* Significant increases in plasma volume are noted within 4 or 5 training sessions. This adaptation may enhance circulatory and thermoregulatory dynamics and facilitate oxygen delivery during exercise.
- *Heart Rate.* Resting and submaximal exercise heart rate decrease with aerobic training, especially for previously sedentary individuals.
- *Stroke Volume.* The heart's stroke volume increases at rest and during exercise. Large stroke volumes are evident among well-trained individuals and generally result from a large ventricular volume accompanied by enhanced myocardial contractility.
- *Cardiac Output.* The most significant change in cardiovascular function with aerobic training is the increase in maximum cardiac output. Because the maximum heart rate may decrease slightly with training, the heart's increased outflow capacity results directly from an improved stroke volume.
- *Oxygen Extraction.* Training produces significant increases in the amount of oxygen extracted from the circulating blood during exercise. An increase in the $a-\bar{v}O_2$ difference results from a more effective distribution of the cardiac output to working muscles as well as an enhanced capacity of the trained muscle cells to use oxygen.
- *Blood Flow and Distribution.* Aerobic training causes large increases in muscle blood flow during maximal exercise owing to (1) improvements in maximal cardiac output, and (2) redistribution of blood from non-active areas that temporarily compromise blood flow in response to all-out effort.

Plasma volume and training. Plasma volume can increase by 10 to 20% within several days of daily vigorous exercise training.

Blood and volume advantage. A larger blood volume provides the trained individual with greater body fluid for heat dissipation as well as a larger vascular volume for the maintenance of stroke volume and cardiac output during exercise. Blood volume returns to near normal levels within a week after training is discontinued.

- *Blood Pressure.* Regular aerobic training tends to reduce both systolic and diastolic blood pressure during rest and submaximal exercise. The largest decreases occur in systolic pressure and are most apparent in hypertensive subjects.
- *Pulmonary Function.* Increased breathing volumes accompany improvements in max $\dot{V}O_2$ as a result of increases in both tidal volume and breathing frequency. In submaximal exercise, the trained person ventilates less than before training. This adaptation is helpful in prolonged exercise because increased ventilatory economy means a greater oxygen availability to the active muscles.

Other Adaptations

- *Body Composition.* For the person who is obese or borderline obese, regular aerobic exercise causes a reduction in body fat and often a slight increase in lean body mass. When exercise is used alone or combined with diet, more of the weight lost is fat compared to dieting only, probably because exercise has a conserving effect on the body's lean tissues.
- *Body Heat Transfer.* Well-hydrated, trained individuals exercise more comfortably in hot environments because of a larger blood volume and a more responsive heat regulatory mechanism. Trained men and women dissipate heat faster and cool the body more effectively. This means that the heat generated by exercise causes less physiologic strain; this prolongs exercise tolerance.

A schema is proposed to summarize adaptive changes that accompany aerobic training. Figure 12-12 illustrates that maximal oxygen uptake increases about 15 to 30% in the first 3 months of intensive training, and may rise by as much as 50% over a 2-year period. When training stops, the aerobic capacity returns toward the pretraining level. The picture is even more impressive for the aerobic enzymes that facilitate carbohydrate and lipid breakdown, which increase rapidly and substantially throughout training in both fiber types. Conversely, a large amount of this metabolic adaptation is lost within a few weeks after training ceases. The number of muscle capillaries increases throughout training. With detraining, this adaptation in blood supply is probably lost at a relatively slow rate.

Intensive training lasting longer than 6 months causes an increase in the mitochondrial respiratory capacity of the trained muscles. This "local" metabolic improvement greatly outstrips the body's ability to circulate, deliver, and use oxygen during intense exercise (as demonstrated by the relatively small further increase in max $\dot{V}O_2$). In this phase of training, however, a muscle's lactate level may be much lower (lower production or greater removal rate) than that observed in submaximal exercise of similar relative intensity before training. These adjustments in cellular function may account for a trained person being able to do prolonged steady-rate exercise at a larger percentage of max $\dot{V}O_2$.

Potential Psychologic Benefits of Regular Exercise
- Reduction in state anxiety
- Decrease in mild to moderate depression
- Reduction in neuroticism (long-term exercise)
- Adjunct to the professional treatment of severe depression
- Improvement in mood, self esteem, and self concept
- Reduction in the various indices of stress

Even cardiac patients benefit. Selected patients with coronary artery disease when trained in excess of normality prescribed exercise intensity show physiologic adaptations much larger than previously believed. The good news is that these adaptations include favorable adjustments in myocardial oxygenation and enhanced ventricular function.

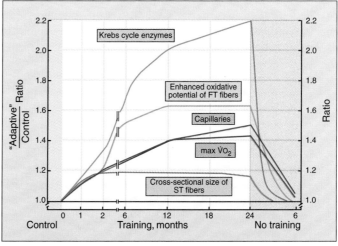

FIGURE 12-12. A generalized summary of adaptations in aerobic capacity and active muscle with endurance training based on longitudinal and cross-sectional studies of humans. (From Saltin, B., et al.: Fiber types and metabolic potentials of skeletal muscles in sedentary man and endurance runners. *Ann. N.Y. Acad. Sci.,* 301: 3, 1977.)

SUMMARY

1. Activities can be classified by their predominant activation of a specific system of energy transfer. An effective training program is one that allocates appropriate time to train the specific energy system(s) involved in the activity.

2. The contribution of anaerobic and aerobic energy transfer depends largely on exercise intensity and duration. During sprint-power activities, for example, the primary means for energy transfer involves the immediate and short-term energy systems. The long-term aerobic system becomes progressively more important in activities that last longer than 2 minutes.

3. Proper physical conditioning is based on four important principles for producing optimum improvements. These are the overload principle, the specificity of exercise principle, the individual difference principle, and the reversibility principle.

4. Anaerobic training increases resting levels of anaerobic substrates and key glycolytic enzymes. This is usually accompanied by concomitant increases in all-out exercise performance.

5. The step test provides a convenient means by which heart rate can be used to evaluate the efficiency of the cardiovascular response to aerobic exercise and training.

6. Aerobic training must be geared to enhance both circulatory function and the metabolic capacity of specific muscles. Peripheral adaptations in active tissues may have a profound effect on exercise performance.

7. The four major factors that affect training improvement are initial fitness level, frequency of training, exercise intensity, and duration of exercise. The most important of these is exercise intensity.

8. Training intensity can be applied either on an absolute basis in terms of exercise load, or on a relative basis geared to an individual's physiologic response. Training levels that correspond to 70 to 90% of maximum heart rate are most desirable for inducing changes in aerobic fitness.

9. Approximately 30 minutes per training session appears to be desirable in terms of exercise duration. Extending the duration can compensate somewhat for reduced exercise intensity.

10. Frequency for effective aerobic training appears to be a minimum of 3 days per week. Optimal frequency levels have not been established.

11. If intensity, duration, and frequency are held constant, training improvements are similar regardless of training mode, as long as large muscle groups are exercised.

12. The frequency and duration of physical activity required to maintain an improved level of aerobic fitness is less than that required to improve it, as long as exercise intensity is maintained.

13. For the physically active, healthy woman who becomes pregnant, moderate aerobic exercise does not appear to compromise fetal oxygen supply. It remains unclear, however, whether extremes of maternal exercise are beneficial to the course of pregnancy or to the child in the early period after birth.

14. Aerobic training causes functional and dimensional changes in the cardiovascular system. These changes include decreases in resting and submaximal exercise heart rate, enhanced stroke volume and cardiac output, and an improved ability of the specifically trained muscles to process oxygen.

American College of Sports Medicine: The recommended quantity and quality of exercise for developing and maintaining cardiorespiratory and muscular fitness in healthy adults. *Med. Sci. Sports Exerc.,* 22: 205, 1990.

Ballor, D. L., et al: Resistance weight training during caloric restriction enhances lean body weight maintenance. *Am. J. Clin. Nutr.,* 47: 19, 1988.

Belman, M. J., and Gaesser, G. A.: Exercise training below and above the lactate threshold in the elderly. *Med. Sci. Sports Exerc.,* 23: 562, 1991.

Bouchard, C., et al.: Long-term exercise training with constant energy intake. I. Effect on body composition and selected metabolic variables. *Int. J. Obesity,* 14: 57, 1990.

Bouchard, C., and Pérusse, L. Heredity, activity level, fitness, and health. In *Physical Activity, Fitness, and Health.* Edited by C. Bouchard, et al., Champaign, IL, Human Kinetics, 1994.

Carpenter, M.W.: Physical activity, fitness, and health of the pregnant mother and fetus. In *Physical Activity, Fitness, and Health.* Edited by C. Bourchard, et al., Champaign, IL, Human Kinetics, 1994.

Clapp, J. F., et al.: Exercise in pregnancy, Med. Sci. Sports Exerc., 24: S294, 1992.

Clifford, P.S., et al.: Arterial blood pressure response to rowing. *Med. Sci. Sports Exerc.,* 26: 715, 1994.

Cureton, K. J., et. al.: Generalized equation for prediction of $\dot{V}O_{2\ peak}$ from 1-mile run/walk performance. *Med. Sci. Sports Exerc.,* 27 (3): 445, 1995.

Dewey, K.G., et al.: A randomized study of the effects of aerobic exercise by lactating women on breast-milk volume and composition. *N. Engl. J. Med.,* 330: 449, 1994.

Franklin, B. A.: Aerobic exercise training programs for the upper body. *Med. Sci. Sports Exerc.,* 21: S141, 1989.

Hartung, G. H., et al.: Estimation of aerobic capacity from submaximal cycle ergometry in women. *Med. Sci. Sports Exerc.,* 27 (3):452, 1995

Holloszy, J. O.: Metabolic consequences of endurance training. In *Exercise, Nutrition, and Energy Metabolism.* Edited by E. S. Horton, and R. L. Terjung. New York, Macmillan, 1988.

Hooper, S.L., et al.: Markers for monitoring overtraining and recovery. *Med. Sci. Sports Exerc.,* 27: 106, 1995.

Jackson, A.J., et al.: Changes in aerobic capacity in men, ages 25-70 yr. *Med. Sci. Sports Exerc.,* 27: 113, 1995.

Jacobs, I.: Sprint training effects on muscle myoglobin, enzymes, fiber types, and blood lactate. *Med. Sci. Sports* Exerc., 19: 368, 1987.

Jones, B. H., et al.: Epidemiology of injuries associated with physical training among young men in the army. *Med. Sci. Sports Exerc.,* 25: 197, 1993.

Joyner, M. J.: Physiological limiting factors and distance running: influence of gender and age on record performances. In *Exercise and Sport Sciences Reviews.* Vol. 21. Edited by J. O. Holloszy. Baltimore MD, Williams & Wilkins, 1993.

King, A. C., et al.: Group- vs. home-based exercise training in healthy older men and women. *JAMA,* 1991.

Kohrt, W. M., et al.: Longitudinal assessment of responses of triathletes to swimming, cycling, and running. *Med. Sci. Sports Exerc.,* 21: 569, 1989.

Lovelady, C.A., et al.: Effects of exercise on plasma lipids and metabolism of lactating women. *Med. Sci. Sports Exerc.,* 27: 22, 1995.

Loy, S.F., et al.: Effects of stairclimbing on VO_2 max and quadriceps strength in middle-aged females. *Med. Sci. Sports Exerc.,* 26: 241, 1994.

Magel, J. R., et al.: Specificity of swim training on maximum oxygen uptake. *J. Appl. Physiol.,* 38: 151, 1978.

McArdle, W. D., et al.: Specificity of run training on $\dot{V}O_2$ max and heart rate changes during running and swimming. *Med. Sci. Sports Exerc.,* 10: 16, 1978.

McMurry, R. G., et al.: Recent advances in understanding maternal and fetal responses. *Med. Sci. Sports Exerc.,* 25: 1305, 1993.

Minotti, J. R., et al.: Training-induced skeletal muscle adaptations are independent of systemic adaptations. *J. Appl. Physiol.,* 68: 289, 1990.

Mitchell, J. H., et al.: Acute response and chronic adaptation to exercise in women. *Med. Sci. Sports Exerc.,* 24: S2589, 1992.

Morgan, D.W., et al: Daily variability in running economy among well-trained male and female distance runners. *Res. Q. Exerc. Sport.,* 65: 72, 1994.

Neufer, P. D., et al.: Effect of reduced training on muscular strength and endurance in competitive swimmers. *Med. Sci. Sports Exerc.,* 19: 486, 1987.

Pollock, M. L., et al.: Effects of mode of training on cardiovascular function and body composition of adult men. *Med. Sci. Sports Exerc.,* 7: 139, 1975.

Riviere, D., et al.: Lipolytic response of fat cells to catecholamines in sedentary and exercise-trained women. *J. Appl. Physiol.,* 66: 330, 1989.

Saasverda, C., et al.: Maximal anaerobic performance of the knee extensor muscles during growth. *Med. Sci. Sports Exerc.,* 23: 1083, 1991.

Swain, D.P., et al.: Target heart rates for the development of cardiorespiratory fitness. *Med. Sci. Sports Exerc.* 26: 112, 1994.

Treadway, J. L., and Young, J. C.: Decreased glucose uptake in fetus after maternal exercise. *Med. Sci. Sports Exerc.,* 21: 140, 1989.

Williams, C.L., Gandy, G.: Physiology and nutrition for sprinting. In: *Physiology and Nutrition for Competitive Sport.* (Eds) Lamb, D.R., et al. Volume 7. Cooper Publishing Group. Carmel, IN. 1994. Pg. 55.

Wolfe, L.A., et al.: Effects of pregnancy and chronic exercise on respiratory responses to graded exercise. *J. Appl. Physiol.,* 76: 1928, 1994.

Wolfe, L.A., et al.: Maternal exercise, fetal well-being and pregnancy outcome. *Exerc. Sport Sci. Rev.,* 22: 145, 1994.

Wolf, L. A., et al.: Physiological interactions between pregnancy and aerobic exercise. In *Exercise and Sport Sciences Reviews.* Vol. 17. Edited by K. B. Pandolf. Baltimore, Williams & Wilkins, 1989.

Woodby-Brown, S., et al.: Oxygen cost of aerobic dance bench stepping at threee heights. *J. Strength and Cond. Res.,* 7:163, 1993.

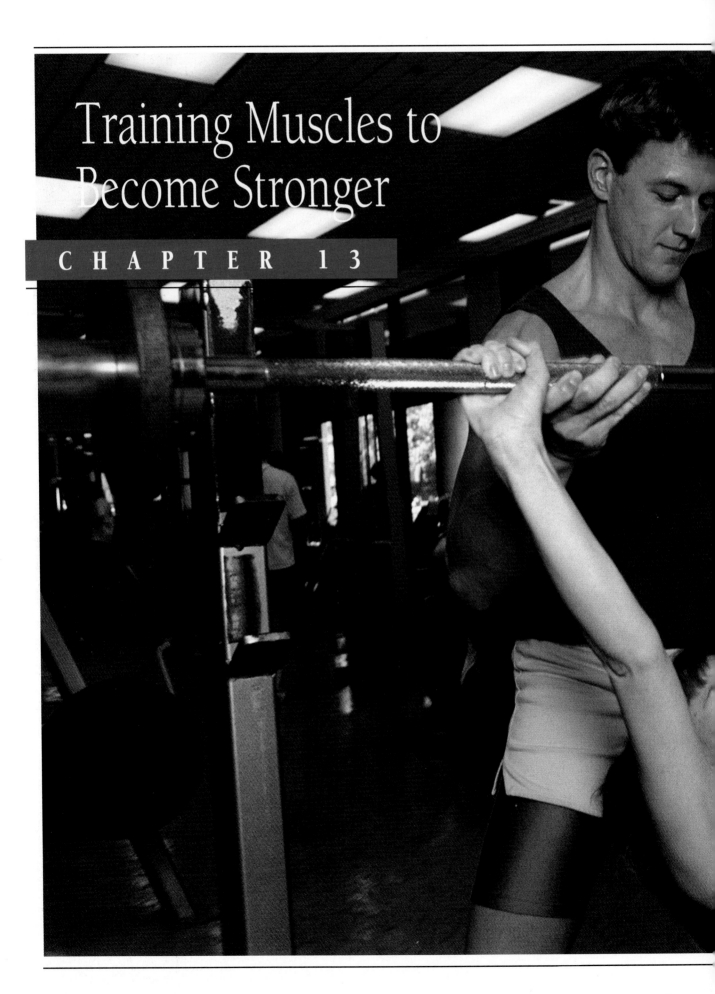

Training Muscles to Become Stronger

CHAPTER 13

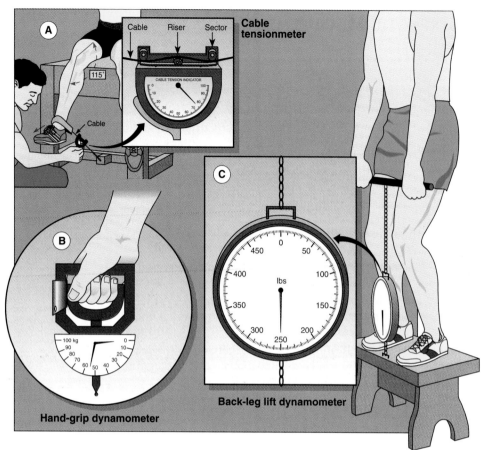

Cable tensionmeter

Cable   Riser   Sector

CABLE TENSION INDICATOR

Hand-grip dynamometer

Back-leg lift dynamometer

FIGURE 13-1. Measurement of static strength by use of (A) cable tensiometer, (B) hand-grip dynamometer, and (C) back-leg lift dynamometer.

external "static" force has been applied to the dynamometer.

One-Repetition Maximum (1-RM)

A dynamic method for measuring the maximum muscular strength makes use of the 1-RM method. This refers to the maximum amount of weight lifted one time with correct form. To test 1-RM for any particular muscle group or groups such as forearm flexors, leg extensors, or shoulders, a suitable starting weight is selected close to but below the subject's maximum lifting capacity. If one repetition is completed, weight is added to the exercise device until maximum lift capacity is achieved. Depending on the muscle group evaluated, the weight increments are usually 5, 2, or 1 kg during the period of measurement. During the 1-RM maneuver, both concentric and eccentric muscle actions are performed, but it is the concentric phase of the action that is used to evaluate 1-RM. Figure 13-2 illustrates two additional "submaxi-

mal" methods for evaluating a muscle's "maximum" force generating capacity. In these tests, the greatest amount of weight that can be lifted either 5 or 10 times is used as the criterion repetition maximum to assess strength. For these methods, less than the maximum is lifted because by definition the 1-RM test requires 100% of maximum. The 5-RM and 10-RM methods serve as convenient markers of "strength," particularly when considering for safety when testing children and older adults.

Computer-Assisted Electromechanical and Isokinetic Determinations

The emergence of microprocessor technology has made possible a rapid way to quantify muscular force during a variety of movements. Sensitive instruments are currently available to measure force, acceleration, and velocity of body segments in various movement patterns. Force platforms can be used to measure the external application of muscular force by a limb, such as in jumping. Other electromechanical devices measure the forces generated during all phases of an exercise movement, such as cycling or during a supine bench press or leg press.

An *isokinetic dynamometer* is an electromechanical instrument that contains a speed-controlling mechanism that accelerates to a preset speed when any force is applied. Once a constant speed is attained, the isokinetic loading mechanism accommodates automatically to provide a counterforce in relation to the force generated by the muscle while maintaining movement speed. *Thus, maximum force (or any percentage of maximum effort) can be applied during all phases of the movement at a constant velocity.*

A load cell inside the dynamometer continuously monitors the immediate level of applied force (and matching resistance) and records this information. An electronic integrator placed in series with the recorder provides a readout of the average force generated for a given time. The voltage output from the integrator can be interfaced directly with a computer to provide almost instantaneous readouts of average force, power output, and total work.

The interface of computer technology with mechanical devices provides the exercise scientist with valuable data for purposes of exercise evaluation and prescription. Such advances in technology, however, are not accepted universally by many who still consider a maximum lift (1-RM) as the best criterion of overall muscular strength. The counterargument of such dogma is that the dynamics of muscle strength involve considerably more than just the final outcome of a 1-RM, 5-RM, or 10-RM. Even if two people have a 1-RM score of 100 kg, for example, the force-time curves could be quite dissimilar. Such differences in force dynamics (e.g., time to peak tension or rate of force development) may reflect an entirely different underlying neuromuscular physiology. Without the aid of the newer technologies, it simply would not be possible to study many of the exciting areas of muscle dynamics.

· · · · · · · · · · · · · · ·
STRENGTH TESTING CONSIDERATIONS

The following considerations are important when testing "strength," whether by cable tensiometry, dynamometry, 1-RM, or computer-assisted methods. This will ensure that fair comparisons can be made among subjects.

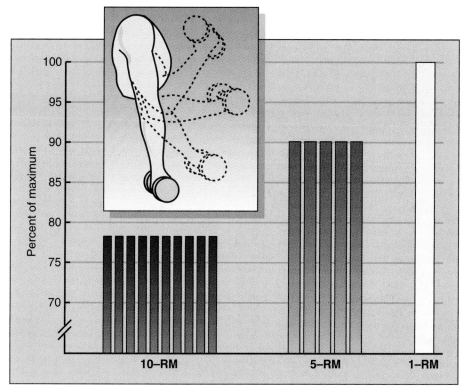

FIGURE 13-2. Three different dynamic methods to assess force- generating capacity in a particular movement.

- Standardized instructions should be given prior to testing
- A "warm-up" should be given that is of uniform duration and intensity
- The subject must have adequate practice before the actual test to minimize a "learning" component that could compromise initial results or the evaluation of true training effects
- Care must be taken to ensure that the measurement angle of the limb is consistent for all subjects
- A minimum number of trials (repetitions) should be determined beforehand to establish a criterion score. In most cases, however, an average of several trials will be more representative of a person's strength or power performance than a single trial
- Use strength tests with established reliability or reproducibility of measurement. This is a crucial aspect of testing that is often overlooked. Unreliability of measure-

ment per se can mask the individual's performance on the test

- Be prepared to consider individual differences in such factors as body size and composition when evaluating strength scores between individuals and groups. For example, is it fair to compare the absolute "strength" of a 120-kg defensive lineman with the "strength" of a 62-kg distance runner? Unfortunately, there is no clear-cut answer to this dilemma, but in the next section we do present some alternatives

GENDER DIFFERENCES IN STRENGTH

Two approaches have been used to determine whether true gender differences exist in terms of muscular strength. Strength has been evaluated in terms of the following: On an *absolute* basis as total force exerted and on a *relative* basis as force exerted in relation to body mass, lean body mass, or muscle cross-sectional area.

Absolute Muscular Strength

When strength is compared on an absolute score basis (that is, total force in pounds or kilograms), men are usually considerably stronger than women for all muscle groups tested, regardless of the device used to measure strength. These strength differences between the genders are particularly apparent in comparisons of upper body strength where women are about 50% weaker than men; in lower body strength, women are about 30% weaker. The exceptions may occur for some strength-trained female track and field athletes and bodybuilders, who significantly increase the strength of specific muscle groups by resistance exercises.

Relative Muscular Strength

Human skeletal muscle can generate approximately 3 to 8 kg of force per cm^2 of muscle cross section, regardless of gender. In the body, however, this force-output capacity varies depending on the arrangement of the bony levers and muscle architecture. Figure 13-3 presents a comparison of the arm flexor strength of men and women in relation to the cross-sectional area of muscle.

Clearly, the greatest force is exerted by individuals with the largest muscle cross section. The linear relationship between strength and muscle size, however, indicates little difference in arm flexor strength for the same size muscle in men and women. This is further demonstrated in the

---

Strength and puberty. Boys maintain about 10% greater muscle strength than girls up to puberty. After age 12, however, boys show a continued increase in strength while the strength scores of girls tend to plateau.

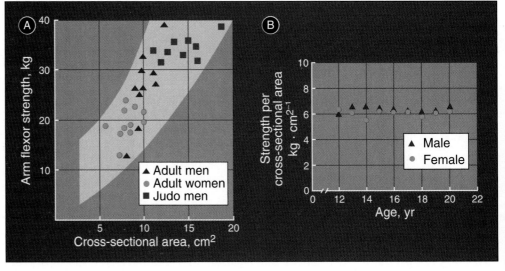

FIGURE 13-3. (*A*) Variability of upper arm flexion strength of men and women in relation to the flexor muscle's cross-sectional area. Absolute strength was computed as the measured strength x 4.90. (*B*) Strength per unit cross-sectional area of muscle in males and females aged 12 to 20 years. (From Ikai, M., and Fukunaga, T.: Calculation of muscle strength per unit cross-sectional area of human muscle by means of ultrasonic measurements. *Arbeitsphysiologie,* 26: 26, 1968.)

insert graph when the strength of males and females is expressed per unit area of muscle cross section.

TRAINING MUSCLES TO BECOME STRONGER

In training for muscular strength, the overload principle is applied by the use of weights (dumbbells or barbells), immovable bars, straps, pulleys, or springs, and water, air, and oil hydraulic devices. There is nothing unique in the use of a barbell or spring, or any heavy object to improve muscular strength. In each case, the muscle responds to the intensity of the overload rather than to the actual form of overload.

In general, muscular overload is applied by increasing the load or resistance, increasing the number of times or repetitions the exercise is performed, increasing the speed of muscular action, or by various combinations of these three factors.

Different Forms of Muscular Action

There are three basic types of muscular actions: concentric, eccentric, and isometric.

- *Concentric action* is the most common type of muscular action and occurs in dynamic activities in which the muscle shortens and joint movement occurs as it develops tension. Figure 13-4A illustrates a concentric muscular action during the raising of a dumbbell from the extended to the flexed elbow position.
- *Eccentric action* occurs when external resistance exceeds muscle force and the muscle lengthens while developing tension. As shown in Figure 13-4B, the weight is slowly lowered against the force of gravity. The muscles of the upper arm increase in length as they contract eccentrically to prevent the weight from crashing to the floor.

- *Isometric action* occurs when a muscle attempts to shorten but is unable to overcome the resistance. Considerable muscular force can be generated during an isometric action with no noticeable lengthening or shortening of the muscle and with no joint movement. Figure 13-4C illustrates an isometric muscular action.

Both concentric and eccentric muscular actions are commonly referred to as isotonic because in both cases movement occurs. The term "*isotonic*" is derived from the Greek word isotonos (iso meaning the same or equal; tonos, tension or strain). Actually this term is imprecise when applied to most dynamic muscular actions that involve movement because the muscle's force-generating capacity varies as the joint angle changes; thus, force output does not

Consider both concentric and eccentric actions. During the recovery phase of a resistance exercise, eccentric muscle action adds to the total work of the exercise repetition. This combination of concentric-eccentric muscle actions contributes to the effectiveness of the exercise in terms of enhanced muscle strength and fiber size.

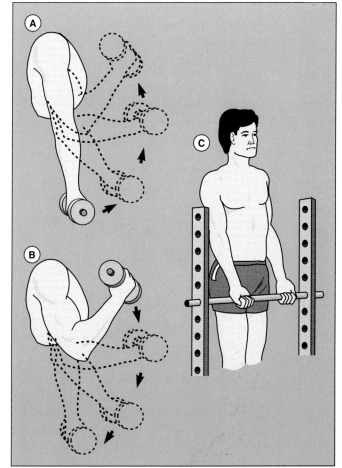

FIGURE 13-4. Muscular force generated during (*A*) concentric (shortening), (*B*) eccentric (lengthening), and (*C*) isometric (static) actions.

remain constant through the range of motion.

Resistance Training for Children

Relatively little is known concerning the benefits and possible risks of resistance training in preadolescents. Because the skeletal system is in the formative stage, obvious concern arises as to the potential for bone and joint injury with heavy muscular overload in growing children. Furthermore, because the hormonal profile is still in progressive development, especially for the tissue-building hormone testosterone, one might question whether resistance training could induce significant strength improvements at a relatively young age. *However, the limited available evidence indicates that closely supervised resistance training programs that employ concentric muscular actions with high repetitions and relatively low resistance can significantly improve the muscular strength of children with no adverse effect on bone or muscle.* Certainly, more studies are warranted before definitive statements can be made regarding the benefit-to-risk ratio and long-term effect on growth and development of regular and more stressful muscular overload.

TYPES OF RESISTANCE TRAINING

Three exercise systems are commonly used to develop muscular strength:

- Weight training
- Isometric training
- Isokinetic training

Weight Training (Dynamic Exercise)

This popular system of resistance training uses weight plates, barbells and dumbbells, or a variety of exercise machines against which muscles exert tension to overcome and move a fixed or variable resistance.

Progressive Resistance Exercise. Researchers in rehabilitation medicine following World War II devised a method of resistance training to improve the force-generating capacity of previously injured limbs. Their method involved three sets of exercises each consisting of 10 repetitions done consecutively without resting. The first set was done with one-half of the maximum weight that could be lifted 10 times or 1/2, 10-RM; the second set was done with 3/4, 10-RM; the final set was done with maximum weight (10-RM). As patients trained and became stronger, it was necessary to increase the 10-RM resistance periodically so strength improvement progressed. This technique of *progressive resistance exercise* (PRE) is a practical application of the overload principle and forms the basis of most strength conditioning programs.

Variations of PRE. Variations of PRE have been studied to determine the optimal number of sets and repetitions, and the frequency and relative intensity of training to improve strength. The findings can be summarized as follows:

- Performing an exercise between 3-RM and 9-RM is the most effective number of repetitions for increasing muscular strength
- PRE training once weekly with only 1-RM for one set increases strength significantly after the first week of training and each week up to at least the sixth week
- No particular sequence of PRE training with different percentages of 10-RM is more effective for strength improvement, as long as one set of 10-RM is performed each training session
- Performing one set of an exercise is less effective for increasing strength than two or three sets, and three sets are more effective than two
- The optimum number of training days per week with PRE is unknown. For beginners, significant strength increases have

Is more better for children? Sports and overuse injuries among children are up sharply. The causes:
- Intensive sports training programs
- Specialty sports camps and longer playing seasons
- Improper training techniques and sports equipment

occurred with training between 1 and 5 days weekly

- When PRE training uses several different exercises, training 4 or 5 days a week may be less effective for increasing strength than training 2 or 3 times weekly. The more frequent training may prevent sufficient recuperation between exercise sessions, which could retard progress in neuromuscular adaptation and strength development
- For a given resistance, a fast rate of movement may generate greater strength improvement than lifting at a slower rate. Furthermore, neither free weights (barbells or dumbbells) nor concentric-eccentric-type weight machines or isotonic devices are inherently superior to the other for strength development

Isometric Training (Static Exercise)

The system of isometric strength training was most popular between 1955 and 1965. Research in Germany during this time showed that an increase in isometric strength of about 5% a week could be achieved by performing a single, maximum contraction of only 1 second duration each day! Repeating this contraction between 5 and 10 times daily produced even greater increases in isometric strength.

Limitations of Isometrics. There are several limitations of isometric-static training. A major drawback of the isometric method is the difficulty in obtaining knowledge of training results. Because there is essentially no movement, it is difficult to determine objectively if the person's strength is actually improving and whether an appropriate overload force is being exerted during training. Furthermore, the measurement of isometric force requires specialized equipment such as a strain gauge or cable tensiometer not available at most exercise facilities. Another limitation is that isometric strength is developed specific to

the angle at which the force is applied. For example, pushing against an immovable object shown in Figure 13-4C will develop isometric strength at the particular joint angle at which the force is applied. *Thus, the muscle trained isometrically is stronger when measured isometrically, and particularly when measured at the specific joint angle at which the isometric overload was applied.*

Benefits of Isometrics. Isometric training is effective for developing the "total" strength of a particular muscle or group of muscles if the isometric force is applied at four or five angles through the range of motion. Isometric training is desirable for special orthopedic applications that require specific strength assessment and rehabilitation. With isometric training, the exact area of muscle weakness can be isolated and strengthening exercises administered at the proper joint angle.

Which is Better, Static or Dynamic Training?

Both static and dynamic resistance training produce significant increases in muscular strength. The training method selected, however, must be determined by the individual's particular needs and governed by the specificity of the training response.

Specificity of the Training Response. The isometrically trained muscle is stronger when measured isometrically, whereas the muscle trained dynamically is stronger when evaluated during the movement of resistance. The specificity of resistance training occurs because strength improvements result from favorable adaptations within the muscle itself, as well as in the neural organization required for a particular movement. Even when muscles are trained in a limited range of motion, they show the greatest strength improvement when evaluated in that specific range of motion. This angle-specific training response is observed for both static and dynamic resistance training.

Isometric strength training is not ideal for sports training. Isometric training can provide a relatively quick and convenient method for overloading and strengthening muscles, especially in rehabilitation medicine. Because of the specificity of the training response, however, this means of strength training is less than optimal for most sports activities that require dynamic rather than static muscle action.

You get what you train for. Not surprisingly, the "strength" you develop will depend upon the type of overload. With low resistance, high repetition, high speed training, muscle power is developed. Conversely, high resistance, low repetition, slow speed training has a greater effect on strength improvement.

Transfer of isometric strength. There is little if any transfer of isometric strength developed at one joint angle to other angles or body positions, even when the same muscles are involved.

FIGURE 13-5.
The force-generating capacity of a muscle or muscle group varies in relation to joint angle throughout the range of motion in both flexion and extension.

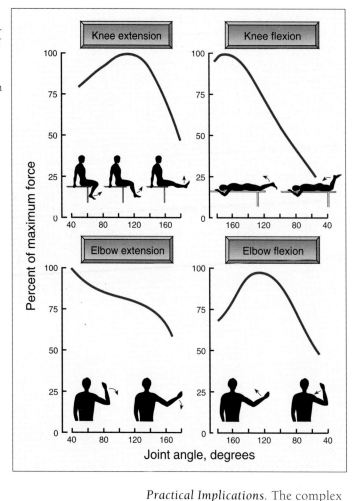

Practical Implications. The complex interaction between the nervous and muscular systems provides some explanation for why the leg muscles, when strengthened using squats or deep knee bends, do not show the same improvement in another leg movement such as jumping. Consequently, strengthening muscles for use in a specific activity such as golf, rowing, swimming, or football requires more than just identifying and overloading the muscles involved in the movement. *Rather, training should be specific to the exact movement.* There is little transfer of newly acquired strength to other patterns of movement, even though the same muscles are involved. This was clearly shown in a study of older men in which a 227% increase in leg extension strength occurred through standard weight training. When peak torque of the leg extensors was evaluated in the same subjects with an isokinetic dynamometer (see next sec-

tion), however, there was only a 10 to 17% improvement!

The importance of the angle-specific training response can be appreciated when one evaluates the "strength curves" for various muscle groups. Figure 13-5 illustrates that there are substantial differences in the maximal force curves for the flexor and extensor leg and arm muscles during maximal actions throughout the range of motion. The shape of a particular strength curve for a given muscle group is affected by two common factors: (1) the amount of force that can be developed at a given muscle length (force is least at a short muscle length), and (2) the perpendicular distance between the direction of the muscle's action and the orientation (axis) of the joint during the action. A greater perpendicular distance produces a greater *torque* or rotational force. The observed differences in the strength curves for the flexion and extension arm and leg movements illustrate the effect of the perpendicular distance between the muscle's line of pull and the resultant forces that can be produced. The "bottom line" for the coach and athlete is to pay careful attention to the muscle group(s) involved in a particular movement, and to gear training to develop maximum force-generating capacity for that muscle group throughout its range of motion at a speed that closely mimics the actual sports performance. This is impossible to accomplish with isometric actions because there is no limb movement; with isokinetic actions, relatively fast velocities of movement are possible because the speed of movement using an electromechanical dynamometers can approach 400 degrees·sec^{-1}. Even moving at this relatively "fast" speed does not approach the velocity of movement during an actual sports skill in which velocity of limb motion can exceed 1,000 degrees·sec^{-1}! During a baseball pitch, the velocity of arm motion measured about the elbow joint routinely exceeds 600-700 degrees·sec^{-1}, and the velocity of the lower limb during a football or soccer kick is nearly double the speed of the fastest electromechanical measuring device.

Isokinetic Training

Isokinetic resistance training is different from both conventional dynamic and static methods. Recall that dynamic training occurs against an external load that generally remains constant throughout the movement, whereas static training is performed at a constant angle against an immovable load. *In contrast, isokinetic training generates force during movement at a preset, fixed speed. This enables the muscle to mobilize its maximum force-generating capacity through the full range of movement while shortening.* This is done with the aid of an isokinetic dynamometer described previously.

A distinction can be made between a muscle loaded isotonically and one loaded isokinetically. Figure 13-6 shows the differences in the force curves between a bench press performed isotonically and a bench press performed isokinetically. As with all joints in the body, the maximal muscle force exerted against an external resistance varies with the bony lever configuration as the joint moves through its normal range of motion. In the bench press weight-lifting exercise with a conventional barbell, the inertia of the load must first be overcome; then execution of the movement progresses. The weight lifted can be no heavier than the maximum force capacity of the muscles at the "weakest" point in the range of motion; otherwise the movement would not be completed. Consequently, the amount of force generated by the muscles during a dynamic action cannot be maximum through all phases of the movement. Note the decrease in force output during the latter stages of the isotonic bench press. In contrast, the force curve for a muscle loaded isokinetically in the bench press (solid curve

at the top) does not decline appreciably until the end of the movement. The green line represents the calculated resistance of the electromechanical device at a preselected velocity of movement. During an isokinetic movement, the desired velocity of the limb(s) occurs almost immediately at the start of the movement, and the muscle is thereafter able to develop and maintain its peak force-generating capacity throughout the movement at the preselected, specific velocity of movement.

Experiments With Isokinetic Exercise and Training. Experiments using isokinetic exercise have been designed to explore the *force-velocity* relationships in various exercises and to relate this to the muscle's fiber composition. Figure 13-7 displays the progressive decline in concentric peak torque output in relation to increasing angular velocity of the knee extensor muscles in two groups of subjects who differed in sports training and muscle fiber composition. In the experiments that involved movement at 180 degrees per second, the power athletes and elite Swedish track and field sprinters and jumpers produced significantly higher torque values per kilogram of body mass than the other group of athletes that included competition walkers and cross-country

A coordinated integration of neuromuscular factors. The effective application of force in relatively complex, learned movements such as the tennis serve or the shot put depends on a series of coordinated neuromuscular patterns, and not simply the strength of the muscle groups required for the movement.

"Sticking point." Weight lifters frequently refer to the weakest point in their range of motion as the "sticking point."

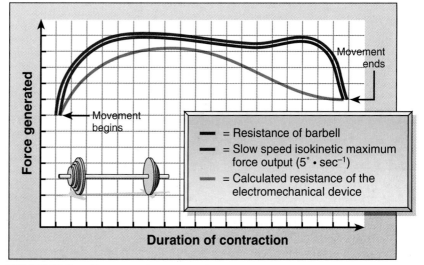

FIGURE 13-6. Differences in force curves for a bench press performed with weights and on an isokinetic dynamometer.

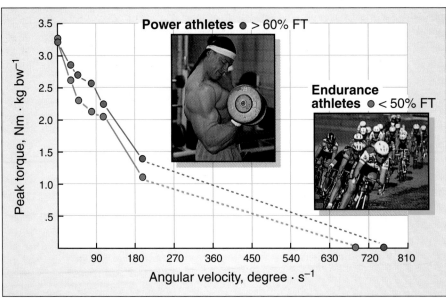

FIGURE 13-7. Peak torque output per unit body mass in relation to angular velocity in two groups of athletes with different muscle fiber composition. The torque-velocity curves were extrapolated (dashed line) to the approximated maximal velocity for knee extension. (From Throstensson, A.: Muscle strength, fiber types, and enzyme activities in man. *Acta Physiol. Scand.,* Suppl. 443, 1976.)

Force-velocity relationship. The faster the velocity of movement the less peak force the muscle can generate.

Advantage of isokinetic training. Theoretically, isokinetic training makes it possible to activate muscles maximally at all points through the range of motion at a particular speed.

Is slow training best? No definitive conclusion can be drawn as to whether fast or slow velocity training is significantly more effective for improving muscular force and power throughout the entire velocity spectrum.

runners. At this angular velocity, the maximal torque was equal to about 55% of the maximal isometric force.

The two curves in Figure 13-7 can also be distinguished in terms of peak torque depending on the group's muscle fiber composition. At zero velocity (isometric contraction), peak force was the same for athletes with relatively high or low percentages of fast-twitch fibers; this indicated that both fast- and slow-twitch motor units were activated in maximal isometric knee extension. As movement velocity increased, greater torque was achieved by individuals with a higher percentage of fast-twitch fibers. This suggests that a high percentage of fast-twitch fibers is desirable for power activities in which success is largely influenced by one's ability to generate large values for muscular torque at rapid velocities of movement.

Fast- Versus Slow-Speed Isokinetic Training. Studies have compared strength and power improvement with isokinetic training at slow and fast limb speeds. Such studies have

provided further support for the principle of specificity applied to both performance and training response. For example, several research studies support the contention that gains in "strength" from slow-speed training are highly specific to the angular velocity of movement used in training. Exercising at fast speeds gives a more general improvement because increases in power output occurred at both fast and slow velocities of movement. In fact, muscular hypertrophy was noted *only* during fast-speed training and this occurred *only* in the fast contracting type II muscle fibers. This hypertrophy possibly accounts for a more general strength improvement with fast-speed training. In the aforementioned studies, however, the greatest improvements in muscular performance occurred at the specific angular velocity and movement pattern at which training took place.

The fundamental basis for isokinetic training is attractive because muscles can be overloaded through a full range of motion at speeds somewhat similar to, but considerably slower than, specific sport and physical activities. It should be remembered that while isokinetic-type training occurs at a relatively slow but constant, preselected angular velocity of movement, there are few physical activities that are performed at a constant, relatively slow speed of joint motion. Also, the present generation of isokinetic-type dynamometers cannot provide effective overload for eccentric muscular actions that are important for limb deceleration and "braking" control of human movements. In addition, the combination of concentric-eccentric muscle actions during heavy resistance training facilitates optimal strength development compared to training that utilizes only the concentric phase of the movement. It is hypothesized that the addition of eccentric muscle action to the performance of a repetition augments neural adaptations with training, and thus facilitates strength gains.

Plyometric Training

Athletes involved in sports that require specific powerful movements such as football, volleyball, sprinting, and basketball have used a special form of exercise training drills termed *plyometrics* or explosive jump training. With plyometric exercise, movements are structured to make use of the inherent stretch-recoil characteristics of skeletal muscle as well as the modulation of a muscle's response via the stretch or myotatic reflex (see Chapter 10, page 294). Essentially with plyometric exercise, overload is applied to skeletal muscle in a manner that rapidly places the muscle on stretch (lengthening phase) immediately before the concentric phase of muscle action. This rapid lengthening phase probably facilitates a more rapid, forceful subsequent movement and hence, might augment the speed-power benefits of training.

Practical Application. A plyometric drill uses one's body mass and the force of gravity to provide the all-

important rapid prestretch or cocking phase to "activate" the muscle's natural elastic recoil elements. This then augments the subsequent concentric muscle action in the opposite direction. An example of a natural form of plyometric movement is an eccentric prestretch brought on by rapidly lowering and dropping the arms to the side before vertical jumping. Specific plyometric drills for the lower body include a standing jump, multiple jumps, repetitive jumping in place, depth-jumps or jumping from a specific height (referred to as drop jumping), single and double leg jumps, and various modifications. It is believed that repetitions of these exercises provide the proper neural and muscular training to enhance the power performance of specific muscles.

Testimonials abound as to the benefits of plyometric training, but carefully controlled evaluation is lacking of both benefits and possible orthopedic risks of such exercise. At this point, research is required to establish the appropriate role, if any, of plyometric drills in a total strength-power training program.

PHYSICAL TESTING IN THE OCCUPATIONAL SETTING: THE ROLE OF SPECIFICITY

The high degree of specificity within various components of physical performance and physiologic function such as aerobic fitness and muscular strength and power, as well as the specific nature of the training response, casts serious doubt on the assumption that broad constructs of physical fitness exist to any significant extent. Clearly, there is no one measure of muscular strength just as there is no one measure of aerobic fitness. An individual possesses an array of muscular "strengths" and "powers." Often, these expressions of physiologic function and performance are poorly related to each other if at all. Likewise, a person has

Isokinetics is widely used for rehabilitation. Isokinetic equipment is used widely in sports medicine and athletic training. Many rehabilitation programs apply isokinetic training to evaluate and improve the muscular strength and power of injured limbs over their full range of motion.

diverse capabilities for expressing aerobic function, depending on the muscle mass used. Certainly, within the occupational setting, the use of a 12-minute run to infer aerobic capacity for fire fighting or lumbering (both requiring significant upper body aerobic function), or the use of static grip or leg strength to evaluate the diverse strengths and powers required in such occupations is physiologically naive in light of current knowledge of performance specificity in exercise physiology. In the occupational setting it is imperative to apply measurement that most closely resembles the actual content of the job, not only in terms of specific tasks, but also in a manner that faithfully reflects physiologic demands in terms of the intensity, duration, and pace of the job.

SUMMARY

PART 1

1. The most common methods for measuring muscular strength are (1) tensiometry, (2) dynamometry, (3) 1-RM testing with weights, and (4) computer-assisted force and work-output determinations including isokinetic-type measurement.

2. Human skeletal muscle can generate between 3 to 8 kg of force per cm^2 of muscle cross section, regardless of gender. On an absolute basis, however, men are usually stronger than women because of the male's larger quantity of muscle mass.

3. Muscles become stronger in response to overload training. Overload is created by either increasing the load, the speed of muscular action, or a combination of these factors.

4. A load that represents 60 to 80% of a muscle's force-generating capacity is usually sufficient overload to produce strength gains.

5. Based on limited data, closely supervised resistance training programs using relatively moderate levels of concentric exercise significantly improve the muscular strength of children with no adverse effects on bone or muscle.

6. The three major systems for developing strength are progressive resistance weight training, isometrics, and isokinetic-type training. Each system results in strength gains that are highly specific to the type of training.

7. Isokinetic-type training, because of the possibility for generating maximum force throughout the full range of motion at different velocities of limb movement, may offer a unique method for resistance training that is applicable to sports performance.

8. Plyometric training drills attempt to use the inherent stretch-recoil characteristics of the neuromuscular system to facilitate the development of muscular power of specific muscles. Determining both the risks and the benefits of such training awaits further research.

9. The high degree of specificity of physiologic and performance measures, as well as their response to training, casts doubt on the wisdom of using broad or general fitness measures to infer one's ability to perform specific tasks or occupations.

Figure 13-8 displays six factors that impact on the development and maintenance of muscle mass. Without doubt, genetics provides the governing frame of reference that influences the effect of each of the other factors on the ultimate training outcome. Muscle activity, however, contributes little to tissue growth without appropriate nutrition to provide essential building blocks. Similarly, specific hormones and patterns of nervous system activation are crucial to the outcome. Without tension overload, however, each of the other factors is relatively ineffective to produce improvement.

subsequent comparisons. In one series of experiments, the researchers measured arm strength while intermittent gunshots were fired behind the subjects just before their exertions. At

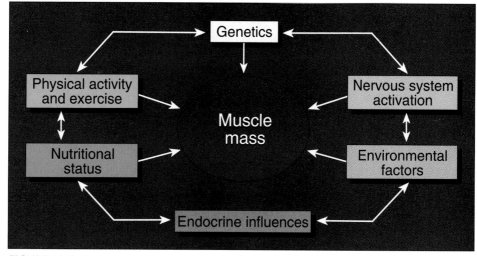

FIGURE 13-8. Six factors that impact on the development and maintenance of the body's muscle mass.

FACTORS THAT MODIFY THE EXPRESSION OF HUMAN STRENGTH

The gross structural and microscopic changes that occur within muscle tissue as a result of overload training are fairly well documented. As shown in Figure 13-9, factors broadly classified as psychological (neural) and muscular influence the expression of human strength. Many of these factors are readily modified by a resistance training program, whereas others appear to be training resistant; these are probably determined by natural endowment or are fixed early in life.

Psychological Factors

A unique series of experiments illustrated clearly the importance of psychologic factors in the expression of muscular strength. The strength of the arm muscles was determined for 17 male and 8 female subjects before various treatments. These strength scores served as the baseline for all

another time they instructed the subjects to shout or scream loudly at the moment force was exerted. Following the "shoot and shout" experiments, the experimenters measured subjects' strength under the influence of two disinhibitory drugs, alcohol and amphetamines or "pep pills." They also measured strength while subjects were in a posthypnotic state and were told their strength would be greater than ever before and they should have no fear of injury. In almost all of the psychologic conditions, arm strength was significantly greater than under normal conditions. The greatest strength increases were observed under hypnosis, the most "mental" of all the treatments.

To explain these observations the researchers suggested that physical factors such as the size and type of muscle fibers and the anatomic lever arrangement of bone and muscle ultimately determine a person's *capacity* for muscular strength. They took the

Strength increases rapidly when beginning training. An enhanced level of neural facilitation probably accounts for the rapid and significant strength increase early in training, which is not associated with an increase in muscle size and cross-sectional area.

position that psychologic or mental factors within the central nervous system exert neural influences that prevent most people from achieving this strength capacity. Neural inhibitions might be the result of social conditioning, unpleasant past experiences with physical activity, or an overprotective home environment. When performing under intense emotional conditions, such as athletic competition, an emergency situation, or posthypnotic suggestion, the inhibitory neural mechanisms are considerably reduced so the person is often capable of a "super performance" that more closely matches the physiologically determined capacity.

Observations such as these help to explain the apparent beneficial effects of "psyching" or the almost self-induced hypnosis of athletes before competition. Excellent examples of such disinhibition can be observed in weightlifters, high-jumpers and other track and field competitors, and self-defense experts who perform nontraditional skills such as smashing cement bricks with their hands and feet. The great feats of strength observed during emotionally laden emergency situations also fit nicely into this explanation. In addition, the rapid improvements in muscular strength made during the first few weeks of a strength training program may largely be due to a learning phenomenon as well as to the lessening of fear and psychologic inhibition as the person becomes more accustomed to performing in the strength activity.

Muscular Factors

Although psychologic inhibitions, as well as learning factors greatly modify ability to express muscular strength, the ultimate limit of strength development is determined by anatomic and

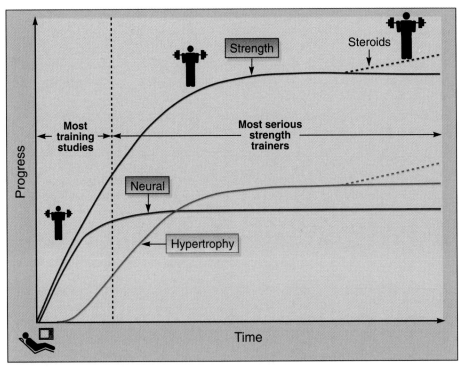

FIGURE 13-9. The relative roles of neural and muscular adaptation to strength training. Note that neural adaptation predominates in the early phase of training. This phase also encompasses most training studies. In intermediate and advanced training, progress becomes limited by the extent of muscular adaptation, notably hypertrophy — hence, there is temptation to use anabolic steroids when it becomes difficult to induce hypertrophy by training alone. (From Sale, D. G.: Neural adaptation to resistance training. *Med. Sci. Sports Exerc.*, 20:135, 1988.)

physiologic factors within the muscle. As shown in Table 13-1, these factors are not immutable but can be modified considerably with resistance training. The gross structural and microscopic changes in muscles that occur as a result of resistance training are generally limited to adaptations in the contractile mechanisms and are usually accompanied by substantial increases in muscular strength and power.

Muscle Hypertrophy. Increases in muscle size with resistance training for both men and women can be viewed as a fundamental biologic adaptation. The large muscle size of weightlifters and body builders results from an enlargement or *hypertrophy* of individual muscle cells, particularly the fast-twitch fibers. This growth results from a synthesis of biologic compounds; there is an increase in the contractile proteins, actin and myosin, as well as an increase in enzymes and stored nutrients.

Muscle Hyperplasia. Whether or not the actual number of muscle cells increases with resistance training in humans, a response called *hyperplasia,* is a question frequently raised. Researchers have reported that some muscle fibers from trained animals undergo a process of longitudinal splitting that results in the development of new fibers. However, this response may be species specific because most animals do not undergo the massive hypertrophy observed in humans with resistance training. Recent studies of bodybuilders with a relatively large muscle mass have failed to show that these athletes possessed a significant hypertrophy of individual muscle fibers. This certainly leaves open the possibility of hyperplasia in humans with resistance training. It suggests either an inherited difference in fiber number or that muscle cells may adapt differently to the high-volume, high intensity training used by body builders compared with the typical low-repe-

tition, heavy-load system favored by strength and power athletes.

Aside from enlarging existing muscle fibers, resistance training also stimulates an increase in bone mineral content as well as a proliferation of connective tissue that surrounds the individual muscle fibers. This thickens and strengthens the muscles' connective tissue harness. Resistance training also improves the structural and functional integrity of both tendons and ligaments. These adaptations provide protection from joint and muscle injury; this supports the use of resistance exercise as preventive and rehabilitative training.

RESISTANCE TRAINING FOR WOMEN

One of the more vivid illustrations of the redefining of women's roles in society has been their present participation in a wide range of competitive sport and physical activities. Although muscular strength is an important factor in achieving optimum sports performance, many women have shied away from strengthening exercises for fear of developing the enlarged muscles so commonly observed in men. This is unfortunate because the failure of some women to learn skills and improve in activities such as tennis, golf, dance, and gymnastics can be attributed to a lack of muscular strength, especially upper-body strength. A proper program of resistance training can usually improve such muscular weakness.

TABLE 13-1. Physiologic adaptations that occur in response to resistance training*

System/Variable	Response
Muscle Fibers	
Number	Equivocal
Size	Increase
Type	Unknown
Capillary Density	
In body builders	No change
In power lifters	Decrease
Mitochondrial	
Volume	Decrease
Density	Decrease
Twitch Contraction Time	Decrease
Enzymes	
Creatine phosphokinase	Increase
Myokinase	Increase
Enzymes of Glycolysis	
Phosphofructokinase	Increase
Lactate dehydrogenase	No change
Aerobic Metabolism Enzymes	
Carbohydrate	Increase
Triglyceride	Not known
Intramuscular Fuel Stores	
Adenosine triphosphate	Increase
Phosphocreatine	Increase
Glycogen	Increase
Triglycerides	Not known
max $\dot{V}O_2$	
Circuit resistance training	Increase
Heavy resistance training	No change
Connective Tissue	
Ligament strength	Increase
Tendon strength	Increase
Collagen content of muscle	No change
Bone	
Mineral content	Increase
Cross-sectional area	No change

*Modified from Fleck, S. J., and Kramer, W. J.: Resistance training: physiological responses and adaptations (Part 2 of 4). *Phys. Sportsmed.*, 16:108, 1988.

Hypertrophy versus hyperplasia. Even if hyperplasia is replicated in other human studies (and even if the response is a positive adjustment), the greatest contribution to muscular size with overload training is made by the enlargement of existing individual muscle cells.

The decline in muscular strength with age is well documented, although the cause of this decline is poorly understood. Certainly biological aging per se, the cumulative effects of disease, a sedentary lifestyle, and nutritional inadequacies are all contributing factors. If the strength decline in the elderly is largely the result of a "disuse syndrome", however, it should be possible to intervene with an appropriate program of resistance training to reverse or at least slow down the loss of muscle function.

Resistance training by the elderly is rare, mainly because of safety considerations, but also because it is widely believed that "old" muscle is not as responsive to overload training as "younger" muscle. Fortunately, recent research has seriously challenged such beliefs. In one study, ten subjects with an average age of 90.2 years participated in an 8 week resistance training program. Both concentric and eccentric muscle actions were used to train the quadriceps and hamstring muscles during a seated leg

extension/flexion movement. Training was conducted 3 days a week, and consisted of 3 sets of 8 repetitions (6 to 9 seconds per repetition) with a 1 to 2 minute rest interval between sets. During the first week of training the resistance equaled

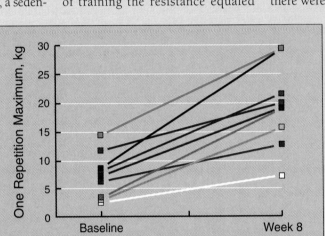

Left knee extensor strength before and after 8 weeks of high intensity training in 9 subjects, 87 to 96 years old. Similar strength gains were seen in the right leg.

50% of 1-RM (measured every 2 wks); by the second week the load was increasd to 80% 1-RM and maintained thereafter for 8 weeks.

The insert figure shows changes in 1-RM strength for the left leg from the pretraining baseline to after 8 weeks of training for each of the 9 subjects. The changes were impressive, averaging 174% (167% for the right leg). The absolute weight lifted

increasd from 8.0 kg to 20.6 kg for the right leg, and 7.6 kg to 19.3 kg for the left leg! The strength increases were progressive throughout the 8 weeks and did not tend to level off as training progressed. Furthermore, there were no differences in strength improvement between male and female subjects. An interesting finding was that each subject increased functional mobility, including ability to raise out of a chair, increased walking speed, and 2 subjects no longer needed a cane to walk. Following the resistance training program, the subjects returned to their sedentary lifestyle. After only 4 weeks of this "detraining", a 32% loss of strength was noted!

The remarkable results of this study indicate that conventional resistance training is possible (and desirable) for older-age adults and literally can reverse the effects of "aging" on muscular strength.

Reference

Fiatarone, M.A., et al: High-intensity strength training in nonagenarians. *J.A.M.A.*, 263:3029, 1990.

Muscular Strength and Hypertrophy

Despite similar percentage improvements in strength with resistance training, increases in muscle girth have been reported to be less for women. Researchers speculated that this was due to hormonal differences between the genders, especially the 20 to 30 times higher testosterone level in men that exerts a strong anabolic or tissue-building effect. It should be noted, however, that testosterone levels are on a continuum for men and women, with some females normally possessing high levels of this hormone. In addition, in several studies low correlations were reported among strength, body composition, and testosterone levels. Thus, while blood levels of testosterone may be elevated following a single weight training session, there appears to be no causal relationship between testosterone level and muscular strength or strength gains.

Experiments using computed tomography (CT) scans to directly evaluate muscle cross-sectional area indicated that the hypertrophic response to resistance training was similar for men and women. The absolute change in muscle size was certainly greater for men (because their total muscle mass was greater), but the enlargement of muscle on a percentage basis was *the same* between genders. Other comparisons between elite male and female bodybuilders have verified these observations. More research is needed before definitive statements can be made concerning similarities and differences in the resistance training responses of men and women. The limited data from relatively short-term studies do suggest that women can use conventional resistance training and gain strength on a similar percentage basis to men without developing overly large muscles.

METABOLIC STRESS OF RESISTANCE TRAINING

Numerous claims have been made concerning the physical benefits to be derived from various forms of resistance training. These include the promise of improved "organic vigor," reduced body fat, and improved aerobic and cardiovascular function. Undoubtedly, a properly planned program of resistance training is highly effective for developing and maintaining muscular strength. It does not appear, however, that traditional methods of resistance training are especially effective for programs of aerobic fitness or weight control, or for modifying risk factors related to cardiovascular disease.

Isometric and Weight-Lifting Exercise

In a series of experiments in one of our laboratories, we studied the immediate physiologic effects of isometric and resistance exercises. The resistance exercises were performed with a weight that enabled the person to complete eight repetitions of a particular movement. Isometric exercise involved a 6-second contraction performed against a bar placed in a position halfway through the range of motion of the corresponding weight-lifting exercise. In this experiment we studied the two-arm curl, two-arm press, bench press, and squat.

The results for heart rate and oxygen uptake indicated that both forms of exercise would be classified as only *light to moderate* in terms of energy expenditure, even though considerable stress is placed on the involved muscle groups. Although a person may perform 15 or 20 different resistance exercises during a 1-hour training session, the time devoted to actual exercise is short, usually no longer than 6 or 7 minutes. This brief activity period that produces only a moderate expenditure of energy indi-

Testosterone. Testosterone is the major male sex hormone responsible for promoting growth and development of the reproductive organs and secondary sex characteristics.

Gender difference. A basic gender difference in the response to resistance training appears to be the absolute amount of muscle hypertrophy.

Not a big calorie burner. Recent research indicates that the excess post-exercise oxygen consumption (EPOC) following light and heavy resistance exercise is relatively small in magnitude and duration. When the EPOC is combined with the energy cost during resistance exercise, the total kcal expended is relatively low.

cates that traditional resistance training programs would not improve endurance capacity for activities such as running or swimming. Furthermore, they would be of limited value as major activities in weight-reducing programs because the caloric expenditure is low during an exercise session.

Circuit Resistance Training

By modifying standard resistance training so that heavy overload is deemphasized, it is possible to increase the caloric cost of exercise and improve more than one aspect of physical fitness. Current research has focused on the energy cost and cardiorespiratory demands of *circuit resistance training* (CRT). In CRT, resistance exercises are performed in a pre-established exercise-rest sequence. In most programs, the circuit consists of 8 to 12 different exercise stations with a prescribed number of repetitions, usually 15 to 20, performed for each exercise. Such exercise requires between 40 and 50% of 1-RM. After a 15-second rest, the participant moves to the next exercise station and so on until the circuit is completed.

In one experiment, the energy expended during CRT was determined for 20 men and 20 women (Table 13-2). They performed three exercise circuits (10 stations per circuit using weight machines); there was a 15-second rest interval between

exercises. The total time to perform the three circuits was 22.5 minutes. The net amount of energy expended (excluding resting metabolism), was 129 kcal for the men and 95 kcal for the women over the total exercise period. The heart rates averaged 142 beats per minute (72% of maximum) for the men and 158 beats per minute (82% of maximum) for the women. This corresponded to about 40% of max $\dot{V}O_2$ for the men and 45% for the women. Because the energy expended during the circuit was related to the participant's body mass, the results in Table 13-2 are presented in terms of body mass. On average, the continuous level of energy expended in CRT was equivalent to a slow jog, hiking in the hills at a moderate pace, playing basketball, playing tennis, or leisurely swimming the crawl stroke.

This modification of standard resistance training is an attractive alternative for those fitness enthusiasts desiring a general conditioning program. It may also be a good supplemental off-season fitness program for athletes involved in sports that require a high level of strength, power, and muscular endurance.

ORGANIZING A RESISTANCE-TRAINING PROGRAM

People without previous resistance-training experience should follow a program designed to produce all-around strength improvements.

TABLE 13-2. Net energy expenditure during circuit resistance training for men and women

	Kcal Expended Per Minute*											
Body Weight, lb	100	110	120	130	140	150	160	170	180	190	200	210
Men			4.1	4.4	4.8	5.1	5.4	5.7	6.0	6.4	6.7	7.0
Women	3.4	3.6	3.7	3.9	4.1	4.3	4.4	4.6	4.8			

* Calculated from data of Wilmore, J.H., et al.: Energy cost of circuit weight training. *Med. Sci. Sports* 10:75, 1978. To determine the total number of calories expended above rest during workouts, multiply the value in the column that corresponds to your body weight by the duration of the circuit. For example, a 160-pound male who exercises on the circuit for 43 minutes would expend 232 kcal (5.4 kcal · min^{-1} x 43 min), excluding resting metabolism.

The Warm Up

The value of *preliminary warm-up exercise* to reduce the chances for muscle and joint injuries, as well as to improve subsequent performance, has been challenged over the years. Although the scientific basis for recommending a warm-up is not conclusive, we believe it would be unwise to ignore warming-up completely . Furthermore, evidence indicates that moderate preliminary exercise improves the cardiovascular response to subsequent strenuous exercise. Adjustments in blood flow within the heart muscle to a sudden, vigorous bout of exercise are not instantaneous and even healthy individuals may show a transient poor oxygen supply to the myocardium under such conditions. However, with a prior warm-up of several minutes of easy jogging, for example, adjustments in myocardial blood flow and oxygen supply are more favorable. Any sequence of calisthenic and flexibility exercises can be used as a warm-up, as well as jogging in place or other moderate rhythmic exercises. The general warm-up exercises illustrated in Figure 13-10 serve this purpose and can be completed in a few minutes. These exercises will gradually increase joint flexibility and general circulation, and may help deter muscle and joint discomfort.

The stretching exercises should be done slowly and smoothly until a mild tension is felt in the muscles. The goal is not to complete many repetitions of the particular movement, but rather to hold the stretch. A reasonable goal is to hold the stretch for 10 seconds in the beginning; as flexibility improves, increase the duration of the static stretch to 30 seconds.

The Lower Back

The lower back is susceptible to injury. Many people lose considerable time at work, suffer chronic discomfort, and spend large amounts of money on orthopedists and chiropractors attempting to alleviate lower-back pain. In fact, it has been estimated that one-half of the work force in the United States will suffer from back problems at some point in their career! The causes for this malady are not always apparent and a cure is elusive. However, many orthopedists believe the prime factors in "low back syndrome" are muscular weakness, especially in the abdominal region, and poor joint flexibility in the back and legs. Both strengthening and flexibility exercises are commonly prescribed for the prevention of and rehabilitation from chronic low back strain.

The use of resistance training exercises poses a dilemma. If done properly, such training provides an excellent means to strengthen the muscles of the abdomen and lower back to support and protect the spine. As is often the case, however, many people, attempting to create too much force, perform an exercise improperly. As a result, additional muscle groups are recruited, the spinal column is placed in improper alignment, especially with the arching of the back, and lower-back strain results. A seemingly simple exercise such as a sit-up, if done improperly with the legs stiff, the back arched and the head thrown back, can place tremendous strain on the lower spine (sit-ups should always be done with the knees flexed and chin tucked to chest). Pressing and curling exercises with weights, if performed with excessive hyperextension or arch to the back may cause muscle strain or spinal pressure that can trigger lower-back pain. For these reasons, those who begin a program of strengthening exercises are urged to do all exercises correctly in the manner described.

Selecting the Proper Load

In the beginning stages of training, one should not attempt to see how much weight can be lifted. This serves little purpose in improving strength

Hold that stretch! Stretching that employs fast bouncing and jerky movement that uses the body's momentum can strain or tear muscles and may create a reflex action that actually resists the muscle's stretching.

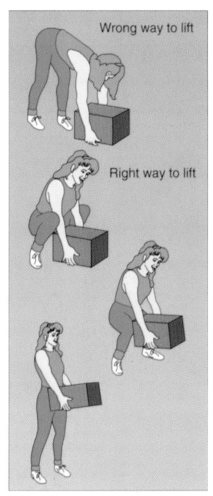

Proper lifting mechanics avoids musculoskeletal injuries. *(Top)* The wrong way to lift an object. *(Bottom)* The right way to lift an object. Maintain a wide base of support by keeping the feet wider apart than shoulder width. After you grasp the object, stand up using the power of the leg muscles and keeping the head up and back straight as you straighten up.

FIGURE 13-10. Calisthenic and flexibility exercises that can be performed as part of general warm-up prior to more vigorous activities.

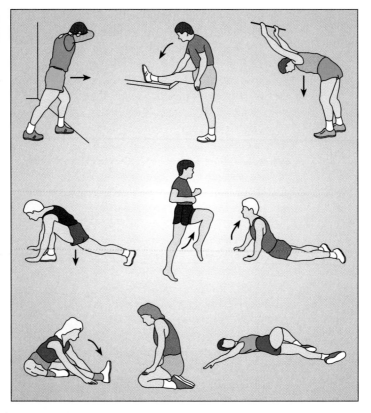

Sit up exercise

Correct

1. Knees bent
2. Chin tucked into chest
3. Rise up to any one of the four trunk angles
4. Maintain control
5. Reverse sequence by uncurling to starting position

Incorrect

1. Legs straight
2. Arched back when raising trunk off surface
3. Bounce

repetitions, the weight is too heavy. This is a trial-and-error process and it may take several exercise sessions before a proper starting weight is selected.

After 5 or 6 training sessions the muscles will begin to adapt and the exerciser will have learned the correct lifting movements. The number of repetitions should now be reduced to between 6 and 8 and the resistance increased accordingly. When the exerciser can complete 8 repetitions, add more weight. This additional weight will undoubtedly reduce the number of repetitions. This is exactly the desired outcome. Eight repetitions should be achieved within several exercise sessions, and again, more weight will have to be added.

The exercises are performed in the same order on each workout day. This is because many exercises involve more than one muscle group, and some fatigue may result from a previous exercise. By maintaining the same order of exercise, the cumulative fatigue effect should remain relatively constant. In scheduling workouts, consistency is the key to successful training. This does not mean that workouts should be scheduled every day. At least 2 or 3 exercise sessions each week are necessary to continue strength improvements. Some people exercise 5 or 6 days a week. With this protocol different muscle groups are usually exercised on alternate days, so in reality, a specific muscle group is still trained only 2 or 3 days a week. Section III of the *Student Study Guide and Workbook* presents selected tests for the measurement of muscular strength and endurance, and joint flexibility.

and greatly increases the likelihood of muscle or joint injury. Also, it is unnecessary to exercise at maximum levels to develop muscular strength. A load that represents between 60 and 80% of a muscle's maximum strength (1-RM) is sufficient overload for improvement. This resistance permits the completion of between 6 and 10 repetitions of a particular exercise when using barbells or exercise machines. Our experience has shown that beginners should aim to complete 12 repetitions of an exercise. If the weight selected for the 12 repetitions feels "too easy," a heavier weight should be used. If the exerciser cannot do 12

MUSCLE SORENESS AND STIFFNESS

Following an extended layoff from exercise, most of us have experienced soreness and stiffness in the exercised muscles and joints. A temporary soreness may persist for several hours immediately after unaccustomed exercise, whereas a residual soreness may appear later and last for 3 to 4 days. Any one of at least five factors may be the causative agent:

* Minute tears in the muscle tissue itself
* Osmotic pressure changes that cause retention of fluids in the surrounding tissues
* Muscle spasms
* Overstretching and perhaps tearing of portions of the muscle's connective tissue harness
* Alterations in the cell's mechanism for calcium regulation

Predominantly with Eccentric Actions

Although the precise cause of muscle soreness remains unknown, the degree of discomfort depends to a large extent on the intensity and duration of effort and the type of exercise performed. *Eccentric and to some extent isometric muscular actions generally cause the greatest postexercise discomfort.* This effect does not relate to lactate build up because level running (concentric contractions) produced no residual soreness despite significant elevations in blood lactate. Downhill running (eccentric actions) caused moderate-to-severe *delayed onset muscle soreness* (DOMS) with no elevation in lactate during or after exercise.

Actual Cell Damage

In a study that used downhill running, significant DOMS developed 42 hours postexercise. There were also corresponding increases for the serum levels of the muscles' specific enzyme, creatine kinase (CK), and

myoglobin (Mb), both of which are used commonly as markers of muscle injury. The subjects were then retested on the same exercise after 3, 6, and 9 weeks. Figure 13-11 shows the perceived soreness rating for the leg muscles as a function of time postexercise for the three study durations. For the 3- and 6-week comparisons, the differences between bouts were significant with diminished DOMS noted in the second trial (open squares). The pattern of results for CK and Mb was similar to the perception of muscle soreness. It is interesting that peak soreness ratings achieved at 48 hours did not correlate with the absolute or relative changes in CK or Mb. That is, individuals reporting the greatest soreness did not necessarily have the highest CK and Mb values.

The first bout of repetitive, high-intensity exercise may disrupt the integrity of the cellular environment and produce temporary ultrastructural muscle damage in a pool of stress-susceptible or degenerating muscle fibers. This damage becomes more extensive several days after exercise than in the immediate postexercise period. Of interest is that a single bout of exercise has a significant prophylactic effect on the development of muscle soreness in subsequent exercise, and this effect appears to last for up to 6 weeks. Such results support the wisdom of initiating a training program with light exercise to protect against the muscle soreness that is almost sure to follow an initial heavy exercise bout that contains an eccentric component. However, even prior lower-intensity exercise of specific muscles does not provide complete protection from subsequent soreness with more intense exercise.

Always use the proper technique. One should never sacrifice proper execution to lift a heavier load or "squeeze out" an additional repetition. The extra weight lifted through improper technique will not facilitate muscle strengthening, and may precipitate lower-back injury.

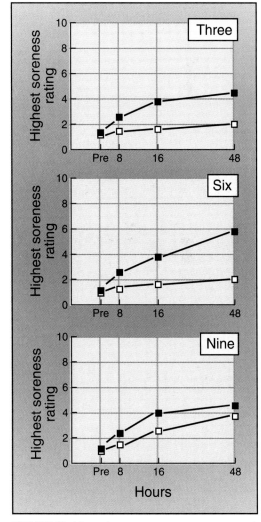

FIGURE 13-11. Highest soreness rating prior to and 6, 18, and 48 hours following bout 1 (closed square) and bout 2 (open square) performed either 3, 6, or 9 weeks later. Similar results were obtained for creatine kinase and myoglobin. (From Byrnes, W. C., et al.: Delayed onset muscle soreness following repeated bouts of downhill running. *J. Appl. Physiol.*, 59:710, 1985.)

Experimental Studies

Four theories have been proposed to explain DOMS.

Spasm Hypothesis. Several experiments provide evidence to support the spasm hypothesis of muscle soreness. In one study, soreness was produced in both arms by repeated wrist hyperextensions against a 4.3-kg resistance. The muscles of one arm were then stretched by the static technique. This was beneficial because significantly greater levels of soreness occurred 24 and 48 hours after exercise in the arm that was not stretched after exercise. In another study, the resting electromyographic (EMG) activity of the anterior lower leg muscles was evaluated as a consequence of static stretching procedures in subjects with shin splints, a musculoskeletal disorder involving severe pain in the anterior portion of the lower leg. Static stretching procedures brought about symptomatic relief and marked reductions in EMG activity. It is noteworthy, however, that postexercise stretching has not consistently been shown to alleviate DOMS.

Tear Theory. As already discussed, the tear theory of muscle soreness proposes that minute tears or ruptures of individual fibers cause the delayed soreness. Because eccentric actions can place greater strain on connective tissue and muscle fibers compared with concentric muscle action, it is likely that these eccentric actions increase the likelihood of structural changes in muscle fibers with a resulting enzyme efflux.

Excess Metabolite Theory. A competing excess metabolite theory proposes that prolonged exercise that follows a layoff causes an accumulation of metabolites in the muscle. This accumulation triggers osmotic changes in the cellular environment and fluid is retained. The edema caused by increased osmotic pressure excites sensory nerve endings and causes pain. This explanation is inadequate. It

should be recalled that muscle soreness was much greater after eccentric exercise than after static or concentric actions. The metabolic stress of concentric (positive) work, however, is usually about 5 to 7 times greater than that of eccentric work. Consequently, one would expect the metabolite buildup and accompanying soreness to be greater in the concentric exercise and not in the eccentric exercise, as is generally reported.

Connective Tissue Damage. In some studies, muscle soreness was induced by repeated bouts of arm-curl, weight-lifting exercise, and bench stepping. Several measures were employed to evaluate the degree of soreness and to shed light on possible causative mechanisms. Surface electrodes recorded the EMG activity of the muscles for durations up to 48 hours. Urine samples were obtained at selected intervals to detect postexercise myoglobinuria, because the presence of myoglobin in the urine is an indicator of trauma to muscle fibers. Urinary levels of hydroxyproline were measured to evaluate connective tissue damage. This assay is useful for determining specific breakdown products of connective tissue and for evaluating collagen metabolism. Subjects also rated the degree of muscle soreness by a subjective rating scale. Analysis of these results showed no relationship between muscle pain and EMG activity in the sore muscles. When static stretching procedures were used to alleviate the soreness, there was no change in EMG activity, although pain was reduced somewhat for 1 to 2 minutes. In fact, slowly flexing and extending the arm relieved the pain to the same extent as the static stretching procedures!

Interesting results were observed for the hydroxyproline excretion rates in relation to muscle soreness produced by bench stepping. As a result of stepping, all subjects reported soreness in both the concentric (quadriceps) and the eccentric (gastrocnemius) active muscles. There were statistically significant increases in the 48-hour postexercise hydroxyproline levels and in the total 4-day average excretion levels for the exercise as compared to the nonexercise condition. The significant increase in hydroxyproline 48 hours after exercise, coupled with the fact that subjects complained of pain in the tendons of the eccentrically exercised muscles, suggests that connective tissue damage in and around the muscles, or an imbalance of collagen metabolism (a degradation process), is somehow involved in exercise-induced muscle soreness. Figure 13-12 is a flow diagram that lists the probable steps in the development of DOMS and subsequent recuperation.

Fiber-type specific. Muscle damage appears to be concentrated in the fast-twitch fibers with low oxidative capacity.

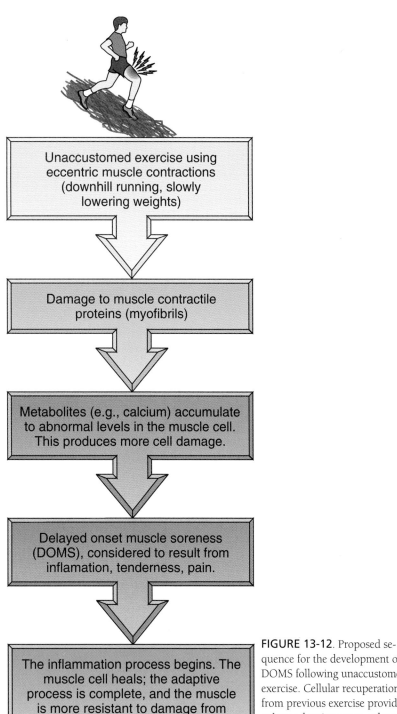

Unaccustomed exercise using eccentric muscle contractions (downhill running, slowly lowering weights)

Damage to muscle contractile proteins (myofibrils)

Metabolites (e.g., calcium) accumulate to abnormal levels in the muscle cell. This produces more cell damage.

Delayed onset muscle soreness (DOMS), considered to result from inflamation, tenderness, pain.

The inflammation process begins. The muscle cell heals; the adaptive process is complete, and the muscle is more resistant to damage from subsequent exercise.

FIGURE 13-12. Proposed sequence for the development of DOMS following unaccustomed exercise. Cellular recuperation from previous exercise provides enhanced resistance to subsequent damage and pain.

PART 2

1. Genetic, exercise, nutritional, hormonal, environmental, and neural factors interact to regulate skeletal muscle mass and corresponding strength development.

2. A person's capacity for muscular strength is largely determined by physiologic factors such as size and type of muscle fibers, as well as by the anatomic-lever arrangement of bone and muscle. This strength capacity is probably greatly affected by neural influences from the central nervous system that activate the prime movers in a specific muscular action.

3. Increases in strength with resistance training result from improved capacity for neuromuscular activation as well as significant alterations in the contractile elements within the muscle cell itself.

4. As muscles are overloaded and become stronger, they normally hypertrophy or grow larger. This process involves increased protein synthesis for the contractile elements within the muscle cell and proliferation of connective tissue cells that thicken and strengthen the muscle's connective tissue harness.

5. Muscular hypertrophy generally involves structural changes within the contractile mechanism of individual fibers, especially the fast-twitch fibers, as well as increases in anaerobic energy stores. If new muscle fibers actually develop, their contribution to muscular enlargement is as yet undetermined.

6. Heavy resistance training does not bring about adaptations in cellular components that would contribute to enhanced local aerobic energy transfer.

7. In short-term training studies, strength improvements for women on a percentage basis are similar to those of men. Research also indicates that women are capable of significant increases in muscle mass as a result of resistance training.

8. Conventional resistance-training exercises per se contribute little to cardiovascular-aerobic fitness. Because of their relatively low caloric cost, they also would not be effective major activities in weight-reducing programs.

9. By use of lower resistance and higher repetitions, circuit resistance training offers an effective alternative for combining the muscle-training benefits of resistance exercise with the cardiovascular caloric-burning benefits of more continuous exercise.

10. Significantly greater delayed-onset muscle soreness occurs in eccentric muscular actions compared with concentric only or isometric exercise.

11. A single bout of exercise has a significant protective effect on the development of muscle soreness and damage in subsequent exercise. This supports the wisdom of gradual progression when beginning an exercise program.

12. There is significant experimental evidence to support the argument for muscle tears and connective tissue damage as the cause for delayed onset muscle soreness. Disruption of the sarcoplasmic reticulum and associated changes in calcium regulation may also contribute to cellular damage.

Abernethy, P. J., and Quigley, B. M.: Concurrent strength and endurance training of the elbow flexors. *J. Strength and Cond. Res.*, 7:234, 1993.

Allerheiligen, W.B.: Speed development and plyometric training. In: *Essentials of Strength Training and Conditioning.* Baechle, T.R. m(ed.). Champaign, IL., Human Kinetics, 1994.

Alway, S. E., et al.: Functional and structural adaptations in skeletal muscle of trained athletes. *J. Appl. Physiol.*, 64:1114, 1988.

Alway, S. E., et al.: Contrasts in muscle and myofibers of elite male and female body builders. *J. Appl. Physiol.*, 67:24, 1989.

Antonio, J., and Gonyea, W.J.: Skeletal muscle fiber hyperplasia. *Med. Sci. Sports Exerc.*, 25: 1333, 1993.

Baker, D., et al: Periodization: the effect on strength of manipulating volume and intensity. *J. Strength. Cond. Res.* 8(4): 235, 1994.

Ballor, D. L., et al.: Metabolic response to nine different exercise:rest protocols. *Med. Sci. Sports Exerc.*, 21:90, 1989.

Bembem, M. G., et al.: Isometric muscle force production as a function of age in healthy 20- to 74-year-old men. *Med. Sci. Sports Exerc.*, 23: 1302, 1992.

Billeter, R. and Hoppeler, H. Muscular basis of strength. In: (ed. Homi, P.). *Strength and Power in Sport.* Blackwell Scientific Publications. London. 1992.

Boocock, M. G., et al.: Changes in stature following drop jumping and post-exercise gravity inversion. *Med. Sci. Sports Exerc.*, 22:385, 1990.

Bulbulian, R, et al.: Effect of downhill running on motoneuron pool excitability. *J. Appl. Physiol.*, 73:968, 1992.

Buroker, K. C., and Schwane, J. A.: Does post-exercise stretching alleviate delayed muscle soreness? *Phys. Sportsmed.*, 17:65, 1989.

Clarkson, P. M., and Trembly, I.: Exercise induced muscle damage, repair, and adaptation in humans. *J. Appl. Physiol.*, 65:1, 1988.

Coggan, A.R., et al.: Skeletal muscle adaptations to endurance training in 60- to 70-yr old men and women. *J. Appl. Physiol.*, 72: 1780, 1992.

Cureton, K. J., et al.: Muscle hypertrophy in men and women. *Med. Sci. Sports Exerc.*, 20:338, 1988.

DeLorme, T. L., and Watkins, A. L.: *Progressive Resistance Exercise.* New York, Appleton-Century-Crofts, 1951.

Dudley, G. A., et al.: Importance of eccentric actions in performance adaptations to resistance training. *Aviat. Space Environ. Med.*, 62:543, 1991.

Evans, W. J., and Cannon, J. G.: The metabolic effects of exercise-induced muscle damage. In *Exercise and Sport Sciences Reviews.* Vol. 19. Edited by J. O. Holloszy. Baltimore, Williams & Wilkins, 1991.

Fiatarone, M.A., et al.: Exercise training and nutritional supplementation for physical frailty in very elderly people. *N. Engl. J. Med.*, 330: 1769, 1994.

Fogelholm, F. M., et al.: Low-dose amino acid supplementation: No effect on serum human growth hormone and insulin in male weight lifters. *Int. J. Sport Nutr.*, 3:290, 1993.

Frontera, W. R., et al.: Strength conditioning in older men: skeletal muscle hypertrophy and improved function. *J. Appl. Physiol.*, 64:1038, 1988.

Gonyea, W. J., et al.: Exercise induced increases in muscle fiber number. *Eur. J. Appl. Physiol.*, 55:137, 1986.

Graves, J. E., et al.: Specificity of limited range of motion variable resistance training. *Med. Sci. Sports Exerc.*, 21:84, 1989.

Haennel, R., et al.: Effects of hydraulic circuit training on cardiovascular function. *Med Sci. Sports Exerc.*, 21:605, 1985.

Heyward, V. H., et al.: Gender differences in strength. *Res. Q. Exerc. Sport,* 57:154, 1986.

Hochschuler, S. *Back in Shape.* Boston, Houghton Mifflin Co., 1991.

Hortobagyi, T., and Katch, F. I.: Role of concentric force in limiting improvement in muscular strength. *J. Appl. Physiol.*, 68:659, 1990.

Hurley, B. F., et al.: Effects of high intensity strength training on cardiovascular function. *Med. Sci. Sports Exerc.*, 16:483, 1984.

Ikai, M., and Steinhaus, A. H.: Some factors modifying the expression of human strength. *J. Appl. Physiol.*, 16:157, 1961.

Katch, F. I., et al.: Evaluation of acute cardiorespiratory responses to hydraulic resistance exercise. *Med. Sci. Sports Exerc.*, 17:168, 1985.

Keleman, M. H.: Resistance training safety and assessment guidelines for cardiac and coronary prone patients. *Med. Sci. Sports Exerc.*, 21:675, 1989.

Kokkinos, P. F., et al.: Strength training does not improve lipoprotein-lipid profiles in men at risk for CHD. *Med Sci. Sports Exerc.*, 23:1134, 1991.

Kraemer, W. J., et al.: Changes in hormonal concentrations after different heavy-resistance exercise protocols in women. *J. Appl. Physiol.*, 75: 594, 1993.

Larson, L., and Tesch, P. A.: Motor unit fibre density in extremely hypertrophied skeletal muscles in man. Electrophysiological signs of muscle fibre hyperplasia. *Eur. J. Appl. Physiol.*, 55:130, 1986.

Lieber, R.L. et al.: In vivo measurement of human wrist extensor muscle sarcomere length changes. *J. Appl. Physiol.* 874, 1994.

Lieber, R.L., and Fridén, J.: Muscle damage is not a function of muscle force but active muscle strain. *J. Appl. Physiol.*, 74: 520, 1993.

Lieber, R.L.: *Skeletal Muscle Structure and Function.* Williams & Wilkins, Baltimore. 1992.

Lowe, D.A., et al.: Eccentric contraction-induced injury of mouse soleus muscle: effect of varying [Ca++]. *J. Appl. Physiol.*, 76: 1445, 1994.

Luthi, J. M., et al.: Structural changes in skeletal muscle tissue with heavy-resistance exercise. *Int. J. Sports Med.*, 7:123, 1986.

MacDougall, J. D., et al.: Muscle fiber number in biceps brachii in body builders and control subjects. *J. Appl. Physiol.*, 57:1399, 1984.

MacDougall, J. D.: Morphological changes in human skeletal muscle following strength training and immobilization. In *Human Muscle Power.* Edited by N. L. Jones, et al., Champaign, IL, Human Kinetics, 1986.

Mayhew, J. L., et al.: Assessing bench press power in college football players: the seated shot put. *J. Strength and Cond. Res.*, 7:90, 1993.

McArdle, W. D., and Foglia, G. F.: Energy cost and cardiorespiratory stress of isometric and weight training exercise. *J. Sports Med. Phys. Fit.*, 9:23, 1969.

McCartney, N., et al.: Weight-training induced attenuation of the circulatory response of older males to weight lifting. *J. Appl. Physiol.*, 74: 1056, 1993.

Nichols, D.L., et al.: Relationship of regional body composition to bone mineral density in college females. *Med. Sci. Sports Exerc.*, 27: 178, 1995.

Olds, T.S., and Abernethy, P.J.: Post exercise oxygen consumption following heavy and light resistance exercise. *J. Strength and Cond. Res.*, 7:147, 1993.

Ozmun, J.C., et al.: Neuromuscular adaptations following prepubescent strength training. *Med. Sci. Sports Exerc.*, 26: 510, 1994.

Ploutz, L.L., et al.: Effect of resistance training on muscle use during exercise. *J. Appl. Physiol.*, 76: 1675, 1994.

Rayment, I., et al.: Structure of the actin-myosin complex and its implications for muscle contraction. *Science*, 261 (July 2): 58, 1993.

Rayment, I., et al.: Three-dimensional structure of myosin subfragment-1: a molecular motor. *Science*, 261 (July 2): 50, 1993.

Rice, C.L., et al.: Strength training alters contractile properties of the triceps brachii in men aged 65-78 years. *Eur. J. Appl. Physiol.*, 66: 275, 1993.

Roy, R.R., and Edgerton, V.R.: Skeletal muscle architecture and performance. In: (ed) Komi, P.V. *Strength and Power in Sport*. Blackwell Scientific. Boston, 1992.

Roundtable: practical considerations for utilizing plyometrics. *NSCA Journal*, 8(3):14, 1986.

Roy, R. R., et al.: The plasticity of skeletal muscle: effects of neuromuscular activity. In *Exercise and Sport Sciences Reviews*. Vol. 19. Edited by J. O. Holloszy. Baltimore, Williams & Wilkins, 1991.

Sale, D. G.: Influence of exercise and training on motor unit activation. In *Exercise and Sport Sciences Reviews*. Vol. 15. Edited by K. B. Pandolf. New York, Macmillan, 1987.

Sipalä, S., and Suominen, H.: Effects of strength and endurance training on thigh and leg muscle mass and composition in elderly women. *J. Appl. Physiol.*, 78: 334, 1995.

Sjöström, M., et al.: Evidence of fiber hyperplasia in human skeletal muscles from healthy young men. *Eur. J. Appl. Physiol.*, 62: 301, 1992.

Smith, L. L.: Acute inflammation: the underlying mechanism in delayed onset muscle soreness. *Med. Sci. Sports Exerc.*, 23:542, 1991.

Sparling, P. S., and Cantwell, J. A.: Strength training guidelines for cardiac patients. *Phys. Sportsmed.*, 17:191, 1989.

Stauber, W. T.: Eccentric action of muscles: Physiology, injury, and adaptation. In *Exercise and Sport Sciences Reviews*. Vol. 17. Edited by K. B. Pandolf. Baltimore, Williams & Wilkins, 1989.

Staron, R.S., et al.: Skeletal muscle adaptations during the early phase of heavy-resistance training in men and women. *J. Appl. Physiol.*, 76: 1247, 1994.

Staron, R.S., et al.: Strength and skeletal muscle adaptations in heavy-resistance-trained women after detraining and retraining. *J. Appl. Physiol.*, 70: 631, 1991.

Tesch, P. A.: Skeletal muscle adaptations consequent to long-term heavy resistance exercise. *Med. Sci. Sports Exerc.*, 20:S132, 1988.

Vailas, A.C., and Vailas, J.C.: Physical activity and connective tissue. In *Physical Activity, Fitness, and Health*. In Bouchard, C., et al., Champaign, IL, Human Kinetics, 1994.

Wathan, D. Periodization: concepts and applications. In: *Essentials of Strength Training and Conditioning*. (ed: Baechle, T.R.) Human Kinetics, Champaign, IL 1994. pages 459-472.

Weir, J.P., et al.: Electromyographic evaluation of joint angle specificity and cross-training after isometric training. *J. Appl. Physiol.*, 77: 1927, 1994.

Weltman, A. W., et al.: The effects of hydraulic resistance strength training in pre-pubertal males. *Med. Sci. Sports Exerc.*, 18:629, 1986.

Yarasheski, K.E., et al.: Acute effects of resistance exercise on muscle protein synthesis in young and elderly adults. *Am. J. Physiol.*, 265: E 210, 1993.

FACTORS AFFECTING PHYSIOLOGIC FUNCTION, ENERGY TRANSFER, AND PERFORMANCE

Coaches and athletes are continually searching for ways to gain the competitive "edge" and improve athletic performance. It is not surprising, therefore, that a variety of substances and procedures are used routinely at almost all competitive levels, often without regard for potential health dangers or lack of scientific evidence to support their effectiveness. Drugs are used most often by college and professional athletes, whereas nutrition supplementation and warm-up procedures are common to men and women who train for fitness and sport activities.

In many instances the environment influences the body's physiology in a way that augments the stress of exercise and impairs performance. Sport activities are held at altitudes that impair the normal oxygenation of blood flowing through the lungs. Above a certain elevation, the capacity to generate aerobic energy for exercise is severely limited. Exercising in a hot, humid environment or under conditions of extreme cold can impose a severe thermal stress. The total effect of each environmental stressor is clearly determined by the degree to which it deviates from neutral conditions as well as by the duration of the exposure. In addition, several environmental stressors operating at the same time (e.g., extreme cold exposure at high altitude) may exceed and override the simple additive effects of each stressor were it imposed singularly.

In chapters 14 and 15, we explore a variety of substances and "treatments" alleged to improve working capacity or athletic performance. Also presented is a discussion of the specific problems encountered at altitude and during exercise in hot and cold environments. This information is presented within the framework of the immediate physiologic adjustments and long-term adaptations as the body strives to maintain internal consistency despite an environmental challenge.

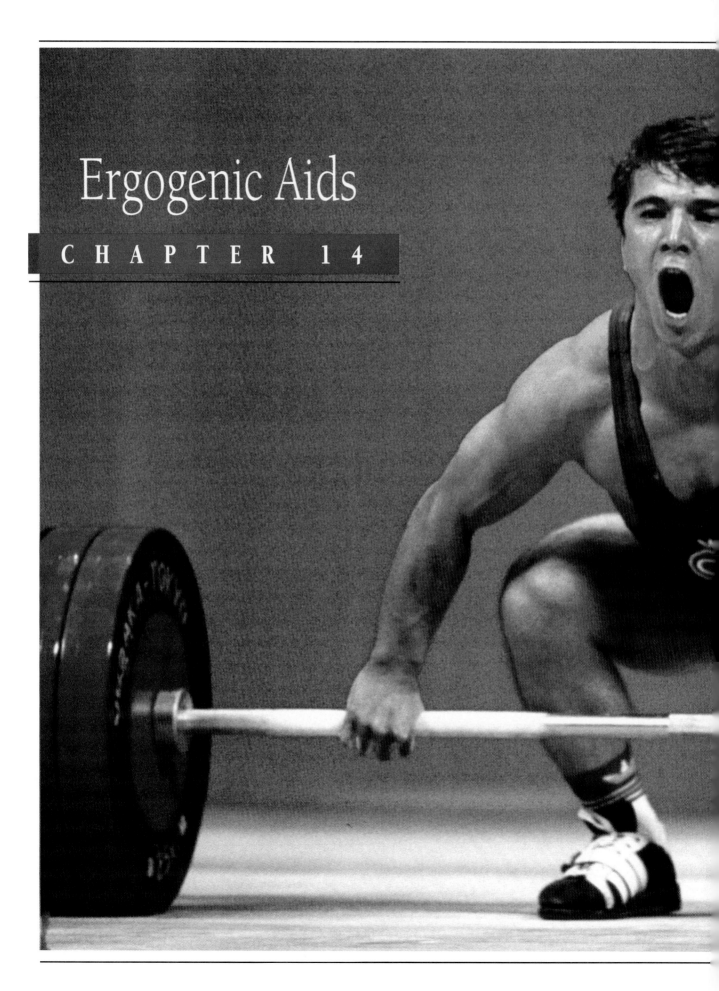

Ergogenic Aids

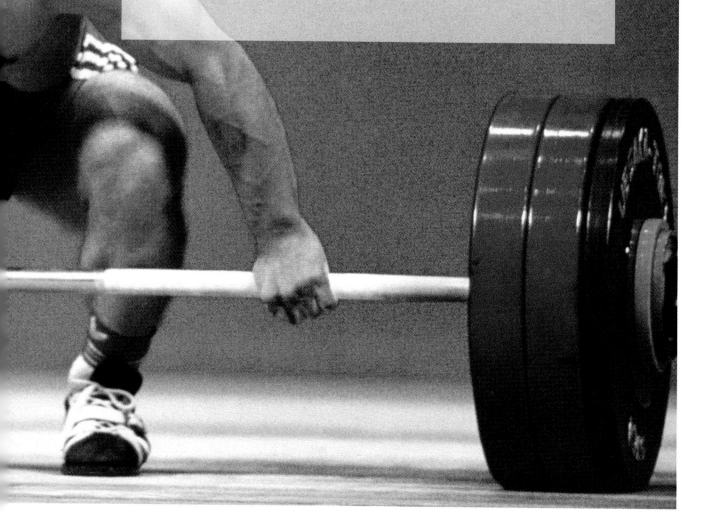

After reading this chapter you should be able to:

- Define the term ergogenic aid.
- Give examples of substances and procedures commonly believed to offer an ergogenic benefit.
- Advise an athlete about taking anabolic steroids to increase muscle mass and sports performance. Discuss the mode of action of anabolic steroids, their effectiveness, and the risks involved for males and females.
- Describe research studies that show the ergogenic benefits and risks of taking amphetamines, caffeine, and buffering solutions.
- Discuss the medical use of human growth hormone, and the potential dangers to healthy athletes using this drug.
- Describe the procedure for red blood cell reinfusion, and why this procedure enhances endurance performance and aerobic capacity.
- Define the terms "general warm-up" and "specific warm-up".
- Describe the potential cardiovascular benefits of prior warm-up.
- Give the rationale for breathing hyperoxic gas mixtures to enhance exercise performance. How much additional oxygen is made available to the body with this procedure?

Considerable literature exists on the topic of ergogenic aids and athletic performance. It includes studies of the potential performance benefits of alcohol, amphetamines, hormones, carbohydrates and proteins, additional red blood cells, caffeine, phosphates, oxygen-rich breathing mixtures, wheatgerm oil, vitamins, minerals, ionized air, music, warm-up, hypnosis, and even marijuana and cocaine. Only a few of these alleged aids, however, are used routinely by athletes and only a few cause real controversy. In this chapter we review the use of anabolic steroids and amphetamines and the unique procedure of "blood doping." Because warm-up and oxygen administration are in common use, we also include their practical implications for human exercise physiology and performance. Evaluation of the ergogenic effects of supplements of the micro- and macronutrients is presented in the specific chapter dealing with these nutrients.

PHARMACOLOGIC AGENTS

Many athletes use a variety of pharmacologic agents in the belief that a specific drug will enhance skill, strength, or endurance. In our drug-oriented, competitive culture, it is not surprising to find drug use for ergogenic purposes on the upswing among high school and even junior high school athletes. When winning becomes all important, one can do little to prevent the use and abuse of drugs by athletes, even if little "hard" scientific evidence exists between drug use and improved athletic performance. It seems ironic that athletes go to great lengths to promote all aspects of their health. They train hard, they eat well-balanced meals, they seek and receive medical advice for various injuries (no matter how minor), and yet they willingly ingest synthetic agents, many of which can precipitate side effects ranging from nausea, hair loss, itching, and nervous irritability, to severe consequences such as sterility, liver disease, drug addiction, and even death caused by liver and blood cancer in an effort to improve performance.

We now take a closer look at two categories of drugs often used by athletes — anabolic steroids and amphetamines.

Anabolic Steroids

Structure and Action. An anabolic steroid is a drug that functions in a manner similar to that of the male hormone testosterone. By binding with special receptor sites on muscle and various other tissues, this hormone greatly contributes to the male secondary sex characteristics, and to the gender differences in muscle mass and strength that begin to develop at the onset of puberty. The hormone's *androgenic* or masculinizing effects can be minimized by synthetically manipulating the chemical structure of the steroid so that the cell's anabolic tissue-building, nitrogen-retaining process is emphasized for purposes of promoting increased muscular growth. Nevertheless, the masculinizing effect is still noticeable, especially when the drug is used by females. Athletes who take these drugs do so usually during their competitive years, often taking a progressively increasing combined steroid dose in both oral and injectable form — called "stacking" — far in excess of the recommended medical dose. The dose is then progressively reduced in the months before competition to reduce chances of detection.

Male and female athletes most frequently take steroids in conjunction with a resistance training program and augmented protein intake. The aim of steroid use is to improve performance in sports that emphasize strength, speed, and power. The fact that many athletes get their steroids on the "black market" raises the fear that misinformed individuals may take a massive, prolonged dose of the

Another drug for abuse. Federal authorities conservatively estimate that the emerging illegal trafficking in steroids exceeds 100 million dollars yearly and is growing rapidly. Particularly worrisome is steroid use among an estimated half million adolescents and its accompanying effects including extreme virilization and premature cessation of bone growth.

drug without any medical monitoring for possible harmful alterations in physiologic function.

Are They Effective? The use of anabolic steroids in sports has generated considerable controversy. Testimonials abound as to the muscular size and performance benefits from steroid use. This situation has been further aggravated by the disqualification and suspension of numerous elite amateur and professional athletes for steroid use. Aside from the moral and ethical issues, this is unfortunate because of the conflicting scientific data as to the degree that they exert a positive influence on muscular growth and performance in normal, healthy athletes.

Much of the confusion as to the ergogenic effectiveness of anabolic steroids has been due to variations in experimental design, poor controls, differences in specific drugs, and dosages (50 to >200 mg per day versus the usual medical dosage of 5 to 20 mg), treatment duration, training intensity, measurement techniques, previous experience as subjects, individual variation in response, and nutritional supplementation. There is also speculation that the relatively small residual androgenic action of the anabolic steroid acts via the central nervous system to facilitate improvements by making the athlete more aggressive, competitive, and fatigue resistant so that he or she trains harder for a longer period of time, or gains the impression that augmented training effects are taking place while using the drug.

The Risks Involved. In our opinion, the infrequent but distinct possibility of harmful side effects from anabolic steroid abuse greatly outweighs any potential performance benefits to be gained from steroid treatment. In addition, high doses of anabolic steroids can lead to a long-lasting impairment of normal testosterone-endocrine function. In fact, a study of five male power athletes showed that the cessation of 26 weeks of

steroid administration brought about a reduction in serum testosterone to levels that were less than half that seen at the beginning of the study; this effect lasted throughout the 12 to 16 week follow-up period. Other accompanying hormonal alterations in males included a seven-fold increased concentration of circulating estradiol, a major female hormone, during steroid administration. This level was representative of average values for normal females and possibly explains the *gynecomastia* (palpable breast tissue) often reported among male users of anabolic steroids. As part of a long-range educational program, the American College of Sports Medicine (ACSM) has taken a stand on the use and abuse of anabolic-androgenic steroids in sports. We endorse their position paper that follows.

ACSM Position Statement on Anabolic Steroids. Based on a comprehensive survey of the world literature and a careful analysis of the claims made for and against the efficacy of anabolic-androgenic steroids in improving human physical performance, it is the position of the ACSM that:

- Anabolic-androgenic steroids in the presence of an adequate diet and training can contribute to increases in body weight, often in the lean mass compartment.
- The gains in muscular strength achieved through high-intensity exercise and proper diet can occur by the increased use of anabolic-androgenic steroids in some individuals.
- Anabolic-androgenic steroids do not increase aerobic power or capacity for muscular exercise.
- Anabolic-androgenic steroids have been associated with adverse effects on the liver (see Table 14-1), cardiovascular system, reproductive system, and psychologic status in therapeutic trials and in limited research on athletes. Until further research is completed, the potential hazards

It's against the law. A new federal law makes it illegal to prescribe, distribute, or possess anabolic steroids for any purpose other than treatment of disease or other medical conditions. First offenders can be sentenced to up to 5 years in prison and fined up to $250,000.

of the use of the anabolic-andro-genic steroids in athletes must include those found in therapeutic trials.

- The use of anabolic-androgenic steroids by athletes is contrary to the rules and ethical principles of athletic competition as set forth by many of the sports governing bodies. The American College of Sports Medicine supports these ethical principles and deplores the use of anabolic-androgenic steroids by athletes.

Steroid Use and Plasma Lipoproteins. Steroid use produces a rapid, profound lowering of high-density lipoprotein cholesterol and elevations in both low-density lipoprotein cholesterol and total cholesterol in healthy, trained men and women. *Each of these changes relates to an increase in one's risk for coronary artery disease.* In one study of weight lifters who used anabolic steroids, the average value for HDL cholesterol was 26 mg · dl^{-1} compared to 50 mg · dl^{-1} for the weightlifters not on the drug! A reduction of this lipoprotein to this low level constitutes a significant heart disease risk to the steroid user.

Steroid Use by Females. There is little information on the use of anabolic agents by female athletes, but hearsay reports and "off-the-record" statements by coaches, physicians, and the athletes themselves give every reason to conclude that this form of drug abuse is on the upswing. In addition to the broad range of side effects discussed previously, women, especially those who have not fully matured, are susceptible to specific dangers. These include masculinization, disruption of normal growth

pattern by premature closure of the plates for bone growth (also for boys), voice changes, altered menstrual function, dramatic increase in sebaceous gland size, acne, hirsutism, and enlargement of the clitoris. The long-term effects on reproductive function are unknown, but anabolic steroid abuse may be harmful in this area.

Growth Hormone: The Next Magic Pill?

Physicians and pharmacologists predict that the anabolic steroid will be obsolete as a training aid, and that it will be replaced by *human growth hormone* (GH), also known as *somatotropic hormone*. This hormone is produced by the adenohypophysis of the pituitary gland and is intimately involved in tissue-building processes and normal human growth. Medically, it is sometimes given to children who are deficient in GH to help them achieve near-normal size. The use of GH is attractive to the athlete because it stimulates amino acid uptake and protein synthesis by muscle, increases lipid breakdown, and decreases the quantity of carbohydrate used by the body. In a double-blind study,

More bad news for steroid users. Research with animals suggests that steroid use may lead to connective tissue damage which can decrease the tensile strength of tendons.

A questionable practice. Many weight lifters and body builders use oral amino acid supplements in the belief that they will boost the body's natural production of growth hormone to improve muscle size and strength. However, recent research shows that supplements of amino acid such as L-arginine, L-ornithine, and L-lysine had no effect on serum growth hormone concentration.

TABLE 14-1. Oral adrenergic-anabolic steroids associated with detrimental side effects[a]

Chemical Name	Trade Name	Daily Dosage (mg)	Duration in Affected Patients (Months)	Complications
Oxymetholone	Ora-Testryl Adroyd Anapolon Anadrol 50	10–250	10–51	Pellosis hepatis[b]
Methyltestosterone	Oreton Methyl Metandren Android	20–50	1–165	Hepatoma[c]
Stanazolol	Winstrol	15	18	Hepatoma[c]
Methandrostenolone	Dianabol	10–15	12–18	Hepatoma[c]
Fluoxymesterone	Halotestin	15–80	4–16	Pellosis hepatis[b]
Norethandrolone	Nilevar	20–30	1.5–9	Pellosis hepatis[b]

[a] Data from Johnson, F.L.: The association of oral androgenic-anabolic steroids and life threatening disease. *Med. Sci. Sports,* 7:284, 1975.
[b] Severe liver malfunction
[c] Liver cancer

six well-trained men were administered either biosynthetic GH or a placebo while maintaining a high-protein diet. During 6 weeks of standard resistance training with GH, percent body fat decreased and fat-free weight increased significantly. No changes in body composition were noted for the group who trained with the placebo.

Because GH occurs naturally in the body, there is as yet no foolproof way to detect its use as an ergogenic aid. At present, the hormone is expensive and usually available to the athlete only on the black market and often in a highly adulterated form. With the techniques of gene splicing, it is now possible to produce a synthetic form of GH at a reasonable price. Undoubtedly, as athletes begin to use this hormone in the hope of attaining a competitive edge, we will see an increased incidence of gigantism in children and acromegalic syndrome — coarsening of the skin, thickening of bones, and overgrowth of soft tissue — in adults.

Amphetamines

Amphetamines or "pep pills" are a group of pharmacologic compounds that exert a powerful stimulating effect on central nervous system function. Amphetamine (Benzedrine) and dextroamphetamine sulfate (Dexedrine) are the compounds used most frequently. Amphetamines are *sympathomimetic* in that their action mimics the sympathetic hormones epinephrine and norepinephrine. Consequently, they cause a rise in blood pressure, pulse rate, cardiac output, breathing rate, metabolism, and blood-sugar level. Five to 20 mg of amphetamine usually exerts its effect for 30 to 90 minutes after ingestion, although its influence can persist for much longer. Aside from bringing about an aroused level of sympathetic function, amphetamines are supposed to increase alertness and wakefulness as well as the capacity to perform increased amounts of work; this is achieved by depressing the sensation of muscle fatigue. It is not surprising, therefore, that athletes frequently use amphetamines with the hope of gaining an ergogenic edge.

Dangers of Amphetamine. The use of amphetamines in athletics is ill-advised for the following medical reasons:

- Continual use can lead to either physiologic or emotional drug dependency. This often brings about a cyclical dependency on "uppers" (amphetamines) or "downers" (barbiturates) — the barbiturates are taken to reduce or tranquilize the "hyper" state brought on by amphetamines.
- General side effects of amphetamines are headaches, tremulousness, agitation, fever, dizziness, and confusion — all of which can have a negative effect on sports performance requiring reaction, judgment, and a high level of steadiness and mental concentration.
- Larger doses are eventually required to achieve the same effect because individual tolerances to the drug increase with prolonged use; this may aggravate and even precipitate certain cardiovascular disorders.
- Agents that inhibit or suppress the body's normal mechanisms for perceiving and responding to pain, fatigue, or heat stress can severely jeopardize the health and safety of the athlete.
- The effects of prolonged intake of high doses of amphetamines are unknown.

Amphetamine Use and Athletic Performance. The major reason athletes take amphetamines is to get "up" for an event and to keep up and be psychologically ready to compete. The day or evening before a contest, however, competitors are often nervous and irritable and have difficulty relaxing. Under these circumstances, a barbiturate is used to induce sleep. The athlete then regains the "hyper" condition by popping an "upper." Not only is this cycle of depressant-to-stimulant undesirable and potentially dangerous, but the stimulant does not act in its normal manner after a barbiturate. Knowledgeable and prudent people urge that amphetamines be banned from sport competition. The International Olympic Committee, the American Medical Association, and most athletic governing groups have rules to disqualify athletes who use amphetamines. Ironically, *almost all studies on the ergogenic effects of amphetamines show little or no effect on exercise performance or on simple psychomotor skills.* Perhaps their greatest influence is in the psychologic realm, in which athletes are easily convinced that any supplement will bring on a superior performance. A placebo containing an inert substance often produces identical results!

Caffeine

A possible exception to the general rule against stimulants is caffeine. Caffeine is one of a group of compounds called methylxanthines found naturally in coffee beans, tea leaves, chocolate, cocoa beans, and cola nuts, and is often added to carbonated beverages and nonprescription medicines. It is absorbed rapidly into the body and reaches peak concentrations in the blood between 30 and 120 minutes after ingestion to exert an influence on the nervous, cardiovascular, and muscular systems.

Although all studies do not support the ergogenic benefits of caffeine it has been shown that consuming the amount of caffeine (330 mg) commonly found in 2.5 cups of regularly percolated coffee (a caffeine dose legal under current International Olympic Committee guidelines) 60 minutes before exercising significantly extended endurance in moderately strenuous exercise. Subjects who drank caffeine were able to exercise for an average of 90.2 minutes compared to 75.5 minutes during a decaffeinated exercise treatment. Even though values for heart rate and oxygen uptake

during the two trials were similar, the caffeine also made the work feel easier. During exercise prior to which caffeine had been ingested, the plasma glycerol and free fatty acid levels and the respiratory exchange ratio indicated a high level of lipid metabolism and a corresponding reduced rate of carbohydrate oxidation. It is likely that this ergogenic effect of caffeine is due to the facilitated use of lipid as a fuel for exercise, perhaps mediated via catecholamine release, thus sparing the body's limited carbohydrate reserves.

Certainly, conserving muscle and liver glycogen would be of considerable benefit in prolonged exercise in which glycogen depletion is intimately related to diminished endurance capacity. It is likely that a lessening of the subjective ratings of effort was due to a central analgesic effect of caffeine, or its effect on neuronal excitability, possibly through a lowering of the threshold for motor-unit recruitment and nerve transmission.

Endurance Effects Are Often Inconsistent. The effect of caffeine ingestion on mobilization of free fatty acids is significantly blunted, and this metabolic mixture is unaltered during prolonged submaximal exercise in individuals who have maintained a high carbohydrate intake prior to exercise. This influence of prior nutrition may partly account for the wide and often inconsistent variation in individual response to exercise following caffeine ingestion. Individual sensitivity and tolerance due to patterns of caffeine consumption are probably also important factors that affect the ergogenic nature of this drug, because benefits are not consistently noted, especially among habitual caffeine users.

Effects on Muscle. Caffeine may also act directly on muscle to enhance its capacity for exercise. By means of a double-blind research design, both voluntary and electrically stimulated muscle contractions were evaluated

The "upper" for the next game. For the competitive collegiate or professional athlete, getting "up" for the next game in a new city after a day of travel is quite difficult on a regular basis. The susceptible athlete will often turn to amphetamine, in the mistaken hope of obtaining a competitive edge.

Rich in caffeine. Depending on preparation, one cup of brewed coffee contains between 50 and 150 mg of caffeine, tea contains between 10 and 50 mg, and caffeinated soft drinks contain about 50 mg.

ALCOHOL: NO ERGOGENIC AID

The use and abuse of alcohol is legendary. Consumption of alcoholic beverages has served social, religious, and medical applications in many cultures. In western society, alcohol is used mostly as a "social drug" and as a means to relax and reduce anxiety. Historically, alcohol has been used as an ergogenic aid. For example, wine was used by ancient warriors to increase strength and endurance. In the 1800s, the British Navy gave rum to its sailors because it was thought to increase their strength prior to battle. Many endurance athletes during the early 1900s consumed wine and beer prior to and even during competition in the belief that it would improve endurance.

The greatest use of alcohol, however, has been related to its supposed psychological effects. Alcohol is thought to positively effect performance through either neural disinhibition or a direct sympathetic stimulating effect, by increasing self-confidence, decreasing sensitivity to pain, or reducing psychological hindrances to performance. Alcohol, because of its ability to reduce anxiety and tremor, is also thought to benefit individuals who require "a steady hand" in performance. For example, in the 1968 Olympics, two pistol shooters were disqualified for consuming alcohol prior to competition.

Alcohol (ethyl alcohol or ethanol) is sometimes classified as a nutrient because it contains about 7 kcal of energy per gram. One drink of alcohol is equivalent to 0.5 oz (14 g) of 100% ethanol, the amount in a 12 oz can of beer, 4 oz of wine, or 1.25 oz of 40% (80 proof) liquor. By volume, beer averages about 4 to 5% alcohol, wine about 12 to 14%, and a mixed drink with liquor is 45%. Nearly 20% of the ingested alcohol is absorbed by the stomach and 80% by the small intestine. After absorption, the alcohol is diluted by the body fluids and distributed to various water-soluble body tissues such as the brain. Between 90 to 97% of the ingested alcohol is metabolized by the liver at a rate of about 10 g per hour. Factors such as body size and composition influence the blood alcohol content or BAC. For the average male, one drink results in a BAC of about 0.025 $g \cdot dl^{-1}$, and 0.05 $g \cdot dl^{-1}$ for two drinks in an hour.

Research findings do not support an ergogenic benefit from alcohol in sports that require strength, speed, power, and local muscular endurance. In addition, it is not used as a major energy source during short or longer duration exercise. Alcohol may be detrimental in prolonged exercise tasks lasting several hours because it can interfere with liver function by decreasing gluconeogenesis and glucose output from the liver. Of additional concern is the effects of alcohol consumption the night before competition. Research suggests that 1 or 2 drinks will not adversely effect performance the following morning. However, alcohol consumption resulting in BACs of 0.10 to 0.20 $g \cdot dl^{-1}$ may significantly impair subsequent exercise performance, particularly tasks requiring fine motor movements or endurance. Because alcohol is a diuretic, excessive intake the evening prior to competition may result in a state of dehydration the following morning. If rehydration is inadequate prior to competition, the athlete may be in a partially dehydrated state during competition. This could impair temperature regulation.

The insert table presents some typical effects of increasing BAC. For most sport participants, alcohol offers no ergogenic potential; the bad news is that it may be detrimental and therefore should be avoided.

Effects of Increasing Blood Alcohol Levels

Drinks in 2 hrs	Blood alcohol level (g/dL)	Effects
2 to 3	0.02 to 0.04	Reduced tension and stress; relaxed feeling
4 to 5	0.06 to 0.09	Euphoria; impaired judgement and fine motor coordination
6 to 8	0.11 to 0.16	Legally drunk; slurred speech; impaired gross motor coordination; staggering gait
9 to 12	0.18 to 0.25	Loss of control of voluntary activity; erratic behavior; impaired vision
13 to 18	0.27 to 0.39	Total loss of coordination
>19	>0.40	Coma; depression of respiratory centers, death

Reference

Williams, M.H.: Alcohol, marijuana and beta blockers. *Perspectives in Exercise Science and Sports Medicine*, Vol. 4: Ergogenics: Enhancement of Performance in Exercise and Sport. Edited by D.R. Lamb, and M. H. Williams, Dubuque, IA, Brown & Benchmark, 1991.

after ingestion. For the susceptible athlete, such a side effect could negate any potential ergogenic benefit.

RED BLOOD CELL REINFUSION — BLOOD DOPING

Red blood cell reinfusion, often called *induced erythrocythemia*, blood boosting, or "blood doping," came into public prominence as a possible ergogenic technique during the 1972 Munich Olympics, when a champion endurance athlete was alleged to have used this in preparation for his eventual gold medal endurance run.

How it Works

With red blood cell reinfusion, usually between 1 and 4 units (1 unit = 450 ml of blood) of a person's blood (referred to as *autologous*) are withdrawn, the plasma is removed and immediately reinfused, and the packed red cells are placed in frozen storage. (With *homologous* transfusion a type-matched donor's blood is infused.) To prevent a dramatic reduction in blood-cell concentration, each unit of blood is withdrawn over a 3 to 8 week period because it generally takes this long for the person to reestablish normal red blood cell levels. The stored blood cells are then reinfused 1 to 7 days before an endurance event. As a result, the red blood cell count and hemoglobin level of the blood are often elevated some 8 to 20%. This hemoconcentration translates to an average increase in hemoglobin for men from a normal of 15 g per 100 ml of blood to 19 g per 100 ml (or from hematocrits of 40 to 60%). It is theorized that the added blood volume contributes to a larger maximal cardiac output, and that the red blood cell packing increases the blood's oxygen-carrying capacity. Thus, the quantity of oxygen available to the working muscles is increased. This would be beneficial to the endurance athlete, especially the marathoner, for whom oxygen transport is often a limiting factor in exercise.

Usually 900 to 1800 ml of freeze-preserved autologous blood is the amount infused to bring about ergogenic benefits. For each infusion of 500 ml of whole blood or its equivalent of 275 ml of packed red cells, about 100 ml of oxygen are theoretically added to the total oxygen-carrying capacity of the blood. (This is because each 100 ml of whole blood carries about 20 ml of oxygen.) Because an athlete's total blood volume circulates five or six times each minute in all-out exercise, the potential "extra" oxygen available to the tissues from red cell reinfusion is about 0.5 liters.

It is also possible that blood doping could have effects opposite to those intended. A large infusion of red blood cells (and resulting increase in cellular concentration or *polycythemia*) could increase blood viscosity and bring about a decrease in cardiac output, a decrease in blood flow velocity, and a reduction in peripheral oxygen content — all of which would reduce aerobic capacity. Certainly any increase in blood viscosity or "thickness" could pose a considerable risk by compromising blood flow through the atherosclerotic vessels of those with significant coronary artery disease.

Does It Work? The more recent research in this area generally supports the findings of the early studies and shows physiologic and performance improvements with red blood cell reinfusion. *The differences among the various research studies are based largely on blood storage methods.* Frozen red blood cells can be stored in excess of 6 weeks without significant loss of cells compared to conventional storage at 4°C (used in earlier studies); at 4°C, substantial hemolysis occurs after only 3 weeks. This is important because, as shown in Figure 14-1, it usually takes a person 5 to 6 weeks to re-establish the blood cells lost after withdrawal of 2 units of whole blood.

Residual effects. The average red blood cell lives about 120 days, so any residual benefits of blood doping could last for up to six weeks.

Potential thermoregulatory benefit. Blood doping may also aid in thermoregulation during exercise. The "extra" oxygen carried in the blood increases tissue oxygenation so more blood is "freed" to be shunted to the skin to be cooled without compromising oxygen delivery to muscles.

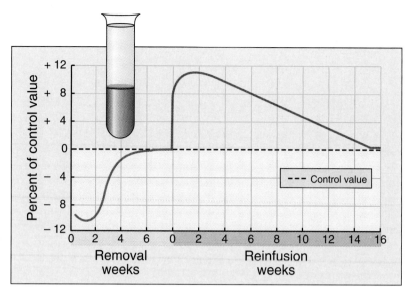

FIGURE 14-1. Time course of hematological changes after removal and reinfusion of 900 ml of freeze-preserved blood. (From Gledhill, N.: Blood doping and related issues: a brief review. *Med. Sci. Sports Exerc.,* 14: 183, 1982.)

The procedure of red blood cell reinfusion has a significant effect in elevating hematologic characteristics for both men and women. This, in turn, translates to a 5 to 13% increase in aerobic capacity, a reduced sub-maximal heart rate and blood lactate for a standard exercise task, and an augmented endurance performance both at altitude and sea level. Table 14-3 illustrates hematologic, physiologic, and performance responses for five adult men during submaximal and maximal exercise before and 24 hours after the comparatively large infusion of 750 ml of packed red blood cells. These response patterns are generally representative of the more recent research in this area.

A New Twist — Hormonal Blood Boosting

In an attempt to eliminate the some-what cumbersome and lengthy process of blood doping, endurance athletes are now experimenting with *erythro-poietin,* a hormone normally produced

TABLE 14-3. Physiologic, performance, and hematologic characteristics prior to and 24 hours after the reinfusion of 750 ml of packed red blood cells

Variable	Pre-Infusion	Post-Infusion	Difference	Difference, %
Hemoglobin, g·100 ml blood^{-1}	13.8	17.6	3.8*	+27.5*
Hematocrit[a], %	43.3	54.8	11.5*	+26.5*
Submaximal $\dot{V}O_2$, 1·min^{-1}	1.60	1.59	−0.01	−0.6
Submaximal HR, b·min^{-1}	127.4	109.2	18.2	−14.3*
Max $\dot{V}O_2$, 1·min^{-1}	3.28	3.70	0.42*	+12.8*
Max HR, b·min^{-1}	181.6	180.0	−1.6	−0.9
Treadmill Run Time, sec	793	918	125*	+15.8

[a] Hematocrit is presented as the percent (%) of 100 ml of whole blood occupied by the red blood cells.
[b] Difference is statistically significant.
(From Robertson, R.J., et al.: Effect of induced erythrocytemia on hypoxia tolerance during exercise. *J. Appl. Physiol.,* 53:490, 1982.)

by the kidneys. This hormone stimulates the bone marrow to produce red blood cells. From a medical standpoint, it has proved quite useful in combating the anemia often observed in patients with severe kidney disease. Normally, when the blood count is low or when the pressure of oxygen in arterial blood decreases (as in severe lung disease or on ascent to high altitude), this hormone is released to stimulate red blood cell production. Unfortunately, if administered exogenously in an unregulated and unmonitored fashion (simply injecting the hormone requires much less sophistication than the procedures for blood doping), hematocrits can increase to dangerous levels, in excess of 60%. Such a significant increase in hemoconcentration, and thus blood viscosity, greatly augments the exercise-induced increase in systolic blood pressure and also increases the likelihood for stroke, heart attack, heart failure, pulmonary embolism, and even death.

WARM-UP (PRELIMINARY EXERCISE)

Engaging in some type of physical activity or warm-up before vigorous exercise is generally accepted as a valid procedure by coaches, trainers, and athletes at all levels of competition. The underlying belief is that this preliminary exercise aids the performer in preparing either physiologically or psychologically for an event and may reduce the chances of joint and muscle injury. With animals, greater forces and increases in muscle length were required to injure a "warmed-up" muscle compared with a muscle in the "cold" condition. It was suggested that the warming-up process stretches the muscle-tendon unit and subsequently allows for greater length and less tension at any given load on the unit.

The warm-up is generally classified under one of two categories, although overlap often exists.

- *General warm-up* involves calisthenics, stretching, and general body movements or "loosening-up" exercises usually unrelated to the specific neuromuscular action of the anticipated performance.
- *Specific warm-up* provides a skill rehearsal in the actual activity for which the participant is preparing. Swinging a golf club, throwing a baseball or football, tennis or basketball practice, and preliminary lead-up in the high jump or pole vault are examples of specific warm-up.

Psychologic Considerations

Competitors at all levels often consider that some prior activity prepares them mentally for their event, so that their concentration and "psych" become clearly focused on the upcoming performance. Evidence supports the contention that a specific warm-up related to the activity itself improves the necessary skill and coordination. Consequently, sports that require accuracy, timing, and precise movements generally benefit from some type of specific or "formal" preliminary practice.

There is also the notion that prior exercise, especially before a strenuous effort, gradually prepares a person to go "all out" without fear of injury. A good example is the ritual warm-up of baseball pitchers. Is it conceivable that a pitcher would ever enter a game, throwing at competitive speeds, without previously warming up? Would any athlete begin competition without first engaging in a particular form, intensity, or duration of warm-up? Although in most instances the answer is a definite "no," it would be nearly impossible to design an experiment with topflight athletes to resolve whether or not warm-up is really necessary and, in fact, whether or not it improves subsequent performance.

In certain situations, peak performance is expected as soon as play

Literally warming-up. A vigorous warm-up has been shown to increase both core and muscle temperature and increase the contribution of aerobic metabolism at the onset of heavy exercise. This potentially beneficial response may be due to the increase in local muscle blood flow brought on by the warm-up.

Psychologic factors. Psychologic factors such as an athlete's ingrained belief in the importance of warming up establish a definite bias in comparing performance in the "no warm-up" condition. It is difficult to obtain maximum effort with no warm-up if a subject believes warm-up is important. In this regard, some researchers have hypnotized their subjects to neutralize preconceived notions about warm-up.

begins, and there is little time for warming up. For example, when a reserve player goes into the last few minutes of a game there is no time for preliminary stretching, vigorous calisthenics, or taking practice shots; the player is expected to go all out with no warm-up, except that done before the game or at intermission. Are more injuries recorded in such cases? Is physical performance such as shooting, rebounding, or basketball defense, for example, poorer during the first few minutes of this "unwarmed" condition than it is following a performance preceded by a warm-up?

Physiologic Considerations

On purely physiologic grounds, the following are possible mechanisms by which warm-up should improve performance owing to subsequent increases in blood flow and muscle and core temperature:

- Increased speed of contraction and relaxation of muscles
- Greater economy of movement because of lowered viscous resistance within the muscles
- Facilitated oxygen utilization by the muscles because hemoglobin releases oxygen more readily at higher temperatures
- Facilitated nerve transmission and muscle metabolism at higher temperatures; a specific warm-up may also facilitate the recruitment of motor units required in a subsequent all-out activity
- Increased blood flow through active tissues as the local vascular bed dilates with higher levels of metabolism and muscle temperatures

Effects on Performance

There is little concrete evidence that warm-up per se directly affects subsequent exercise performance. That is not to say that warm-up is unimportant for such purposes.

Rather, there is simply little justification from laboratory studies to support such practices. Because of the strong psychologic component and possible physical benefits of warming up, however, whether it be passive (massage, heat applications, and diathermy), general (calisthenics, jogging), or specific (practice of the actual movements), we recommend that such procedures be continued. Until there is substantial evidence justifying its elimination, a brief warm-up is certainly a comfortable way to lead up to more vigorous exercise. *The warm-up should be gradual and sufficient to increase muscle and core temperature without causing fatigue or reducing energy stores.* This consideration is highly individualized; adequate warm-up in terms of intensity and duration for an Olympic swimmer would totally exhaust the average recreational swimmer. To reap the possible benefits from increased body temperature, the actual event or activity should begin within several minutes from the end of the warm-up. In warming up, the specific muscles should be used in a way that mimics the anticipated activity and brings about a full range of joint motion.

Sudden Strenuous Exercise

Several studies have evaluated the effects of preliminary exercise on cardiovascular response to sudden, strenuous exercise. The findings provide an essentially different physiologic framework for justifying warm-up that is important to those involved in adult fitness and cardiac rehabilitation, as well as in occupations and sports requiring a sudden burst of high-intensity exercise.

In one study, 44 men, free from overt symptoms of coronary heart disease, ran on a treadmill at an intense workload for 10 to 15 seconds without prior warm-up. Evaluation of the post-exercise electrocardiogram (ECG) revealed that 70% of the subjects displayed abnormal electrocardiographic changes that could be attributed to inadequate oxygen supply to the heart muscle. These changes were not related to age or fitness level. To evaluate the effect of a warm-up, 22 of the men jogged in place at moderate intensity (heart rate about 145 beats per minute) for 2 minutes before the treadmill run. With warm-up, 10 men who had previously shown abnormal ECG responses to the treadmill run now had normal tracings and 10 men had improved their ECGs, whereas only two subjects still showed significant ischemic changes (poor oxygen supply). The blood pressure response also improved with warm-up. For seven subjects with no warm-up, systolic blood pressure averaged 168 mm Hg immediately after the treadmill run. This was reduced to 140 mm Hg with the 2-minute jog-in-place warm-up.

These observations indicate that the adaptation of coronary blood flow to a sudden and vigorous cardiac workload is not instantaneous and that transient myocardial ischemia may occur in apparently healthy and fit individuals. *The effect of prior warm-up (at least 2 minutes of easy jogging) on the electrocardiogram and blood pressure appears to be significant in establishing a more favorable relationship between myocardial oxygen supply and demand.*

Although warm-up preceding strenuous exercise is probably a prudent practice for all people, it is most important for those who have cardiovascular problems that limit the heart's oxygen supply. Brief, prior exercise provides for more optimal blood pressure and hormonal adjustment at the onset of subsequent strenuous exercise. This warm-up would serve two purposes: (1) reduce the myocardial workload and thus the myocardial oxygen requirement, and (2) provide adequate coronary blood flow in sudden, high-intensity exercise.

OXYGEN INHALATION (HYPEROXIA)

It is common to observe athletes breathing oxygen-enriched or *hyperoxic* gas mixtures during times out, at half-time, or following strenuous exercise. The belief is that this procedure significantly enhances the blood's oxygen-carrying capacity and thus facilitates oxygen transport to the exercising muscles. The fact is, however, that when healthy people breathe ambient air at sea level, the hemoglobin in arterial blood leaving the lungs is about 95 to 98% saturated with oxygen. Thus:

- Breathing high concentrations of oxygen could increase oxygen transport by hemoglobin to only a small extent, i.e., about 10 ml of extra oxygen for every 1000 ml of whole blood.
- The oxygen dissolved in plasma when breathing a hyperoxic mixture would also increase slightly from its normal quantity of 3 ml to about 7 ml per 1000 ml of blood.

Consequently, the blood's oxygen-carrying capacity under hyperoxic conditions would be increased potentially by approximately 14 ml of oxygen for every 1000 ml of blood — 10 ml extra attached to hemoglobin and 4 ml extra dissolved in plasma.

Pre-Exercise

A 70-kg person has about 5000 ml of blood. A hyperoxic breathing mixture could therefore potentially add or "store" about 70 ml of oxygen in the total blood volume (5000 ml blood x 14.0 ml "extra" O_2 per 1000 ml blood = 70 ml O_2). Thus, despite the potential psychologic benefit of the athlete believing that pre-exercise oxygen breathing helps performance, this procedure might confer only a slight performance advantage owing to the oxygen per se. This, however, could occur *only* if the subsequent exercise took

Psychologic effects play a role. The potential positive psychologic influence of oxygen breathing should not be discounted, however, for it may provide a useful rationale for continuing this practice.

Environmental Factors and Exercise

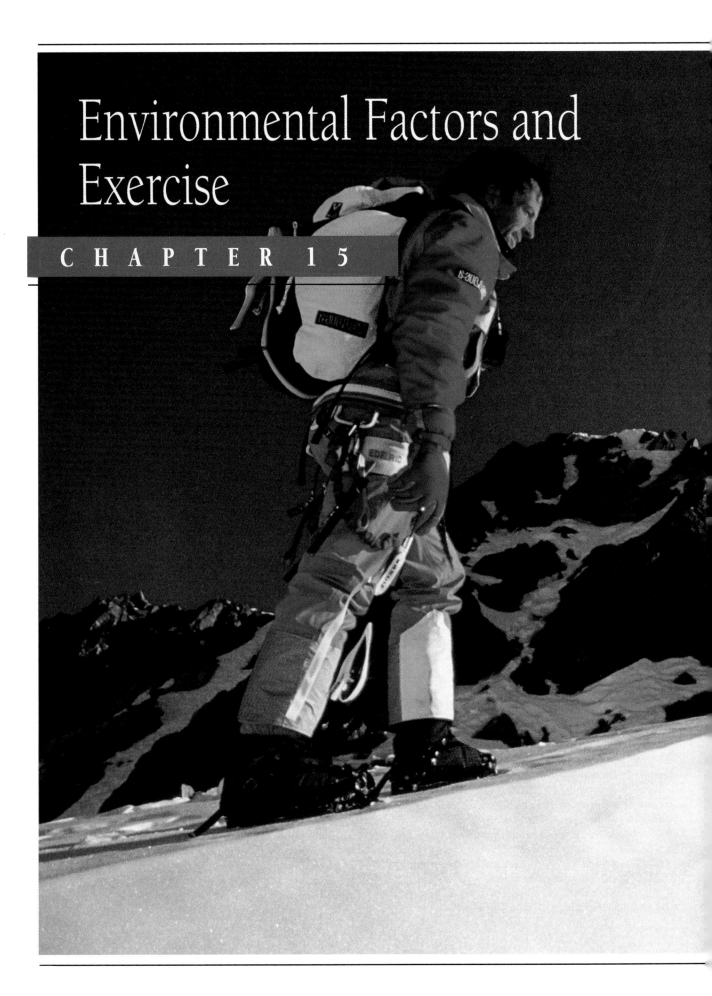

After reading this chapter, you should be able to:

- Discuss the following statement: "The central regulatory hypothalamic center plays the most important role in maintaining the body's thermal balance."
- Explain the four physical factors that can contribute to heat gain and heat loss by the body.
- Discuss how the circulatory system serves as a "workhorse" to maintain thermal balance.
- List the desirable characteristics for clothing designed for exercise in (a) cold weather, and (b) warm weather.
- Discuss the response of cardiac output, heart rate, and stroke volume during exercise in the heat.
- Describe the circulatory adjustments that maintain blood pressure during exercise in the heat.
- Indicate how much fluid can be lost during exercise in the heat. What are the physiological consequences of such dehydration?
- Discuss how the following factors modify a person's heat tolerance during exercise: acclimatization, training, age, gender, and body fat.
- Describe the factors that make up the Heat Stress Index.
- Discuss the purpose of the Wind Chill Index.
- Indicate what physiologic adjustments the body makes in response to cold stress.
- Outline the effects of increasingly higher altitudes on the: (a) partial pressure of oxygen in ambient air, (b) saturation of hemoglobin with oxygen in the pulmonary capillaries, and (3) max $\dot{V}O_2$.
- Discuss the immediate and the longer-term physiologic adjustments to altitude exposure.
- Discuss whether training at altitude is more effective than sea-level training on subsequent sea-level performance.

The requirements for thermoregulation can be considerable; the price for failure is death. A drop in deep body temperature of 10°C (18°F) and an increase of only 5°C (9°F) can be tolerated. Consider this grim statistic; between 1960 and 1983, 70 football players died as a direct result of excessive heat stress during practice or actual competition! Heat injury is also an unfortunate common occurrence in a variety of longer duration athletic events. Such tragedies are avoidable with the proper understanding of thermoregulation and the best ways to support these mechanisms. A major part of this responsibility rests with the people who organize and guide sport and physical activity programs.

THERMAL BALANCE

As shown in Figure 15-1, body temperature or, more specifically, the temperature of the deeper tissues or *core*, is in dynamic equilibrium as a result of a balance between factors that add and subtract body heat. This balance is maintained by the integration of mechanisms that alter heat transfer to the periphery or *shell*, regulate evaporative cooling, and vary the body's rate of heat production. If heat gain outstrips heat loss, as can readily occur in vigorous exercise in a warm environment, core temperature rises. In the cold, on the other hand, heat loss often exceeds heat production and core temperature falls.

HYPOTHALAMIC REGULATION OF TEMPERATURE

The hypothalamus contains the coordinating center for the various processes of temperature regulation. This group of specialized neurons at the floor of the brain acts as a "thermostat" (usually set and carefully regulated at 37° C ± 1° C) that makes thermoregulatory adjustments to deviations from a temperature norm. Unlike our home thermostat, however, the hypothalamus cannot "turn off" the heat; it can only initiate responses to protect the body from a buildup or loss of heat.

Peripheral thermal receptors or sensors responsive to rapid changes in heat and cold are distributed predominantly as free nerve endings in the skin. These receptors act as an "early warning system" that relays sensory information to the hypothalamus and cortex to bring about appropriate heat-conserving or heat-dissipating adjustments, and to cause the individual consciously to seek relief from a thermal challenge.

The central regulatory hypothalamic center plays the most important role in maintaining thermal balance. Cells in

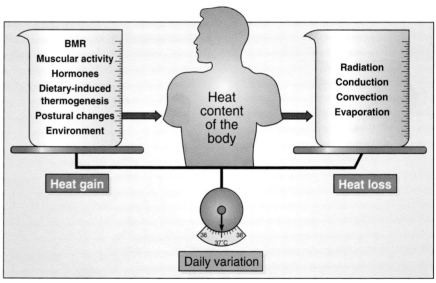

Figure 15-1. Factors that contribute to heat gain and heat loss as the body attempts to regulate core temperature at approximately 37° C.

the anterior portion of the hypothalamus are themselves capable of detecting changes in blood temperature. These cells then activate other hypothalamic regions to initiate coordinated responses for heat conservation (posterior hypothalamus) or heat loss (anterior hypothalamus). In contrast

Fatness

Excessive body fat is a liability when working in the heat. Because the specific heat of fat is greater than for muscle tissue, excess fat increases the insulatory quality of the body shell and retards conduction of heat to the periphery. The large, overfat person also has a relatively small body surface for the evaporation of sweat compared to a leaner, smaller person.

In addition to thwarting effective heat exchange, excess body fat directly adds to the metabolic cost of activities where the body mass must be moved. When this effect is compounded by the additional weight of equipment such as football gear, intense competition, and a hot, humid environment, the overfat person is at a distinct disadvantage in terms of thermoregulation and exercise performance. In fact, fatal heat stroke occurs 3.5 times more frequently in excessively overweight young adults than in individuals whose body weight is within reasonable limits.

HOW HOT IS "TOO HOT"?

The most effective way to control heat stress injuries is to prevent their occurrence. For one thing, acclimatization and appropriate fluid replacement greatly reduce the chance for heat injury. Another consideration is to evaluate the environment in terms of its potential heat challenge. This can be done with the use of a heat stress index; this was developed by the military and was derived from measures of ambient temperature, relative humidity, and radiant heat. The index, termed the *wet bulb-globe temperature or WB-GT index,* is calculated as:

$$WB\text{-}GT = 0.1 \times DBT + 0.7 \times WBT + 0.2 \times GT$$

where DBT is the dry-bulb or air temperature recorded by an ordinary mercury thermometer used for recording air temperature. WBT is the wet-bulb temperature recorded by a similar thermometer except that a wet wick

Heat Stress Index

Air temperature (°F)

Heat sensation

Relative humidity	70°	75°	80°	85°	90°	95°	100°	105°	110°	115°	120°
0%	64°	69°	73°	78°	83°	87°	91°	95°	99°	103°	107°
10%	65°	70°	75°	80°	85°	90°	95°	100°	105°	111°	116°
20%	66°	72°	77°	82°	87°	93°	99°	105°	112°	120°	130°
30%	67°	73°	78°	84°	90°	96°	104°	113°	123°	135°	148°
40%	68°	74°	79°	86°	93°	101°	110°	123°	137°	151°	
50%	69°	75°	81°	88°	96°	107°	120°	135°	150°		
60%	70°	76°	82°	90°	100°	114°	132°	149°			
70%	70°	77°	85°	93°	106°	124°	144°				
80%	71°	78°	86°	97°	113°	136°					
90%	71°	79°	88°	102°	122°						
100%	72°	80°	91°	108°							

Heat sensation	Risk of heat injury
90°–105°	Possibility of heat cramps
105°–130°	Heat cramps or heat exhaustion likely Heat stroke possible
130°+	Heatstroke a definite risk

How hot is hot? It's more than just the thermometer reading.

surrounds the mercury bulb that is exposed to rapid air movement. When the relative humidity is high, little evaporative cooling occurs from the wetted bulb so the temperature of this thermometer is similar to that of the dry–bulb. On a dry day, however, significant evaporation occurs from the wetted bulb and the difference between the two thermometer readings is maximized. A small difference between readings indicates a high relative humidity, whereas a large difference indicates little air moisture and a high rate of evaporation and subsequent cooling. GT is the globe temperature recorded by a thermometer whose bulb is enclosed in a metal sphere painted black. The black globe absorbs radiant energy from the surroundings to provide a measure of this important source of heat gain.

Figure 15-6 (top) presents WB-GT guidelines that can be applied to athletic activities to reduce the chance of heat injury. These standards apply to lightly clothed humans, but do not take into account the specific heat load imposed by uniforms or equipment such as that used in football. For this activity, the lower end of each temperature range serves as a more prudent guide.

A simple indication of the ambient heat load can also be obtained from the wet-bulb thermometer. This reading evaluates both temperature and humidity. The thermometer is relatively inexpensive and can be purchased at most industrial supply companies. The bottom of Figure 15-6 presents recommendations based on wet-bulb temperature.

. . . .
EXERCISE IN THE COLD

Water is an excellent medium to study physiologic adjustment to cold because body heat is lost about two to four times as fast in cool water as in air at the same temperature. Shivering is frequently observed if people remain inactive in a pool or ocean environment because of a large con-

WB-GT Range		Recommendations
°F	°C	
80–84	26.5–28.8	• Use discretion, especially if unconditioned or unacclimatized
85–87	29.5–30.5	• Avoid strenuous activity in the sun
88	31.2	• Avoid exercise training

WBT Range		Recommendations
°F	°C	
60	15.5	• No prevention necessary
61–65	16.2–18.4	• Alert all participants to problems of heat stress and importance of adequate hydration
66–70	18.8–21.1	• Insist that appropriate quantity of fluid be ingested
71–75	21.6–23.8	• Rest periods and water breaks every 20 to 30 minutes; limits placed on intense activity
76–79	24.5–26.1	• Practice curtailed and modified considerably
80	26.5	• Practice cancelled

Figure 15-6. WB-GT for outdoor activities and wet-bulb temperature (WBT) guide. (Modified from Murphy, R.J., and Ashe, W.F.: Prevention of heat illness in football players. *JAMA*, 194:650, 1965.)

ductive heat loss. Swimming at a submaximal pace at 18° C (64° F) requires about 500 ml of oxygen more per minute than swimming at the same speed in 26° C (79° F) water. This additional oxygen uptake is directly related to the added energy cost of shivering as the body attempts to combat heat loss. This additional metabolic heat, however, is often insufficient to counter the large thermal drain and core temperature drops.

Body Fatness, Exercise, and Cold Stress

To a large extent, the stress from "cold" is relative. The physiologic strain imposed by the cold depends not only on the environmental temperature per se, but also on the level of metabolism and the resistance to heat flow provided by body fat. Successful distance swimmers, for example, usually possess a relatively large amount of subcutaneous fat. This greatly increases their effective insulation when peripheral blood is redirected to the body's core in cold water. With this advantage, these athletes can swim in cool ocean waters with almost no fall in core temperature.

Optimal water temperature. For most people, water temperatures between 26° C and 30° C provide for effective heat dissipation in exercise, yet are not excessively cold so that exercise capacity is compromised.

Physical fitness and cold stress. Although not specifically a form of cold acclimatization, improved fitness, as reflected by a high aerobic capacity and muscle mass, enhances a person's thermoregulatory defense against cold stress. This manifests itself in a larger shivering response as well as an earlier or more sensitive onset of this response with cold exposure.

Acclimatization to the Cold

Humans possess much less capacity for adaptation to regular cold exposure than to exposure to heat. Indeed, the basic response of Eskimos and Lapps is to avoid the cold or minimize its effect. For example, the clothing of these cold weather inhabitants provides a near-tropical microclimate, and the temperature inside an igloo is generally maintained at about 21° C (70° F).

Some indication of cold adaptation has been provided from studies of the Ama, the women divers of Korea and southern Japan. These women can tolerate daily prolonged exposure to diving for food in cold water, which in winter is about 10° C (50° F). In addition to an apparent psychologic "toughness," the capability of these women to tolerate extreme cold has been attributed to an elevated resting metabolism. In winter, this is increased by about 25% compared to nondiving women of the same community. Interestingly, the body fat of these women is no greater than their nondiving female counterparts. It is possible, therefore, that circulatory adaptations also aid these divers by retarding heat transfer from the core to the skin.

Wind speed, mph	Ambient temperature, °F**															
	40	35	30	25	20	15	10	5	0	–5	–10	–15	–20	–25	–30	
	Equivalent temperature, °F															
Calm	40	35	30	25	20	15	10	5	0	–5	–10	–15	–20	–25	–30	Calm
5	37	33	27	21	16	12	6	1	–5	–11	–15	–20	–26	–31	–35	5
10	28	21	16	9	4	–2	–9	–15	–21	–27	–33	–38	–46	–52	–58	10
15	22	16	11	1	–5	–11	–18	–25	–36	–40	–45	–51	–58	–65	–70	15
20	18	12	3	–4	–10	–17	–25	–32	–39	–46	–53	–60	–67	–76	–81	20
25	16	7	0	–7	–15	–22	–29	–37	–44	–52	–59	–67	–74	–83	–89	25
30	13	5	–2	–11	–18	–26	–33	–41	–48	–56	–63	–70	–79	–87	–94	30
35	11	3	–4	–13	–20	–27	–35	–43	–49	–60	–67	–72	–82	–90	–98	35
*40	10	1	–6	–15	–21	–29	–37	–45	–53	–62	–69	–76	–85	–94	–101	40*

☐ Little danger ☐ Danger ■ Great danger

* Convective heat loss at wind speeds above 40 mph has little additional effect on body cooling.
** °C = 0.556 (°F –32)

Figure 15-7. The Wind Chill Index.

A type of general cold adaptation appears to occur following regular and prolonged cold-air exposure. As a result, heat loss is not compensated for by increased heat production and individuals "regulate" at a lower rectal temperature in response to cold. Some peripheral adaptations also reflect a form of acclimation with severe local cold exposure. Repeated cold exposure to the hands or feet brings about an increased blood flow through these areas when they are subjected to cold stress. This is readily apparent in cold-water fisherman who handle nets and fish in extreme cold. Although this local adaptation would actually result in a loss of body heat from the periphery, it does represent a form of "self-defense" because a vigorous circulation in the exposed areas aids in preventing tissue damage due to hypothermia.

How Cold Is "Too Cold"?

Cold injuries from overexposure are on the upswing because of increased interest in outdoor winter activities such as ice skating, cross-country skiing, snowmobiling, ice fishing, and all-season jogging. Owing to the pronounced peripheral vasoconstriction during severe cold exposure, the temperature of the skin and the extremities may fall to dangerous levels. Early warning signs of cold injury include a tingling and numbness in the fingers and toes, or a burning sensation of the nose and ears. If these signs are not heeded, overexposure can lead to tissue damage in the form of frostbite; in extreme cases the damage is irreversible and the tissue must be surgically removed.

The Wind Chill Index. One dilemma in evaluating the thermal quality of an environment is that ambient temperature alone is not always a valid indication of "coldness." All too often we have experienced the chilling winds of a spring day even though the temperature was well above freezing. On the other hand, a calm subfreezing day may feel quite comfortable.

The important factor is the wind; on a windy day air currents magnify heat loss as the warmer insulating air layer surrounding the body is continually replaced by cooler ambient air.

The cooling effect of wind is clearly shown in the *Wind Chill Index* presented in Figure 15-7. This figure illustrates the effects of wind velocity on bare skin for different temperatures and velocities. For example, a 30° F reading is equivalent to 0° F when the wind speed is 25 mph, while a 10° F reading is equivalent to –29° F when the wind speed is 25 mph. In addition, if a person runs, skis, or skates into the wind the effective cooling from the wind is increased in direct relation to the exerciser's velocity. Thus, running at 8 mph into a 12 mph headwind is the equivalent of a 20 mph wind speed. Conversely, running at 8 mph with a 12 mph wind at your back creates a relative wind speed of only 4 mph. In the lightly- shaded zone on the left there is relatively little danger from cold exposure for a properly clothed person. In contrast, in the medium-shaded zone, which generally begins at about 22° F, there is increasing danger to exposed flesh, especially the ears, nose, and fingers. In the heavily shaded zone on the right, the equivalent temperatures pose a serious danger to the freezing of exposed flesh within a matter of minutes.

The Respiratory Tract During Cold–Weather Exercise

Cold ambient air generally does not pose a special danger in terms of damage to the respiratory passages. Even in extreme cold, the incoming air is generally warmed to between 26° C and 32° C by the time it reaches the bronchi. When the incoming breath of air is warmed, its capacity to hold moisture increases greatly and humidification occurs at the expense of water from the respiratory passages. Thus, significant amounts of water and heat can be lost from the respiratory tract, especially during exercise when ventilatory volumes are quite large. This often contributes to respiratory complaints during exercise in the cold. A general dehydration can accompany exercise, as well as a dryness of the mouth, a burning sensation in the throat, and an irritation of the respiratory passages. These symptoms can be greatly reduced by wearing a scarf or mask–type "baklava" that covers the nose and mouth and that traps the water in the exhaled air. This action subsequently warms and moistens the next breath of incoming air.

1. Core temperature normally increases during exercise with the magnitude of the rise in temperature determined by the relative stress of a particular work load. This well-regulated temperature adjustment probably creates a favorable environment for physiologic function.

2. Sweating places demands on the body's fluid reserves and creates a relative state of dehydration. If sweating is excessive and fluids are not continually replaced, blood volume falls and core temperature may rise to lethal levels.

3. Exercise in hot, humid environments poses a great challenge to temperature regulation because the large sweat loss in high humidity contributes little to evaporative cooling.

4. Relatively small degrees of dehydration impede heat dissipation and compromise cardiovascular function and work capacity.

5. The primary aim of fluid replacement is to maintain plasma volume so that circulation and sweating progress at optimal levels. For the ideal replacement schedule during exercise, fluid intake should match fluid loss. This can be monitored effectively by changes in body weight.

6. Electrolytes lost through sweating are readily replaced by adding a small amount of salt to the food in the daily diet.

7. Repeated heat stress initiates thermoregulatory adjustments that result in improved exercise capacity and less discomfort on subsequent heat exposure. This heat acclimatization brings about a favorable distribution of cardiac output and a greatly increased capacity for sweating. Full acclimatization generally occurs in about 10 days of heat exposure.

8. The ability to tolerate and acclimatize to moderate heat stress probably does not appreciably deteriorate with age.

9. Women seem to be at least as efficient in temperature regulation as men, although they produce less sweat while maintaining the same temperature.

10. Various practical heat stress indices make use of ambient temperature, radiant heat, and relative humidity to evaluate the potential heat challenge of an environment to an exercising subject.

11. Because heat conduction in water is about 25 times greater than in air, immersion in water of only 28 to 30° C can provide a considerable thermal stress and bring about thermoregulatory adjustments in a relatively short time period.

12. Subcutaneous fat provides excellent body insulation against cold stress. It greatly enhances the effectiveness of vasomotor adjustments and enables fat individuals to retain a large percentage of metabolic heat. This is apparent in cold water where relatively fat individuals show proportionately smaller thermal and cardiovascular adjustments and greater exercise tolerance in comparison to leaner counterparts.

13. The body is much less capable of adapting physiologically to prolonged cold stress than to prolonged heat exposure. In most instances, appropriate clothing enables humans to tolerate even the coldest climates on earth.

14. The "coldness" of an environment is influenced by the ambient temperature and the wind. The cooling effect of the wind can be determined by the Wind Chill Index.

15. Although considerable water can be lost from the respiratory passages when exercising on a cold day, the temperature of the inspired ambient air generally does not pose a danger to the respiratory tract.

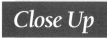

THE UNDERWATER ENVIRONMENT: NOT WITHOUT ITS DANGERS

The pleasures of underwater diving are countless. Just ask the nearly 4.5 million scuba divers in the United States and the 200,000 new ones being trained to dive each year. Underwater exploration offers discoveries of new and colorful species of plants and fish, old-world relics, and a feeling of self-awareness unknown to most. But the lure of the deep is not without its hazards.

As one descends into the sea, the pressure of the water against the body becomes substantial. For each 33 feet below the surface, for example, water exerts a force equivalent to one sea- level atmosphere or 760 mmHg (14.7 lb per in^2). This external water pressure against the diver has little effect on the body's fluid-filled spaces. The effect on the air-filled cavities (lungs, respiratory passages, the sinus and middle-ear spaces) can be rapid and substantial, leading to pain, injury and death unless adjustments are made to equalize pressure.

Swimming at the surface of the water with fins, mask, and snorkel is a common form of recreation and sport. If a person takes a full inspiration of ambient air, about 1000 ml of oxygen is brought into the lungs. If the breath is then held, 600 to 700 ml of O_2 in the lungs can be used to sustain metabolism before the partial pressures of arterial O_2 and CO_2 signal the need for renewed breathing. With some training, individuals can breathhold for 1 minute or longer. During this time, arterial Po_2 drops to about 60 mmHg, whereas arterial Pco_2 rises to 50 mmHg. During exercise, breathhold time is greatly reduced because oxygen uptake and carbon dioxide production increase with the severity of exercise. Breathhold diving, preceded by hyperventilation,

can extend the breathhold period, yet can significantly increase the danger of the dive.

A sudden loss of consciousness or blackout during attempts to extend the duration of time underwater while breathholding is not unique to the unskilled or novice diver. Most reports of blackout during underwater activity involve men (97% of all incidences) between the ages of 16 and 20, all known to be good or excellent swimmers. In most cases, the person was in competition with himself or others to see how far he could swim underwater or stay below the surface. Surprisingly, in about 80% of the cases, the accident occurred in a pool with a lifeguard on duty. For people who survived underwater blackout and were able to recount their story, most reported that they had an urge to breathe but lost consciousness without recognizable warning signs. In several instances the victim did not remember any feelings associated with reaching the "breaking point" before passing out.

The break point for breathhold usually corresponds to an increase in arterial Pco_2 to about 50 mmHg. For some people, however, it is possible to ignore this stimulus and continue to breathhold until CO_2 reaches levels that cause severe disorientation and blackout.

With hyperventilation prior to breathhold, arterial Pco_2 may decrease from its normal value of 40 mmHg to15 mmHg. This elimination of CO_2 significantly extends the duration of breathhold until the arterial Pco_2 increases to a level that stimulates ventilation. The longest breathhold recorded while breathing air without prior hyperventilation is 270 seconds. Breathholds of 15 to 20 minutes have been reported with hyperventilation followed by several breaths of pure oxygen immediately prior to breathholding. However, this procedure is risky. Alveolar oxygen continually moves into the blood to be delivered to the working muscles. With prior hyperventilation, carbon dioxide levels remain low and the diver is free from the urge to breathe. Concurrently, as the diver goes deeper, the external water pressure compresses the thorax. This increased pressure maintains a relatively high Po_2 within the alveoli. Thus, even though the absolute quantity of oxygen in the lungs is lowered (as oxygen moves into the blood), adequate pressure is maintained to load hemoglobin as the dive progresses. Now, as the diver senses the need to breathe and begins the ascent, significant reversals occur in pressure. As water pressure on the thorax decreases and lung volume expands, the partial pressure of alveolar oxygen is reduced proportionately. In fact, as the diver nears the surface, the alveolar Po_2 may be so low that dissolved oxygen actually leaves the blood and flows into the alveoli! In this situation, the diver can suddenly lose consciousness before reaching the surface.

Depth		Atmosphere	Pressure	Lung Volume
Feet	Meters		mmHg	ml
Sea level		1	760	6000
33	10	2	1520	3000
66	20	3	2280	2000
99	30	4	3040	1500
133	40	5	3800	1200
166	50	6	4560	1000
200	60	7	5320	857

Relationship of depth in water to pressure and volume of a gas. If divers fill their lungs with 6 liters of air at sea level and descend to a depth of 33 feet, the lung volume is compressed to 3 liters; diving an additional 33 feet, the original 6 liter lung volume is reduced one third to 2 liters. When the diver returns to the surface, the air volume re-expands to its original 6 liter volume.

Reference

Craig, A. B. Summary of 58 cases of loss of consciousness during underwater swimming and diving. *Med. Sci. Sports.* 8:171, 1976.

Hyperventilation. The immediate first line of defense of the native lowlander to altitude exposure is hyperventilation brought on by the reduced arterial Po_2. Special receptors sensitive to reduced oxygen pressure are located in the aortic arch and at the branching of the carotid arteries in the neck. Any significant reduction in arterial Po_2 progressively stimulates these chemoreceptors. This in turn increases alveolar ventilation and causes alveolar oxygen concentration to increase toward the level in ambient air — the greater the hyperventilation, the more closely alveolar air resembles inspired air. The increase in alveolar Po_2 with hyperventilation facilitates oxygen loading in the lungs.

Accelerated Circulatory Response. In the early stages of altitude acclimatization, submaximal heart rate and cardiac output may increase 50% above sea-level values, whereas the heart's stroke volume remains essentially unchanged. Because the oxygen cost of exercise at altitude is essentially unchanged compared to sea level, the increase in submaximal blood flow compensates for the reduced oxygen in arterial blood. In maximal exercise, however, the circulatory adjustments to acute altitude exposure cannot compensate for the lower oxygen content of arterial blood and max $\dot{V}O_2$ and exercise capacity are dramatically reduced.

Fluid Loss. Because the air in mountainous regions is usually cool and dry, considerable body water can be lost through evaporation as air is warmed and moistened in the respiratory passages. This fluid loss often leads to moderate dehydration and accompanying symptoms of dryness of the lips, mouth, and throat. This is particularly true for active people for whom the daily total sweat loss and

TABLE 15-2. Immediate and longer-term adjustments to altitude hypoxia

System	Immediate	Longer-Term
Pulmonary Acid-Base	Hyperventilation	Hyperventilation
	Body fluids become more alkaline due to reduction in CO_2 with hyperventilation	Excretion of base via the kidneys and concommitant reduction in alkaline reserve
Cardiovascular	Increase in submaximal heart rate	Submaximal heart rate remains elevated
	Increase in submaximal cardiac output	Submaximal cardiac output falls to or below sea-level values
	Stroke volume remains the same or is slightly lowered	Stroke volume is lowered
	Maximum cardiac output remains the same or is slightly lowered	Maximum cardiac output is lowered
Hematologic		Decrease in plasma volume Increased hematocrit Increased hemoglobin concentration Increased total number of red blood cells
Local		Possible increased capillarization of skeletal muscle Increased red-blood-cell 2.3-DPG Increased mitochondria Increased aerobic enzymes

pulmonary ventilation (and hence water loss) are large. For these active people, body weight should be checked frequently and easy access to water provided at all times.

Longer-Term Adjustments

Hyperventilation and increased submaximal cardiac output provide a rapid and relatively effective counter to the acute challenge of altitude. Concurrently, other slower acting physiologic adjustments are set in motion during a prolonged altitude stay. The most important of these involve:

Acid-Base Readjustment. Although hyperventilation at altitude favorably increases alveolar oxygen concentration, it has the opposite effect on carbon dioxide. Because ambient air contains essentially no carbon dioxide, the increased breathing at altitude tends to "wash out" or dilute this gas in the alveoli. This creates a larger-than-normal gradient for the diffusion of carbon dioxide from the blood to the lungs, and arterial carbon dioxide is reduced considerably. During a prolonged high-altitude stay, the pressure of alveolar carbon dioxide often falls as low as 10 mm Hg compared to its sea-level value of 40 mm Hg.

The loss of carbon dioxide from the body's fluids at altitude causes the pH to rise as the blood becomes more alkaline. (Recall from Chapter 8, that the largest amount of carbon dioxide is carried combined with water as carbonic acid.) The control of respiratory alkalosis is accomplished by the kidneys which slowly excrete base (HCO_3^-) through the renal tubules.

The establishment of acid-base equilibrium with acclimatization occurs at the expense of a loss of alkaline reserve. Thus, although the pathways of anaerobic metabolism are unaffected at altitude, the blood's buffering capacity for acids is gradually decreased and the critical limit is lowered for the accumulation of acid metabolites such as lactic acid.

Hematologic Changes. The most important long-term adaptation to altitude is an increase in the blood's oxygen-carrying capacity.

- *Decrease in plasma volume:* Red blood cells become more concentrated during the first few days at altitude because of a decrease in plasma volume. This rapid adjustment in plasma volume and accompanying hemoconcentration causes the oxygen content of arterial blood to increase significantly above values observed immediately on ascent to altitude.

- *Increase in red cell mass:* The reduced arterial oxygen pressure at altitude stimulates an increase in the total number of red blood cells. This response, termed *polycythemia,* directly translates into a large increase in the blood's capacity to transport oxygen.

The response for polycythemia is mediated by an erythrocyte-stimulating factor, *erythropoietin,* released from the kidneys and other tissues within 15 hours after altitude ascent. In the weeks that follow, the production of erythrocytes in the marrow of the long bones increases considerably and remains elevated during residence at altitude. For example, the oxygen-carrying capacity of blood for high-altitude residents of Peru is 28% above sea-level averages. For well-acclimatized mountaineers, 25 to 31 ml of oxygen are carried per 100 ml of blood (at sea-level Po_2) compared to about 19.7 for lowland residents. Thus, even with the reduced saturation of hemoglobin at altitude, the actual quantity of oxygen in arterial blood approaches or even equals sea-level values.

The general trend for increases in hemoglobin and hematocrit during altitude acclimatization is illustrated in Figure 15-9. These data were obtained for eight young women at the University of Missouri (altitude 213 m) who lived and worked for 10 weeks at the 4267 m summit of Pikes Peak. Upon reaching Pikes Peak, red blood cell concentration increased

Loss of muscle mass. During long-term exposure to high altitude, a significant loss of body mass is generally observed that is generally derived from the muscle component of the fat-free body mass.

rapidly. This increase was caused by a reduction in plasma volume during

the first 24 hours at altitude. In the month that followed, hemoglobin concentration and hematocrit continued to increase and then stabilized for the remainder of the stay. Prealtitude values were established 2 weeks after the women returned to Missouri.

Cellular Adaptations. Peripheral changes take place during acclimatization process that facilitate the process of aerobic metabolism.

- Capillaries become more concentrated in skeletal muscle. This modification in local circulation reduces the distance for oxygen diffusion between the blood and tissues.
- Muscle myoglobin increases by as much as 16% after acclimatization. This is complemented by an increase in the number of mitochondria and the concentration of enzymes required for aerobic energy transfer. These adaptations would increase the "storage" of oxygen in specific muscles and facilitate intracellular oxygen delivery and utilization, especially at low tissue Po_2.
- An increase in the concentration of the metabolic intermediate, 2,3-diphosphoglycerate in red blood cells occurs during long-term altitude residence. This adaptation favors the release of available oxygen to the tissues for a given drop in cellular Po_2.

Acute Mountain Sickness

Despite the body's rapid defense against the stress of altitude, many people experience the acute discomfort of mountain sickness during the first few days at altitudes of about 3048 m (10,000 ft) or higher. These symptoms usually include headache (most frequent symptom probably due to dilation of cerebral blood vessels), dizziness, nausea, vomiting, dimness of vision, insomnia, and generalized weakness. For people suffering the effects of mountain sickness, even moderate exercise can be intolerable. With acclimatization, symp-

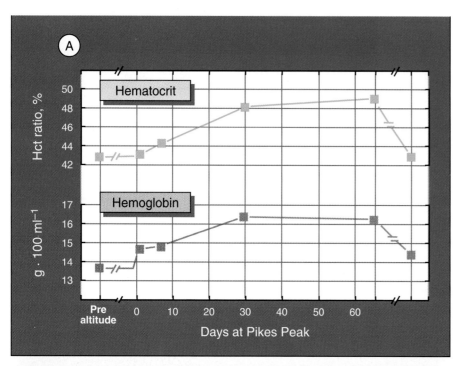

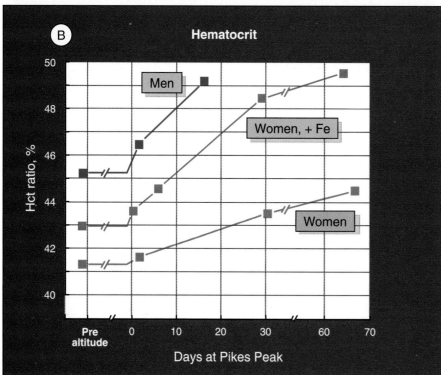

Figure 15-9. (A) Effects of altitude on hemoglobin and hematocrit levels of 8 young women prior to, during, and 2 weeks after exposure to altitude of 4267 m. (From Hannon, J. P., et al.: Effects of altitude acclimatization on blood composition of women. *J. Appl. Physiol.,* 26: 540, 1968.) (B) Hematocrit response of young women receiving supplemental iron (+ Fe) prior to and during altitude exposure compared to groups of male and female subjects receiving no supplemental iron. (Courtesy of Dr. J. P. Hannon.)

toms subside and many disappear. Mountain sickness can usually be prevented by acclimatizing slowly to moderate altitudes, followed by a slow progression to higher altitudes.

EXERCISE CAPACITY AT ALTITUDE

The stress of high altitude imposes significant restrictions on exercise capacity and physiologic function. Even at lower altitudes, the body's adjustments do not fully compensate for reduced oxygen pressure, and exercise performance is compromised.

Aerobic Capacity

Aerobic capacity shows a progressive and somewhat linear decrease with increases in altitude. One can generally expect a 1.5 to 3.5% reduction in max $\dot{V}O_2$ (for both the trained and untrained) for every 305 m (1000 ft.) above 1524 m (5000 ft.) altitude. Consequently, the maximum aerobic capacity of a relatively fit man atop Mt. Everest would be about 1000 ml of oxygen per minute.

Circulatory Factors

Even after several months of acclimatization, aerobic capacity still remains significantly below sea-level values. This occurs because the benefits of acclimatization are offset by a reduction in circulatory efficiency in moderate and strenuous exercise.

Submaximal Exercise. Although the immediate altitude response involves an increase in submaximal cardiac output, the exercise cardiac output in the days and weeks of acclimatization that follow is reduced and does not improve with longer altitude exposure. This is caused by a decrease in stroke volume as altitude progresses.

Maximal Exercise. Reduction in maximum cardiac output occurs after about a week at altitudes above 3048 m. This reduction in blood flow dur-

ing all-out exercise, that persists through one's altitude stay, is generally the combined effect of a decrease in maximum heart rate and stroke volume.

Performance Measures. A 2 to 13% decrement in exercise performance is observed for fit subjects in 1- and 3-mile runs at the medium altitude of 2300 m. At higher altitudes the effects are more pronounced. Even after 4 weeks of acclimatization, significant decrements in endurance performance at altitude are noted compared to sea-level values.

ALTITUDE TRAINING AND SEA-LEVEL PERFORMANCE

Without doubt, altitude acclimatization improves one's capacity to exercise at altitude. What is not clear, however, is the effect of prior altitude exposure and altitude training on aerobic power and endurance performance immediately on return to sea level. Certainly, altitude adaptations in local circulation and cellular function as well as the compensatory increase in the blood's oxygen-carrying capacity should facilitate sea-level performance. Unfortunately, much of the previous altitude research has not been designed to evaluate adequately this possibility. Often, the activity level of the subjects is poorly controlled, so it is difficult to determine whether an improved max $\dot{V}O_2$ or performance score on return from altitude represents a training effect, an altitude effect, or a synergism between altitude and training.

Max $\dot{V}O_2$ on Return to Sea Level

When max $\dot{V}O_2$ is used as the criterion, sea-level performance is not significantly improved after living at altitude. For example, there was no significant change in the aerobic capacity of young runners on return to sea level after 18 days at an altitude of 3100 m compared to the prealtitude measures. In addition, training

Competing at altitude. For athletes desiring to compete at altitude, intense training should commence as soon as possible during the acclimatization period. This will minimize any detraining effects because it is difficult to engage in hard training in the early days of one's altitude stay.

Blood doping. Within a physiologic context, the controversial use of blood doping mimics the hematologic benefits of a stay at altitude without the potential negative effects of altitude on cardiovascular dynamics and body composition.

Gender, iron, and acclimatization. For women, iron supplementation enhances the rate of hematocrit increase at altitude to a level similar for men at the same location. This indicates that athletes who have borderline iron stores may not respond to the acclimatization process as wel as individuals who have adequate iron reserves to sustain an increase in red blood cell production.

in chambers designed to simulate altitude provided no additional benefit to sea-level performance compared to similar training at sea level. As expected, the "altitude-trained" group showed significantly higher physical performance in the "altitude" experiments compared to their sea level counterparts.

Some of the physiologic changes that occur during prolonged altitude exposure may actually negate adaptations that possibly could improve exercise performance upon return to sea level. The residual effects of a loss in muscle mass and a reduced maximum heart rate and stroke volume frequently observed at altitude certainly would not enhance sea-level performance. Any reduction in maximum cardiac output would offset the benefits derived from the blood's greater oxygen-carrying capacity.

Can Training Be Maintained at Altitude?

Exposure to altitudes of 2300 m and higher makes it nearly impossi-

ble for athletes to train at the same intensity as that engaged in at sea level. At 4000 m, for example, runners are only able to train at about 40% of their sea level max $\dot{V}O_2$ compared to an intensity of about 80% when training at sea level. This reduction in training intensity is possibly of such magnitude that an athlete may be unable to maintain peak condition for sea-level competition.

Is Altitude Training More Effective Than Sea–Level Training?

To answer this question, highly trained middle-distance runners were trained at sea level for 3 weeks at 75% of sea level max $\dot{V}O_2$, whereas another group of six runners trained an equivalent distance at the same percentage of the max $\dot{V}O_2$ at 2300 m. The groups then exchanged training sites and continued training for 3 weeks at an intensity similar to that of the preceding group. Initially, 2-mile run times were 7.2% slower at altitude than at sea level. This improved about 2.0% for both groups after altitude training, but post–altitude performance at sea level was unchanged when compared to prealtitude sea-level runs. As shown in Figure 15-10, max $\dot{V}O_2$ for both groups at altitude was reduced initially by about 17%. This improved only slightly after 20 days of altitude training. When the runners were then measured at sea level, aerobic power was 2.8% below prealtitude sea level values! Clearly, for these well-conditioned runners, there was no synergistic effect of hard aerobic training at medium altitude over equivalently severe training at sea level.

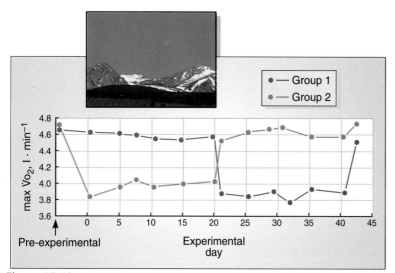

Figure 15-10. Maximal oxygen uptakes of two equivalent groups during training for 3 weeks at altitude and 3 weeks at sea level. Group 1 trained first at sea level and then continued training for 3 weeks at altitude. For Group 2, the procedure was reversed as they trained first at altitude and then at sea level. (From Adams, W. C., et al.: Effects of equivalent sea-level and altitude training on $\dot{V}O_2$ max and running performance. *J. Appl. Physiol.*, 39:262, 1975.)

SUMMARY

1. The progressive reduction in ambient Po_2 upon ascent to altitude eventually leads to inadequate oxygenation of hemoglobin. This produces noticeable performance decrements in aerobic activities at altitudes of 2000 m and higher.

2. The reduced Po_2 and accompanying hypoxia at altitude stimulate physiologic responses and adjustments that improve one's tolerance during rest and exercise. The primary immediate responses are hyperventilation and increased submaximal cardiac output via an elevated heart rate.

3. The longer term acclimatization process involves physiologic adjustments that greatly improve tolerance to altitude hypoxia. The main adjustments involve (1) reestablishing the acid-base balance of the body fluids, (2) increased formation of hemoglobin and red blood cells, and (3) changes in local circulation and cellular function. Adjustments (2) and (3) significantly facilitate oxygen transport and utilization.

4. The rate and magnitude of acclimatization depends on the altitude. Noticeable improvements are observed within several days, and the major adjustments require about 2 weeks, although 4 to 6 weeks may be required to acclimatize to high altitudes.

5. For acclimatized men at a simulated altitude that approaches the summit of Mt. Everest, alveolar Po_2 is about 25 mm Hg. This results in a 70% reduction in max $\dot{V}O_2$. Unacclimatized individuals at this altitude would become unconscious within 30 seconds.

6. Acclimatization does not fully compensate for the stress of altitude. Even after acclimatization, the max $\dot{V}O_2$ is decreased about 2% for every 300 m about 1500 m. This is paralleled by a drop in performance in endurance-related activities.

7. The inability to achieve sea-level max $\dot{V}O_2$ values at altitude is partially explained by the fact that the beneficial effects of acclimatization are offset by altitude-related decrements in maximum heart rate and stroke volume.

8. Although acclimatization to altitude would certainly seem to enhance aerobic power and endurance performance upon return to sea level, research results generally do not support this contention.

9. Training at altitude provides no additional benefit to sea-level performance compared to equivalent training at sea level.

SELECTED REFERENCES

American College of Sports Medicine position stand on prevention of thermal injuries during distance running. *Sports Med. Bull.*, 19:8, 1984.

Anderson, R. K., and Kenney, W. L.: Effect of age on heat-activated sweat gland density and flow during exercise in dry heat. *J. Appl. Physiol.*, 63:1089, 1987.

Armstrong, L. E., and Pandolf, D. B.: Physical training, cardiorespiratory physical fitness and exercise-heat tolerance. In *Human Performance Physiology and Environmental Medicine at Terrestrial Extremes.* Edited by K. B. Pandolf, et al. Indianapolis, Benchmark Press, 1988.

Bar-Or, O.: Temperature regulation during exercise in children and adolescents. In *Perspectives in Exercise Science and Sports Medicine.* Vol. 2. Edited by C. V. Gisolfi and D. R. Lamb. Indiana, Benchmark Press, 1989.

Brouns, F.: Nutritional aspects of health and performance at lowland and altitude. *Int. J. Sports Med.*, 13, Suppl 1:S100, 1992.

Buono, M. J., and Sjoholm, N. T.: Effect of physical training on peripheral sweat production. *J. Appl. Physiol.*, 65:811, 1988.

Carter, J. E., and Gisolfi, C. V.: Fluid replacement during and after exercise in the heat. *Med. Sci. Sports Exerc.*, 21:532, 1989.

Convertino, V., et al.: Plasma volume, renin, and vasopressin responses to graded exercise after training. *J. Appl. Physiol.*, 54:508, 1983.

Coyle, E. F., and Coyle, E.: Carbohydrates that speed recovery from training. *Phys. Sportsmed.*, 21 (2):111, 1993.

Cymerman, A., et al.: Operation Everest II: maximal oxygen uptake at extreme altitude. *J. Appl. Physiol.*, 66:2446, 1989.

Deschamps, A., et al.: Effect of saline infusion on body temperature and endurance during heavy exercise. *J. Appl. Physiol.*, 66:2799, 1989.

DeSouza, M. J., et al.: Menstrual status and plasma vasopressin, renin and aldosterone exercise responses. *J. Appl. Physiol.*, 67:736, 1989.

Falk, B., et al.: Thermoregulatory responses of pre-, mid-, and late pubertal boys to exercise in dry heat. *Med. Sci. Sports Exerc.*, 24: 688, 1992.

Falk, B., et al.: Response to rest and exercise in the cold: effects of age and aerobic fitness. *J. Appl. Physiol.*, 76: 72, 1994.

Feblruio, M.A., et al.: Muscle metabolism during exercise and heat stress in trained men: effect of acclimatization. *J. Appl. Physiol.*, 76: 589, 1994.

Ferretti, G. et al.: Oxygen transport system before and after exposure to chronic hypoxia. *Int. J. Sports Med.*, 11:S15, 1990.

Francesconi, R. P.: Endocrine and physiological responses to exercise in stressful environments. In *Exercise and Sport*

Sciences Reviews. Vol. 16. Edited by K. B. Pandolf. New York, Macmillan, 1988.

Green, H. J., et al.: Operation Everest II: adaptations in human skeletal muscle. *J. Appl. Physiol.,* 66:2454, 1989.

Haymes, E. M.: Physiological responses of female athletes to heat stress: a review. *Phys. Sportsmed.,* 12:45, 1984.

Hiller, W. B. D.: Dehydration and hyponatraemia during triathlons. *Med. Sci. Sports Exerc.,* 21:219, 1989.

Honigman, B., et al.: Acute mountain sickness in a general tourist population at moderate altitude. *Ann. Intern. Med.,* 188: 587, 1993.

Jacobs, I., et al.: Thermoregulatory thermogenesis in humans during cold stress. *Exerc. Sport Sci. Rev.,* 22: 221, 1994.

Krasney, J.A.: Brief review: a neurogenic basis for acute altitude sickness. *Med. Sci. Sports Exerc.,* 26: 195, 1994.

LeBlanc, J.: Factors affecting cold acclimation and thermogenesis in man. *Med. Sci. Sports Exerc.,* 20:S193, 1988.

Mack, G.W., et al.: Body fluid balance in dehydrated healthy older men: thirst and renal osmoregulation. *J. Appl. Physiol.,* 76: 1615, 1994.

Mack, G.W., et al.: Influence of exercise intensity and plasma volume on active cutaneous vasodilatation in humans. *Med. Sci. Sports Exerc.,* 26: 209, 1994.

Malconian, M.K. and Rock, P.B. Medical problems related to altitude. In: *Human Performance Physiology And Environmental Medicine At Terrestrial Extremes.* (Eds: Pandolf, K. et al.). Cooper Publishing Group. Carmel, IN. 1994. p. 545-563.

McArdle, W. D., et al.: Thermal responses of men and women during coldwater immersion: influence of exercise intensity. *Eur. J. Appl. Physiol.,* 65:265, 1992.

McArdle, W.D., et al.: Thermal responses of men and women during cold-water immersion: influences of exercise intensity. *Eur. J. Appl. Physiol.,* 65: 265, 1992.

Maugham, R. F.: Fluid and electrolyte loss and replacement in exercise. In *Foods, Nutrition and Sports Performance.* Edited by C. Williams, and J. T. Devlin. London, E. & F. N. Spon, 1992.

Mazzeo, R., et al.: Adrenergic blockade does not prevent the lactate response to exercise after acclimatization to high altitude. *J. Appl. Physiol.,* 76: 629, 1994.

Mizuano, M., et al.: Limb skeletal muscle adaptation in athletes after training at altitude. *J. Appl. Physiol.,* 68:496, 1990.

Montain, S. J., et al.: Fluid ingestion during exercise increases skin blood flow independent of increases in blood volume. *J. Appl. Physiol.,* 73:903, 1992.

Nadel, E, R., et al.: Influence of fluid replacement beverages on body fluid homeostasis during exercise and recovery. In *Perspectives in Exercise Science and Sports Medicine.* Vol. 3. Edited by C. V. Gisolfi and D. R. Lamb. Carmel, Benchmark Press, 1990.

Noakes, T. D., et al.: The danger of an inadequate water intake during prolonged exercise. A novel concept revisted. *Eur. J. Appl. Physiol.,* 57:210, 1988.

Noakes, T. D.: Fluid replacement during exercise. In *Exercise and Sport Sciences Reviews.* Vol. 21. Edited by J. O. Holloszy. Baltimore, MD, Williams & Wilkins, 1993.

Nose, H. et al.: Involvement of sodium retention hormones during rehydration in humans. *J. Appl. Physiol.,* 65:332, 1988.

Pandolf, K. B., et al.: Thermoregulatory responses of middle-aged and young men during dry-heat acclimatization. *J. Appl. Physiol.,* 65:65, 1988.

Pandolf, K. et al. (Eds:): *Human Performance Physiology And Environmental Medicine At Terrestrial Extremes.* Cooper Publishing Group. Carmel, IN. 1994.

Reeves, J. T.: Operation Everest II; preservation of cardiac function at extreme altitude. *J. Appl. Physiol.,* 63:531, 1987.

Rennie, D. W.: Tissue heat transfer in water: lessons from the Korean divers. *Med. Sci. Sports Exerc.,* 20:S177, 1988.

Rose, M. S., et al.: Operation Everest II: nutrition and body composition. *J. Appl. Physiol.,* 65:2545, 1988.

Rowell, L. B.: *Human Circulation.* New York, Oxford University Press, 1986.

Sawka, M. N., and Wegner, C. B.: Physiological responses to acute-exercise heat stress. In *Human Performance Physiolo-gy and Environmenmtal Medicine at Terrestrial Extremes.* Edited by Kent B. Pandolf, et al. Indianapolis, Benchmark Press, 1988.

Schoene, R. B.: High-altitude pulmonary edema: the disguised killer. *Phys. Sportsmed.,* 16:103, 1988.

Stephenson, L. A., and Kolka, M. A.: Thermoregulation in women. In *Exercise and Sport Sciences Reviews.* Vol. 21. Edited by J. O. Holloszy. Baltimore MD, Williams & Wilkins, 1993.

Stephenson, L.A., and Kolka, M.A.: Effect of gender, circadian period and sleep loss on thermal responses during exercise. In: *Human Performance Physiology And Environmental Medicine At Terrestrial Extremes.* (Eds: Pandolf, K. et al.). Cooper Publishing Group. Carmel, IN. 1994. p. 267-304.

Stephenson, L.A., and Kolka, M.A.: Thermoregulation in women. *Exerc. Sport Sci. Rev.,* 21: 231, 1993.

Toner, M. M., and McArdle, W. D.: Physiological adjustments of man to the cold. In *Human Performance Physiology and Environmental Medicine at Terrestrial Esxtremes.* Edited by K. B. Pandolf, et al. Indianapolis, Benchmark Press, 1988.

Welch, H. G.: Effects of hypoxia and hyperoxia on human performance. In *Exercise and Sport Sciences Reviews.* Vol. 15. Edited by Kent B. Pandolf. New York, Macmillan, 1987.

Wolfel, E.E., et al.: Systemic hypertension at 4,300 m is related to sympathoadrenal activity. *J. Appl. Physiol.,* 76: 1643, 1994.

Young, A. J. Energy substrate utilization during exercise in extreme environments. In *Exercise and Sport Sciences Reviews.* Vol. 18. Edited by Kent B. Pandolf and J. O. Holloszy. Baltimore, Williams & Wilkins, 1990.

Young, A. J., and Young, P. M.: Human Acclimatization to high terrestrial altitude. In *Human performance Physiology and Environmental Medicine at Terrestrial Extremes.* Edited by K. B. Pandolf, et al. Indianapolis, Benchmark Press, 1988.

Body Composition, Weight Control, and the Age- and Health-Related Aspects of Exercise

SECTION VI

An excess accumulation of body fat is undesirable for a variety of reasons. From a health standpoint, medical problems exist for which obesity or "overfatness" is a risk and for which a fat reduction is desirable. Also, being too fat is often accompanied by social and professional discrimination as well as changes in personality and behavior frequently shown as depression, withdrawal, self-pity, and aggression. Thus, it is small wonder that about $50 billion is spent annually by more than 60 million men, women, and children attempting to achieve permanent weight loss.

The first step in evaluating body weight and size as well as in formulating an effective program of weight control is to appraise body composition objectively. It is possible to be heavy and even overweight according to established charts, yet possess only a moderate amount of body fat. Many athletes, for example, are quite muscular but are otherwise lean in terms of their overall body composition. A weight loss program for such people may be unnecessary. Such an approach would be prudent, however, for others who may be 5 to 10 kg overfat. Of even greater importance is the need for effective weight control among the increasingly large segment of the population afflicted with "creeping obesity". During the adult years, body mass and body fat can increase insidiously to the point that body fat exceeds even the most liberal limits for normalcy. It is at this point that the health-related aspects of obesity become a serious concern. Unfortunately, correction of adult acquired obesity through dietary intervention or exercise is much more difficult than its early prevention.

In terms of aging effects, there is no question that the physiologic and exercise capacities of older people are generally below those of younger counterparts. What is uncertain is the degree to which these differences are caused by true biologic aging or are simply the result of disuse brought on by alterations in lifestyle and activity opportunities as people age. No longer can older men and women be stereotyped as sedentary with little or no initiative for active pursuits. There is currently a tremendous upswing in participation by "senior citizens" in a broad range of physical activities and exercise programs. Research clearly demonstrates that if an active lifestyle is continued into later years, a relatively high level of function is retained and vigorous activities can be engaged in safely and successfully. In addition, regular exercise throughout life offers significant protection against a variety of diseases and risk factors, particularly those related to the cardiovascular system.

Chapter 16 discusses the underlying rationale for evaluating body composition in terms of body fat and lean body mass. Also presented are average values for body composition as well as the extremes in body composition often observed in champion male and female sports competitors. In Chapter 17, we define "overweight" in terms of acceptable limits of body fat for a particular age range for men and women, and explore the various criteria for obesity. We discuss the interrelated factors often associated with obesity as well as the efficacy of diet and exercise as a treatment for the overfat condition. Chapter 18 explores several aspects of the aging process with special emphasis on exercise and its relation to cardiovascular disease.

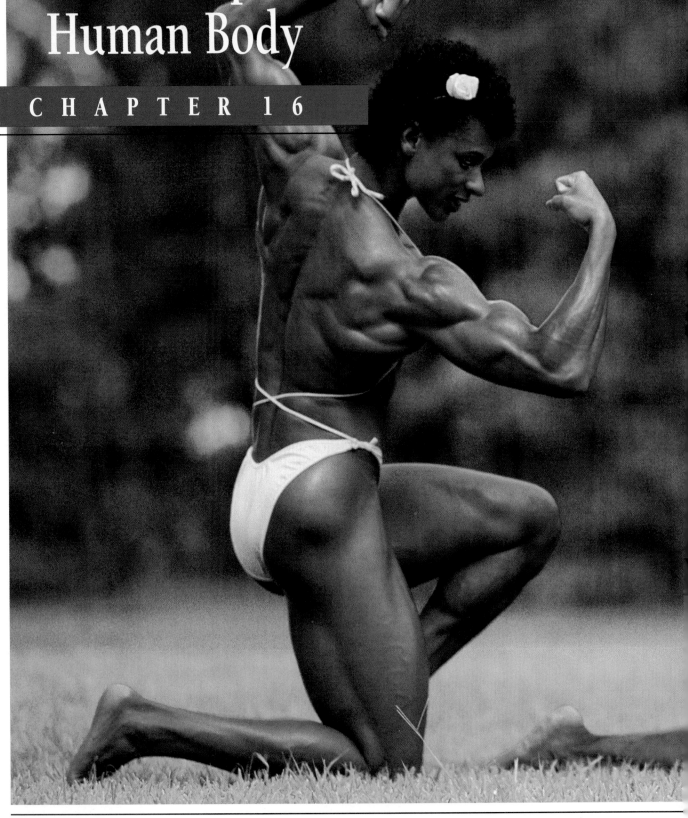

The Composition of the Human Body

CHAPTER 16

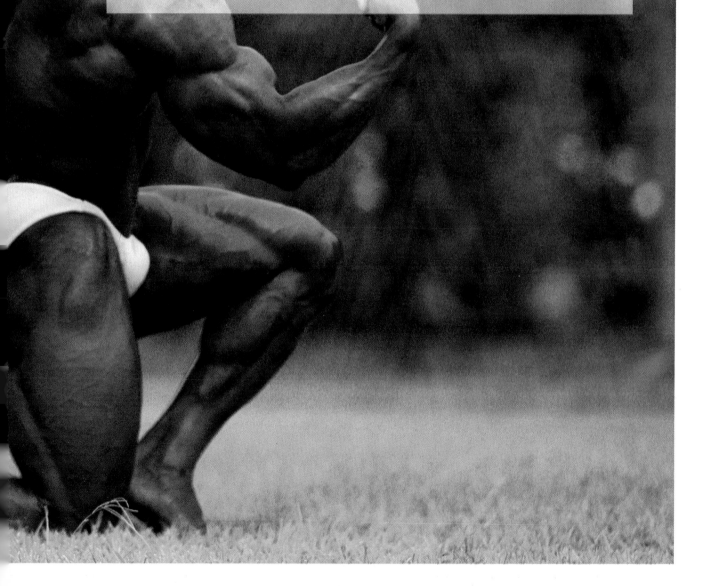

TOPICS COVERED IN THIS CHAPTER

After reading this chapter, you should be able to:

- Give an overview of the early research by Dr. Albert Behnke that pointed up the inadequacies of the "height-weight" tables.
- Outline the specific characteristics of the "Reference man" and "Reference woman". Include specific values for storage fat, essential fat, and gender-specific essential fat.
- Define the terms lean body mass, fat-free body mass, and minimal weight.
- Discuss what factors may trigger menstrual irregularities among certain groups of female athletes.
- Describe Archimedes' principle of water displacement applied to the measurement of density.
- Discuss the assumptions in computing percent body fat from body density.
- Outline the specific procedures for hydrostatic weighing. Why is it important to know the subject's residual lung volume?
- Describe the anatomic location for six frequently measured fatfold sites and girth sites.
- Discuss how fatfolds and girths can provide meaningful information on body fat and its distribution.
- Explain what is meant by the statement: "Fatfold and girth equations to predict body fat are population specific."
- Compare the average body composition values of young men and women to elite competitors in endurance sports, football, and weight lifting and body building.

In the early 1940s, Dr. Albert Behnke, a U.S. Navy physician and the foremost authority on body composition, made detailed measurements of the size, shape, and structure of 25 professional football players, many of whom had achieved All-American status while in college. According to military standards at that time, a person whose body mass was 15% above the average "weight-for-height," as determined from insurance company statistics, was designated as overweight and rejected for entry into the military. When these standards were applied to the football players whose body mass ranged from 72.3 to 118.2 kg (159 to 261 lb), 17 of them were classified as too fat and unfit for military service. However, a more careful evaluation of each player's *body composition* revealed that 11 of the 17 overweight players actually had a relatively low percentage of body fat — the excess weight resulted primarily from their large muscular development.

These data illustrated clearly that the popular height-weight tables provided little information about the quality or composition of an individual's body mass. A football player may indeed weigh much more than some "average," "ideal," or "desirable" body mass based on the height-weight tables, but more than likely this athlete is not excessively fat or in need of reducing body mass. *Thus, "overweight" refers only to body mass in excess of some standard, usually the average mass for a specific stature.* The use of height–weight tables can be misleading for a person who actually wants to know: How fat or "overfat" am I?

In this chapter, we analyze the gross composition of the human body and present the rationale underlying various indirect methods for partitioning the body into two basic compartments, body fat and fat-free body mass. In addition, simple methods are presented for analyzing an individual's body composition to estimate percent body fat, pounds of fat, and lean body mass.

GROSS COMPOSITION OF THE HUMAN BODY

Three major structural components of the human body are muscle, fat, and bone. Because there are marked gender differences in these parameters, a convenient basis for comparison is to employ the concept developed by Dr. Behnke of a *Reference man* and *Reference woman* as depicted in Figure 16-1.

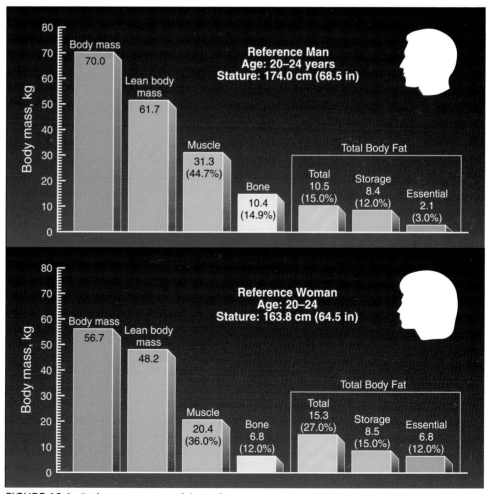

FIGURE 16-1. Body composition of the Reference man and Reference woman.

Not all excess weight is bad weight. If football players followed the height-weight guidelines, it's a good bet that they would cease playing football and might even jeopardize their overall health by undertaking a crash or bizarre diet regimen.

Reference man and woman. The Reference man and Reference woman are theoretical models based on average physical dimensions from detailed measurements of thousands of individuals who were subjects in large-scale anthropometric and nutrition-assessment surveys. The reference models provide a useful frame of comparison when making inter-individual and intra- individual assessments of body composition.

Gender-specific essential fat. The contribution of breast fat has been estimated to be no higher than 4% of body mass for women whose total body fat content varied from 14 to 35%. This means that sites other than the breasts contribute a large proportion of gender-specific essential fat (perhaps the lower body region that includes the pelvis and thighs).

Lean body mass. In normally hydrated healthy adult males, the only difference between lean body mass and fat-free body mass is that lean body mass includes the "essential" lipid-rich stores in bone marrow, brain, spinal cord, and internal organs.

Reference Man and Reference Woman

Compared with the Reference female, the Reference male is taller by 10.2 cm and heavier by 13.3 kg, his skeleton weighs more (10.4 vs. 6.8 kg), and he has a larger muscle mass (31.3 vs. 20.4 kg) and lower total fat content (10.5 vs. 15.3 kg). These gender differences exist even when the amount of fat, muscle, and bone are expressed as a percentage of body mass. This is particularly true for body fat, which represents 15% of total body mass for the Reference man and 27% for his female counterpart. The concept of reference standards does not mean that men and women should strive to achieve this body composition, nor that the Reference man and woman are in fact "average" or desirable.

Essential and Storage Fat

According to the Reference model, total body fat exists in two depots or storage sites.

Essential Fat. The first depot, termed *essential fat*, is the fat stored in the marrow of bones as well as in the heart, lungs, liver, spleen, kidneys, intestines, muscles, and lipid-rich tissues of the central nervous system. *This fat is required for normal physiologic functioning.* In the female, essential fat includes additional *gender- specific essential fat.* It is not at all clear whether this fat is expendable or serves as reserve storage. More than likely, this additional fat is biologically important for childbearing and other hormone-related functions. The mammary glands and pelvic region are probably primary sites for this component of essential fat, although the precise amounts are unknown. The essential body fat appears to represent a biologic lower limit beyond which a person's body mass cannot be reduced without impairing health status.

Storage Fat. The other major depot, the *storage fat*, consists of fat that accumulates in adipose tissue. This nutri-ent energy reserve includes the fatty tissues that protect the various internal organs as well as the larger *subcutaneous fat* volume beneath the skin surface. The percentage of body fat that is storage fat in males and females is similar (approximately 12% of body mass in males and 15% in females).

Lean Body Mass (Men). In men, the lower limit beyond which a person's body mass cannot be reduced without impairing health status is referred to as *lean body mass*; it is calculated as body mass minus the mass of storage fat. For the Reference man, lean body mass is equivalent to 61.6 kg, which includes approximately 3% or 1.9 kg of essential fat. Body fat values approaching this 3% "lower limit" have been obtained for champion male athletes in various sports. The fat content of world-class marathon runners, for example, ranges from about 3 to 8%. This is just about the quantity of essential fat that apparently cannot be reduced without health consequences. The low fat content and body mass for these athletes reflects, to some degree, a positive adaptation to the severe energy requirements of distance training. Also, a low percentage of body fat facilitates heat loss during high-intensity exercise and reduces the load of excess weight to be transported while running.

There is considerable variation in the lean body mass of different groups of male athletes, with values ranging from a low of 48 kg in some jockeys to a high of 116 kg for an Olympic champion discus thrower. Table 16-1 presents data on the physique and body composition of selected professional male athletes who could be classified as "underfat" or "overweight" There are striking differences between these groups in body size as well as in body fat, lean body mass, and the lean-to-fat ratio. The defensive backs and offensive backs are "underfat" in relation to the Reference man (or any other nonathletic standard), whereas the linemen and shot putters are clearly "overweight" for their stature (their

TABLE 16-1. Physique and body composition of "underfat" professional Football Players and "Overweight" offensive and defensive professional football linemen and shot-putters

Variable	Defensive Backs (All-Pro)				Offensive Back (All-Pro, N= 1)	Offensive Linemen (Dallas, 1977, N = 10)	Defensive Linemen (Dallas, 1977, N = 5)	Shot Putters (Olympic, N = 13)
	1	2	3	4				
Age, yr	27.1	30.2	29.4	24.0	32.0	—	—	24.0
Stature, cm	184.7	181.9	187.2	181.5	184.7	193.8	197.6	187.0
Mass, kg	87.9	87.1	88.4	88.9	90.6	116.0	116.5	112.3
Relative fat, %	3.9	3.8	3.8	2.5	1.4	18.6	13.2	14.8
Absolute fat, kg	3.4	3.3	3.4	2.2	1.3	21.6	15.4	16.6
Lean body mass, kg	84.5	83.8	85.0	86.7	89.3	94.4	101.1	95.7
Lean/fat ratio	24.8	25.3	25.0	39.4	68.7	4.37	6.57	5.77

(From Katch, V.I., and Katch, V.L.: The body composition profile: Techniques of measurement applications. *Clin. Sports Med.*, 3:31, 1984.)

mass per unit stature exceeds the 90th percentile for nonathletic males).

Minimal Weight (Women). In contrast to the lower limit of body mass for males that includes about 3% essential fat, the lower limit of body mass for the Reference female, termed *minimal weight*, includes 12 to 14% essential fat (essential fat plus gender- specific fat). For the Reference female, minimal weight is equivalent to 48.2 kg. In general, body fat levels in the leanest women in the population do not fall below about 12% of body mass. This probably represents the lower limit of fatness for most women in good health.

Underweight and Thin. The terms underweight and thin are not necessarily synonymous. In some cases they describe physical characteristics that differ considerably. In one study, structural characteristics were compared between thin or "skinny" females and women who were either normal in body fat or obese to determine if body frame size (as measured by bone widths) differed among these diverse three groups. The results were unexpected. While the thin females were indeed relatively low in body fat— 18.2% compared with 25% body fat for the normal-size women and 32% for the obese group — there were *no differences* in average structural dimensions (trunk and extremity bone dimensions) among the three groups! What this means is that for women of approx-

imately the same stature, the level of body fat is not necessarily predictive of a small, medium, or large frame size as assessed from bone widths.

Leanness, Exercise, and Menstrual Irregularity

Physically active females in general, as well as females in specific sports associated with excessive leanness, increase their chances of either a delayed onset of menstruation, an irregular menstrual cycle (*oligomenorrhea*), or complete cessation of menses (*amenorrhea*). For example, female ballet dancers as a group are quite lean and report a greater incidence of menstrual irregularity, eating disorders, and higher age at menarche compared to age-matched females who are not dancers. The speculation is that the body in some way "senses" when energy reserves are inadequate to sustain pregnancy, and thus ceases ovulation to prevent conception. Maintenance of at least 17% body fat is often cited as the "critical level" for the onset of menstruation and is required to maintain a normal cycle. Some have argued that hormonal and metabolic disturbances that affect the menses are triggered if body fat falls below these levels.

Leanness Is Not the Only Factor. Although the lean-to-fat ratio does appear to be important for normal menstrual function (perhaps through

Minimal weight. The concept of minimal weight in females, which incorporates about 12% essential fat, is equivalent to lean body mass in males that includes 3% essential fat.

Light is not necessarily lean. Appearing thin or skinny does not necessarily mean that skeletal frame size is diminutive or that the body's total fat content is excessively low.

Menstrual irregularity is prevalent among athletic women. One-third to one-half of female athletes in certain sports have some menstrual irregularity.

the role of peripheral fat in converting androgens to estrogens), other factors must be considered. There are many outstanding female distance runners, dancers, gymnasts, and body builders engaged in highly structured and vigorous training programs who have normal menses and who compete at a body fat level below 17%. In a study from one of our laboratories, 30 female athletes and 30 nonathletes with body fat below 20% were compared for menstrual cycle regularity. For women who ranged between 11 and 15% body fat, 4 athletes and 3 nonathletes had regular cycles, whereas 7 athletes and 2 nonathletes had irregular cycles or were amenorrheic. For the total sample, 14 athletes and 21 nonathletes had regular cycles. These data corroborate other findings and cast doubt on the hypothesis of a critical fat level of 17%.

In addition, when the menstrual cycle returns to normal, it is not always associated with an increase in body mass or body fat. These observations have led researchers to focus on the role of *physiologic and psychologic stress,* including that provided by exercise training, in influencing normal menstrual function. More recently, *nutritional inadequacy and energy imbalance* among athletes with irregular menstrual function have also been identified as possible predisposing factors.

Consideration also must be given to the complex interplay of physical, nutritional, genetic, hormonal, psychologic, and environmental factors, as well as regional fat distribution, as they affect menstrual function. Research shows that for active women, an intense bout of exercise triggers the release of an array of hormones some of which have anti-reproductive properties. It remains to be determined whether regular bouts of heavy exercise have a cumulative effect sufficient to alter normal menses. When young amenorrheic ballet dancers sustained injuries that prevented them from exercising, normal menstruation resumed although body mass remained unchanged. For most women, exercise-associated distur-

bances in menstrual function can be reversed with changes in lifestyle without serious consequences. If a critical fat level does exist, it is probably specific for each woman and may change throughout life.

In light of current knowledge on the topic of body fat and menstrual irregularities, approximately 13 to 17% body fat should be regarded as the lower range of body fatness associated with regularity of menstrual function. The risks of sustained amenorrhea on the reproductive system are undetermined; the well-documented danger to bone mass is presented in Chapter 6. Failure to menstruate or cessation of the normal cycle should be evaluated by a gynecologist or endocrinologist because it may reflect a significant medical condition such as pituitary or thyroid gland malfunction or premature menopause.

Delayed Onset of Menstruation and Cancer Risk. Researchers now suggest that the delayed onset of menarche generally observed in chronically active young females provides a positive health benefit. Female college athletes who started training in high school or earlier show a lower lifetime occurrence of cancer of the breast and reproductive organs, as well as cancers not involving the reproductive system, compared to their nonathletic counterparts. This lower cancer risk with delayed onset of menstruation may be linked to the production of less total estrogen or a less potent form of estrogen over a lifetime. Lower body fat levels may also be involved because fatty tissues convert androgens to estrogen.

Body Frame-Size

One of the more interesting areas in the study of body composition is the concept of "frame size". Most of us are familiar with this concept because the standard height-weight tables list different weights at a given height for people with small, medium, or large body frames. These tables, however, gave no indication as how to measure frame size, or exactly what is meant by frame size. To the physical anthropologist (who among other things studies body size and shape), frame size reflects the overall size of an individual's skeletal mass. This includes not only an estimate of bone width, but also bone length. Figure 16-2 displays the theoretical components of frame-size. Note the two different lines that set the boundaries for small, medium, or large frame-size. A person who has long bones would obviously be tall in stature, yet may possess a small, medium or large frame-size, depending on the width of the bones. Likewise, a person who is short in stature, yet who possesses a wide bony structure (particularly in the shoulders, chest, and hips) could have the same overall frame-size as the tall person. The common practice of measuring the wrist or elbow bone width, while giving some information about bony structure, does not give sufficient information to determine overall body frame-size.

It is interesting to consider whether those individuals with a large frame size are generally fatter than persons who have a small or medium bony frame. Certainly, many people justify their larger body mass on the basis of possessing a large bony structure. Although the research is limited, when individuals are appropriately classified into frame-size and their body fat is evaluated, there is no clear indication that bigger frame-sizes are related to increased adiposity. Similarly, when individuals are grouped into low, medium, and high percent fat level, there is no clear indication that these groupings are linked to a specific body frame-size. The one exception is the child-onset obese female who tends to fall into the large frame size grouping.

. . . .

COMMON LABORATORY METHODS TO ASSESS BODY COMPOSITION

The fat and lean components of the human body have been determined by two general procedures:

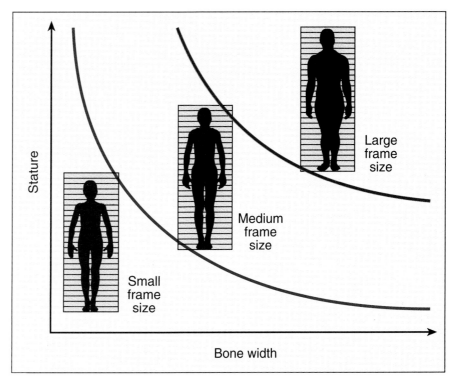

FIGURE 16-2. Theoretical components of body frame size include stature and an estimate of average bone width. The insert graphs provide an outline of a body type that would represent a typical person of small, medium, and large frame size.

- Directly by chemical analysis
- Indirectly by hydrostatic weighing or with simple circumferences and fatfold measurements, or other procedures.

Direct Assessment

Although there is considerable research on the *direct* chemical assessment of body composition in various species of animals, few studies have chemically determined human fat content. Such analyses are time-consuming and tedious, require specialized laboratory equipment, and involve many ethical and legal problems in obtaining cadavers for research purposes.

While there is considerable individual variation in total body fatness, the composition of the skeletal mass and lean and fat tissues remains relatively stable. The constancy of these

Direct analysis. Two approaches have been used in the direct assessment of body composition. In one technique the body is literally dissolved in a chemical solution and the fat and non-fat components of the mixture determined. The other technique involves the physical dissection of a variety of body components such as fat, fat-free adipose tissue, muscle, and bone.

tissues has enabled researchers to develop mathematical equations to determine the body's fat percentage. This is indeed fortunate, as the direct method for assessing the fat content of cadavers, while of considerable theoretical importance, obviously cannot be used with live subjects.

Indirect Assessment

Three *indirect* procedures are commonly used to assess body composition. The first involves Archimedes' principle as applied to *hydrostatic weighing* (also referred to as *underwater weighing*). With this method, percent body fat is computed from body density (the ratio of body mass to body volume). The second approach assesses body composition through estimates of subcutaneous body fat; in the third procedure, body fat is predicted from circumference (girth) measurements. Both circumference and fatfold measurements are of practical significance because body fat can be predicted simply and accurately.

Hydrostatic Weighing (Archimedes' Principle).

About 2000 years ago, the Greek mathematician Archimedes discovered a basic principle that is currently applied in the evaluation of body composition. An itinerant scholar of that time described the interesting circumstances surrounding the event:

> "King Hieron of Syracuse suspected that his pure gold crown had been altered by substitution of silver for gold. The King directed Archimedes to devise a method for testing the crown for its gold content without dismantling it. Archimedes pondered over this problem for many weeks without succeeding, until one day, he stepped into a bath filled to the top with water and observed the overflow. He thought about this for a moment, and then, wild with joy, jumped from the bath and ran naked through the streets of Syracuse

shouting eureka, eureka, I have discovered a way to solve the mystery of the King's crown."

Archimedes reasoned that a substance such as gold must have a volume proportionate to its mass, and the way to measure the volume of an irregular object such as the crown was to submerge it in water and collect the overflow. Archimedes took a lump of gold and silver, each having the same mass as the crown, and submerged each in a container full of water. To his delight, he discovered that the crown displaced more water than the lump of gold and less than the lump of silver. What this meant was that the crown was indeed composed of both silver and gold, as the King had suspected.

Essentially, what Archimedes evaluated was the *specific gravity* of the crown (ratio of the mass of the crown to the mass of an equal volume of water) compared to the specific gravities for gold and silver. Archimedes probably also reasoned that an object submerged in water is buoyed up by a counterforce that equals the weight of the water it displaces. This buoyancy force supports an object in water against the downward pull of gravity, causing the object to lose weight in water. *Because the object's loss of weight in water equals the weight of the volume of water it displaces, we can redefine specific gravity as the ratio of the weight of an object in air divided by its loss of weight in water.* Thus,

> **Specific gravity =**
> **Weight in air ÷**
> **Loss of weight in water.**

In this case, the loss of weight in water is equal to the weight in air *minus* the weight in water.

In practical terms, suppose a crown weighed 2.27 kg in air and 0.13 kg less, or 2.14 kg, when weighed underwater (Figure 16-3). The specific gravity of the crown would then be computed by dividing the weight of the crown (2.27 kg) by its loss of weight

---

Assess the composition of the body. It is the indirect, noninvasive procedures that enable us to assess the fat and nonfat components of living persons.

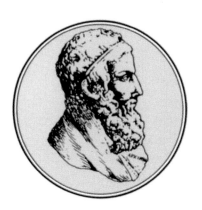

Fat-free tissues. The assumed densities for the components of the fat-free mass at body temperature of 37°C are: water, 0.933 g/cc; mineral, 3,000 g/cc; protein, 1.340 g/cc.

in water (0.13 kg), which results in a specific gravity of 17.5. Because this ratio is considerably different than the specific gravity of gold that has a value of 19.3, we too can conclude: "Eureka, the crown is a fraud!"

The physical principle Archimedes discovered can be applied to the assessment of body composition in humans. This is achieved by determining the body's volume by water submersion. We can then compute the density of the body once the mass and volume are known.

Determining Body Density. For illustrative purposes, suppose a 50 kg person weighs 2 kg when submerged completely underwater. According to Archimedes' principle, the buoyancy or counterforce of the water equals 48 kg. The 48 kg loss of body weight in water equals the weight of the displaced water. Because the density of water at any temperature is known (the exact values can be found in the Handbook of Chemistry), we can compute the volume of water displaced. In this example, 48 kg (48,000 g) of water is equal to a volume of 48 liters or 48,000 cc (1 g water = 1 cc by volume, or 1 g/cc at 39.2° F). If the person were measured at the cold-water temperature of 39.2°F, no density correction for water would be necessary. In practice, researchers use warmer water and apply the appropriate density value for water at the particular temperature. The density of the subject, computed as mass ÷ volume, would be 50,000 g (50 kg) ÷ 48,000 cc, or 1.0417 g/cc. The next step is to estimate the percentage of body fat and the mass of fat and lean tissue.

Computing Percent Body Fat and Mass of Fat and Lean Tissue. The relative percentage of fat in the human body can be estimated with a simple equation that incorporates body density. This equation was derived from the theoretical premise that the densities of fat and fat-free tissues remain relatively constant (fat tissue = 0.90 g/cc; fat-free tissue = 1.10 g/cc), even

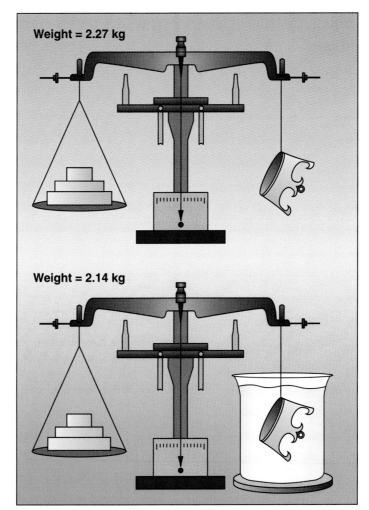

Figure 16-3. Archimedes' solution for determining the volume and subsequently the specific gravity of the king's crown.

with large variations in both total body fat and the lean tissue components of bone and muscle. The following equation, derived by Berkeley scientist Dr. William Siri, is used to compute percent body fat by incorporating the determined value of body density:

Siri Equation
Percent body fat = 495 ÷ body density - 450

The body density value of 1.0417 g/cc determined for the subject in the previous example can now be substituted in the Siri equation for percent body fat as follows:

Percent body fat = 495 ÷ 1.0417 −450
= 25.2% fat

The mass of body fat can then be calculated by multiplying body mass by percent fat:

> **Fat mass (kg)** = Body mass (kg) X [Percent fat ÷100]
> 12.6 kg = 50 kg x 0.252

Lean body mass is calculated by subtracting the mass of fat from body mass:

> **Lean body mass (kg)** = Body mass (kg) - Fat mass (kg)
> 37.4 kg = 50 kg–12.6 kg

In this example, 25.2% or 12.6 kg of the 50 kg body mass is fat. The remaining 37.4 kg is the lean body mass. For simplicity we will use the term lean body mass, although we realize that by subtracting out the total body fat yields a remainder that is "fat-free." The true calculation of lean body mass in males includes the essential fat; in females, the lean body mass (termed minimal weight) also includes gender-specific essential fat.

Possible Limitations. The generalized density values of 1.10 g/cc for lean tissue and 0.90 g/cc for fat tissue are average values for young and middle-aged adults. Although these values are assumed to be constants, this may not be the case. For example, the density of the lean body mass is estimated to be significantly greater for blacks than for whites (1.113 vs. 1.100 g/cc). The existing equations to calculate body composition from body density in whites, therefore, would tend to *overestimate* the lean body mass (and *underestimate* percent fat) when applied to blacks.

In addition to racial differences, applying constant density values for the various tissues to growing children or aging adults could also add uncertainty in predicting body composition. For example, the density of the skeleton is probably in continual change during growth as well as during the well-documented demineralization of osteoporosis with aging. This would make the actual density

of the fat-free tissue of young children and the elderly lower than the assumed constant of 1.10 g/cc and result in *overestimation* of percent body fat. With highly trained and select groups of male athletes such as professional football players and champion distance runners and body builders, the density of the fat-free component could theoretically exceed 1.10 g/cc. This would cause an *underestimation* of relative fat in males.

Measurement of Body Volume. Determining body mass and calculating body density, percent body fat, and lean body mass are quite simple. The more difficult task is the accurate assessment of body volume, which is usually measured by the procedure of hydrostatic weighing. Figure 16-4 illustrates the procedure for measuring body volume by hydrostatic weighing.

A diver's belt is usually secured around the waist so the subject does not float toward the surface during submersion. While seated with the head out of the water, the subject makes a forced maximal exhalation as the head is lowered beneath the water. The breath is held for several seconds while the underwater weight is recorded. Eight to twelve repeated weighings are made to obtain a dependable underwater weight score. This amount of practice is given because there is a predictable "learning curve" in making a forced exhalation during submersion. Even when achieving a full exhalation, a small volume of air, the *residual lung volume*, remains in the lungs. This air volume, however, is measured for each subject just before, during, or following the underwater weighing and its buoyant effect is subtracted in the calculation of body volume.

Examples of Calculations. Let us put theory into practice by showing the sequence of steps to compute body density, percent fat, mass of fat, and lean body mass. The subjects are two professional football players: an offensive guard and a quarterback. The following measurements were made:

Resting and total daily energy expenditure predicted from lean body mass.
Use the following equations to estimate resting energy expenditure (REE) and total daily energy expenditure (TDEE) from lean body mass (LBM) using the following equations:

(1) **REE (kcal/d)** = 21.6 (LBM, kg) + 370

If, for example, LBM = 70 kg, then:

> REE = 21.6(70) + 370
> = 1882 kcal/d

(2) **TDEE(kcal/d)** = 26.0 (LBM, kg) + 682

If, for example, LBM = 70 kg, then:

> TDEE = 26.0(70) + 682 = 2502 kcal/d

TDEE can vary greatly depending on physical activity level.

Effect of residual volume on computed body density. If the residual lung volume is not accounted for, the computed body density value will decrease because the lungs' air volume contributes to buoyancy. Failure to properly account for the residual air volume would indeed make a person "fatter" when converting body density to percent body fat.

	Offensive Guard	Quarterback
Body weight	110 kg	85 kg
Underwater weight	3.5 kg	5.0 kg
Residual lung volume	1.2 L	1.0 L
Water temperature correction factor	0.996	0.996

Because the loss of weight in water is equal to volume, the body volume of the offensive guard is 110 kg – 3.5 kg = 106.5 kg or 106.5 liters; for the quarterback, body volume is 85 kg – 5.0 kg = 80.0 kg or 80 liters. Dividing body volume by the water temperature correction factor of 0.996 increases body volume slightly for both players (106.9 liters for the guard and 80.3 liters for the quarterback). Because residual lung volume also contributes to buoyancy, this volume is subtracted. The body volume of the offensive guard then becomes 105.7 liters (106.9 liters - 1.2 liters); for the quarterback, 79.3 liters (80.3 liters - 1.0 liters).

Body density is then computed as mass ÷ volume. For the offensive guard, body density is 110 kg ÷ 105.7 liters = 1.0407 kg/liter or 1.0407 g/cc. For the quarterback, body density is 85.0 kg ÷ 79.3 liters = 1.0719 g/cc.

The percentage of fat is computed from the Siri equation:

Percent body fat = 495 ÷ Body density – 450
Offensive guard: 495 ÷ 1.0407– 450 = 25.6%
Quarterback: 495 ÷ 1.0719– 450 = 11.8%

The total mass of the body fat is calculated as follows:

Fat mass = Body mass x (Percent fat ÷ 100)
Offensive guard: 110 kg x 0.256 = 28.2 kg
Quarterback: 85 kg x 0.118 = 10.0 kg

Lean body mass is calculated as follows:

Lean body mass: = **Body mass – Fat mass**
Offensive guard: 110 kg – 28.2 kg = 81.8 kg
Quarterback: 85 kg - 10.0 kg = 75.0 kg

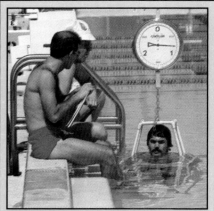

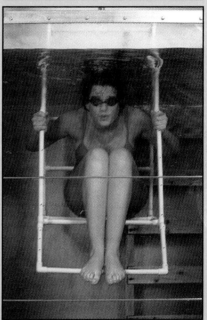

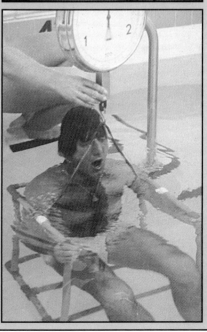

FIGURE 16-4. Measuring body volume by the procedure of underwater weighing. The residual lung volume can be measured either before, during, or after the underwater weighing. Top, in a swimming pool; middle, in a stainless steel pool with Plexiglas front in the laboratory; bottom, seated in a therapy pool. For any of the methods, a snorkel and nose clip can be used by subjects who are apprehensive about submersion.

This analysis of body composition illustrates that the offensive guard possesses more than twice the percentage body fat as the quarterback (25.6% vs. 11.8%) and almost three times as much total fat (28.2 kg vs. 10.0 kg). On the other hand, lean body mass, which provides a good indication of muscle mass, is also much larger for the guard than for the quarterback. Although the guard is 25 kg heavier than the quarterback, similar differences in body composition occur for people of the same body mass, especially between physically active and sedentary people. These results point up the crucial role of body composition analysis in determining the fat and lean components of the body.

Fatfold Measurements. Hydrostatic weighing is a widely used indirect method for assessing body composition. When laboratory facilities are unavailable, simpler alternative procedures can be used to *predict* body fatness. Two of these procedures, the measurement of fatfolds and girths or circumferences, require relatively inexpensive equipment. The rationale for fatfold measurements to estimate total body fat is that a relationship exists between the fat located directly beneath the skin (referred to as *subcutaneous fat*) and internal fat, and that both of these measures are related to body density.

By 1930, a special pincer-type caliper was used to measure subcutaneous fat at selected sites on the body with relative accuracy. The caliper works on the same principle as the micrometer used to measure distance between two points. The procedure for measuring fatfold thickness is to grasp a fold of skin and subcutaneous fat firmly with the thumb and forefingers, pulling it away from the underlying muscle tissue following the natural contour of the fatfold. The caliper is applied with its jaws exerting constant tension of 10 g/mm^2 at their point of contact with the skin. The thickness of the double layer of skin and subcutaneous tissue is then read directly from the caliper dial and recorded in millimeters, within several seconds after applying the caliper. This avoids undue compression of the fatfold when measuring (see Close Up).

The most common areas for measuring fatfolds are at triceps, subscapular, suprailiac, abdominal, chest, and upper thigh sites. All measures are taken on the right side of the body with the subject standing. A minimum of two or three measurements are made at each site, and the average value is used as the fatfold score. Figure 16-5 shows the anatomic location of the most frequently measured fatfold sites:

- **Triceps:** Vertical fold measured at the midline of the upper arm halfway between the tip of the shoulder and tip of the elbow
- **Subscapular:** Oblique fold measured just below the bottom tip of the scapula
- **Suprailiac:** Slightly oblique fold measured just above the hip bone; the fold is lifted to follow the natural diagonal line at this point
- **Abdominal:** Vertical fold measured 1 inch to the right of the umbilicus
- **Thigh:** Vertical fold measured at the midline of the thigh, two-thirds of the distance from the middle of the patella (knee cap) to the hip
- **Chest:** Fold with its long axis directed towards the nipple. Measured on the anterior axillary fold as high as possible

Usefulness. Fatfold measurements provide meaningful information concerning body fat and its distribution. There are basically two ways to use fatfolds. The first is to sum the scores as an indication of relative fatness among individuals. This "sum of fatfolds" as well as the individual fatfold values, also can be used to reflect *changes* in fatness before and after a physical conditioning regimen. Changes in individual fatfold values as well as the total fatfold score can then be evaluated on either an absolute or percentage basis.

The following observations can be made from the fatfold data shown in Table 16-2 obtained from a 22-year-old female college student before and after a 16-week exercise program:

- The largest changes in fatfold thickness occurred at the suprailiac and abdominal sites
- The triceps showed the largest decrease and the subscapular the smallest decrease when changes were expressed as percentages
- The total reduction in subcutaneous fatfolds at the five sites was 16.6 mm, or 12.6% below the starting condition

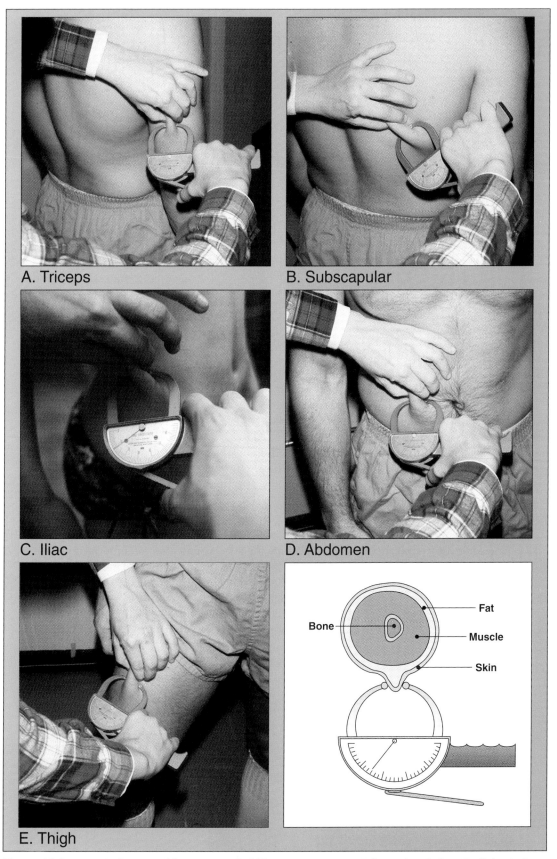

Figure 16-5. Anatomic location of five common fatfold sites: *A.* Triceps. *B.* Subscapular. *C.* Iliac. *D.* Abdominal. *E.* Thigh. Measurements are in the vertical plane except at the subscapular and suprailiac sites where they are diagonal.

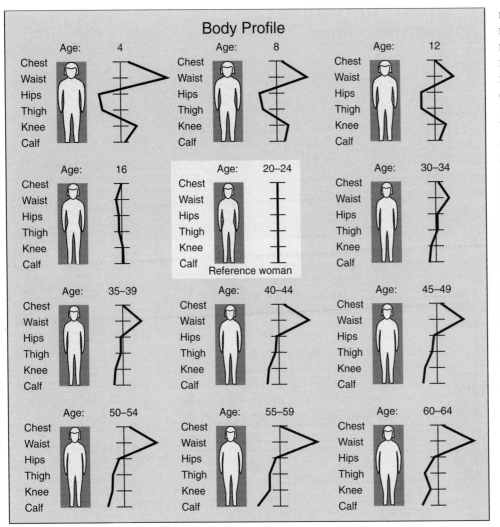

Body Profile

Body Profile Analysis. Another useful application of the girth technique, is the body profile analysis that displays the muscular and non-muscular areas of the body in relation to standards established for the reference man and woman.The accompanying graphics displays the age-trend in the pattern of girth measurements for females from age 4 to age 64. Note that the waist (designated a non-muscular region) increases progressively in dimension from age 30 to age 64! If all of the girths were to remain in relative proportion as individuals aged, there would be no positive deviations in the body profile and all of the measurements would plot as a vertical line as it does for the Reference woman at age 20-24.

to next section) for older men and women. Section III in the *Study Guide and Workbook* presents normative standards for percent body fat based on data from a number of studies of young adult women and men. Also presented are the fatfold sites and percent fat conversion tables for a commonly used and validated generalized prediction equation.

Not For All People. Although fatfolds have been widely used in physical education and the allied health professions to predict percent body fat, a major drawback is that the person taking the measurements must have considerable experience with the proper techniques to obtain consistent values. With extremely obese people, the thickness of the fatfold often exceeds the width of the caliper's jaws! The particular caliper used also

may contribute to measurement error. Because there are no standards to compare results between different investigators, it is difficult to determine which sets of fatfold data are "best" to use. Thus, prediction equations developed by a particular researcher (which may be highly valid for the sample measured) may result in large errors in prediction when another person takes the measurements. This is an important factor to consider when making decisions about how to use prediction equations to assess body composition.

Girth Measurements. The measurement of circumferences (or girths) provides another indirect assessment of body fat. A linen or plastic measuring tape is applied lightly to the skin surface so that the tape is taut but not tight. This procedure avoids skin compression that produces artificially low scores. Duplicate measurements are taken at each site and the average is used. Figure 16-6 displays the anatomic landmarks for the various girths used to assess body fatness:

- **Abdomen:** One inch above the umbilicus

- **Buttocks:** Maximum protrusion with the heels together

- **Right thigh:** Upper thigh just below the buttocks

- **Right upper arm:** Arm straight, palm up and extended in front of the body, measured at the midpoint between the shoulder and the elbow

- **Right forearm:** Maximum girth with the arm extended in front of the body with palm up

- **Right calf:** Widest girth midway between the ankle and knee

Usefulness. The girth-based predictions are most useful in ranking individuals within a group according to their relative fatness. If one uses the equations and constants presented in Appendix 4 for young and older men and women, the error in predicting an individual's percent body fat is generally between ± 2.5 and 4.0%. These relatively low prediction errors make the equations particularly useful to those without access to laboratory facilities, because the measurements are easy to take and a tape measure is inexpensive. Keep in mind, however, that the equations are *population specific* and should *not* be used to predict fatness in individuals who appear very thin or very fat or have been involved for a number of years in strenuous sports or resistance training.

In addition to predicting percent body fat, girth measures are well suited for determining patterns of fat distribution on the body as well as changes in the pattern of fat distribution following weight loss.

Predicting Body Fat from Girths. From the appropriate tables in Appendix 4, we can substitute the corresponding constants A, B, and C in the formula shown at the bottom of each table. One addition and two subtraction steps are required. The following five-step example shows how to compute percent fat, fat mass, and lean body mass for a 21-year-old man who weighs 79.1 kg:

Step 1. The upper arm, abdomen, and right forearm girths are measured with a cloth tape and recorded to the nearest 1/4 inch: upper arm = 11.5 in (29.21 cm); abdomen = 31.0 in (78.74 cm); right forearm = 10.75 in (27.30 cm)

Step 2. The three constants A, B, and C corresponding to the three girths are determined from the Appendix: Constant A, corresponding to 11.5 in = 42.56; Constant B, corresponding to 31.0 in = 40.68; Constant C, corresponding to 10.75 in = 58.37

Step 3. Percent body fat is computed by substituting the appropriate constants in the formula for young men shown at the bottom of Chart 1 in Appendix 4 as follows:

> **Percent fat =**
> **Constant A +**
> **Constant B −**
> **Constant C − 10.2**

Percentile Ranking for Triceps Fatfolds in Children				
Boys				
Age	15th	50th	85th	95th
6	6.2	8.4	11.1	14.1
8	6.1	8.8	13.7	17.2
10	6.0	9.1	16.0	20.7
12	5.8	9.4	17.3	23.3
14	5.6	8.9	16.4	23.5
16	5.5	8.5	15.8	21.5
18	5.6	8.5	16.6	21.8
Girls				
6	6.8	10.1	13.4	15.6
8	7.6	11.4	16.4	20.2
10	8.4	12.7	19.0	24.4
12	9.3	14.1	21.3	28.0
14	10.4	15.5	23.3	30.9
16	11.3	26.6	25.1	33.2
18	11.7	17.0	25.8	33.8

Source: Must, J., et al.: Reference data for obesity: 85th and 95th percentiles of body mass index (wt/ht^2) and triceps skinfold thickness. *Am. J. Clin. Nutr.*, 53:839, 1991.

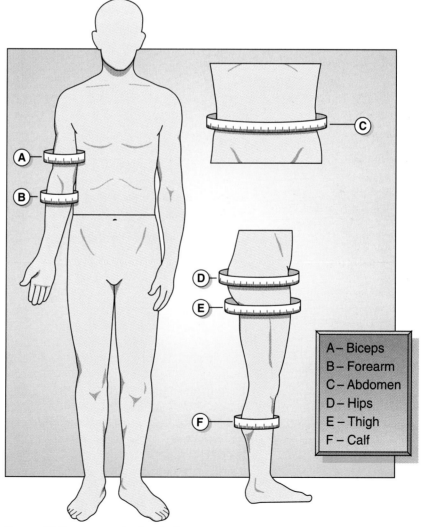

A– Biceps
B– Forearm
C– Abdomen
D– Hips
E – Thigh
F – Calf

Figure 16-6. Anatomic landmarks for measuring various girths.

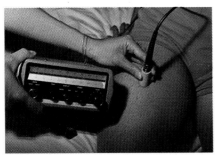

Ultrasound meter for recording fat and muscle thickness. The ultrasound technique operates by emitting high-frequency sound waves that penetrate the skin surface. The sound waves pass through adipose tissue until they reach the muscle layer, where they are reflected from the fat-muscle interface to produce an echo that returns to the ultrasound unit. The time for sound waves to be transmitted through the tissues and back to the receiver is converted to a distance score that is displayed on an easy to see readout. Ultrasound can be used to "map" muscle and fat thickness at various body sites, as well as estimate total body fat based on age and gender specific regression equations.

$= 42.56 + 40.68 - 58.37 - 10.2$
$= 83.24 - 58.37 - 10.2$
$= 24.87 - 10.2$
$= 14.7\%$

Step 4. Next, the mass of body fat is calculated:

$$\text{Fat mass} = \text{Body mass} \times [\% \text{ fat} \div 100]$$

$= 79.1 \text{ kg} \times [14.7 \div 100]$
$= 79.1 \text{ kg} \times 0.147$
$= 11.63 \text{ kg}$

Step 5. Lean body mass is determined as:

$$\text{LBM} = \text{Body mass} - \text{Fat mass}$$

$= 79.1 \text{ kg} - 11.63 \text{ kg}$
$= 67.5 \text{ kg}$

Other Indirect Procedures. There are alternative indirect procedures that enable the researcher to gain valuable information about body composition.

Bioelectric Impedance Analysis (BIA). The principle underlying BIA is based on the fact that the flow of electricity is facilitated through hydrated fat-free tissue and extracellular water compared to fat tissue. This occurs because of the greater electrolyte content (and thus lower electrical resistance) of the fat-free component. Consequently, impedance to the flow of electric current is directly related to the level of body fat. With the BIA technique, electrodes are placed on the hands and feet, a painless electric signal is introduced, and the impedance or resistance to current flow is determined. The value for impedance is then converted to body density (adding body mass, stature, and sometimes several girths to an equation), which in turn is converted to percent body fat by use of the Siri equation (page 459).

A factor that affects the accuracy of BIA is the need for the subject to maintain a normal hydration level, because either dehydration or over-

hydration affects the body's electrolyte concentration, independent of real changes in body fat. *More specifically, loss of body water decreases the impedance measure to yield a lower percent fat, whereas overhydration produces the opposite effect.* Even under conditions of normal hydration, the prediction of body fat may be questionable in relation to values obtained from hydrostatic weighing. In fact, the technique may be less accurate than the anthropometric methods that use girths and fatfolds to predict body fat. Skin temperature, which is influenced by ambient conditions, also affects whole-body resistance. Thus, the predicted body fat value is significantly lower in a warm compared to a cold environment. *At best, BIA is another noninvasive, indirect means to assess body composition provided that measurements are made under conditions strictly standardized for both ambient temperature and level of hydration.*

Computed Tomography (CT), Magnetic Resonance Imaging (MRI), and Dual-Energy X-ray Absorptiometry (DEXA). The CT and MRI scanning procedures produce radiographic images of sections of the body. By use of appropriate computer software, the scan provides pictorial and quantitative information for total tissue area, total fat area, and intra-abdominal fat area. Figure 16-7A-C, shows CT scans of both upper legs and a cross section at the midthigh in a professional walker who completed an 11,200 mile walk through the 50 United States in 50 weeks.

A comparison of CT scans prior to and after the walk showed a significant increase in the total cross section of muscle area and corresponding decrease in subcutaneous fat in the midthigh region. In recent studies using CT scans, scientists have been able to determine the relationship between the outer thickness of fat at the abdomen and visceral fat within the abdominal cavity. Surprisingly, there is little relation in both males and females between these "external" and "internal" fat depots.

BIA technique: proceed with caution. A recent study has questioned the validity of using BIA to evaluate change in body composition. Researchers studied the individual data from seven experiments with adults who incurred a change in body mass and lean body mass resulting from a diet or diet and exercise program. The results were quite clear; the mathematical equations that form the foundation of the BIA technique were unable to successfully predict the change in body composition even when there was a 20% change in body mass or lean body mass!

The newer technology of MRI shown in Figure 16-7D provides valuable information about the body's tissue compartments. In MRI, electromagnetic radiation in the presence of a strong magnetic field is used to excite the hydrogen nuclei of water and lipid molecules. This causes the nuclei to give off a detectable signal that can then be rearranged under computer control to provide a visual representation of body tissues. The MRI procedure can be used effectively to evaluate changes in a tissue's lean-to-fat components. This has been done to evaluate changes in the cross-sectional area of muscle following resistance exercise training and during growth and aging.

Dual-energy x-ray absorptiometry (DEXA) is another high-technology procedure that permits quantification of fat and muscle not only around the bony areas of the body, but also in areas where there is no bone present. The DEXA procedure is an accepted clinical tool for assessment of spinal osteoporosis and related bone disorders. The underlying principle of DEXA is that the bone and soft tissue areas of the body can be penetrated to a depth of about 30 cm by two distinct x-ray energies. Specialized computer software then reconstructs an image of the underlying tissues. A whole scan of the body takes approximately 12 minutes, and

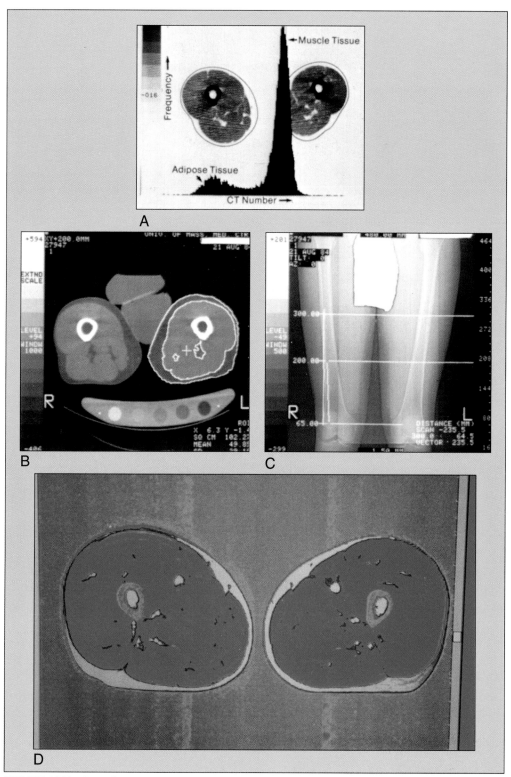

FIGURE 16-7. CT and MRI scans. (*A*) Plot of pixel elements (CT scan) illustrating the extent of adipose and muscle tissue in a cross-section of the thigh. The two other views show a cross-section of the midthigh (*B*) and an anterior view of the upper legs, (*C*) prior to a one-year walk across the U.S. in a champion walker. *D*. MRI scan of the midthigh of a 30-year-old male middle-distance runner. (CT scans are courtesy of Dr. Steven Heymsfeld and the Department of Radiology, University of Massachusetts Medical School, Worcester, MA; MRI scan courtesy of J. Staab, Department of the Army, USARIEM, Natick, MA)

TABLE 16–3. Average values of body fat for younger and older women and men from selected studies

Study	Age Range	Stature, cm	Mass, kg	% Fat	68% Variation Limits
Younger Women					
North Carolina, 1962	17 - 25	165.0	55.5	22.9	17.5 - 28.5
New York, 1962	16 - 30	167.5	59.0	28.7	24.6 - 32.9
California, 1968	19 - 23	165.9	58.4	21.9	17.0 - 26.9
California, 1970	17 - 29	164.9	58.6	25.5	21.0 - 30.1
Air Force, 1972	17 - 22	164.1	55.8	28.7	22.3 - 35.3
New York, 1973	17 - 26	160.4	59.0	26.2	23.4 - 33.3
North Carolina, 1975		166.1	57.5	24.6	—
Army Recruits, 1986	17 - 25	162.0	58.6	28.4	23.9 - 32.9
Massachusetts, 1994	17 - 30	165.3	57.7	21.8	16.7 - 27.8
Older Women					
Minnesota, 1953	31 - 45	163.3	60.7	28.9	25.1 - 32.8
	43 - 68	160.0	60.9	34.2	28.0 - 40.5
New York, 1963	30 - 40	164.9	59.6	28.6	22.1 - 35.3
	40 - 50	163.1	56.4	34.4	29.5 - 39.5
North Carolina, 1975	33 - 50	—	—	29.7	23.1 - 36.5
Massachusetts, 1993	31 - 50	165.2	58.9	25.2	19.2 - 31.2
Younger Men					
Minnesota, 1951	17 - 26	177.8	69.1	11.8	5.9 - 11.8
Colorado, 1956	17 - 25	172.4	68.3	13.5	8.3 - 18.8
Indiana, 1966	18 - 23	180.1	75.5	12.6	8.7 - 16.5
California, 1968	16 - 31	175.7	74.1	15.2	6.3 - 24.2
New York, 1973	17 - 26	176.4	71.4	15.0	8.9 - 21.1
Texas, 1977	18 - 24	179.9	74.6	13.4	7.4 - 19.4
Army Recruits, 1986	17 - 25	174.7	70.5	15.6	10.0 - 21.2
Massachusetts, 1994	17 - 30	178.2	76.3	12.9	7.8 - 18.9
Older Men					
Indiana, 1966	24 - 38	179.0	76.6	17.8	11.3 - 24.3
	40 - 48	177.0	80.5	22.3	16.3 - 28.3
North Carolina, 1976	27 - 50	—	—	23.7	17.9 - 30.1
Texas, 1977	27 - 59	180.0	85.3	27.1	23.7 - 30.5
Massachusetts, 1993	31 - 50	177.1	77.5	19.9	13.2 - 26.5

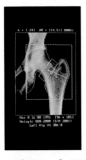

Proximal view of a DEXA scan of the femur. (Photo courtesy of Hologic, Inc., 590 Lincoln Street, Waltham, MA)

the computer-generated report quantifies bone mineral, total fat mass, lean mass and lean mass. Selected regions of the body can also be pinpointed for more in-depth analysis.

• • • • • • • • • • • • • • •

AVERAGE VALUES FOR BODY COMPOSITION

Average values for body fat in samples of men and women throughout the United States are presented in Table 16-3.

Also included are values representing plus and minus one standard deviation to give some indication of the amount of variation or spread from the average: the column headed "68% Variation Limits" indicates the range of values for percent body fat that includes one standard deviation, or about 68 of every 100 persons measured. As an example, the average percent body fat of young men from the New York sample is 15.0%, and the 68% variation limits are from 8.9 to 21.1% body fat. Interpreting this statistically, it could be expected that for 68 of every 100 young men measured, values for percent fat would range between 8.9 and 21.1%. Of the remaining 32 young men, 16 would possess more than 21.1% body fat, while for the other 16 men, body fat would be less than 8.9%. In the next chapter we discuss what is considered abnormal or excessive fatness.

Representative Samples Are Lacking.

Although considerable data are available concerning average body composition for many groups of men and women of different ages and fitness levels, there has been no systematic evaluation of the body composition of representative samples from the general population that would warrant setting up precise norms or desirable values of body composition. At this time, the best we can do is to present the average values from various studies of different age groups.

A general conclusion based on these data is that with increasing age, the percentage of body fat tends to rise in both men and women. This average change does not necessarily mean the trend should be interpreted as desirable or "normal." Changes in body composition with age could occur because the aging skeleton becomes demineralized and porous; such a process reduces body density because of the decrease in bone density. Another reason for the relative increase in body fat with age is a reduction in the level of daily physical activity. A more sedentary lifestyle could increase the deposition of storage fat and reduce the quantity of muscle mass. This would occur even if the daily caloric intake remained unchanged.

Desirable Body Mass Although an excess of body fat is undesirable for good health and fitness, an optimum level of body fat or body mass for a particular individual cannot be precisely stated. More than likely, this optimum varies from person to person and is greatly influenced by genetic factors. Based on data from physically active young adults, it would be desirable in our opinion to strive for a body fat content of 15% for men (certainly less than 20%) and about 25% for women (certainly less than 30%). An "optimal" or "desirable" body mass can be computed using a desired level of body fat as follows:

> **Desirable body mass =**
> Lean body mass ÷
> (1.00 –% fat desired)

Suppose a 91 kg (200 lb) man, who has 20% body fat, wishes to know the weight he should attain so that this new lower body weight would contain 10% body fat. The computations would be as follows:

Fat mass
> = 91.0 kg x 0.20
> = 18.2 kg

Lean body mass
> = 91.0 kg – 18.2 kg
> = 72.8 kg

Desirable body mass
> = 72.8 kg ÷ (1.00 - 0.10)
> = 72.8 kg ÷ 0.90
> = 80.9 kg (178 lb)

> **Desirable fat loss = Present body mass –Desirable body mass**

> = 91.0 kg - 80.9 kg
> = 10.1 kg (22.2 lb)

If this man lost 10.1 kg of body fat, his new body mass of 80.9 kg would have a fat content equal to 10% of body mass.

We believe that the notion of an upper and lower limit around the desired weight, rather than a precise value, is the best recommendation when prescribing optimal levels of body composition. Furthermore, weight loss should always be accompanied by a planned, systematic program of increased physical activity. This will reduce reliance on drastic dieting and increase the likelihood that the lost weight will be mostly fat and not lean tissue.

BODY COMPOSITION OF CHAMPION ATHLETES

High levels of physical activity and athletic performance are often associated with specific body composition characteristics. Among successful athletes, differences in physique are often pronounced when comparisons are made among sports participants of the same gender.

Body fat in children. In boys, percent body fat increases from an average of 11% at age 6 to 16% at age 11; in girls, body fat increases progressively from 14% at age 6 to 27% at age 11.

A desirable range for goal weight. For practical purposes, a desirable weight range is recommended rather than one specific goal weight. In most instances, this range should lie within 1 or 2 kg of the computed "desirable body mass." For example, if the desirable body mass is 135 lb, one should strive for a body mass that ranges from 133 to 137 lb.

Keep active and keep lean. Research indicates the participation in vigorous physical activities after age 35 can retard the "average" increase in body fatness so common in middle age. Even at ages 70 and older, if former athletes keep physically active, their bone mass also will be superior, compared to average individuals of the same age.

TABLE 16-4. Body composition of elite male and female endurance runners

Group	N	Stature cm	Mass kg	LBM kg	Body Fat %
Runners					
Male[a]	19	176.4	62.6	59.6	3.0
Female[b]	11	169.4	57.2	48.1	15.2
Untrained[c]					
Male	54	176.4	71.4	60.5	15.3
Female	69	160.4	59.0	43.5	26.2

a Data from Pollock, M.L., et al.: Body composition of elite class distance runners. *Ann. N.Y. Acad.Sci.*, 301:361, 1977.
b From Wilmore, J.H., and Brown, C.H.: Psychological profiles of women distance runners. *Med. Sci. Sports*, 6:178, 1974.
c Data from Katch, F.I., and McArdle, W.D.: Prediction of body density from simple anthropometric measurements in college-age men and women. *Hum. Biol.*, 45:445, 1973.

· ·

The making of a champion. In the best endurance runners, a lean and relatively light physique is blended with a highly developed aerobic system. When this is combined with a proper psychologic attitude for prolonged training, the ingredients certainly exist for a champion!

Long-Distance Runners

Table 16-4 presents data for body mass, stature, and body composition (determined by underwater weighing) for elite male and female distance runners. For comparative purposes, data are presented for a typical sample of untrained young adult men and women. The female runners averaged 15.2% body fat which is similar to reports of female high school cross-country runners and considerably lower than the average value of about 26% reported for females of the same age, stature, and body mass. Compared to other female athletes, the runners have a lower average fat value than collegiate basketball players (20.9%), competitive gymnasts (15.5%), swimmers (20.1%), or tennis players (22.8%)

Interestingly, the average body fat for the female runners is the same as the 15% average generally reported for males and is close to the quantity of essential fat proposed by Behnke in his model for the Reference woman.

For the male endurance runners, body fat values were extremely low, considering that the quantity of essential fat is probably about 3% of body mass. Clearly, these endurance runners are at the lower end of the lean-to-fat continuum for topflight athletes. Apparently, this physique characteristic is a prerequisite for success in distance running. This makes sense for several reasons. First, the body's ability to dissipate heat during running is of primary importance in maintaining thermal balance during competition. Excess fat thwarts heat dissipation. Second, excess body fat is "dead weight" that adds directly to the energy cost of running.

Football Players

Table 16-5 shows the average values for body mass, percent body fat, and lean body mass of college and professional football players grouped by position. The "pro" group consists of 164 players from 14 teams in the National Football League (NFL). Also included is a professional group of 107 members of the 1976-1978 Dallas Cowboys and New York Jets football teams. For comparison, three groups of collegiate players are represented: (1) the St. Cloud State College, Minnesota, players who were candidates for spring practice, (2) players from the University of Massachusetts (U Mass.) who were also candidates for spring practice, and (3) teams from the University of Southern California (USC 1973-1992), who were National Champions and participants in two Rose Bowls.

One would generally expect modern day professional players to be larger in body size at each position than a representative collegiate group. Although this was generally true for the comparison with the St. Cloud and U Mass. players, the USC players were similar in physique to the professionals. With the exception of defensive linemen, the USC players at each position had almost the same body fat content, although they tended to weigh less than the current players at each position. For the all-important component of lean body mass, the USC players were no more than 4.4 kg lighter than the "pros" at each position. In fact, the average defensive lineman in the NFL outweighed his USC counterpart in lean tissue by only 1.8 kg. The total body mass of the pro linemen, however, was significantly heavier than that of the USC players. This

TABLE 16-5. Comparison of body composition between collegiate and professional football players grouped by position[a]

Position	Level	N	Stature (cm)	Mass (kg)	Body Fat (%)	LBM (kg)
Defensive backs	St. Cloud[b]	15	178.3	77.3	11.5	68.4
	U Mass[c]	12	179.9	83.1	8.8	76.8
	USC[d]	15	183.0	83.7	9.6	75.7
	Pro, current[e]	26	182.5	84.8	9.6	76.7
	Pro, older[g]	25	183.0	91.2	10.7	81.4
Offensive backs and receivers	St. Cloud	15	179.7	79.8	12.4	69.6
	U Mass	29	181.8	84.1	9.5	76.4
	USC	18	185.6	86.1	9.9	77.6
	Pro, current	40	183.8	90.7	9.4	81.9
	Pro, older	25	183.0	91.7	10.0	87.5
Linebackers	St. Cloud	7	180.1	87.2	13.4	75.4
	U Mass	17	186.1	97.1	13.1	84.2
	USC	17	185.6	98.8	13.2	85.8
	Pro, current	28	188.6	102.2	14.0	87.6
Offensive linemen and tight ends	St. Cloud	13	186.0	99.2	19.1	79.8
	U Mass	23	187.5	107.6	19.5	86.6
	USC	25	191.1	106.5	15.3	90.3
	Pro, current	38	193.0	112.6	15.6	94.7
Defensive linemen	St. Cloud	15	186.6	97.8	18.5	79.3
	U Mass	8	188.8	114.3	19.5	91.9
	USC	13	191.1	109.3	14.7	93.2
	Pro, current	32	192.4	117.1	18.2	95.8
	Pro, older	25	185.7	97.1	14.0	83.5
Total	St. Cloud	65	182.5	88.0	15.0	74.2
	U Mass	91	184.9	97.3	13.9	83.2
	USC	88	186.6	96.6	11.4	84.6
	Pro, current	164	188.1	101.5	13.4	87.3
	Pro, older	25	183.1	91.2	10.4	81.3
	Dallas-Jets[f]	107	188.2	100.4	12.6	87.7

[a] Grouping according to Wilmore, J. H., and Haskel, W. L.: Body composition and endurance capacity of professional football players. *J. Appl. Physiol.*, 33:564, 1972.
[b] Data from Wickkiser, J.D., and Kelly, J.M.: The body composition of a college football team. *Med. Sci. Sports*, 7:199, 1975.
[c] U Mass. data courtesy of Coach Robert Stull and F. Katch. University of Massachusetts. Data collected during spring practice, 1985; % fat by densitometry.
[d] USC data courtesy of Dr. Robert Girandola, University of Southern California, Los Angeles, 1978, 1993.
[e] Data from Wilmore, J.H., et al.: Football pros' strengths — and CV weakness — charted. *Phys. Sportsmed.*, 4:45, 1976.
[f] Data from Katch, F.I., and Katch, V.L.: Body composition of the Dallas Cowboys and New York Jets Football teams. Unpublished data, 1978.
[g] Data from Dr. A.R. Behnke.

difference occurred because the professional linemen possessed 18.2% body fat whereas collegians were leaner at 14.7%.

High School Wrestlers

Wrestlers represent a unique group of athletes who undergo both severe training and acute weight loss. Despite warnings from medical and professional groups regarding rapid and repetitive weight loss, most high school and college wrestlers lose considerable weight a few days before or on the day of competition. This is done in the hope of gaining a competitive advantage by wrestling at a lower weight category. This process of "making weight" usually occurs by combining food restriction and dehydration, either through fluid depriva-

TABLE 16-6. Anthropometric comparisons between certified and champion Iowa and Minnesota high school wrestlers[a] and comparison to Nebraska wrestlers[b]

| Measurement | Certified Wrestlers | | Champion Wrestlers | | Nebraska Wrestlers |
	Iowa (N = 484)	Minn (N = 245)	Iowa (N = 382)	Minn (N = 164)	(N = 409)
Age, yr	15.9	16.8	17.8	17.4	16.4
Stature, cm	169.9	172.0	171.7	172.5	171.0
Body mass, kg	64.3	65.3	64.6	64.7	63.2
Chest diameter, cm	26.8	26.5	27.7	26.6	27.9
Chest depth, cm	19.0	16.8	19.2	17.3	18.9
Bitrochanteric diameter, cm	31.0	31.4	31.1	31.5	31.0
Ankles diameter, cm	14.3	14.3	14.0	14.3	13.8
Fatfolds, mm					
Scapular	8.4	7.9	6.4	6.8	8.8
Triceps	8.6	9.1	6.0	5.6	8.9
Suprailiac	13.3	12.3	9.1	7.5	11.8
Abdominal	13.1	12.2	8.6	8.3	11.6
Thigh	10.8	13.6	7.7	8.3	9.4
Sum of 5 fatfolds	54.2	55.1	37.8	36.5	50.5

[a] From Clarke, K.S.: Predicting certified weight of young wrestlers; a field study of the Tcheng-Tipton method. *Med. Sci. Sports*, 6:52, 1974.

[b] From Housh, T.J., et al.: Validity of anthropometric estimations of body compositions in high school wrestlers. *Res. Q. Exec. Sport*, 60:239, 1989.

College vs. pro players. At the highest levels of collegiate competition, the body size and compositions of college and professional players are similar.

tion or exercising in a hot environment while wearing plastic or rubber garments. To reduce the possibility of injury from acute weight loss and dehydration, the American College of Sports Medicine recommends that each wrestler's body composition be assessed several weeks prior to the competitive season to determine an acceptable minimal wrestling weight. *A lower limit of 5 to 7% body fat is proposed as the lowest acceptable level for safe wrestling competition.*

The physical characteristics of three groups of high school wrestlers are presented in Table 16-6. The "certified" Iowa and Minnesota wrestlers were assigned to wrestle at one of 12 different weight categories; the "champion" wrestlers competed in the State or Conference finals. Except for age and fatfolds, there was little difference in the physical characteristics of the certified and champion wrestlers. As reflected by the fatfold measures, however, the champions were considerably leaner than their less successful teammates.

Because differences in body mass were small among groups, the elite wrestlers actually competed at a heavier lean body mass. This may have contributed greatly to their success in a particular weight class. The last column in the table presents additional data on 4089 Nebraska high school wrestlers. Their anthropometric characteristics are most similar to the Iowa and Minnesota certified wrestlers. Their percent body fat was 11.0% (range 1.5-26.0%) while their minimal wrestling weight at 5% body fat averaged 59.1 kg.

Weight Lifters and Body Builders

Men and women who engage in resistance training often exhibit remarkable muscular development, although quantification of this hypertrophy has been limited. Bodybuilders are a group of athletes who lift weights solely to improve body configuration and form, with little concern for subsequent sports performance. This group differs from the other types of weight lifters who train for the purpose of increasing the amount of weight lifted with less concern for muscle size and definition.

Males. Excess muscular development and lean body mass have been quantified in competitive male body builders, Olympic weight lifters, and power weight lifters. For percent body fat, the values were quite similar averaging 9.3% for the body builders, 9.1% for the power lifters, and 10.8% for the Olympic competitors. This degree of leanness existed even though each group of athletes was classified as being between 14 to 19% "overweight" from the "height-weight" tables! Estimation of excess muscle revealed that the body builders possessed nearly 16 kg of excess muscle, while power lifters had 15 kg and Olympic lifters had 13 kg.

Females. A study of the body composition of 10 competitive female body builders revealed that these athletes were quite lean averaging 13.2% body fat (range 8.0–18.3%) with an average lean body mass of 46.6 kg. Their body mass averaged 53.8 kg, stature 160.8 cm, and age 27.1 years. With the exception of champion gymnasts who also average about 13% body fat, the body builders were shorter in stature by about 3%, lower in body mass by 5%, and possessed 7 to 10% less total mass of body fat compared with other top female athletes. The most striking compositional characteristic of the female body builders was their dramatically large lean-to-fat ratio of 7:1 (weight of the lean mass relative to the weight of fat mass) in comparison to 4.3:1 for other female athletic groups. This occurred without the use of steroids as reported by the women in a questionnaire. It is interesting to note that menstrual function was reported as normal by eight of ten body builders in this study, despite their relatively low level of body fat.

Minimal wrestling weight. The recommended minimum percent body fat is 7% for wrestlers under 16 years of age and 5% for those who are older. A fatfold equation for use with interscholastic wrestlers is:

Body Density = 1.0982 - (0.000815 x [triceps + abdominal fatfolds]) + (0.00000084 x [triceps + abdominal skinfolds]^2)

% Fat = ([4.570 ÷ Body Density] −4.142) x 100

Minimal Wrestling Weight = Fat-Free Body Weight ÷ 1.00 −% Fat Recommended

If the wrestler's body weight is above the "minimal wrestling weight," a gradual fat loss program can begin with a realistic and prudent loss of 1 to 2 pounds of body fat per week through diet and exercise. Source: Thorland, W., et al.:New equations for prediction of a minimal weight in high school wrestlers. *Med. Sci. Sports Exerc.* 21:S72, 1989.

S U M M A R Y

1. Standard "height-weight" tables reveal little about an individual's body composition that can vary considerably at any given body mass and stature. A person can be overweight without being overfat.

2. Total body fat consists of essential fat and storage fat. Essential fat is that present in bone marrow, nerve tissue, and the various organs; it is generally required for normal physiologic function. Storage fat is the energy reserve that accumulates mainly as adipose tissue beneath the skin.

3. True gender differences exist for quantities of essential fat. Although storage fat values for men and women average 12% and 15% of body mass, respectively, the essential fat differences are large and amount to 3% for men and 12% for women. This difference is probably related to childbearing and hormonal functions.

4. In terms of maintaining good health, a person should not reduce below the essential fat level.

5. Menstrual irregularities occur among some groups of female athletes, especially among women who train hard and maintain low levels of body fat. The precise interaction between the physiologic and psychologic stress of intense, regular training, hormonal balance, energy and nutrient intake, and body fat requires further study.

6. A positive aspect may exist between the delayed onset of menarche observed in chronically active young females and health because of a lower lifetime occurrence of cancer of the reproductive organs and other types of cancer.

7. The two most popular indirect methods to assess body composition are hydrostatic weighing and anthropometry (prediction methods from fatfolds and circumferences). Hydrostatic weighing involves the determination of body density and subsequent estimation of percent body fat.

Obesity, Exercise, and Weight Control

CHAPTER 17

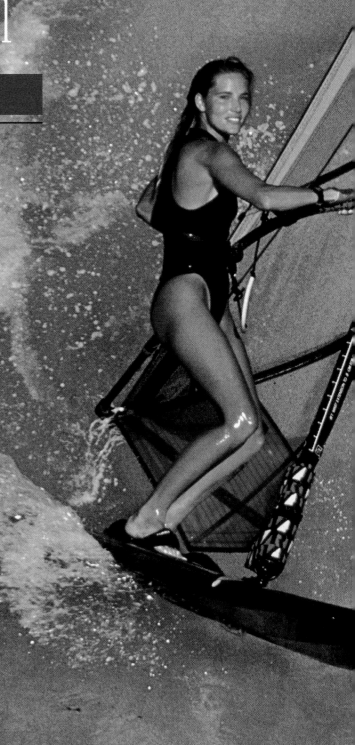

TOPICS COVERED IN THIS CHAPTER

After reading this chapter you should be able to:

- List 10 significant health risks of obesity.
- Discuss each of the following as a criterion for obesity: (a) percent body fat, (b) body fat distribution, and (c) fat cell size and fat cell number.
- Define fat cell hypertrophy and fat cell hyperplasia, and discuss how each contributes to obesity.
- Compare fat cell size and fat cell number between individuals with average body fat and those who are massively obese.
- Describe the general effects of weight gain and weight loss in adults on the size and number of fat cells.
- Outline how changes in the Energy Balance Equation can affect a change in body weight.
- Summarize why proponents of the "set-point theory" argue that dieting is generally ineffective for long-term weight loss.
- Discuss what is meant by the term weight cycling.
- Recommend the optimal amount of weekly weight loss and type of dietary plan to assure successful weight loss.
- Give the rationale for including exercise when attempting to lose weight.
- Discuss the effects of variations in daily exercise on (a) daily food intake, and (b) daily energy expenditure.
- Provide information about the effectiveness of "spot" reducing exercise.
- Advise a person who wishes to gain weight to improve their appearance, or enhance their image in sports performance.

Americans consume more fat per capita than any nation in the world. We also consume more than 90% of the foods high in saturated fats and processed sugars. The end result of this national preoccupation with food and effortless living is that about 110 million men and women (and 10 to 12 million teenagers) are "too fat" and need to reduce. If these overfat men and women consumed 600 fewer calories each day to reduce to a "normal" body fat value (achievable in 68 days for men and 101 days for women), the reduced caloric intake would equal 5.7 trillion calories. This energy could supply the yearly residential electricity demands of Boston, Chicago, San Francisco, and Washington, DC, or 1.3 billion gallons of gasoline to fuel about 1 million autos for a year!

Part 1 OBESITY

OBESITY: OFTEN A LONG-TERM PROCESS

Obesity often begins in childhood. When this occurs, the chances for adult obesity are three times greater compared to children of normal body mass. Simply stated, a child generally does not "grow out of" an obesity problem. When body weight is "tracked" through generations, the data indicate that the obese parent is likely to give birth to an overweight child who will grow into an obese adult whose offspring are likely to become obese.

Excessive fatness also develops slowly during adulthood with ages 25 to 44 being the years of greatest fat accretion. In one longitudinal study, the fat content of 27 adult men increased an average of 6.5 kg over a 12-year period from ages 32 to 44. This was equal to the group's total weight gain over the duration of the study. Women are the biggest weight gainers with about 14% putting on more than 13.6 kg between the ages of 25 and 34. The extent to which this "creeping obesity" during adulthood reflects a normal biologic pattern is unknown.

NOT NECESSARILY OVEREATING

If obesity were truly a unitary disorder, and gluttony and overindulgence were the only factors associated with an increase in body fat, the easiest way to reduce permanently would surely be to cut back on food. Obviously, other influences are operating such as genetic, environmental, social, and perhaps racial. Research also suggests specific factors may predispose a person to excessive weight gain. These include: eating patterns, eating environment, food packaging, body image, biochemical differences related to resting metabolic rate, dietary-induced thermogenesis, level of spontaneous activity or "fidgeting", and basal body temperature, levels of cellular adenosine triphosphatase, lipoprotein lipase and other enzymes, the metabolically active brown adipose tissue, and the level of daily physical activity.

It is difficult to partition the causes of obesity into distinct categories because they probably overlap. It seems fairly certain that the treatment procedures devised so far — whether diets, surgery, drugs, psychological methods, or exercise, either alone or in combination — have not been particularly successful in solving the problem on a long-term basis. There is optimism, nonetheless, that as researchers continue to investigate the many facets of obesity and its treatment, significant progress will be made to conquer this major health problem.

A gradual process. In the Western world, the average 35-year-old male gains between 0.2 and 0.8 kg of fat each year until the sixth decade of life despite a progressive decrease in food intake.

Obesity in children continues to increase. Childhood and adolescent obesity constitutes a major health problem and is increasing in prevalence. Over the past 15 years the prevalence of obesity has increased by about 40 to 50% in both children and adolescents regardless of race or gender — and as many as 30% of American children may average less than one-half hour of daily physical activity.

Genetics sets the stage. Our genetic makeup does not necessarily cause the obesity, but it does influence susceptibility. In the right disease-producing environment (sedentary and stressful, with easy access to food), the susceptible individual will gain weight — and possibly lots of it.

Metabolism, the body's defense against weight change. Caloric restriction brings about significant depression of resting metabolism as the body defends against weight loss. Even when a person attempts to gain weight above normal level by means of overeating, the body resists this change through an increase in resting metabolism.

Disconcerting news. Although being overweight clearly raises the chances for heart trouble, the failure to keep weight off might be even worse. Repeated bouts of weight loss and weight gain further increase the risk of dying from a heart attack. In fact, the risk is almost 70% higher in those who take weight off and put it on again, compared to people whose weight stays reasonably steady.

Weight loss in the '90s. Nutrition experts are encouraged about a gradual shift away from crash diets and rigid weight loss programs and a movement toward more sensible eating and regular exercising. Good advice for the '90s:
- Be realistic in your weight loss goals
- Consume more fruits and vegetables
- Exercise regularly
- Reduce intake of dietary fat

There are no magic potions. There is simply no compelling evidence that popular "fad" diets have any advantage over a calorically restricted, well-balanced diet. No magic metabolic mixture will assure more effective weight loss than can be achieved with a well-balanced, low-calorie diet.

Recent research provides further disconcerting news for those desiring permanent fat loss. It now appears that when obese people lose body mass, the adipocytes increase their level of lipoprotein lipase, the enzyme that facilitates fat synthesis and storage. The effect of these high enzyme levels is to make it easier for the formerly obese to regain fat — and the fatter people are before their weight loss, the more lipoprotein lipase they produce when they reduce. This suggests that the fatter people are originally, the more vigorously their bodies attempt to regain lost weight. Such findings provide an additional biologic mechanism to explain the great difficulty the obese encounter in maintaining weight loss.

Although the set-point theory may be unwelcome news for those who possess a set-point that is tuned "too high," the good news is that regular exercise may lower the set-point toward a more desirable level. Concurrently, regular exercise conserves and even increases lean body mass, stabilizes or slightly raises resting metabolism, and brings about enzymatic changes that facilitate fat breakdown in the tissues, all of which would make dieting more effective. For overweight men and women who exercise regularly, food intake tends to drop initially despite the increase in energy output, and body fat decreases. Eventually, as an active lifestyle is maintained, caloric intake balances the daily energy requirement so body mass is stabilized at a new, lower level.

How to Select a Diet Plan

The most difficult aspect of dieting is deciding exactly what foods to include in the daily menu. There are literally hundreds of diet plans to choose from: water diets, drinker's diets, fruit or vegetable diets, egg diets, meat diets, fast-food diets, ice cream diets, "eat to win" diets, and diets named for cities — the New York City or Beverly Hills diet — not to mention the potentially dangerous varieties of high-fat, low-carbohydrate, and high-protein diets. Some authors have even preached that it is not total calories that contribute to weight loss, but the order in which foods are eaten! Of course, such claims are ludicrous, but for those desperate to shed excess weight, such misinformation reinforces negative eating behaviors. As a result, it is easy to repeat a vicious cycle of failures. Table 17-1 summarizes the principles and the main advantages and disadvantages of some of the popular dietary approaches to weight loss.

Well Balanced But Less of It. A calorie-counting approach to weight loss should provide a well-balanced diet containing all of the essential nutrients. The general recommendation is that reducing diets should contain the RDA for the micronutrients and protein with reduced amounts of cholesterol and saturated fats and the remainder consisting predominantly of unrefined, fiber-rich, complex carbohydrates. *Calories do count*; the trick is to keep within the daily limit specified by the rate of fat loss desired. Recall from the previous section that our daily energy expenditure is largely determined by two factors: the resting energy requirement, and the energy expended in daily physical activities. As long as a diet is nutritionally sound, it really is not important what we eat, but rather how many calories are consumed. If a true caloric deficit exists and input is less than output, weight loss will occur independent of the diet's composition of carbohydrate, lipid, or protein. During weight loss, the initial decrease in body mass occurs primarily from water loss and some depletion of carbohydrate reserves. As the diet progresses, a larger amount of body fat is metabolized to make up the energy deficit created by dieting.

Maintenance of Goal Weight Is A Difficult Task. A review of the scientific literature dealing with weight loss reveals that people who have initial success are usually unsuccessful in permanently maintaining their desired body size.

TABLE 17–1. Principles and main advantages and disadvantages of some popular weight loss methods

Method	Principle	Advantages	Disadvantages	Comments
Surgical procedures	Alteration of the gastrointestinal tract changes capacity or amount of absorptive surface	Caloric restriction is less necessary	Risks of surgery and post-surgical complications can include death	Radical procedures include stapling of the stomach and removal of a section of the small intestine (a jejunoileal bypass)
Fasting	No energy input assures negative energy balance	Weight loss is rapid (which may be a disadvantage) Exposure to temptation is reduced	Ketogenic A large portion of weight lost is from lean body mass Nutrients are lacking	Medical supervision is mandatory and hospitalization is recommended
Protein-sparing modified fast	Same as fasting except protein or protein with carbohydrate intake assumedly helps preserve lean body mass	Same as in fasting	Ketogenic Nutrients are lacking Some unconfirmed deaths have been reported, possibly from potassium depletion	Medical supervision is mandatory Popular presentation was made in Linn's *The Last Chance Diet*
One-food-centered diets	Low-caloric intake favors negative energy balance	Being easy to follow has initial psychologic appeal	Being too restrictive means that nutrients are probably lacking Repetitious nature may cause boredom	No food or food combination is known to "burn off" fat Examples include the grapefruit diet and the egg diet
Low-carbohydate/ high-fat diets	Increased ketone excretion removes energy-containing substances from the body Fat intake is often voluntarily decreased; a low caloric diet results	Inclusion of rich foods may have psychologic appeal Initial rapid loss of water may be an incentive	Ketogenic High-fat intake is contraindicated for heart and diabetes patients Nutrients are lacking	Popular versions have been offered by Taller and Atkins; some have been called the "Mayo", "Drinking Man's", and "Air Force" diets
Low-carbohydrate/ high-protein diets	Low caloric intake favors negative energy balance		Expense and repetitious nature may make it difficult to sustain	If meat is emphasized, the diet becomes one that is high in fat The Pennington diet is an example
High-carbohydrate/ low-fat diets	Low caloric intake favors negative energy balance	Wise food selections can make the diet nutritionally sound	Initial water retention may be discouraging	The Pritikin diet is an example

Modified and reprinted by permission from Reed, P.B.: *Nutrition: An Applied Science.* Copyright © 1980 by West Publishing Co. All Rights Reserved.

This has been pointed out in numerous follow-up studies of patients who participated in weight loss programs in which caloric intake was carefully regulated. In an early survey of the effectiveness of obesity clinics during a 10-year period, the dropout rate varied between 20 and 80%. Of those who remained in a program, no more than 25% lost as much as 9 kg, and only 5% lost 18 kg or more.

In a follow-up study of 121 patients, illustrated in Figure 17-6, much of the reduced weight was maintained for the first 12 to 18 months. The tendency to regain weight was

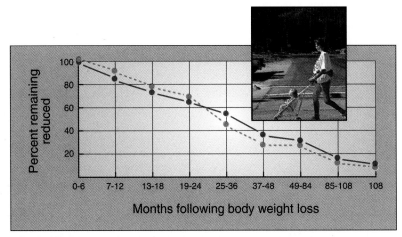

Figure 17-6. Percent of patients remaining at reduced body weights at various time intervals following accomplished weight loss. The solid line represents 60 subjects with obesity onset before age 21; dashed line, 42 subjects with obesity onset after age 21. (From Johnson, D, and Drenick, E.J.: Therapeutic fasting in morbid obesity. *Arch. Intern. Med.*, 137: 1381, 1977.)

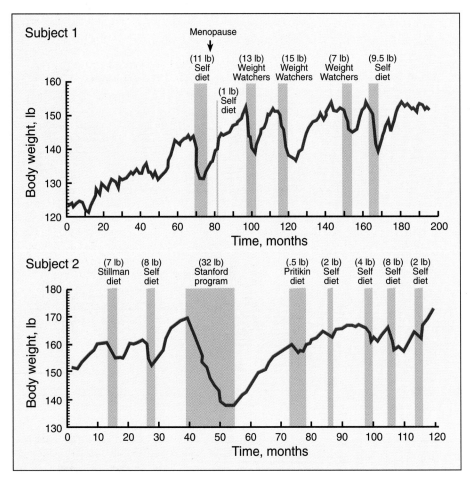

Figure 17-7. Tracking of weekly body weights of 2 females over a prolonged time. Subject 1 gained about 30 lb over a 16 year period; subject 2 gained 22 lb over the 10 years of measurement. (From Black, D.R. et al.,: A time series analysis of longitudinal weight changes in two adult women. *Int. J. Obes.*, 15:623, 1991.)

independent of the length of the fast, extent of weight lost, or age at onset of obesity. Return to original weight occurred in one-half of the subjects within 2 or 3 years, and only 7 patients remained at their reduced weight after 7 years.

While most weight reduction attempts are disappointing, relatively little is known about long term maintenance. Figure 17-7 presents data on body weights of 2 females who recorded their weight weekly. Subject 1 gained about 30 lb over a 16 year period, while subject 2 gained 22 lb over 10 years.

Subject 1 participated in 6 weight loss programs during the 16 years she recorded her weight. Her efforts lasted from 1 to 6 months. The three formal programs of weight loss lasted about 5 months, while the three self-directed efforts lasted approximately 2 months. The average weight lost for all programs was 9.2 lbs and this woman regained an average of 12 lbs over about 12 months following each weight loss attempt.

Subject 2 participated in 8 weight loss programs during her 10 years of recording body weight. Her weight loss attempts lasted between 2 to 16 months, and the average weight lost for all programs was 8 lbs. As was the case with subject 1, she regained weight following each weight loss attempt with an average gain of 9.9 lb over an average of 9 months.

For both women, significant gains in body weight occurred in spite of interruptions due to dieting; these gains could not be attributed to menopause, alterations in exercise patterns, pregnancy, changes in smoking status, or seasonal variation. Each weight loss attempt was followed immediately by weight increases towards obesity. Body weights increased to original or higher levels in time intervals approximately 2 to 3 times longer than the time required for weight loss. Finally, the steady weight gain observed for both females when they were not on a weight loss regimen speaks against the idea of a fixed set-point, but rather supports the hypothesis that aging results in physiologic changes that facilitate weight gain (and perhaps "resetting" of the set-point) even with attempts to lose weight.

EXERCISING TO TIP THE ENERGY BALANCE EQUATION

The precise contributions of sedentary living and excessive caloric intake to obesity are not clearly understood. What is clear is that an increased level of daily physical activity can impact significantly on energy balance.

Not Simply a Problem of Gluttony

In the past, it was generally accepted that obesity was the result of excessive food intake. Clearly, then, the proper approach to weight loss would be some form of caloric restriction by dieting. This view of obesity is overly simplistic, as *evidence indicates that excess weight gain often parallels reduced physical activity rather than an increase in energy intake.* In fact, among active young and middle-aged endurance-trained men, body fat was inversely related to energy expenditure; no relationship existed between body fat and food intake. Among the physically active, those who eat the most often weigh the least and are the most fit! In the United States, per capita caloric intake has steadily decreased over the past 80 years, yet body mass and body fat have slowly increased. Americans now eat 5 to 10% fewer calories than they did 20 years ago, yet they weigh an average of 2.3 kg more. Certainly, if food intake were the culprit, this reduction in caloric intake should bring the national body mass to a lower, not higher level!

This pattern holds for children too. Obese infants do not characteristically consume more calories than the recommended dietary standards. Physically active children tend to be leaner than less active counterparts. Time-in-motion photography to document activity patterns of elementary school students clearly showed that overweight children were considerably less active than their normal-weight peers, and their excess weight was not related to food intake. The caloric intake of obese high school girls and boys was actually below that of their nonobese peers. This observation that fat people often eat the same or even less than thinner ones is also true for adults over a broad age range as they become less active and slowly begin to add weight. Consequently, reducing caloric intake is inappropriate as the only method to combat the overfat condition.

Increased Energy Output is Worth Considering

It is increasingly clear that men and women of all ages who maintain a physically active lifestyle or become involved in aerobic exercise programs maintain a desirable level of body composition. Increased caloric output with exercise provides a significant option for unbalancing the energy balance equation. Only recently, however, has this approach to bring about desirable weight loss and body composition changes come into prominence. Two arguments have generally been raised against the exercise option. One is the belief that exercise inevitably increases the appetite so that any caloric deficit is rapidly made up by proportionately greater food intake. The second argument is that the calorie-burning effects of exercise are so small that a reasonable use of exercise would only "dent" the body's fat reserves compared to using starvation or semi-starvation. Let's take a closer look at these two misconceptions.

Effects of Exercise on Food Intake. Sedentary people do not always maintain a fine balance between energy expenditure and food intake. For them, the daily caloric intake generally exceeds their low energy requirement. This lack of precision in regulating food intake at the low end of the physical activity spectrum may account for the "creeping obesity"

A lot of money but limited results. In 1991 nearly 8 million people enrolled in commercial weight loss programs (not including those that use liquid diets like *Optifast* or *Medifast* that require medical supervision) generating more than $2 billion dollars in revenues for these plans. Although data are limited, it appears that for those men and women that complete commercial diets many will regain one third of their lost weight after one year and almost all of this weight within 3 to 5 years.

Childhood obesity and food intake. Research indicates that children age 6 to 17 years have shown about a 4% decline in caloric intake over the past 20 years. Consequently, an increase in energy intake does not appear to be the primary factor for the increasing prevalence of childhood obesity.

Balance between energy intake and energy expenditure. Regular physical activity contributes to the normal functioning of the brain's feeding control mechanisms to bring about a balance between energy intake and energy expenditure.

Exercise does not always stimulate appetite. Short-term increases in physical activity do not always increase caloric intake in proportion to the calories expended during exercise. In fact, some individuals show no increase in food intake with moderate daily exercise.

The prevalence and persistence of childhood obesity is now recognized as a national health problem. As many as 25% of children in the United States can be classified as obese. Indeed, the prevalence of obesity is approaching epidemic proportions. Over the last 15 years there has been a 54% increase in obesity and a 98% increase in extreme obesity in children age 6 to 11 years. As with adults, the prevention and treatment of childhood obesity has proven to be extremely difficult, independent of treatment modality. Eighty to 90% of children who lose weight typically return to their previous body weight percentiles in a short time, and this is complicated by the growth process.

Both increased energy intake and reduced energy output have been investigated as possible causes for excessiwe weight gain in children. The data are often conflicting as to whether the obese child eats more or exercises less than the child with good control of body weight. An interesting line of research has focused on the role television watching has on the development of obesity in children. Children in the U. S. spend as much time watching TV each year as they do attending school!

In 1985, the last time estimates were made, 6 to 11 year-old children watched about 26 hours of TV each week, and adolescents watched 22 hours weekly. The amount of television viewing also has been related to obesity; each hourly increment of TV watching by adolescents is associated with a 2% increase in the prevalence of obesity. The same is true for adults; men who viewed more than 3 hours of daily TV were twice as likely to be obese as men who viewed less than 1 hour a day. Many researchers believe that individuals are obese because they watch more TV, not that they watch more TV because they are obese.

The reason why TV watching contributes to the development of obesity is unclear, but the results of a recent study may provide a clue. The metabolic rate of 15 obese and 16 normal-weight girls (average age 10.2 yrs) was assessed during rest and

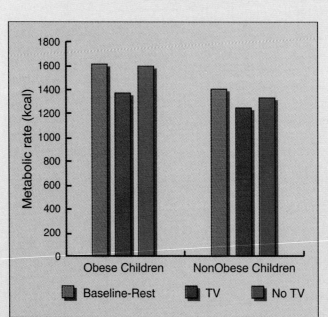

while resting for 25 minutes when viewing TV. The results are shown in the insert graph. The metabolic rate was depressed by 15% in the obese girls and by 17% in the nonobese girls during TV viewing. However, because obese children watch more TV per day than their normal weight peers, the cumulative effect of a lowered metabolic rate during TV viewing has a greater impact on the obese. Thus, children who watch too much TV are at greater risk for becoming obese because their resting energy expenditure is lower than if they did nothing at all!

The acute decrease in metabolism during TV viewing provides support for a causal relationship between the time spent watching TV and excessive weight gain. A vicious cycle is also created because children who watch an excessive amount of TV are not involved in more energy demanding activities; they tend to snack while watching TV, and these snacks are more likely to be high in caloric density. Such results emphasize the importance of controlling the amount of TV watched by children at risk for obesity.

Reference
Klesges, R. C. et al.: Effects of television on metabolic rate: potential implications for childhood obesity. *Pediatrics*. 91:281, 1993.

common in highly mechanized and technically advanced sedentary societies. On the other hand, for individuals who regularly exercise, appetite control is in a "reactive zone" where it is simpler to match food intake with daily energy expenditure.

In considering the effects of exercise on appetite and food intake, a distinction must be made between the type and duration of exercise. There is no question that lumberjacks, farm laborers, and certain athletes who regularly perform hard physical labor often consume about twice the daily calories (4000 to 6000 kcal) as more sedentary people (2000 to 3000 kcal). Endurance athletes such as marathon runners, cross-country skiers, and cyclists consume about 4000 to 5000 kcal daily, yet these men and women are among the leanest in the world. Obviously, this extreme food intake is required just to meet the energy demands of training!

Effects of Exercise on Energy Expenditure. The second misconception concerns the number of calories expended through regular exercise — the idea that a person must perform an extraordinary amount of exercise to lose body fat. We have all heard the statistics that a person has to chop wood for 10 hours, golf for 20 hours, perform mild calisthenics for 22 hours, play ping-pong for 28 hours or volleyball for 32 hours, or run 35 miles just to reduce body fat by 0.45 kg (1.0 lb). Understandably, such a commitment is overwhelming to the overweight person who plans to reduce by 10 or 15 kg or more. Looking at it from a different perspective, however, if a person played golf only 2 hours (about 350 kcal per day) for 2 days a week (700 kcal), it would take about 5 weeks, or 10 golfing days, to lose 0.45 kg of fat (3500 kcal). Assuming golf was played year-round, golfing 2 days a week would result in a 4.5 kg loss of fat during the year provided food intake remained fairly constant. While most of us would probably not play golf this frequently (nor are we likely to play golf for 20

consecutive hours), the point is that *the calorie-expending effects of exercise are cumulative:* a caloric deficit of 3500 kcal is equivalent to a 0.45 kg fat loss whether it occurs rapidly or systematically over time.

The caloric expenditure values for the physical activities presented in Appendix 3 and in Section III of the *Student Study Guide and Workbook* should not be considered absolute. These are "average" values, applicable under "average" conditions when applied to the "average" person of a given body mass. However, these values do provide a good approximation of energy expenditure and are useful in establishing the caloric cost of an exercise program.

Exercise Is Effective

Regular aerobic exercise, with or without dietary restriction, brings about favorable changes in body mass and body composition. Even conventional resistance training combined with caloric restriction results in maintenance of lean body mass compared to a weight loss program that relies exclusively on dieting. As a general rule, persons who are obese lose weight and fat more readily through exercising than do their normal-weight counterparts. In addition, exercise provides significant positive "spin-off" because it alters body composition (reduced fat with maintenance or even small increase in lean tissue) in such a way that the resting metabolism is maintained or even slightly increased. This reduces the body's tendency to store calories.

A person planning to exercise for weight control should consider factors such as frequency, intensity, and duration as well as the specific form of exercise. Ideal activities are continuous, big muscle aerobic activities that have a moderate to high caloric cost, such as walking, running, rope skipping, cycling, and swimming. Many recreational sports and games are also effective in reducing body weight, although precise quantification of energy expenditure is difficult during such activities. Aerobic exercises burn considerable calories, stim-

It's what's burned during exercise that counts. With moderate exercise as performed by most people for weight control, the contribution of recovery metabolism — the so-called afterglow — to total energy expenditure is probably quite small because recovery from such exercise is rapid.

Work with parents. A study that followed children from age 6 months to 16 years found that the overfat teenagers did not necessarily eat more than normal weight children. However, their daily physical activity levels were lower. A desirable treatment is to have parents become more physically active with their child.

Keep on walking. For individuals desiring to use walking as the sole means for exercise training and weight loss, hand, wrist, or ankle weight as well as a race walking technique can be used to increase exercise intensity and caloric output as the program progresses.

The fatter you are, the more you'll lose. The effectiveness of exercise for weight loss is linked to the degree of obesity at the start.

> **The effects are additive.** A small decrease in food intake and a small increase in physical activity can, over time, create a significant deficit in the energy balance equation.

> **There's no one "best" aerobic exercise.** There is generally no selective effect of running, walking, or bicycling; each is equally effective in altering body composition, provided the duration, frequency, and intensity of exercise are similar.

ulate lipid metabolism, reduce body fat, establish favorable blood pressure responses, and generally promote cardiovascular fitness. An extra 300 kcal expended with moderate jogging daily for 30 minutes causes a 0.45 kg fat loss in about 12 days. Over a year's time, this theoretically represents a total caloric deficit equivalent to about 13.6 kg (30 lb) of body fat!

A Dose-Response Relationship. A direct dose-response relationship has been demonstrated between weight loss and time spent exercising. *In fact, the total energy expended is probably the most important factor that influences the effectiveness of an exercise program for weight loss.* Thus, an overfat person who begins exercising lightly with slow walking, for example, can accrue a considerable caloric expenditure simply by extending the duration of the exercise. This effect of duration offsets the inability (and inadvisability) of a previously sedentary, obese person beginning an exercise program at high intensity. Furthermore, because the energy cost of weight-bearing exercise such as walking is proportional to body mass, the overweight person expends considerably more calories to perform these tasks as someone of normal weight.

The importance of exercise duration for weight loss was illustrated in a study of three groups of men who exercised for 20 weeks by walking and running for either 15, 30, or 45 minutes per session. Compared to a sedentary control group, the three exercise groups significantly decreased their total body fat, fatfolds, and waist girth. When comparisons were made between the three groups, the 45-minute training group lost more body fat than either the 30- or 15-minute group. This was directly attributed to the greater caloric expenditure of the longer exercise period.

Start Slowly. A person beginning an exercise program for weight loss should adopt long-term goals, exert personal discipline, and restructure both eating and exercise behaviors. It is often counterproductive to include unduly rapid training progressions because many obese men and women initially are psychologically resistant to physical training. During the first few weeks, slow walking is replaced by intervals of walking and jogging that eventually lead to continuous jogging. Allow at least 6 to 8 weeks for observable changes to occur. Behavioral approaches should also be applied to cause meaningful lifestyle changes that will increase physical activity. For example, walking or bicycling can replace use of the auto, stair climbing can replace the elevator, and manual tools can replace power tools.

Table 17-2 shows the effectiveness of regular exercise for weight loss. In this study, 6 sedentary, obese young men exercised 5 days a week for 16 weeks by walking for 90 minutes at each session. The men lost nearly 6 kg of body fat; this represented a decrease in body fat from 23.5 to 18.6%. In addition, physical fitness and work capacity improved, as did the level of high-density lipoprotein (15.6%) and the high- to low-density lipoprotein ratio (25.9%).

Regularity Is the Key. It appears that at least 3 days of training per week is required to bring about favorable body

TABLE 17-2. Effectiveness of regular exercise for eliciting changes in body composition and blood lipids in six obese young adult men with a sixteen-week walking program[a]

Variable	Pre-Training[b]	Post-Training	Difference
Body mass, kg	99.1	93.4	- 5.7[c]
Body density, g · ml⁻¹	1.044	1.056	+ 0.012[c]
Body fat, %	23.5	18.6	- 4.9[c]
Fat mass, kg	23.3	17.4	- 5.9[c]
Lean body mass, kg	75.8	76.0	+ 0.2
Sum of fatfolds, mm	142.9	104.8	- 38.1[c]
HDL cholesterol, mg · 100 ml⁻¹	32	37	+ 5.0[c]
HDL/LDL cholesterol	0.27	0.34	+ 0.07[c]

[a] From Leon, A.S., et al.: Effects of a vigorous walking program on body composition, and carbohydrate and lipid metabolism of obese young men. *Amer. J. Clin. Nutr.*, 33:1776, 1979.
[b] Values are means.
[c] Statistically significant.

weight changes through exercise. More frequent exercise is even more effective. This frequency effect is most likely the direct result of the added calories burned by the extra exercise. Although it is difficult to precisely determine a threshold energy expenditure for weight and fat loss, the calorie-burning effect of each exercise session should be at least 300 kcal. This can be achieved with 30 minutes of moderate to vigorous running, swimming, or bicycling, or less intense walking for at least 60 minutes.

DIET PLUS EXERCISE

Combinations of exercise and diet offer considerably more *flexibility* for achieving a negative caloric balance than either exercise alone or diet alone. Research indicates that adding regular exercise to the program of weight control facilitates a more permanent fat loss than does total reliance on caloric restriction.

If weight reduction is attempted only by reducing food intake, then one must consider how many calories to consume. While there are no hard and fast rules, considerable experimental and clinical data show that adverse psychological changes can occur if caloric intake is reduced too severely over an extended period. In addition, prolonged dieting increases the chances of developing a variety of nutritional deficiencies. A prudent alternative is to blend diet with exercise. Certainly it is easier to create a daily caloric deficit of 1000 kcal by combining diet and exercise than using either one alone.

Most nutrition experts agree that a loss in body fat of up to 0.9 kg (2 lb) each week is within acceptable limits, although a steady 0.5 to 1.0 lb a week loss may be even more desirable. This guideline for an acceptable limit of weight loss is partially based on the observation that people who have been successful losing weight lost no more than about 0.9 kg a week during the period of caloric deficit.

Setting a Target Time

Suppose the target time selected to achieve a 9 kg (20 lb) fat loss is 20 weeks. The average weekly deficit must therefore be 3500 kcal; the daily caloric deficit is then 500 kcal (3500 ÷ 7). To achieve this deficit by dieting, daily caloric intake must be reduced by 500 kcal. Remember, this level of caloric restriction needs to be maintained for 5 months to achieve the desired fat loss of 0.45 kg per week or 9 kg total. However, if the dieter performed a half hour of moderate exercise equivalent to 350 "extra" kcal 3 days a week, then the weekly caloric output would increase by 1050 kcal (3 days per week x 350 kcal per exercise session). With this additional exercise, the caloric restriction necessary to lose 0.45 kg of fat each week would now only have to reach 2450 kcal instead of 3500. The additional 1050 kcal is "burned" during the weekly exercise. Instead of excluding 500 kcal from the daily diet, the caloric intake need only be reduced by 350 kcal, because the daily contribution of exercise averages 150 kcal (1050 kcal per week ÷ 7). If the same exercise were undertaken 5 days a week, the daily food intake could be increased an additional 100 calories and the 0.45 kg per week fat loss would still be attained. If the duration of the 5 day per week workouts was extended from 30 minutes to 1 hour, then no reduction in food intake would be necessary to lose weight, because the required 3500 kcal deficit would be created entirely through extra physical activity.

If the intensity of the 1-hour exercise performed 5 days a week was then increased by only 10% (cycling at 22 instead of 20 miles per hour, running a mile in 9 instead of 10 minutes, swimming each 50 yards in 54 seconds instead of 60 seconds), the number of exercise calories burned each week would increase an additional 350 kcal (3500 kcal/wk x 10%). This new weekly deficit of 3850 kcal, or 550 kcal per day, would actually per-

Exercise keeps muscle and burns fat. Exercise provides protein-sparing effect that causes a greater portion of the caloric deficit to be made up from the breakdown of body fat.

The heart may also suffer. With extremes of dieting, there is the distinct possibility that lean tissue loss may occur disproportionately from critical organs such as the heart.

Good news for exercisers. When exercise is part of a weight loss program, either alone or in combination with dieting, a smaller reduction in resting metabolism occurs than when weight loss relies solely on dieting. This makes it easier for people who exercise to take weight off and keep it off.

Some fat is more easily removed. Fat stores on the central trunk region may be more responsive to exercise training than fat in the extremities.

mit the dieter to increase daily food intake by 50 calories and still lose a pound of fat each week!

Clearly, physical activity can be used effectively by itself or in combination with mild dietary restriction to trigger weight loss. Perhaps equally important, the feelings of intense hunger and other psychological stress may be minimal compared with a similar weight loss program that relies exclusively on food restriction. Furthermore, exercise protects against the usual lean tissue loss when weight reduction is achieved by diet alone. Lean tissue is preserved because regular exercise enhances the breakdown of fat from the body's adipose depots. In addition, exercise increases protein buildup in skeletal muscle, while at the same time retarding its rate of breakdown.

Summary of Results on Caloric Imbalance

The results of research that has evaluated various approaches to establish a caloric imbalance can be summarized as follows:

- Exercise combined with dietary restriction is a more effective approach for achieving a long-term negative caloric balance as compared with exercise or diet alone.

- During the first few days of weight reduction, the rapid weight loss is due primarily to loss in body water and carbohydrate; longer periods of weight reduction are associated with a substantially greater loss of fat per unit of weight loss.

- Water intake should not be restricted when beginning weight reduction because this can precipitate dehydration with no additional fat loss.

- Undesirable psychological and medically related problems may occur with prolonged caloric restriction maintained below minimal energy requirements.

- Weight loss by diet alone causes significant loss of muscle mass. Exercise protects against lean tissue losses; thus, more of the weight lost is fat.

Spot Reduction: Does It Work?

The underlying basis for the notion of spot reduction is that an increase in a muscle's activity facilitates relatively greater fat mobilization from the fat storage areas in proximity to the muscle. Therefore, by localized exercise of a specific body area, more fat will be selectively reduced from that area than if exercise of the same caloric intensity is performed by a different muscle group. For example, advocates of spot reduction would recommend large numbers of sit-ups or side bends for a person with excessive abdominal fat. Whereas the promise of spot reduction with exercise is attractive from an aesthetic and health risk standpoint, a critical evaluation of the research does not support this notion.

To examine the claims for spot reduction critically, comparisons were made of the girths and subcutaneous fat stores of the right and left forearms of high-caliber tennis players. As expected, the dominant or playing arm was significantly larger than the nondominant arm because of the modest muscular hypertrophy associated with the exercise overload provided by tennis. Measurements of fat-fold thickness, however, showed no difference in the quantity of subcutaneous fat in the two forearms. Clearly, prolonged exercise was not accompanied by reduced fat deposits in the playing arm.

There is no doubt that the negative caloric balance created through regular exercise can significantly contribute to a reduction in total body fat. This fat, however, is not reduced selectively from the exercised areas but rather from total body fat reserves, and usually from the areas of greatest fat concentration.

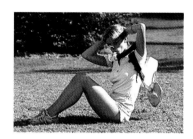

Spot reduction doesn't work. Exercise stimulates mobilization of fat through hormones that act on fat depots throughout the body. Areas of greatest fat concentration or enzyme activity likely supply the greatest amount of this energy. No evidence shows that fatty acids are released more from fat pads directly over the exercising muscle.

GAINING WEIGHT

Gaining weight for athletes poses a unique problem that is not easily resolved. Weight gain per se is a relatively easy and often enjoyable task brought about by unbalancing the body's energy balance in favor of a greater caloric intake. For a sedentary person, an excess intake of 3500 kcal results in a weight gain of about 0.5 kg. This is because the excess calories are stored as body fat. Weight gain for athletes, however, should be in the form of lean tissue, specifically muscle mass. It is generally agreed that this form of weight gain can only be accomplished if an increased caloric intake is accompanied by an appropriate exercise program.

Heavy muscular overload (resistance training) supported by prudent diet can effectively increase muscle mass and strength. If all the "extra" calories consumed in the diet were used for muscle growth during resistance training, then 2000 to 2500 extra kcal from a well-balanced diet are required for each 0.5 kg increase in lean tissue. In a practical sense, 700 to 1000 kcal added to the daily diet will supply the nutrients to support a weekly 0.5- to 1.0-kg gain in lean tissue as well as the energy requirements of the training. This ideal situation presupposes that all extra calories beyond the daily requirement are used to synthesize lean tissue. Variation from this ideal depends on many factors including the type, intensity, and frequency of training as well as the hormonal and muscle fiber characteristics of the athlete. Athletes with a relatively high androgen- to- estrogen ratio and a greater percentage of fast-twitch muscle fibers show the greatest increases in lean tissue with resistance training.

Monitor both body weight and body fat. One means to verify whether the combination of training and increased food intake is increasing lean tissue (and not body fat) is to regularly monitor both body weight and body fat. This can be accomplished in the laboratory with hydrostatic weighing or in the field through appropriate anthropometric and fatfold measurements.

S U M M A R Y

1. Long-term maintenance of weight loss through dietary restriction generally is unsuccessful for most participants in such programs.
2. There are three ways to unbalance the energy balance equation and bring about weight loss: reduce caloric intake below daily energy expenditure, maintain regular food intake and increase energy output, and combine both methods by decreasing food intake and increasing energy expenditure.
3. A caloric deficit of 3500 kcal created through either diet or exercise is the equivalent to the calories in 1 lb (0.45 kg) of adipose tissue.
4. Dieting for weight loss can be effective if done properly. The disadvantages of semistarvation, however, are significant including loss of lean body tissue, lethargy, possible malnutrition and metabolic disorders, and a decrease in the basal energy expenditure. Some factors actually conserve energy and cause the diet to be less effective.
5. Repeated cycles of weight loss and weight gain cause the body to increase its ability to conserve energy. This ultimately leads to greater difficulty in achieving weight loss with subsequent dieting, and makes regaining the lost weight easier.
6. The calorie-expending effects of exercise are cumulative, so that a little exercise performed routinely has a dramatic effect over time. The role of exercise in appetite suppression or stimulation is unclear. Over time, most athletes eventually consume enough calories to counterbalance caloric expenditure—but many of these athletes are the leanest in the world.
7. Exercise and diet offer a flexible and effective approach to weight control. Exercise enhances the mobilization and use of lipids, thus increasing the loss of fat, and retards lean tissue loss.
8. Rapid weight loss during the first few days of caloric deficit is caused by loss in body water and carbohydrate. Continued weight reduction is associated with a greater loss of fat per unit of weight loss.
9. Selective reduction of fat at specific body areas by "spot exercise" does not work.

American College of Sports Medicine: Position statement on proper and improper weight loss programs. *Med. Sci. Sports Med.*, 15(1):ix, 1983.

Atkinson, R. L., and Pi-Sunyer, F. X.: Very-low-calorie diets. *Am. J. Clin. Nutr.*, 56:175S, 1992.

Bahr, R., et al.: Effect of supramaximal exercise on excess postexercise O_2 consumption. *Med. Sci. Sport Exerc.*, 24:66, 1992.

Ballor, D. L., et al.: Resistance weight training during caloric restriction enhances lean body weight maintenance. *Am. J. Clin. Nutr.*, 47:19, 1988.

Ballor, D. L., and Keesey, R. E.: A meta-analysis of the factors affecting exercise-induced changes in body mass, fat mass and fat-free mass in males and females. *Int. J. Obesity*, 15:717, 1991.

Ballor, D. L., and Poehlman, E. T.: Exercise training enhances fat-free mass preservation during diet-induced weight loss: a meta-analytical finding. *Int. J. Obes.*, 18: 35, 1994.

Björntorp, P.: Adipose tissue distribution and function. *Int. J. Obesity*. 15:67, 1991.

Blackburn, G. L., et al.: Weight cycling: the experience of human dieters. *Am. J. Clin. Nutr.*, 49:1105, 1989.

Bouchard, C., et al.: The response to long term feeding in identical twins. *N. Engl. J. Med.*, 322: 1477, 1990.

Bouchard, C.: Genes and body fat. *Am. J. Hum. Biol.*, 5:425, 1993.

Brownell, K. D., et al. (Eds).: *Eating, Body Weight and Performance in Athletes.* Philadelphia, Lea & Fegiber, 1992.

Brownell, K. D., et al.: Weight regulation practices in athletes: analysis of metabolic and health effects. *Med. Sci. Sports Exerc.*, 19:546, 1987.

Campaigne, B. N.: Body fat distribution: metabolic consequences and implications for weight loss. *Med Sci. Sports Exerc.*, 22:291, 1990.

Colditz, G. A.: Economic costs of obesity. *Am. J. Clin. Nutr.*, 55: 503S, 1992.

Després, J-P.: Physical activity and adipose tissue. In *Physical Activity, Fitness, and Health.* Edited by Bouchard, C., et al., Champaign, IL, Human Kinetics, 1994.

Donnelly, J. E., et al.: Effects of a very-low-calorie diet and physical-training regimens on body composition and resting metabolic rate in obese females. *Am. J. Clin. Nutr.*, 54: 56, 1991.

Drenick, E. J., and Johnson, D.: Therapeutic fasting in morbid obesity — long term follow-up. *Arch. Int. Med.*, 137:1381, 1977.

Dullo, A. G., and Girardier, L.: Adaptive changes in energy expenditure during refeeding following low-calorie intake: evidence for a specific metabolic component favoring fat storage. *Am. J. Clin. Nutr.*, 52:415, 1990.

Elliot, D. L., et al.: Sustained depression of the resting metabolic rate after massive weight loss. *Am. J. Clin. Nutr.*, 49:93, 1989.

Emery, E. M., et al.: A review of the association between abdominal fat distribution, health outcome measures, and modifiable risk factors. *Am. J. Health Promotion*, 7: 342, 1993.

Folsom, R., et al.: Body fat distribution and 5-year risk of death in older women. *JAMA*, 269: 483, 1993.

Frank, A., et al.: Fatalities on the liquid-protein diet: an analysis of possible causes. *Int. J. Obesity*. 5:243, 1981.

French, S. A., et al.: Predictors of weight change over two years among a population of working adults: the Healthy Worker Project. *Int. J. Obes.*, 18: 145, 1994.

Gartmaker, S. L., et al.: Increasing pediatric obesity in the United States. *Am. J. Dis. Child.*, 141:535, 1987.

Herring, J. L., et al.: Effect of suspending exercise training on resting metabolic rate in women. *Med. Sci. Sports Exerc.*, 24:59, 1992.

Hill, J. O., et al.: Exercise and moderate obesity. In *Physical Activity, Fitness, and Health.* Edited by C. Bouchard, et al., Champaign, IL, Human Kinetics, 1994.

Hill, J. O., et al.: Effects of exercise and food restriction on body composition and metabolic rates in obese women. *Am. J. Clin. Nutr.*, 46:622, 1987.

Horswill, C. R.: Weight loss and weight cycling in amateur wrestlers: implications for performance and resting metabolic rate. *Int. J. Sport Nutr.*, 3:245, 1993.

Jeffrey, R., et al.: Weight cycling and cardiovascular risk factors in obese men and women. *Am. J. Clin. Nutr.*, 55:641, 1992.

Johnson, M. L., et al.: Relative importance of inactivity and overeating in energy balance in obese high school girls. *Am. J. Clin. Nutr.*, 44:779, 1986.

Kern, P. A., et al.: The effects of weight loss on the activity and expression of adipose-tissue lipoprotein lipase in very obese humans. *N. Engl. J. Med.*, 322:1053, 1990.

Kessey, R. E.: A set-point theory of obesity. In *Handbook of Eating Disorders.* Edited by K. D. Brownell and J. P. Foreyt. New York, Basic Books, 1986.

Keys, A., et al.: *The Biology of Human Starvation.* Minneapolis, University of Minnesota Press, 1970.

King, M. A., and Katch, F. I.: Changes in body density, fatfolds, and girths at 2.3 kg increments of weight loss. *Hum. Biol.*, 58:709, 1986.

Kissileff, H. R., et al.: Acute effects of exercise on food intake in obese and nonobese women. *Am. J. Clin. Nutr.*, 52:240, 1990.

Kuczmarski, R. J., et al.: Increasing prevalence of overweight among US adults. *JAMA*, 272: 205, 1994.

Kuczmarski, R. J.: Prevalence of overweight and weight gain in the United States. *Am. J. Clin. Nutr.*, 55: 495S, 1992.

Lee, I-M., et al.: Body weight and mortality. *JAMA*, 270: 2823, 1993.

Leibel, R., and Hirsch, J.: Metabolic characterization of obesity. *Ann. Intern. Med.*, 103:1000, 1985.

Lissner, L., et al.: Variability of body weight and health outcomes in the Framingham population. *N. Engl. J. Med.*, 324:1839, 1991.

Manore, M. M., et al.: Energy expenditure at rest and during exercise in nonobese female cyclical dieters and in nondieting control subjects. *Am. J. Clin. Nutr.*, 54:41, 1991.

Manson, J. E., et al.: A prospective study of obesity and risk of coronary heart disease in women. *N. Engl. J. Med.*, 322:822, 1990.

McArdle, W. D., and Toner, M. M.: Application of exercise for weight control: the exercise prescription. In *Eating Disorders Handbook: Complete Guide to Understanding and Treatment.* Edited by R. Frankle and M.-U. Yang. Rockville, MD, Aspen Publishers, 1988.

Meredith, C. N., et al.: Body composition and aerobic capacity in young and middle aged endurance-trained men. *Med. Sci. Sports Exerc.*, 19:557, 1987.

Miller, W. C., et al.: Predicting max HR and HR-V0$_2$ relationship for exercise prescription in obesity. *Med. Sci. Sports Exerc.*, 25: 1077, 1993.

Molé , P., et al.: Exercise versus depressed metabolic rate produced by severe caloric restriction. *Med. Sci. Sports Exerc.*, 21:29, 1989.

Must, V., et al.: Long-term morbidity and mortality of overweight adolescents. *N. Engl. J. Med.*, 327: 1350, 1992.

National Institutes of Health Consensus Development Conference Statement: *Health implications of obesity*. Vol. 5, No. 9. Washington, DC, US Government Printing Office, 1985.

National Task Force on the Prevention and Treatment of Obesity: Weight cycling. *JAMA*, 272: 1196, 1994.

Ostlund, R. E., et al.: The ratio of waist-to-hip circumference, plasma insulin level, and glucose intolerance as independent predictors of the HDL2 cholesterol level in older adults. *N. Engl. J. Med.*, 332:229, 1990.

Pavlou, K. N., et al.: Exercise as an adjunct to weight loss and maintenance in moderately obese subjects. *Am. J. Clin. Nutr.*, 49:1115, 1989.

Phinney, S. D.: Exercise during and after very-low-calorie dieting. *Am. J. Clin. Nutr.*, 56:190S, 1992.

Pi-Sunyer, F. X.: Medical hazards of obesity. *Ann. Intern. Med.*, 119: 655, 1993.

Poehlman, E. T., et al.: The impact of exercise and diet restriction on daily energy expenditure. *Sports Med.*, 11: 78, 1991.

Prentice, A. M., et al.: Effects of weight cycling on body composition. *Am. J. Clin. Nutr.*, 56:209S, 1992.

Ravussin, E., et al.: Reduced rate of energy expenditure as a risk factor for body-weight gain. *N. Engl. J. Med.*, 318:467, 1988.

Roberts, S. B., et al.: Energy expenditure and intake in infants born to lean and overweight mothers. *N. Engl. J. Med.*, 318:461, 1988.

Rodin, J., et al.: Weight cycling and fat distribution. *Int. J. Obesity*, 14:303, 1990.

Schelkun, P. H.: Treating overweight patients: don't weigh success in pounds. *Phys. Sportsmed.*, 21(2):148, 1993.

Scott, J. R. et al.: Acute weight gain in collegiate wrestlers following a tournament weigh-in. *Med. Sci. Sports Exerc.* 26(9): 1181, 1994.

Segal, K. R., et al.: Body composition, not body weight, is related to cardiovascular disease risk factors and sex hormone levels in man. *J. Clin. Invest.*, 80:1050, 1987.

Segal, K. R., et al.: Thermic effects of food and exercise in lean and obese men of similar lean body mass. *Am. J. Physiol.*, 252:E110, 1987.

Staten, M. A.: The effect of exercise on food intake in men and women. *Am. J. Clin. Nutr.*, 53:27, 1991.

Stefanik, M. L.: Exercise and weight control. In *Exercise and Sport Sciences Reviews*. Vol. 21. Edited by J. O. Holloszy. Baltimore, MD, Williams & Wilkins, 1993.

Stefanick, M. L.: Exercise and weight control. *Exerc. Sport Sci. Rev.*, 21: 363, 1993.

Sweeney, M. E., et al.: Severe versus moderate energy restriction with and without exercise in the treatment of obesity. Am. J. Clin. Nutr., 5:491, 1993.

Thorland, W. G., et al.: Estimation of body composition in black adolescent male athletes. *Pediatric Exer. Sci.*, 5: 116, 1993.

Thornton, J. S.: Feast or famine: eating disorders in athletes. *Phys. Sportsmed.*, 18:116, 1990.

Tipton, C. M., and Oppliger, R. A. Nutritional and fitness considerations for competitive wrestlers. In: Simopoulos, A. P., and Pavlou, K. N. (eds). *Nutrition and Fitness for Athletes. World Rev. Nutr. Diet.* Karger, Basal. 71: 84, 1993.

Trembly, A., et al.: Exercise training with constant energy intake. 2: Effect on glucose metabolism and resting energy expenditure. Int. J. Obesity, 14:75, 1990.

Troisi, R. J., et al.: Cigarette smoking, dietary intake, and physical activity: effects on body fat distribution - The Normative Aging Study. *Am. J. Clin. Nutr.*, 53:1104, 1991.

Van Dale, D., et al.: Weight maintenance and resting metabolic rate 18-40 months after a diet/exercise treatment. *Int. J. Obesity*, 14:347, 1990.

Wadden, T. A., et al.: Long-term effects of dieting on resting metabolic rate in obese outpatients. *JAMA*, 264:707, 1990.

Wallace, J. P., et al.: Variation in the anthropometric dimensions for estimating upper and lower body obesity. *Am. J. Hum. Biol.* 6: 699, 1994.

Willet, W. C., et al.: Weight, weight change, and coronary heart disease in women: risk within the "normal" weight range. *JAMA*. 273: 461, 1995.

Willett, W. C., et al.: New weight guidelines for Americans: justified or injudicious? (editorial). *Am. J. Clin. Nutr.*, 53:1102, 1991.

Williams, D. P., et al.: Body fatness and risk for elevated blood pressure, total cholesterol, and serum lipoprotein ratios in children and adolescents. *Am. J. Public Health*, 82: 358, 1992.

Young, J. C., et al.: Prior exercise potentiates the thermic effect of a carbohydrate load. *Metabolism*, 35:1048, 1986.

Zang, Y., et al.: Positional cloning of the mouse *obese* gene and its human homologue. *Nature*, 372: 425, 1994.

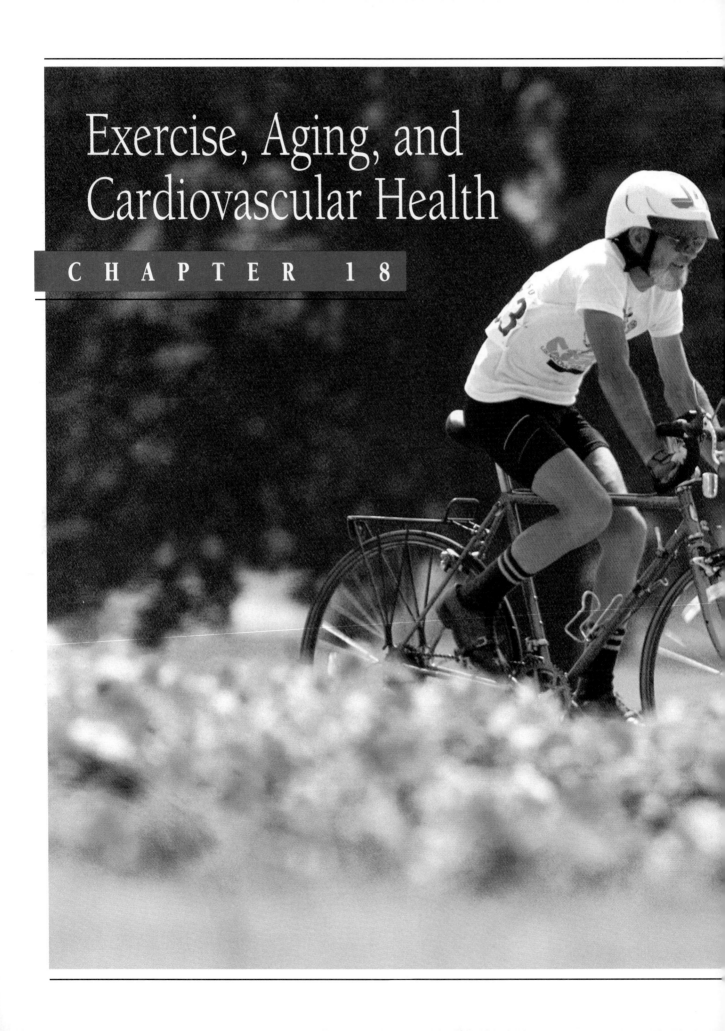

Exercise, Aging, and Cardiovascular Health

After reading this chapter you should be able to:

- Describe the level of regular physical activity of the average American man and woman.

- Respond to the question: "Is exercising safe?"

- Compare the major differences in physiologic response to exercise between children and adults.

- Discuss age-related changes in the following physiologic components: (a) muscular strength, (b) joint flexibility, (c) nervous system function, (d) pulmonary function, and (e) body composition.

- Discuss the following statement: "There is an impressive plasticity in physiologic and performance characteristics, and a marked training response can be obtained at least into the eighth decade of life."

- Describe research that shows that regular physical activity enhances the quality of life and may even contribute to a longer life.

- Discuss the age-related progression of heart disease risk for women.

- List the major risk factors for coronary heart disease. How is each factor affected by regular exercise?

- List the factors that affect the level of blood cholesterol.

- Discuss the ways that physical activity can reduce the risk of coronary heart disease.

- List important reasons why stress testing should be included in an overall evaluation for coronary heart disease.

- Outline a classification system for screening and supervisory procedures for exercise stress testing.

- Discuss objective indicators of coronary heart disease during an exercise stress test.

- Define the following terms for stress test results: true-positive, false-negative, true-negative, and false-positive.

- List the reasons for stopping a stress test.

- Outline an approach for individualizing an "exercise prescription".

Aside from the positive effects of exercise in maintaining physiologic function, it is clear that regular physical activity protects against the ravages of this nation's greatest killer, coronary heart disease (CHD). Individuals in physically active occupations have a two- to threefold lower risk of heart attack than those in sedentary jobs. Furthermore, the chances of surviving a heart attack are much greater for those with a physically demanding job or lifestyle. Regular physical activity can also favorably modify some of the important CHD risk factors. Elevated blood pressure can be lowered by regular aerobic exercise; similarly, body mass, body fat, and blood lipids are lowered with prudent exercise and diet. The blood clotting mechanism can be normalized with exercise training; this would reduce the chances of a blood clot forming on the roughened surface of a coronary artery. Research with animals has demonstrated an improved blood supply to the myocardium as a result of regular exercise. If this adaptation in coronary circulation takes place in humans, then regular exercise may retard the heart disease process, or at least maintain adequate blood supply to the heart muscle to compensate for the channels already narrowed by fatty deposits on their vascular walls.

From a practical standpoint, an active lifestyle is often effective in blunting the cumulative effects of the highly atherogenic American diet and accompanying life of inactivity and stress. Regardless of genetics, age, and life circumstances, individuals can significantly enhance their chances for a healthy life by adapting sound habits that include regular exercise.

PARTICIPATION IN PHYSICAL ACTIVITY

The current status of exercise participation for American adults is not encouraging, as the "exercise boom" appears to be leveling off. According to data from the U.S. National Center for Health Statistics on the physical activity of non-institutionalized adults aged 18 years and older, only 8% of men and 7% of women reported that they engaged in regular *vigorous* exercise. Regular but less intense activity was done by 36% of the men and 32% of the women, indicating that only about 44% of males and 39% of females engage in some regular physical activity. Furthermore, available data indicate that generally about half of those who start exercising give it up within the first 6 months.

Figure 18-1 illustrates the findings for exercise participation from a large-scale study of over 15,000 adults enrolled in exercise programs that included aerobic and muscle-strengthening activities.

With increasing age there was a progressive decline in participation in fitness activities, with the smallest percentage of participation noted for the oldest group. Sadly, these are the men and women who might benefit

The graying of America. The elderly represent the fastest growing segment of the American population with the average life expectancy for men and women rapidly approaching 80 years. By the year 2020, 18% of the population will be over age 65!

Inactivity is a disease. Considered alone, sedentary living probably is to blame for as many as 200,000 preventable cardiovascular deaths in the United States each year. Nearly 60% of adults have reported little or no leisure-time activity. "Risk factors" other than age for inactivity include being female, African-American, poorly educated, overweight, or having a history of a sedentary lifestyle.

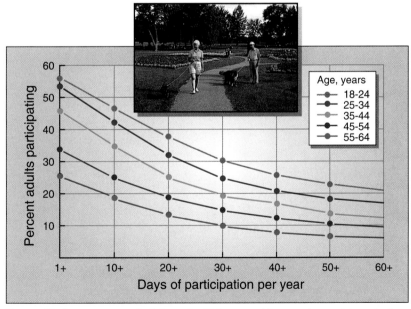

Figure 18–1. Percentage of adults in the U.S. grouped by age who participate in fitness activities. (Courtesy of C. Brooks, Department of Sports Management and Communication, University of Michigan, Ann Arbor, MI)

the most from regular exercise. In fact, an alarmingly large number of older citizens have such poor functional capacity that they cannot do relatively simple physical tasks without assistance.

Is Exercising Safe?

Many people have raised the question of the safety of exercise largely because of several well-publicized reports of sudden death during exercise. In actuality, sudden death rates during exercise have *declined* over the past 20 years even though there has been an overall *increase* in exercise participation. In one report of cardiovascular episodes during a little more than 5 years, 2935 exercisers recorded 374,798 hours of exercise that included 2,726,272 km (1.7 million miles) of running and walking. There were *no deaths* during this time and only 2 nonfatal cardiovascular complications. By gender, there were 3 complications per 100,000 hours of exercise for men and 2 for women. Certainly, there is a small increased risk of a cardiovascular

episode during exercise compared to resting. *However, the total reduction in heart disease risk to be derived from engaging in regular physical activity (compared to leading a sedentary life) far outweighs any slight increase in risk during the actual activity period.*

Perhaps not surprisingly, the most prevalent exercise complications are musculoskeletal in nature. In a study of aerobic dance injuries for 351 participants and 60 instructors at six dance facilities, 327 medical complaints were reported during nearly 30,000 hours of activity. Only 84 of the injuries resulted in disability (2.8 per 1000 person-hours of participation), and just 2.1% of the injuries required medical attention. For jogging and running activities, the orthopedic injury potential is greatest among those who exercise for extended periods of time. In this sense, more is certainly not better!

Aging and Bodily Function

Figure 18-2 shows that the various measures of bodily function generally improve rapidly during childhood to reach a maximum between age 20 and 30 years; thereafter, there is a gradual decline in functional capacity with advancing years. While the trend with age is generally similar for the physically active, physiologic function is about 25% *higher* for each age category, so that an active 50-year-old man or woman often maintains the functional level of a 20-year-old. Although all measures eventually decline with age, not all do so at the same rate and there is considerable variation from person to person and from system to system within the same person.

Nerve conduction velocity, for example, declines only 10 to 15% from 30 to 80 years of age, whereas resting cardiac index (ratio of cardiac output to surface area) and joint flexibility decline 20 to 30%; maximum breathing capacity at age 80 is about 40% that of a 30-year-old. Brain cells die at a constant rate until age 60, while the liver and kidneys lose about

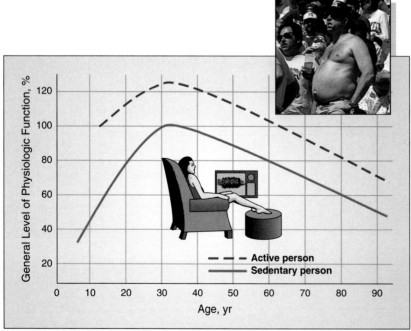

Figure 18–2. Generalized curve to illustrate changes in physiologic function with age. All of the comparisons are made against the 100% value achieved by the 20-to-30-year-old sedentary person.

40 to 50% of their function between ages 30 and 70, and the average female has lost 30% of her bone mass, while men at this age have lost only about 15%.

Some Differences in Exercise Physiology Between Children and Adults.

- During weight bearing exercise like walking and running, the oxygen uptake of children (ml·kg^{-1} min^{-1}) is 10 to 30% higher than adults at a designated submaximal pace. This lower economy, perhaps due to the shorter stride length and greater stride frequency of children, makes a standard walking or running pace physiologically more stressful (and their performance scores poorer) for children than adults, even though on average children have equal or somewhat higher aerobic capacities than adults.
- Because of their smaller body size, children have lower absolute values (L · min^{-1}) for aerobic capacity than larger-sized adults. Thus, when exercising against a standard external resistance that is independent of body size (e.g., stationary cycling, arm cranking) children will be disadvantaged. This is because the fixed oxygen cost (L · min^{-1}) of the exercise represents a greater percentage of the child's smaller capacity. In weight bearing exercise, such as walking, the energy cost is directly related to body weight so children are not disadvantaged by their smaller body size.
- Children do less well than adults on sprint tests of anaerobic power. This is perhaps due to their inability to generate a high level of blood lactate (a marker for the glycolytic process) during exhaustive exercise. Also, their significantly lower levels of the glycolytic enzyme phosphofructokinase compared to adults

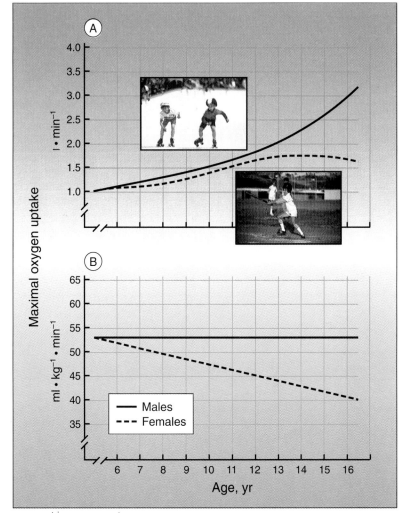

A. Max $\dot{V}O_2$ (L · min^{-1}) for boys and girls is similar to about age 12; at age 14 the boys are about 25% higher and by age 16 the difference exceeds 50%. This difference is generally attributed to the development of a greater muscle mass in boys as well as gender differences in daily physical activity. B. For boys, max $\dot{V}O_2$ (ml · kg^{-1} · min^{-1}) remains level at about 52 ml · kg^{-1} · min^{-1}) from age 6 to 16; for females, the line slopes downward with age reaching about 40 ml · kg^{-1} · min^{-1} at age 16, a value that is 32% below their male counterparts. This difference is probably due to the greater accumulation of body fat in females; this extra fat must be transported but does not contribute to an enhanced capacity for aerobic metabolism. (From: Krahenbuhl, G. S., et al.: Developmental aspects of maximal aerobic power in children. In *Exercise and Sport Sciences Reviews.* Vol. 13, Edited by R. L. Terjung. Macmillan, New York, 1985.)

may explain their poor anaerobic capacity.
- During submaximal exercise children tend to breathe more (greater ventilatory equivalent) than adults at any level of oxygen uptake.
- Children, like adults, can adapt and significantly increase muscular strength in response to

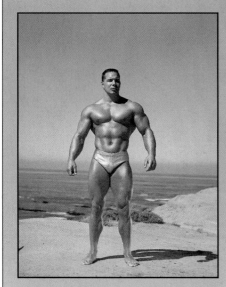

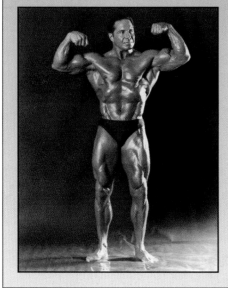

Fifty-one consecutive years of resistance training! Bill Pearl, currently age 63, is one of the greatest body building champions of all time. Holder of four Mr. Universe titles (1956, 1961, 1967, 1971), he still trains about 2.5 hours daily (beginning at 4:30 AM). *Top.* 1967 Mr. Universe, age 37. *Bottom.* Last formal pose at age 59. Photo courtesy of Bill Pearl.

resistance training. Unlike pubescent children and adults, however, prepubescent children have greater difficulty increasing skeletal mass. This may be due partly to the relatively low androgen levels in this age group.

Muscular Strength

Maximum strength of men and women is generally achieved between 20 and 30 years of age, when muscular cross-sectional area is usually the largest. Thereafter, strength progressively declines for most muscle groups so that by age 70 there is 30% less overall strength.

Decrease in Muscle Mass. Reduced muscle mass is a primary factor responsible for the age-associated strength decrease. This reflects loss of total muscle protein brought about by inactivity, aging, or both. There is also probably some loss in the number of muscle fibers with aging. For example, the biceps muscle of a newborn contains about 500,000 individual fibers while the same muscle for a man in his 80s has about 300,000 fibers.

Muscle Trainability Among the Elderly. Regular physical training facilitates protein retention and delays the decrement in lean body mass and muscular strength with aging. Healthy men between the ages of 60 and 72 years were trained for 12 weeks with a standard resistance training program similar to that outlined in Chapter 13. As shown in Figure 18-3, muscle strength increased progressively throughout the training to average about 5% per training session — a training response similar to that noted for young adults. In addition, these dramatic strength improvements were accompanied by significant muscular

hypertrophy. Such improvement in muscular strength by resistance training may be the best way to prevent or reduce the incidence of injury with older individuals.

Flexibility

With advancing age, connective tissue (cartilage, ligaments, and tendons) becomes stiffer and more rigid, which reduces joint flexibility. What is uncertain is whether these changes are the result of biologic aging per se or rather the impact of sedentary living or degenerative disease on the tissues that make up a specific joint. What is clear, however, is that appropriate exercises that move joints through their full range of motion can increase flexibility by as much as 20 to 50% in men and women at all ages.

Nervous System Function

The cumulative effects of aging on central nervous system function are exhibited by a 37% decline in the number of spinal cord axons, and a 10% decline in nerve conduction velocity. Such changes partially explain the age-related decrements in neuromuscular performance. When reaction time is partitioned into central processing time and muscle contraction time, it is processing time that is most affected by the aging process. This suggests that aging mainly affects the ability to detect a stimulus and process the information to produce a response. Since reflexes such as the knee jerk reflex do not involve processing in the brain, they are less affected than voluntary responses by the aging process. *While aging has a definite effect on the nervous system in terms of reaction and movement time, physically active groups (be they young or old) move significantly faster than a corresponding age group that is less active. It is tempting to speculate that the biologic aging of certain neuromuscular functions can be somewhat retarded by regular participation in physical activity.*

Pulmonary Function

Measures of lung function generally deteriorate with age. How regular exercise throughout one's lifetime can override this "aging" of the pulmonary system is unknown, but older endurance-trained athletes do have greater dynamic pulmonary capacity than sedentary peers. Such findings are encouraging because they indicate that regular physical activity may retard the decline in pulmonary function associated with aging.

Cardiovascular Function

Maximal oxygen uptake and endurance performance decline steadily after age 20, and aerobic fitness has decreased by about 35% at age 65. For both active and sedentary people, the decline in aerobic capacity is influenced by age-related decrements in central and peripheral functions linked to oxygen transport and utilization. One clear change is the progressive decline in maximum heart rate with age. A rough approximation of this decline is expressed by the relationship:

$$\text{Max HR (beats} \cdot \text{min}^{-1}\text{)} = 220 - \text{age (years)}$$

Also contributing to diminished blood flow capacity with age is a reduction in the heart's stroke volume that may reflect changes in myocardial contractility. Other age-related cardiovascular changes include reduction in blood flow capacity to peripheral tissues, narrowing of the arteries that supply blood to the heart (by middle age the coronary arteries are about 30% obstructed), and a decrease in the elasticity of major blood vessels.

The Aerobic System Is Responsive to Training at Any Age. Research indicates a high degree of trainability among older men and women, with adaptations similar to those in

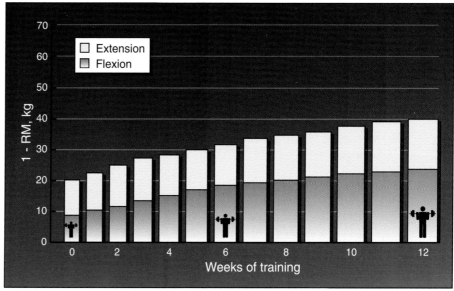

Figure 18–3. Weekly measurement of dynamic muscle strength (1-RM) of left knee extension (yellow) and flexion (red). (From Frontera, W.R., et al.: Strength conditioning in older men: skeletal muscle hypertrophy and improved function. *J. Appl. Physiol.*, 64:1038, 1988.)

younger individuals. Both low- and high-intensity regular exercise enables older individuals to retain a level of cardiovascular function much above that of age-paired sedentary subjects. In fact, when middle-aged men trained regularly over a 10-year period, the usual 10 to 15% decline in exercise capacity and aerobic fitness was forestalled. At age 55, these active men had maintained the same values for blood pressure, body mass, and max $\dot{V}O_2$ as at age 45.

Endurance Performance. The dramatic effects of exercise training on the preservation of cardiovascular function throughout life can be observed by comparing the performance times on endurance events for individuals of different ages. Figure 18-4 shows the age-group, world-record marathon times for males and females starting at about age 4 and into the eighth decade of life. The world record of 2 hr 7 min 11 sec by Carlos Lopes (age 37) of Portugal (recorded in April 1985) corresponds

Not much difference. If the training stimulus is adequate, the skeletal muscles of older men and women adapt (fiber size, capillarization, glycolytic and respiratory enzymes) to both endurance and strength training exercise in a manner similar to young people.

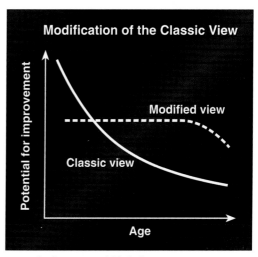

A new look at some old beliefs

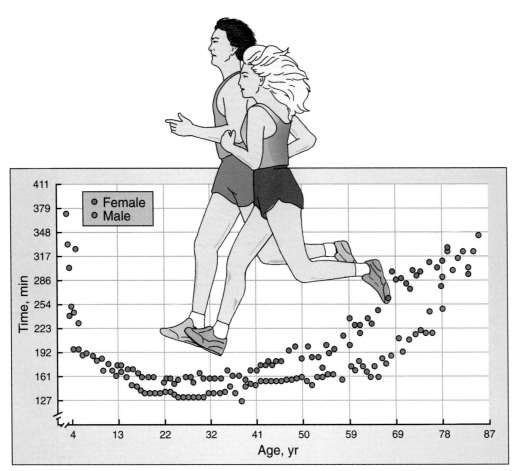

Figure 18–4. Plot of world record times for the marathon for men and women of different ages.

the same stature — and this weight difference is accounted for by differences in body fat. What remains unknown is the extent to which such gains in body fat during adulthood represent a normal biologic pattern. However, observations of physically active older individuals suggest that although it is common to see most "normal" individuals grow fatter as they become older, those who remain physically active retain lean body mass and a reduced level of body fat.

REGULAR EXERCISE: A FOUNTAIN OF YOUTH?

While exercise may not necessarily be a "fountain of youth," researchers are finding that regular physical activity not only retards the decline in functional capacity associated with aging and disuse, but often reverses this loss regardless of when in life a person becomes active.

Does Exercise Improve Health and Extend Life?

Over the years, medical experts have debated whether a lifetime of regular exercise contributes to good health and perhaps longevity compared to the sedentary "good life." Because older fit individuals have many of the functional characteristics of younger people, one could argue that improved physical fitness and a vigorous lifestyle may retard the aging process and confer some protection to health in later life.

One group of researchers studied the diseases and longevity of former college athletes. Because collegiate athletes usually have a longer involvement in habitual physical activity prior to entering college than nonathletes, and since they *may* remain more

to a running speed of 4 min 51 sec per mile (12.4 mph). As can be seen, with the very young and as people get older, endurance performance sharply decreases. Whereas from age 30 to 86 a decrease in performance is progressive, the world record time for the 86-year-old male of 340.2 minutes corresponds to a 12.9 min per mile pace, and for the 80-year-old female the world record time is 328.6 and corresponds to a 12.5 min per mile pace. This rate of running for 26.2 miles is truly remarkable for men and women in their eighth decade of life and attests to the tremendous cardiovascular capabilities of healthy older individuals who continue to train on a regular basis as they grow older.

Body Mass and Body Fat

The accumulation of excess fat usually begins in childhood or develops slowly during adulthood. Middle-aged men and women invariably weigh more than college-age counterparts of

physically active after college, this seemed to be an excellent group to study to provide insight concerning exercise and longevity.

Figure 18-5 shows there was essentially *no difference* in the longevity of the ex-athletes compared to nonathletes. Some degree of equality in genetic background existed between the groups because there was similarity in the average age at death of grandparents, parents, and siblings of ex-athletes and nonathletes. *These and more recent findings suggest that participation in athletics as a young adult does not necessarily ensure significant longevity.*

Enhanced Quality to a Longer Life: A Study of Harvard Alumni. Research concerning the *current* lifestyles and exercise habits of 17,000 Harvard alumni who entered college between 1916 and 1950 indicates that only moderate aerobic exercise, equivalent to jogging 3 miles a day, promotes good health and may actually add some time to life. Men who expended about 2000 kcal in weekly exercise had death rates one-quarter to one-third lower than classmates who did little or no exercise. To achieve this 2000 kcal output weekly requires moderate activity such as a daily 30-minute brisk walk, run, cycle, swim, cross-country ski, or aerobic dance. The specific results of these long-term studies can be summarized as follows:

Regular exercise counters the life-shortening effects of cigarette smoking and excess body weight. Even for people with high blood pressure (a primary heart disease risk), those who exercised regularly reduced their death rate by one-half. Moreover, genetic tendencies toward an early death were countered by regular exercise. For individuals who had one or both parents die before age 65 (another significant risk), a lifestyle that included regular exercise reduced the risk of death by 25%. A 50% reduction in mortality rate was

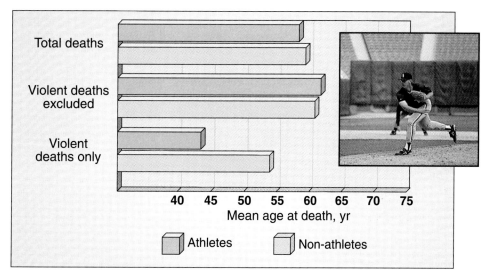

Figure 18–5. Age at death of athletes and nonathletes. None of the differences between the groups were statistically significant. (From Montoye, H.J., et al.: *The Longevity and Morbidity of College Athletes.* Indianapolis, IN. Phi Epsilon Kappa, 1957.)

observed for those whose parents lived beyond 65 years.

As shown in Figure 18-6, a person who exercises more has an improved health profile. For example, mortality rates were 21% lower for men who walked 9 or more miles a week than for those who walked 3 miles or less. Exercising in light sports activities increased life expectancy 24% over men who remained sedentary. From a perspective of energy expenditure, the life expectancy of Harvard alumni increased steadily from a weekly exercise energy output of 500 kcal to 3500 kcal, the equivalent of 6 to 8 hours of

Less structure and more movement. From a Public Health perspective, it may be of benefit to take a less technical approach to physical fitness when recommending physical activity. The message to the public should be to simply strive to become more active in one's daily life — go for a walk, garden more, watch less television, take the stairs, and do whatever is practical to upgrade daily caloric output.

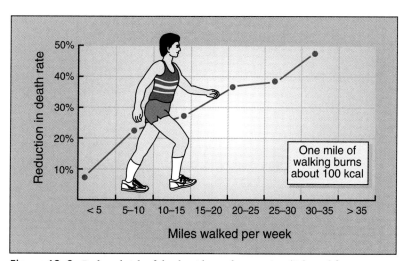

Figure 18–6. Reduced risk of death with regular exercise. (Adapted from Paffanbarger, R.S., Jr., et al.: Physical activity, all-cause mortality, and longevity of college alumni. *New Eng. J. Med.,* 314, 605, 1986.)

strenuous weekly exercise. In addition, active men lived an average of 1 to 2 years longer than sedentary classmates. (More recent research estimates an increase of about 10 months in a life with regular exercise.)

Beyond weekly exercise of 3500 kcal, there were no additional health or longevity benefits. In fact, when exercise was carried to extremes, the men had higher death rates than their less active colleagues — another example of more not necessarily being better!

Epidemiologic Evidence. A critique of 43 studies of the relationship between physical inactivity and CHD concluded that lack of regular exercise contributes to heart disease in a cause-and-effect manner, with the sedentary person at almost twice the risk as the most active individual. The strength of this protective association was essentially the same as that observed between heart disease and hypertension, cigarette smoking, and high serum cholesterol. *In the researchers' opinion, this placed physical inactivity as the greater heart disease risk, considering that more people lead sedentary lives than possess one or more of the other risks.* Although vigorous exercise does entail a small risk of

sudden death during the activity, the significant longer-term health benefits of regular activity far outweigh any potential acute risk.

From available data, it appears that if life-extending benefits of exercise exist, they are associated more with preventing early mortality than with improving overall life span. While the maximum life span may not be greatly extended, more active people tend to survive to a "ripe old age." That only moderate exercise is needed to achieve these benefits is further good news.

Improved Fitness: A Little Goes a Long Way

A recent study of more than 13,000 men and women followed for an average of 8 years indicates that even modest amounts of exercise substantially reduce the risk of dying from heart disease, cancer, and other causes. This was one of the few studies that looked directly at fitness performance rather than verbal or written reports of regular physical activity habits. To isolate the effect of fitness per se, the study considered such factors as smoking, cholesterol and blood sugar levels, blood pressure, and family history of CHD. Based on age-adjusted death rates per 10,000 person-years, Figure 18-7 illustrates that the death rate of the least fit group was more than 3 times that of the most fit subjects.

The most striking finding was that the greatest health benefit occurred in the group rated just above the most sedentary category. For men, the drop in death rate from the least fit to the next category was more than 38 (64.0 vs. 25.5 deaths per 10,000 person-years), whereas the drop in moving from the second group up to the most fit category was only 7. Similar benefits were found for women. The amount of exercise required to move from the most sedentary category to the next most fit — the jump that showed the greatest health benefits — occurred for moderate-intensity

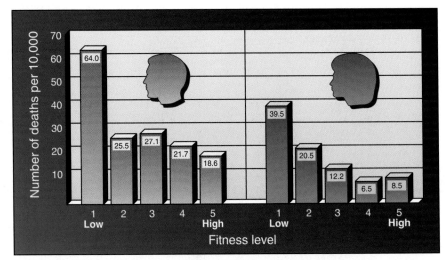

Figure 18–7. Physical fitness and longevity: a little goes along way. The greatest reduction in death rate risk occurs when going from the most sedentary category to a moderate level of fitness. (From Blair, S.N., et al.: Physical fitness and all-cause mortality: a prospective study of healthy men and women. *JAMA,* 262: 2395, 1989.)

exercise such as walking briskly for 30 minutes several times a week.

CORONARY HEART DISEASE

Figure 18-8 illustrates that 50% of total deaths in the United States are caused by diseases of the heart and blood vessels.

Stated somewhat more graphically, as many as 1.5 million Americans will have a heart attack this year and about one-third of them will die. While deaths from CHD have declined more than one-third since 1970, heart disease still remains the leading cause of death in the Western world. Between ages 55 and 65, about 13 of every 100 men and 6 of every 100 women die from CHD. Although the death rates for women lag about 10 years behind those for men, the gap is closing fast, especially with the upswing in cigarette smoking by women. For every American who dies of cancer, nearly 3 die of heart-related disease. The economic cost of this health disaster — medical costs, loss of earnings and productivity — is staggering ($120 billion in 1992). And this does not include the emotional impact of loss of a loved one in the prime of life!

Women at Risk. Not surprisingly, present day women are also at increased risk of developing coronary heart disease. In fact, since 1910 more American women have died of heart disease than any other cause! Because women develop heart disease 10 to 15 years later than men, they are more likely to have heart attacks when they are past middle age, rather than at an early age as do men. Only 1 percent of women under age 45 will develop CHD, while 13 percent of those above age 75 will develop CHD. This age difference makes CHD appear as a more general and dramatic problem in men than in women, because a heart attack for a 75 year-old is a less shocking statistic than a "wage earner" in the prime of life who suffers a heart attack. This

increased CHD occurrence for women in later years is related in part to a loss of protection offered by the sex hormone estrogen that drops markedly after menopause. Although research studies on women are scarce, available evidence suggests that the symptoms, disease progression, and outcome are different in women and men. For example, women are more likely than men to die soon after a heart attack; if they survive, they are more likely to have a second heart attack, and more apt to be sidelined by pain and disability than men. Furthermore, women who have by-pass surgery are less likely to survive, and there may even be gender differences in the risk factors for CHD.

The basic process by which CHD develops is probably the same in men and women, that is, fatty deposits narrow the coronary arteries and reduce blood flow to the myocardium. But hormonal differences may affect the formation of blood clots or the tendency of the coronary vascular wall to go into spasm in the final steps leading to a heart attack. Moreover, the diagnosis of CHD in women is different than in men. Many diagnostic tests, like the treadmill stress test and ECG response, have limited usefulness with women, mostly because the tests were validated only with men. Another reason for the diagnostic gap is that physicians do not take the signs of heart disease in women as seriously as they do in men. Consequently, they do not prescribe a coronary angiograph which is the most valid way to diagnose CHD.

Even though premenopausal women are at a lower CHD risk, they are not

Heart disease is an equal-opportunity killer. According to the American Heart Association, heart attack is the number one killer of women. Each year, women are struck down with just about half of the 520,000 heart attack deaths and more than 90,000 strokes, compared to 40,500 deaths from breast cancer and 41,000 from lung cancer.

Heart attack versus cardiac arrest. The difference is:

- Heart attack—caused by blockage in one or more arteries supplying the heart, thus cutting off the hearts' blood supply, or sudden spasms or constrictions of a coronary vessel, causing part of the heart muscle to die (necrosis)
- Cardiac arrest — caused by irregular neural-electrical transmission within the heart muscle, causing chaotic, unregulated beating in the heart's upper chambers (atrial fibrillation) or lower chambers (ventricular fibrillation)

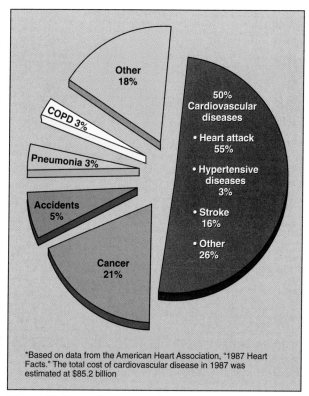

Figure 18–8. Leading causes of death in the United States.

from heart disease, particularly if they smoke. Research indicates that almost one half of all heart attacks in women before age 55 could be traced to cigarette smoking. Smoking as few as 4 cigarettes daily doubles a women's risk of developing CHD! Hypertension also is present in more than one-half the women over age 55 who suffer a heart attack; after age 65 it affects two-thirds of female victims. High blood sugar affects women more often than men. Both Type I and Type II diabetes raise a woman's CHD risk to that of an average nondiabetic man of the same age, and make her risk of dying from a heart attack even greater. In addition, birth-control pills raise a woman's CHD risk.

Women may be able to reduce their CHD risk in one of two ways: estrogen replacement therapy and low-dose aspirin. Women who take replacement estrogen after menopause cut their CHD risk almost in half. But the negative side is that estrogen alone increases the risk of developing uterine and breast cancer. Thus, estrogen therapy usually is supplemented with the hormone progestin to counter the cancer risk; it is not known, however, if progestin blunts the heart disease protection of estrogen replacement. Regular low-dose aspirin has been shown to help lower CHD risk in both men and women.

A Life-Long Process. Almost all people show some evidence of CHD, and it can be severe in seemingly healthy young adults. Actually, this degenerative process probably starts early in life because fatty streaks are common in the coronary arteries of children by the age of 5 years! There seems to be little harm, however, unless the arteries are markedly narrowed. As shown in Figure 18-9, CHD involves long-term degenerative changes in the inner lining of the arteries that supply the heart muscle.

Changes on the Cellular Level. The action and chemical modification of various compounds, including the cholesterol in low-density lipoproteins, initiate a complex process that ultimately causes bulging lesions in the walls of the coronary arteries. These changes initially take the form of fatty streaks, the first signs of atherosclerosis. With further damage and proliferation of underlying cells, the vessel becomes progressively congested with lipid-filled *plaques,* fibrous scar tissue, or both. This change progressively reduces the capacity for blood flow and causes the myocardium to become ischemic — that is, poorly supplied with oxygen because of the reduced blood supply. The roughened, hardened lining of the coronary artery frequently causes the slowly flowing blood to clot. This blood clot, or *thrombus,* may plug one of the smaller coronary vessels. In such cases, a portion of the heart muscle dies and the person is said to have suffered a heart attack, or myocardial infarction. If the blockage is not too severe but blood flow is at times reduced below the heart's requirement, the person may experience temporary chest pains termed *angina pectoris.* These pains are

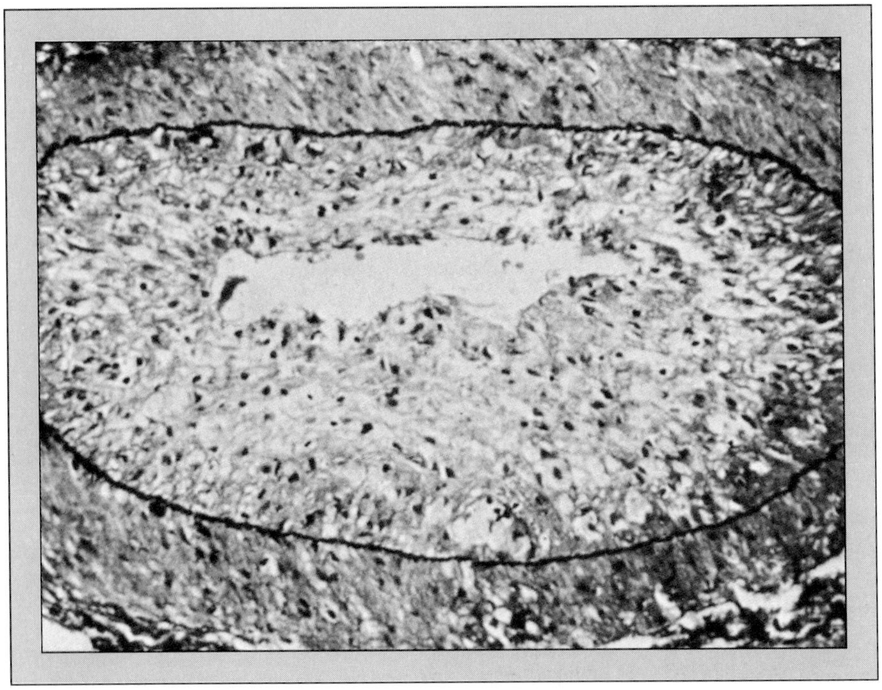

Figure 18–9. Deterioration of a coronary artery is seen as atherosclerosis develops with the beginning of the deposits of fatty substances that roughen the vessel's center. A clot then forms and plugs the artery, depriving the heart muscle of vital blood. The result is a myocardial infarction or heart attack.

usually felt during exertion, because this causes the greatest demand for myocardial blood flow. Anginal attacks provide vivid evidence of the importance of adequate oxygen supply to this vital organ.

Risk Factors for Coronary Heart Disease

Various personal characteristics and environmental factors have been identified over the past 40 years that indicate a person's susceptibility to CHD. The relative importance of each of these factors has been established. In general, the greater the *risk factor*, the more likely it is that the coronary arteries are diseased or will become diseased in the near future. This is not to say that a specific risk factor is the cause of the disease, as numerous factors may be acting and interacting in a cause-and-effect manner. However, based on the total evidence presently available, it is prudent to assess these factors on a personal basis and make efforts to modify each within reasonable limits.

The heart disease risk factors, including those that can and cannot be modified are:

Modifiable

- Diet
- Elevated blood lipids
- Hypertension
- Personality and behavior patterns
- Cigarette smoking
- High uric acid levels
- Physical inactivity
- Pulmonary function abnormalities
- Obesity
- Diabetes mellitus
- ECG abnormalities
- Tension and stress

Non-Modifiable

- Age and gender
- Heredity
- Race
- Male pattern baldness

It is difficult to determine quantitatively the importance of a single CHD risk factor in comparison to any other, because many of the factors are interrelated. For example, blood lipid abnormalities, diabetes, heredity, and obesity often go hand-in-hand. Compounding such observations is the finding that physical training generally lowers body weight, body fat, blood lipids, and the risk of developing diabetes. Also, certain groups, independent of other risk factors, are generally exposed to less psychological stress because of the nature of their occupation or cultural setting.

The risk factors of age, race, gender, and heredity are predetermined and cannot be controlled or remedied. However, four "treatable" factors — serum lipids, blood pressure, physical inactivity, and cigarette smoking — stand out as *potent* CHD risk factors. Of somewhat less predictive value than these *primary risk factors* are the risk factors of obesity and personality type. Although risk factors are closely associated with CHD, the associations do not necessarily infer causality. In many instances it remains to be shown that risk factor modification offers effective protection from the disease. Until definite proof is demonstrated, however, it is prudent to assume that eliminating or reducing one or more risk factors will contribute to a decrease in the probability of contracting CHD.

Age, Gender, and Heredity. Age is a risk factor largely because other associated risk factors such as hypertension, elevated blood lipids, and glucose intolerance become more prevalent in older years. As shown in Figure 18-10, after age 35 in males and age 45 in females, the chances of dying from CHD increase progressively and dramatically.

Between ages 55 and 65, about 13 of every 100 men and 6 of 100 women die from CHD. At most ages women fare much better than men. For example, in middle age, a man stands about a sixfold greater chance of dying from

Now it's the "Big Four." Physical inactivity has now joined high blood cholesterol, cigarette smoking, and hypertension on the American Heart Association's list of primary, yet modifiable, heart disease risks.

Risk factors in children. Multiple CHD risk factors are often observed in young children with obesity, elevated blood lipids, and a family history of heart disease being the most frequently occurring risks. In addition, the fattest children generally have the highest levels of cholesterol and triglycerides. School-based programs aimed at reducing risk factors in children and adolescents should be pursued. Such "risk intervention" will hopefully improve the child's health outlook and substitute positive behaviors that can be carried into adulthood to improve overall health.

TABLE 18-1. Desirable levels of total cholesterol (mg/dl), including HDL and LDL cholesterol, and levels above which adults should receive treatment

Age	Goal	Moderate Risk (75th percentile)	High Risk (90th percentile)
20–29	< 180	>200	>220
30–39	<200	>220	>240
40 and over	<200	>240	>260

UNDESIRABLE LEVELS		
HDL Cholesterol	<	35 mg/dl
LDL Cholesterol	>	130 mg/dl

Source: Adapted from National Institutes of Health Consensus Development Conference Statement: Lowering blood cholesterol to prevent heart disease. *JAMA,* 253:2080, 1985.

Cholesterol levels in children. About 25% of children in the U.S. have blood cholesterol levels above 170 mg · dl^{-1}, a value considered acceptable.

a heart attack. However, American women still lead all other countries in heart disease and the specific "gender advantage" is greatly reduced after the age of menopause. This has led to speculation that some of the CHD protection for women is provided by hormonal differences between the genders. Although the cause is not known, heart attacks that strike at an early age appear to run in families.

Blood Lipid Abnormalities. The precise mechanism by which plasma lipids affect the development of CHD is not fully understood. Nevertheless,

overwhelming evidence links high blood lipid levels with an increased heart disease risk.

Cholesterol and Triglycerides. Table 18-1 presents levels of serum cholesterol above which young and older adults should seek advice on treatment. In general, a cholesterol level of 200 mg/dl or lower is considered desirable.

A cholesterol value of 230 mg/dl increases the risk of heart attack to about twice that of a person with 180 mg/dl, and a value of 300 mg/dl increases the risk fourfold. An increased lipid level in the blood plasma is termed *hyperlipidemia*.

The Forms of Cholesterol Are Also Important. Cholesterol and triglycerides are the two most common lipids associated with CHD risk. Recall from Chapter 6 that these lipids are not soluble in water so they do not circulate freely in the blood plasma. Rather, they are transported in combination with a carrier protein to form a lipoprotein. This lipoprotein can vary in size depending on how much protein and lipid it contains. Although it is proper to refer to an elevation in blood lipids as hyperlipidemia, it is more meaningful to evaluate and discuss the different types of *hyperlipoproteinemia*. Table 18-2 lists the four different lipoproteins, their approximate density, and their percentage composition in the blood. *Serum cholesterol represents a composite of the total cholesterol contained in the different lipoproteins.*

The distribution of cholesterol among the various types of lipoproteins is a more powerful predictor of heart disease than simply the total quantity of plasma lipids (Figure 18-11). This partially explains how one person with a high total serum cholesterol may not develop CHD, while it develops in another with a lower cholesterol level. Specifically, a high level of high-density lipoprotein (HDL), which comprises the smallest portion of the lipopro-

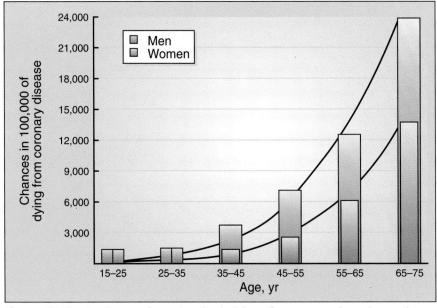

Figure 18-10. The chances of a single individual dying from coronary heart disease. (Data from the American Heart Association)

teins but contain the largest quantity of protein and least amount of cholesterol, is associated with a lower heart disease risk. In contrast, an elevated level of the cholesterol-rich low-density lipoprotein (LDL) represents an increased risk.

It is generally believed that LDL is the means for transporting lipids throughout the body for delivery to the cells, including those of the smooth muscle walls of the arteries. Here it is oxidized and ultimately contributes to the artery-narrowing process of atherosclerosis. Whereas LDL carries cholesterol to the tissues and is associated with arterial damage, HDL acts as a scavenger, gathering cholesterol from cells (including those of the arterial wall) and returning it to the liver, where it is metabolized and excreted in the bile.

Research is progressing to clarify how HDL is protective and what factors can raise its levels. For one thing, cigarette smoking has adverse effects on the HDL pattern. This may account for the significant CHD risk with smoking. It is encouraging from an exercise perspective that HDL levels are elevated in endurance athletes and are favorably altered in sedentary people who engage in either moderate or vigorous aerobic training. Concurrently, LDL is lowered with exercise so the net result is a considerably improved ratio of HDL to LDL or HDL to total cholesterol. This exercise effect appears to be independent of the lipid content of the

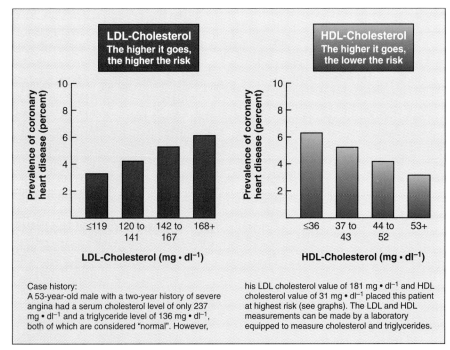

diet or the leanness of the exerciser. A moderate consumption of alcohol (equivalent to about 2 oz or 30 g of 90 proof alcohol, three 6 oz. glasses of wine, or a bit less than three 12 oz cans of beer) has been reported to reduce an otherwise healthy person's risk of heart attack. Although the protective mechanism is unclear, it may be that moderate alcohol intake increases HDL and lowers LDL. Excessive alcohol consumption offers no lipoprotein benefit and greatly increases the risk of liver disease and cancer.

Figure 18-11. Coronary heart disease prevalence and lipoproteins. The risk increases as the LDL-cholesterol level increases; conversely, the risk decreases when the HDL-cholesterol level rises. (Courtesy of CPC International, Best Foods Division)

Family history is important. Should children have their cholesterol measured? Guidelines issued by the National Cholesterol Education Program say yes if there is a family history of high cholesterol or heart disease (particularly if a parent suffered a heart attack before age 50). Shockingly, this parental "cardiac proneness" includes up to one-fourth the adult population of the United States!

TABLE 18-2. Approximate composition of lipoproteins in the blood

	Chylomicrons	Very Low Density Lipoproteins (VLDL: Prebeta)	Low Density Lipoproteins (LDL: Beta)	High-Density Lipoproteins (HDL: Alpha)
Density, g.cc^{-1}	0.95	0.95–1.006	1.006–1.019	1.063–1.210
Protein, %	0.5–1.0	5–15	25	45–55
Lipid, %	99	95	75	50
Cholesterol, %	2–5	10–20	40–45	18
Triglyceride, %	85	50–70	5–10	2
Phospholipid, %	3-6	10–20	20–25	30

ty, hypertension, diabetes, and elevated lipid profiles.

BEHAVIORAL CHANGES THAT CAN IMPROVE THE OVERALL HEALTH PROFILE

Health-promoting habits can be effective in areas other than related to one's risk for heart attack. Table 18-3 ranks the value of several health-saving tactics that reduce risk or bolster resistance to the major diseases of cancer, heart attack, stroke, and diabetes

For example, a low-fat diet is highly effective in protecting against adult-onset diabetes, heart attack, and cancers of the breast and colon (and moderately effective in preventing other cancers as well). A diet rich in vegetables and fruits is most effective against colon cancer, as well as throat cancer, and offers some protection against diabetes and cardiovascular disease. Smoking is our country's single deadliest habit and is the primary cause of lung cancer and a major factor in heart attacks. Regular exercise and weight control are most effective in reducing the risk of heart disease, stroke, and adult-onset diabetes, and they offer some protection against certain cancers.

EXERCISE STRESS TESTING

The potential therapeutic and fitness benefits of exercise should be viewed in perspective. For a sedentary person with significant, undetected coronary heart disease, a sudden burst of strenuous exercise could place an inordinate strain on the cardiovascular system. This risk can be reduced considerably with proper medical evaluation that should minimally include a thorough personal health and family history, and physical examination. The physical examination should emphasize signs and symptoms of cardiovascular disease and include blood pressure, resting 12-lead ECG, cardiac murmurs and abnormal heart rhythms, edema, blood analysis, and chronic lung disease. For many people, an important part of the medical evaluation is the exercise stress test.

Why Stress Test?

There are many reasons to include stress testing in an overall CHD evaluation:
- *To establish*, from ECG observations, a diagnosis of overt heart disease and also to screen for possible "silent" coronary disease in

TABLE 18–3. Preventing major diseases: a checklist of health-saving tactics

	No Tobacco	Low-Fat Diet	High-Fiber Diet	Avoid Alcohol	Avoid Salted, Pickled Foods	Diet High In Vegetables and Fruits	Exercise, Weight Control
Cancer							
Lung	√√√	√				√	
Breast		√√√	√			√√	√
Colon		√√√	√√√			√√√	√
Liver				√√√	√	√√	
Heart Attack	√√√	√√√				√√	√√√
Stroke	√				√√√	√√	√√
Adult Diabetes		√√√	√			√√	√√

√√√ Highly Effective   √√ Moderately effective   √ Somewhat effective
Modified from American Medical Foundation.

seemingly healthy men and women. Approximately 30% of the people with confirmed coronary artery disease have normal resting electrocardiograms. During relatively intense exercise, however, about 80% of these abnormalities are uncovered.

- *To reproduce* and assess exercise-related chest symptoms. In many instances, individuals over the age of 40 suffer chest or related pain in the left shoulder or arm on physical exertion. Proper electrocardiographic analysis during exercise provides a more precise diagnosis of exercise-induced pain.
- *To screen* candidates for preventive and cardiac rehabilitative exercise programs. Stress test results can then be used to design an exercise program that is within the person's current functional capacity and health status, with emphasis on intensity, frequency, duration, and type of exercise. Repeated testing aids in evaluating progress in the exercise intervention program as well as in

determining the need for safe program modification.

- *To detect* an abnormal blood pressure response. It is not uncommon to find individuals with a normal resting blood pressure who show higher than normal increases in systolic blood pressure with exercise. Exercise hypertension may signify developing cardiovascular complications.
- *To monitor* responses to various therapeutic interventions (drug, surgical, and dietary) designed to improve cardiovascular functioning. For example, the success of coronary bypass surgery can be detected by a patient's adjustment to exercise and ability to successfully reach a target exercise heart rate without complications.
- *To define* the functional aerobic capacity and evaluate its degree of deviation from normal standards.

Who Should Be Stress-Tested?

Table 18-4 shows a classification system by age and health status for

Not enough of a good thing. At best, no more than 20% and possibly less than 10% of the adults in the United States obtain sufficient regular physical activity to impart discernible health and fitness benefits. Conservatively, 40% are completely sedentary, and 40% exercise below recommended levels.

TABLE 18-4. Classification by age and health status for men and women who require different screening and supervisory procedures prior to and during a stress test

Age	Patient Health Status	Evaluation and Required Medical Clearance	12-Lead Resting ECG	Personnel Involved During Stress Test
<35	No known primary CHD risk factors;[a] may have secondary CHD risk factors[b]	During past 2 years, signed statement	Not required	No test required
35–40	No known primary CHD risk factors; may have secondary CHD risk factors	During past 2 years, signed statement	Required	Exercise technician; exercise physiologist; M.D. in area
>40	No known primary CHD risk factors; may have secondary CHD risk factors	During past 2 years, signed statement	Required	Exercise technician; exercise physiologist; M.D. in area
Any age	Documented CHD; hypertension; suspected CHD	During past 2 years, signed statement	Required	Exercise technician; exercise physiologist; M.D. conducting test

[a]Primary risk factors: Hypertension, hyperlipidemia, cigarette smoking, and physical inactivity.
[b]Secondary risk factors: Family history, obesity, and diabetes mellitus.

screening and supervisory procedures for use in conjunction with an exercise stress test.

These standards conform to policies and practices of the American College of Sports Medicine and the American Medical Association. The prudent rules are:

- If a person is less than 35 years of age and has no previous history of cardiovascular disease and no known primary risk factors (and has had a medical evaluation within the past 2 years), it is generally acceptable to begin an exercise program without special medical clearance. These people may also be stress tested for purposes of functional evaluation and for preparing the exercise prescription by a trained exercise specialist
- If a person is less than 35 years of age but has evidence of CHD or a significant combination of risk factors, he or she should be medically cleared prior to embarking on an exercise program. This should include a physician supervised graded exercise test
- For all adults above 35 years of age, medical evaluation is advised prior to any major increase in exercise habits. This medical evaluation should include an ECG monitored before, during, and in recovery from a graded exercise test and supervised by a physician

Exercise-Induced Indicators of CHD

Several clues to CHD become apparent during exercise because exercise creates the greatest demand on coronary blood flow.

Angina Pectoris. Approximately 30% of the initial manifestations of CHD during exercise take the form of chest-related pain called angina pectoris. This is a temporary but painful condition that indicates that coronary blood flow and hence oxygen supply has momentarily reached a critically low level. This *myocardial ischemia* (usually the result of restricted coronary circulation brought about by coronary atherosclerosis) stimulates sensory nerves in the walls of the coronary arteries and myocardium itself. The resulting pain or discomfort is generally felt in the upper chest region, although it is frequently characterized by a sensation of pressure or constriction in the left shoulder, neck, jaw, or left arm. After a few minutes of rest, the pain usually subsides with no permanent damage being done to the heart muscle.

ECG Disorders. Alterations in the heart's normal pattern of electric activity are often indicative of extensive obstruction of the coronary arteries, insufficient oxygen supply to the myocardium, and an increased risk of death from CHD. These electric "clues," however, are rarely observed until the metabolic (and blood flow) requirements are increased above the resting level.

The ECG tracing illustrated in Figure 18-13 is a plot of the dynamic electric activity of the heart muscle in millivolts (mV). Normal ECG paper is divided into small 1-mm squares and larger 5-mm squares. Horizontally, each small square is equivalent to 0.04 seconds (with standard paper speed of 25 mm per sec); each large square represents 0.2 seconds.

On the vertical axis each small square indicates a 0.1-mV deflec-

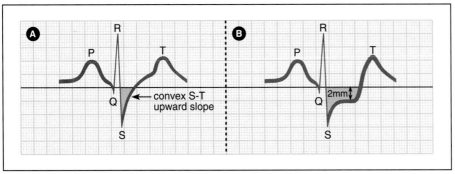

Figure 18-13. *A.* Tracing that illustrates the normal ECG complex. The arrow points to the slightly convex and upward sloping S-T segment. *B.* Tracing shows an abnormal horizontal S-T segment depression (shaded area) of 2 mm measured from a stable baseline.

tion with a calibration of 10 mm per mV. A normal single heart beat or cardiac cycle consists of five major electric waves: *P, Q, R, S, and T.*(Figure 18-13A). The P wave is the electric impulse or wave of depolarization associated with atrial contraction. The Q, R, and S waves are considered as a unit that represents the depolarization and subsequent contraction of the ventricles. Collectively this is known as the *QRS complex.* The T wave is generated by the repolarization of the ventricles. Although it is not known why the S-T segment becomes depressed, this deviation from normal is closely correlated with other indicators of CHD including coronary artery narrowing.

Cardiac Rhythm Abnormalities. Although exercise can induce abnormalities in the S-T segment of the electrocardiogram, it also provides an effective way to observe both normal and abnormal cardiac rhythm. One significant alteration in cardiac rhythm (*arrhythmia*) with exercise is the occurrence of *premature ventricular contractions* or PVCs. In this situation, the ventricles demonstrate disorganized electric activity. They are not stimulated by the normal passage of the wave of depolarization through the atrioventricular node. Rather, portions of the ventricle become spontaneously depolarized. This shows up on the electrocardiogram as an "extra-ventricular beat" or QRS complex that occurs without being preceded by a P wave that indicates atrial depolarization.

Premature ventricular contractions in exercise generally herald the presence of severe ischemic atherosclerotic heart disease, often involving two or more major coronary vessels. Individuals with frequent PVCs are at high risk of sudden death owing to *ventricular fibrillation*, an electrical instability in which the ventricles are unable to contract in a unified manner. As a result, blood is not pumped effectively and cardiac output falls dramatically.

Other Indices of CHD. Two useful non-electrocardiographic indices of possible CHD are the blood pressure and heart rate responses to exercise.

- *Hypertensive response:* During a graded exercise test, there is a normal, progressive increase in systolic blood pressure from about 120 mmHg to 160 to 190 mmHg at peak exercise. The change in diastolic pressure is generally less than 10 mmHg. For some individuals, however, strenuous exercise may cause the systolic blood pressure to rise well above 200 mmHg, whereas the diastolic pressure can increase to 100 to 150 mmHg. This abnormal hypertensive response can be a significant clue to cardiovascular disease.

- *Hypotensive response:* The inability of blood pressure to increase with exercise can also reflect cardiovascular malfunction. For example, failure of the systolic blood pressure to increase by at least 20 or 30 mmHg during graded exercise may reflect diminished cardiac reserve.

- *Heart rate response:* A rapid, large increase in heart rate (*tachycardia*) early in exercise is often a harbinger of cardiac problems. Likewise, abnormally low exercise heart rates (*bradycardia*) may reflect unhealthy function of the heart's sinus node. Also, the inability of the heart rate to increase during exercise, especially when accompanied by extreme fatigue, may be indicative of cardiac strain and heart disease.

Stress Test Protocols

There are many different stress test protocols. In a national survey of 1400 exercise stress test centers, the treadmill was the most common mode of testing. Seventy-one percent of the facilities reported using the treadmill whereas 17% used the bicycle ergometer.

The Balke and Bruce Treadmill Tests.
The Balke and Bruce tests (see Chapter 5, Figure 5-10 for these and other treadmill test descriptions) are two popular treadmill protocols. Both protocols start at relatively high levels of exercise, especially for cardiac patients. Because of this, both tests have undergone modifications. For the Bruce protocol, lower exercise levels were added, whereas for the Balke test, a preliminary 2 to 3 minute stage (2 mph, 0% grade) was included.

It is sometimes difficult to decide which treadmill protocol to use for testing. Choice of protocol must be made based on the particular population studied, and their health status, age, and fitness level. In general, a graded stress test for ECG evaluation should start at a low level and have increments in exercise intensity approximately every 2 to 3 minutes. It is also advisable to use a warm-up, either separately or incorporated into the test itself. The total duration of the test should be at leas 8 minutes. On the other hand, a test that is much longer than 15 minutes is not needed as most important cardiac and physiologic data can be obtained within this time period.

Bicycle Ergometer Tests. Bicycle ergometers are also a good means for exercise stress testing. In contrast to the treadmill, power output on the ergometer is independent of the person's body mass and is easily calculated and regulated. Also, the bike is portable, safe, and relatively inexpensive.

The same general guidelines used for treadmill testing apply for graded exercise tests on the bicycle ergometer. Most bicycle ergometer rates of power output are expressed in kgm·min^{-1} or in watts (1 W = 6.12 kgm·min^{-1}). Bicycle ergometer test protocols have 2- to 4- minute stages of graded exercise with an initial resistance between zero and 15 or 30 watts; power output is generally increased by 15 to 30 watts per stage. Pedaling rate for mechanically braked ergometers is usually set at 50 or 60 revolutions per min.

Outcomes of a Stress Test

The value of stress testing depends directly on how well results on a particular test predict the existence of heart disease. The *sensitivity* of a stress test refers to the percentage of people with disease who have an abnormal test result. No test is ever perfect for diagnosing heart disease. There are four possible outcomes from a graded exercise stress test:

- *True-Positive:* In this condition, the test results are correct in diagnosing a person with heart disease (the stress test is a success)
- *False-Negative:* In this condition, the test results are normal yet the person actually has heart disease (unsuccessful test)
- *True-Negative:* In this condition, the test results are normal and the person does not have heart disease (the test is a success)
- *False-Positive:* In this condition, the test results are abnormal yet the person has no heart disease (the test is unsuccessful)

Both a false-negative and a false-positive test can have dramatic ramifications, especially a false-negative result. Whenever a stress test indicates the presence of heart disease, secondary tests are performed to confirm the diagnosis. Similarly, just because results from graded stress tests are normal does not necessarily rule out the occurrence of heart disease; the predictive value of an abnormal test is much greater than the predictive value of a normal stress test.

Guidelines for Stress Testing

The following guidelines should be used for stopping a stress test. Each of these symptoms generally indicates extreme cardiovascular strain that could be dangerous to the patient.

- Repeated presence of premature ventricular contractions (PVCs)

- Progressive angina pain regardless of the presence or absence of ECG abnormalities consistent with ischemia
- ECG changes that include the presence of S-T segment depression of 2 mm or more, continuous PVCs, and evidence of atrioventricular conduction disturbances (A-V block)
- An extremely rapid increase in heart rate that may reflect a severely compromised cardiovascular response
- Failure of heart rate or blood pressure to increase with progressive exercise or a progressive drop in systolic blood pressure with increasing work load
- An increase in diastolic pressure of 20 mmHg or more, or a rise above 110 mmHg
- Headache, blurred vision, pale, clammy skin, or extreme fatigue
- Dizziness or near fainting
- Nausea

Persons who exhibit these responses require further medical evaluation and should be excluded from unsupervised exercise programs pending such a study. Those patients who complete the stress test without significant ECG responses or other evidence of CHD can be medically cleared for unsupervised exercise that does not exceed the intensity of exercise reached during the test.

The Exercise Prescription

Heart rate and oxygen uptake data obtained during the stress test are used to formulate the *exercise prescription*; this is an individualized exercise program based on the person's current fitness and health status, with emphasis on intensity, frequency, duration, and type of exercise. This is important because many people who start exercising do not recognize their limitations and may exercise above a prudent level. Even group exercise programs that require medical clearance are limited because members exercise at about the same work level (walk, jog, or swim at the same speed) with little attention paid to individual differences in fitness.

Practical Illustration. Figure 18-14 illustrates a practical approach that permits the functional translation

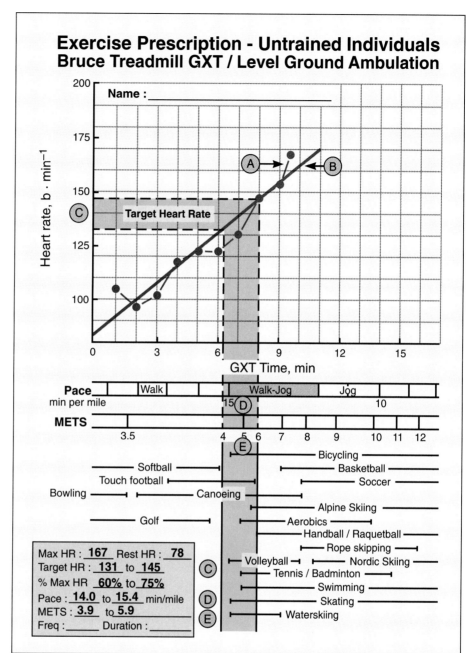

Figure 18-14. Exercise prescription based on functional translation algorithm for level ground ambulation. (Used with permission Dr. Carl Foster, Dept. of Medicine, Cardiovascular Disease Section, Sinai Samaritan Center, Milwaukee, WI)

Benefits to the cardiac patient. Selected patients with coronary artery disease when trained in excess of normally prescribed exercise intensity show physiologic adaptation much larger than previously believed possible. The good news is that these adaptations include favorable adjustments in myocardial oxygenation and enhanced ventricular function.

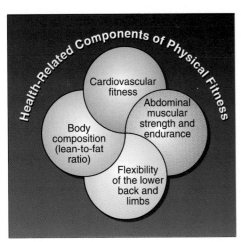

of treadmill or cycle ergometer exercise test responses to the exercise prescription.

The results depicted are for a male cardiac patient and were generated from an algorithm that used exercise test responses from the Bruce treadmill protocol for level-ground ambulation. During the Bruce test, the heart rate (A) was plotted as a function of time. A mathematical line of "best fit" was then applied to the heart rate data, and line B was drawn through the data points. A target zone for heart rate was calculated as 60 to 75% based on the maximum heart rate of 167 beats per minute (shaded portion represented as C). The individualized prescription is then detailed in terms of pace (14.0 to 15.4 min per mile; D) and METs (3.9 to 5.9; E). The acceptable range of exercise intensity in area C, based on heart rate response during the graded exercise test, includes the following recreational activities; bicycling, touch football, canoeing, alpine skiing, aerobics, volleyball, tennis and badminton, swimming, skating, and water-skiing. This quantitative method of exercise prescription may improve the specificity and precision of exercise prescription for the healthy previously sedentary individual as well as the patient with known cardiovascular disease.

Improvements in CHD Patients. With a properly prescribed and monitored exercise program many cardiac patients can expect to safely improve their functional capacity to a degree comparable to a healthy person of the same age. In some instances, even clinical symptoms such as ECG abnormalities are improved or even eliminated. This occurs because many individuals respond to exercise training with physiologic adjustments that actually reduce the work of the heart at any given external work load. For example, reduced exercise heart rate and blood pressure (two major determinants of myocardial oxygen uptake) and improved myocardial

contractility reduce myocardial effort. This delays the onset of anginal pain allowing work of greater intensity and duration. For individuals whose occupations predominantly require arm work, this musculature should be exercised in training because many of the benefits of physical conditioning are highly specific to the muscles trained and generally not transferable from one muscle group to another.

The Program. Exercise programs for preventive and rehabilitative purposes are most effective when they are individualized. Some heart disease patients have a reduced heart rate response to exercise with a corresponding reduction in maximum heart rate. For these individuals, the use of target heart rates based on an age-predicted maximum for the general population will grossly overestimate the proper training intensity. These observations argue for exercise testing each patient to a symptom-limited maximum and then formulating the exercise prescription based on the patient's actual heart rate data.

The guidelines for making decisions concerning frequency, duration, and intensity of training were discussed in Chapter 12. For physical conditioning of adult groups, exercise should generally be performed at least three times a week for 20 to 40 minutes each exercise session. Big muscle endurance activities should be performed at 50 to 75% of the person's working capacity or oxygen uptake capacity as measured on the stress test. This "target zone" puts individuals at or above the threshold level for a training effect, yet ensures that they are not unduly stressed by the training program. Ideally, the personalized exercise prescription should include a recommendation for weight loss and dietary modification (if necessary), as well as warm-up and cool-down exercises and a developmental strength program.

Level of Supervision. The American College of Sports Medicine has categorized several types of exercise programs with specific criteria for entry and supervision as shown in Table 18-5.

They are classified as unsupervised and supervised with 4 subdivisions of the supervised category. Unsupervised programs are for asymptomatic participants of any age with functional capacities of at least 8 METS, and with no known major risk factors. The supervised exercise programs are geared to people with different and specific needs. These include asymptomatic physically active or inactive persons of any age with CHD risk factors but no known disease (B-4) and symptomatic individuals (B1-3) including those with recent onset of CHD and those who report a change in disease status.

TABLE 18-5. Types of Exercise Programs

Type	Participants	Entry MET Level	Supervision
A. Unsupervised	Asymptomatic	8+	None
B. Supervised			
1. Inpatient	All symptomatics—post MI, post op, pulmonary disease	3	Supervised ambulatory therapy
2. Outpatient	All symptomatics—post MI, post op, pulmonary disease	3+	Exercise specialist, physician on call
3. In-Home	Symptomatic + asymptomatic	>3–5	Unsupervised; periodic hospital re-evaluation
4. Community	Symptomatic + asymptomatic, 6–8 wk post infarct, 4–8 wk post operative	>5	Exercise program director + exercise specialist

SUMMARY

1. Physiologic and performance capability generally declines after about 30 years of age. The rates of decline in the various functions differ and are significantly influenced by many factors, including level of physical activity. Regular physical training enables older persons to retain higher levels of functional capacity, especially cardiovascular function.

2. Regardless of age, regular physical activity produces measurable physiologic improvements. The magnitude of these improvements depends on many factors including initial fitness status, age, and type, intensity, and amount of training.

3. Participation in vigorous physical activity early in life probably contributes little to increased longevity or health in later life. However, a physically active lifestyle throughout life confers significant health benefits.

4. Coronary heart disease is the single largest cause of death in the Western world. The pathogenesis of this disease involves degenerative changes in the inner lining of the arterial wall that result in progressive occlusion.

5. Numerous factors have been identified that make individuals more susceptible to developing CHD. The major risk factors are age and gender, elevated blood lipids, hypertension, cigarette smoking, obesity, physical inactivity, diet, heredity, and ECG abnormalities during rest and exercise.

6. In general, a cholesterol level of 200 mg or lower is considered desirable with many experts recommending the lower values as being most healthful.

7. The distribution of the various lipoproteins, especially HDL and LDL cholesterol, is a more powerful predictor of heart disease risk than simply the total quantity of plasma cholesterol.

8. The risk of death from heart disease is almost twice as great for smokers as for nonsmokers. One mechanism for risk may be the adverse effect of smoking on lipoprotein levels.

9. The interaction of CHD risk factors significantly magnifies their individual effect in predicting one's chances for disease.

10. Many CHD risk factors can be modified by proper programs of nutrition, exercise, and weight control. This "risk intervention" generally improves an individual's health outlook.

11. Stress testing is relatively safe provided appropriate guidelines are followed. Graded exercise testing provides valuable information for clearing individuals to begin exercising and also for individualizing the exercise prescription.

12. No one stress test is perfect for diagnosing heart disease. The four possible outcomes of a stress test are: True-Positive (the test is a success); False-Negative (a person with heart disease is not diagnosed); True-Negative (the test is a success); and False-Positive (a healthy person is diagnosed with heart disease).

13. Cardiac patients can often improve their functional capacity to the same extent as healthy people of the same age.

SELECTED REFERENCES

Abbott, R. F., et al.: Cardiovascular risk factors and graded treadmill exercise endurance in healthy adults: The Framingham Offspring Study. *Am. J. Cardiol.*, 63: 342, 1989.

American College of Sports Medicine: *Guidelines for Exercise, Testing and Prescription*. 3rd ed. Philadelphia, Lea & Febiger, 1986.

Becque, M. D., et al.: Coronary risk incidence of obese adolescents: Reduction by exercise plus diet intervention. *Pediatrics*, 81: 605, 1988.

Blair, S. N., et al.: Physical activity and health: a lifestyle approach. *Med. Exerc. Nutr. Health*, 1: 54, 1992.

Blair, S. N., et al.: Physical fitness and all-cause mortality: a prospective study of healthy men and women. *JAMA*, 262: 2395, 1989.

Blair, S.N.: Physical activity, physical fitness, and health. *Res. Q. Exerc. Sport*, 64: 365, 1993.

Both, F.W., et al.: Effect of aging on human skeletal muscle and motor function. *Med. Sci. Sports Exerc.*, 26: 556, 1994.

Bouchard, C., and Shephard, R.J.: Physical activity, fitness, and health: The model and key concepts. In *Physical Activity, Fitness and Health*, Edited by C. Bouchard, and R.J. Shepherd. Champaign, IL, Human Kinetics, 1994.

Bovens, A. M., et al.: Physical activity, fitness, and selected risk factors for CHD in active men and women. *Med. Sci. Sports Exerc.*, 25:572, 1993.

Brooks, S.V., and Faulkner, J.A.: Skeletal muscle weakness in old age: underlying mechanisms. *Med. Sci. Sports Exerc.*, 26: 432, 1994.

Burke, G. L., et al.: Trends in serum cholesterol levels from 1980 to 1987 —

The Minnesota Heart Survey. *N. Engl. J. Med.*, 324: 941, 1991.

Cartee, G.D.: Aging skeletal muscle: response to exercise. *Exerc. Sport Sci. Rev.*, 22: 91, 1994.

Cartee, G.D.: Influence of age on skeletal muscle glucose transport and glycogen metabolism. *Med. Sci. Sports Exerc.*, 26: 577, 1994.

Casazza, G.A., et al.: Exercise training and reduction in some coronary risk factors in female cigarette smokers. *Am. J. Cardiol.*, 75: 85, 1995.

Caspersen, C. J.: Physical activity epidemiology: concepts, methods, and applications to exercise science. In *Exercise and Sport Sciences Reviews*. Vol. 17. Edited by K. B. Pandolf. Baltimore, Williams & Wilkins, 1989.

Consensus statement. *Physical Activity, Fitness, and Health*. Edited by C. Bouchard, et al., Champaign, IL, Human Kinetics, 1994.

Corbin, C. B., and Pangrazi, R. B.: Are American children and youth fit? Res. *Q. Exerc. Sport*, 63: 96, 1992.

Cress, M.E., et al.: Effect of training on VO_2 max, thigh strength, and muscle morphology in septuagenarian women. *Med. Sci. Sports Exerc.*, 23: 752, 1991.

Després, J-P., et al.: Physical activity and coronary heart disease risk factors during childhood and adolescence. In *Exercise and Sport Sciences Reviews*. Vol. 18. Edited by K. B. Pandolf, and J. O. Holloszy, Baltimore, Williams & Wilkins, 1990.

Douglas, P. S., et al.: Exercise and atherosclerotic heart disease in women. *Med. Sci. Sport Exerc.*, 24: S266, 1992.

Durstine, J.L., and Haskell, W.L.: Effects of exercise training on plasma lipids and lipoproteins. *Exerc. Sport Sci. Rev.*, 22: 477, 1994.

Ehsani, A. A.: Cardiovascular adaptations to endurance exercise training in ischemic heart disease. In *Exercise and Sport Sciences Reviews*. Vol. 15. Edited by K. B. Pandolf. New York, Macmillan, 1987.

Eaton, C.B., et al.: Physical activity, physical fitness, and coronary heart disease risk factors. *Med. Sci. Sports Exerc.*, 27(3): 340, 1995.

Emery, E.M., et al.: A review of the association between abdominal fat distribution, health outcome measures, and modifiable risk factors. *Am. J. Health Promotion*, 7: 342, 1993.

Fiatarone, M.A., et al.: Exercise training and nutritional supplementation for physical frailty in very elderly people. *N. Engl. J. Med.*, 330: 1769, 1994.

Folsom, R., et al.: Body fat distribution and 5-year risk of death in older women. *JAMA*, 269: 483, 1993.

Foster, C.: Translation of exercise test responses to exercise prescription. In *Cardiac Rehabilitation and Clinical Exercise Programs: Theory and Practice*. Edited by N. B. Oldridge, et al. Ithaca, NY, Movement Publications, 1989.

Franklin, B.A., et al.: Exercise and cardiac complications: do the benefits outweigh the risks? *Phys. Sportsmed.*, 22(2): 56, 1994.

Franklin, B. A., et al.: Additional diagnostic tests: special populations. In *Resource Manual for Guidelines for Exercise Testing and Prescription*. Edited by S. Blair, et al., Philadelphia, Lea & Febiger, 1988.

Frontera, W. R., et al.: Strength conditioning in older men: skeletal muscle hypertrophy and improved function. *J. Appl. Physiol.*, 64: 1038, 1988.

Gaziano, J.M., et al.: Moderate alcohol intake, increased levels of high-density lipoprotein and its subfractions, and decreased risk of myocardial infarction. *N. Engl. J. Med.*, 329: 1829, 1993.

Gudat, V., et al.: Physical activity, fitness, and non-insulin-dependent (Type II) diabetes mellitus. In *Physical Activity, Fitness, and Health*. Edited by Bouchard, C., et al., Champaign, IL, Human Kinetics, 1994.

Hagberg, J. M., et al.: Metabolic responses to exercise in young and older athletes and sedentary men. *J. Appl. Physiol.*, 65: 900, 1988.

Hagberg, J. M., et al.: Cardiovascular responses of 70- to 79-yr old men and women to exercise training. *J. Appl. Physiol.*, 66: 2589, 1989.

Hanson, P.: Exercise testing and training in patients with chronic heart failure. *Med. Sci. Sports Exerc.*, 26: 527, 1994.

Helmrich, S. P., et al.: Physical activity and reduced occurrence of non-insulin-dependent diabetes mellitus. *N. Engl. J. Med.*, 325, 147, 1991.

Health and Human Services, *The Surgeon General's Report on Nutrition and Health*. U.S. Dept. of Health and Human Services, Washington, DC, 1988.

Higginbotham, M. B., et al.: Physiologic basis for the age-related decline in aerobic work capacity. *Am. J. Cardiol.*, 57: 1374, 1986.

Johnson, C.L., et al.: Declining serum total cholesterol levels among US adults. *JAMA*, 269: 3002, 1993.

Kakka, T.A., et al.: Relation of leisure-time physical activity and cardiorespiratory fitness to the risk of acute myocardial infarction in men. *N. Engl. J. Med.*, 330: 1549, 1994.

Kasch, F. W., et al.: The effect of physical activity and inactivity on aerobic power in older men (a longitudinal study). *Phys. Sportsmed.*, 18: 73, 1990.

Klag, M.J., et al.: Serum cholesterol in young men and subsequent cardiovascular disease. *N. Engl. J. Med.*, 328: 313, 1993.

King, A. C., et al.: Group- vs. home-based exercise training in healthy older men and women. *JAMA*, 266: 1535, 1991.

Killen, J. D., et al.: Cardiovascular disease risk reduction for tenth graders. A multiple-factor school-based program. *JAMA*, 260:1728, 1988.

Lacroix, A. Z., et al.: Smoking and mortality among older men and women in three communities., *N. Engl, J. Med.*, 324: 169, 1991.

Lakatta, E.G.: Cardiovascular regulatory mechanisms in advanced age. *Physiol. Rev.*, 73: 413, 1993.

Lee, I-M., et al.: Body weight and mortality. *JAMA*, 270: 2823, 1993.

Levy, D., et al.: Stratifying the patient at risk from coronary disease: New insights from the Framingham Heart Study. *Am. Heart J.*, 119:712, 1990.

Lexell, J.: Aging and human skeletal muscle: observations from Sweden. *Can. J. Appl. Physiol.*, 18:2, 1993.

McGinnis, J. M.: The public health burden of a sedentary lifestyle. Med. Sci. Sports Exerc., 24:S196, 1992.

Meredith, C. N., et al.: Body composition and aerobic capacity in young and middle-aged endurance-trained men. *Med. Sci. Sports Exerc.*, 19:557, 1987.

Mittleman, M.A., et al.: Triggering of acute myocardial infarction by heavy physical exertion. *N. Engl. J. Med.*, 329: 1677, 1993.

Moore, L.L., et al.: Influence of parent's physical activity levels on young children. *J. Pediatr.*, 118: 215, 1991.

Morris, J.N.: Exercise in the prevention of coronary heart disease: today's best bet in public health. *Med. Sci. Sports Exerc.*, 26: 807, 1994.

Morris, J. N., et al.: Exercise in leisure time: coronary attack and death rates. *Br. Heart J.*, 63:325, 1990.

NIH Consensus Development Conference: Lowering blood cholesterol to prevent heart disease. *JAMA*, 253:2080, 1985.

Paffenbarger, R. S., Jr.. et al: Physical activity, all-cause mortality, and longevity of college alumni. *N. Engl. J. Med.,* 314:605, 1986.

Paffenbarger, R.S., Jr., et al.: Changes in physical activity and other lifeway patterns influencing longevity. *Med. Sci. Sports Exerc.,* 26: 857, 1994.

Paffenbarger, R. S., Jr., et al.: The association between changes in physical-activity level and other lifestyle characteristics with mortality among men. *N. Engl. J. Med.,* 328: 538, 1993.

Poehlman, E.T., et al.: Endurance exercise in aging humans: effects on energy metabolism. *Exerc. Sport Sci. Rev.,* 22: 751, 1994.

Poulin, M. J., et al.: Endurance training of older men: responses to submaximal exercise. *J. Appl. Physiol.,* 73:452, 1992.

Powell, K. E., et al.: Physical activity and the incidence of coronary heart disease. *Ann. Rev. Public Health,* 8:253, 1987.

Powell, K.E., and Blair, S.N.: The public health burdens of sedentary living habits: theoretical but realistic estimates. *Med. Sci. Sports Exerc.,* 26: 851, 1994.

Public Health Service. *Healthy People 2000: National Health Promotion and Disease Prevention Objectives.* Washington DC: US Dept. of Health and Human Services; 1990, US Dept. of Health and Human Services publication PHS 90-50212.

Pyörälä, K.: Dietary cholesterol in relation to plasma cholesterol and coronary heart disease. *Am. J. Clin. Nutr.,* 45:1176, 1987.

Rivera, A. M., et al.: Physiological factors associated with lower maximal oxygen consumption of master runners. *J. Appl. Physiol.,* 66:949, 1989.

Rogers, M.A., et al.: Decline in VO$_2$ max with aging in master athletes and sedentary men. *J. Appl. Physiol.,* 68:2195, 1990.

Rogers, M. A., and Evans, W. J.: Changes in skeletal muscle with aging: effects of exercise training. In *Exercise and Sport Sciences Reviews.* Vol. 21. Edited by J. O. Holloszy. Baltimore, MD, Williams & Wilkins, 1993.

Sandvik, L., et al.: Physical fitness as a predictor of mortality among healthy, middle-aged Norwegian men. *N. Engl. J. Med.,* 328: 533, 1993.

Schulman, S. P., and Gerstenblith, G.: Cardiovascular changes with aging. The response to exercise. *J. Cardiopulmonary Rehab.,* 9:12, 1989.

Seals, D. R., et al.: Endurance training in older men and women. I. Cardiovascular response to exercise. *J. Appl. Physiol.,* 57:1024, 1984.

Seals, D.R., et al.: Exercise and aging: autonomic control of the circulation. *Med. Sci. Sports Exerc.,* 26: 568, 1994.

Siscovick, D. S., et al.: The incidence of primary cardiac arrest during vigorous exercise. *N. Engl. J. Med.,* 311:874, 1984.

Sipalä, S., and Suominen, H.: Effects of strength and endurance training on thigh and leg muscle mass and composition in elderly women. *J. Appl. Physiol.,* 78: 334, 1995.

Spina, R.J., et al.: Differences to cardiovascular adaptations to endurance exercise training between older men and women. *J. Appl. Physiol.,* 75:849, 1993.

Spina, R.J., et al.: Effect of exercise training on left ventricular performance in older women free of cardiopulmonary disease. *Am. J. Cardiol.,* 71: 99, 1993.

Stamford, B. A.: Exercise and the elderly. In *Exercise and Sport Sciences Reviews.* Vol. 16. Edited by K. B. Pandolf. New York, Macmillan, 1988.

Stampfer, M.J., et al.: Vitamin E consumption and the risk of coronary heart disease in women. *N. Engl. J. Med.,* 328: 1444, 1993.

Stampfer. M. J., et al.: A prospective study of cholesterol apolipoproteins and the risk of myocardial infarction, *N. Engl. J. Med.,* 325:373, 1991.

Stefanick, M.L., and Wood, P.D.: Physical activity, lipid and lipoprotein metabolism, and lipid transport. In *Physical Activity, Fitness, and Health.* Edited by C. Bouchard, et al. Champaign, IL, Human Kinetics, 1994.

Straton, J.R., et al.: Cardiovascular responses to exercise: effects of aging. *Circulation,* 89: 1648, 1994.

Sytkowski, P. A., et al.: Changes in risk factors and the decline in mortality from cardiovascular disease. *N. Engl. J. Med.,* 322:1635, 1990.

Tate, C.A., et al.: Mechanism for the responses of cardiac muscle to physical activity in old age. *Med. Sci. Sports Exerc.,* 26: 561, 1994.

Wannamethee, G., and Shaper, A.G.: Physical activity and stroke in British middle-aged men. *Brit. Med. J.,* 304: 597, 1992.

Watson, R. R., and Eisinger, M.: *Exercise and Disease.* Boca Raton, FL, CRC Press, 1992.

Woods, J.A., and Davis, J.M.: Exercise, monocyte/macrophage function, and cancer. *Med. Sci. Sports Exerc.,* 26: 147, 1994.

APPENDICES

Equation (11) can be simplified to:

$$\dot{V}O_2 = \dot{V}_E \left\{ \left(\frac{\%N_{2_E}}{79.04\%} \right) \times 20.93\% \right) - \%O_{2_E} \right\} \tag{12}$$

The final form of the equation is:

$$\dot{V}O_2 = \dot{V}_E \left[(\%N_{2_E} \times .265) - \%O_{2_E} \right] \tag{13}$$

The value obtained within the brackets in equations (12) and (13) is referred to as the *true O_2*; this represents the "oxygen extraction" or, more precisely, the percentage of oxygen consumed for any volume of air *expired*.

Although equation (13) is the equation used most widely compute oxygen uptake from measures of expired air, it is also possible to calculate $\dot{V}O_2$ from direct measurements of both $\dot{V}_I$ and $\dot{V}_E$. In this case, the Haldane transformation is not used, and oxygen uptake is calculated directly as

$$\dot{V}O_2 = (\dot{V}_I \times 20.93) - (\dot{V}_E \times \%O_{2_E}) \tag{14}$$

In situations in which only V_I is measured, the V_E can be calculated from the Haldane transformation as

$$\dot{V}_E = \dot{V}_I \frac{\%N_{2_I}}{\%N_{2_E}}$$

By substitution in equation (14), the computational equation is:

$$\dot{V}O_2 = \dot{V}_I \left[\%O_{2_I} - \left(\frac{\%N_{2_I}}{\%N_{2_E}} \times \%O_{2_E} \right) \right] \tag{15}$$

CALCULATION OF CARBON DIOXIDE PRODUCTION

The carbon dioxide production per minute ($\dot{V}CO_2$) is calculated as follows:

$$\dot{V}CO_2 = \dot{V}_E (\%CO_{2_E} - \%CO_{2_I}) \tag{16}$$

where $\%CO_{2_E}$ = percent carbon dioxide in expired air determined by gas analysis, and $\%CO_{2_I}$ = percent carbon dioxide in inspired air, which is essentially constant at 0.03%.

The final form of the equation is:

$$\dot{V}CO_2 = \dot{V}_E (\%CO_{2_E} - 0.03\%) \tag{17}$$

CALCULATION OF RESPIRATORY QUOTIENT

The respiratory quotient (RQ) is calculated in one of two ways:

1. RQ = $\dot{V}CO_2 / \dot{V}O_2$ \hfill (18)

   or

2. RQ = $\dfrac{\%CO_{2_E} - 0.03\%)}{\text{"true" } O_2}$ \hfill (19)

SAMPLE METABOLIC CALCULATIONS

The following data were obtained during the last minute of a steady-rate, 10-minute treadmill run performed at 6 miles per hour at a 5% grade.

$\dot{V}_E$: 62.1 liters, ATPS
Barometric pressure: 750 mmHg
Temperature: 26°C
%O_2 expired: 16.86 (O_2 analyzer)
%CO_2 expired: 3.60 (CO_2 analyzer)
%N_2 expired: [100 − (16.86 + 3.60)] = 79.54

Determine the following:
1. $\dot{V}_E$, STPD
2. $\dot{V}O_2$, STPD
3. $\dot{V}CO_2$, STPD
4. RQ
5. kcal · min^{-1}

71 157	74 163
6.1	6.3
9.4	9.7
6.6	6.8
8.3	8.6
4.5	4.7
7.1	7.4
12.0	12.5
8.9	9.3
3.8	4.0
2.3	2.4
11.5	12.0
11.6	12.1
12.6	13.1
14.0	14.6
12.6	13.2
13.7	14.3
17.9	18.5
3.8	4.0
9.1	9.5
5.7	5.9

Not
*Co
prot

1. $\dot{V}_E$, STPD (use equation 4 or STPD correction factor in Table 2-2).

$$\dot{V}_E\text{, STPD} = \dot{V}_E\text{, ATPS}\left(\frac{273}{273 + T°C}\right)\left(\frac{P_B - P_{H_2O}}{760}\right)$$

$$= 62.1\left(\frac{273}{299}\right)\left(\frac{750 - 25.2}{760}\right)$$

$$= 54.07 \text{ liters} \cdot \text{min}^{-1}$$

2. $\dot{V}O_2$, STPD (use equation 13)

$$\dot{V}O_2\text{, STPD} = \dot{V}_E\text{, STPD } [(\%N_{2E} \times .265) - \%O_{2E}]$$
$$= 54.07\ [(.7954 \times .265) - .1686]$$
$$= 54.07\ (.0422)$$
$$= 2.281 \text{ liters} \cdot \text{min}^{-1}$$

3. $\dot{V}CO_2$, STPD (use equation 17)

$$\dot{V}CO_2\text{, STPD} = \dot{V}_E\text{, STPD } (CO_{2E} - 0.03\%)$$
$$= 54.07\ (.0360 - .0003)$$
$$= 54.07\ (.0357)$$
$$= 1.930 \text{ liters} \cdot \text{min}^{-1}$$

4. RQ (use equation 18 or 19)

$$RQ = \dot{V}CO_2/\dot{V}O_2$$

$$= \frac{1.930 \text{ liters } CO_2/\text{min}}{2.281 \text{ liters } O_2/\text{min}}$$

$$= 0.846$$

or

$$RQ = \frac{(\%CO_{2E} - 0.03\%)}{\text{"true" } O_2}$$

$$= \frac{3.60 - .03}{4.22}$$

$$= 0.846$$

Because the exercise was performed in a steady rate of aerobic metabolism, the obtained RQ of 0.846 can be applied in Table 8-1 to obtain the appropriate caloric transformation. In this way, the exercise oxygen consumption can be transposed to kcal of energy expended per minute as follows:

5. Energy expenditure ($\text{kcal} \cdot \text{min}^{-1}$) = $\dot{V}O_2$ ($\text{liters} \cdot \text{min}^{-1}$) x caloric equivalent per liter O_2 at the given steady-rate RQ

$$\text{Energy expenditure} = 2.281 \times 4.862$$
$$= 11.09 \text{ kcal} \cdot \text{min}^{-1}$$

Assuming that the RQ value reflects the nonprotein RQ, a reasonable estimate of both the percentage and quantity of fat and carbohydrate metabolized during each minute of the run can be obtained from Table 8-1.

Percentage kcal derived from fat = 50.7%
Percentage kcal derived from carbohydrate = 49.3%
Grams of fat utilized = 0.267 g per liter of oxygen or approximately 0.61 g per minute (0.267 x 2.281 L O_2)
Grams of carbohydrate utilized = 0.580 g per liter of oxygen or approximately 1.36 g per minute (0.580 x 2.281 L O_2)

CHART 4-2. CONVERSION CONSTANTS TO PREDICT PERCENT BODY FAT FOR OLDER MEN*

BUTTOCKS			ABDOMEN			FOREARM		
in	cm	Constant A	in	cm	Constant B	in	cm	Constant C
28.00	71.12	29.34	25.50	64.77	22.84	7.00	17.78	21.01
28.25	71.75	29.60	25.75	65.40	23.06	7.25	18.41	21.76
28.50	72.39	29.87	26.00	66.04	23.29	7.50	19.05	22.52
28.75	73.02	30.13	26.25	66.67	23.51	7.75	19.68	23.26
29.00	73.66	30.39	26.50	67.31	23.73	8.00	20.32	24.02
29.25	74.29	30.65	26.75	67.94	23.96	8.25	20.95	24.76
29.50	74.93	30.92	27.00	68.58	24.18	8.50	21.59	25.52
29.75	75.56	31.18	27.25	69.21	24.40	8.75	22.22	26.26
30.00	76.20	31.44	27.50	69.85	24.63	9.00	22.86	27.02
30.25	76.83	31.70	27.75	70.48	24.85	9.25	23.49	27.76
30.50	77.47	31.96	28.00	71.12	25.08	9.50	24.13	28.52
30.75	78.10	32.22	28.25	71.75	25.29	9.75	24.76	29.26
31.00	78.74	32.49	28.50	72.39	25.52	10.00	25.40	30.02
31.25	79.37	32.75	28.75	73.02	25.75	10.25	26.03	30.76
31.50	80.01	33.01	29.00	73.66	25.97	10.50	26.67	31.52
31.75	80.64	33.27	29.25	74.29	26.19	10.75	27.30	32.27
32.00	81.28	33.54	29.50	74.93	26.42	11.00	27.94	33.02
32.25	81.91	33.80	29.75	75.56	26.64	11.25	28.57	33.77
32.50	82.55	34.06	30.00	76.20	26.87	11.50	29.21	34.52
32.75	83.18	34.32	30.25	76.83	27.09	11.75	29.84	35.27
33.00	83.82	34.58	30.50	77.47	27.32	12.00	30.48	36.02
33.25	84.45	34.84	30.75	78.10	27.54	12.25	31.11	36.77
33.50	85.09	35.11	31.00	78.74	27.76	12.50	31.75	37.53
33.75	85.72	35.37	31.25	79.37	27.98	12.75	32.38	38.27
34.00	86.36	35.63	31.50	80.01	28.21	13.00	33.02	39.03
34.25	86.99	35.89	31.75	80.64	28.43	13.25	33.65	39.77
34.50	87.63	36.16	32.00	81.28	28.66	13.50	34.29	40.53
34.75	88.26	36.42	32.25	81.91	28.88	13.75	34.92	41.27
35.00	88.90	36.68	32.50	82.55	29.11	14.00	35.56	42.03
35.25	89.53	36.94	32.75	83.18	29.33	14.25	36.19	42.77
35.50	90.17	37.20	33.00	83.82	29.55	14.50	36.83	43.53
35.75	90.80	37.46	33.25	84.45	29.78	14.75	37.46	44.27
36.00	91.44	37.73	33.50	85.09	30.00	15.00	38.10	45.03
36.25	92.07	37.99	33.75	85.72	30.22	15.25	38.73	45.77
36.50	92.71	38.25	34.00	86.36	30.45	15.50	39.37	46.53
36.75	93.34	38.51	34.25	86.99	30.67	15.75	40.00	47.28
37.00	93.98	38.78	34.50	87.63	30.89	16.00	40.64	48.03
37.25	94.61	39.04	34.75	88.26	31.12	16.25	41.27	48.78
37.50	95.25	39.30	35.00	88.90	31.35	16.50	41.91	49.53
37.75	95.88	39.56	35.25	89.53	31.57	16.75	42.54	50.28
38.00	96.52	39.82	35.50	90.17	31.79	17.00	43.18	51.03
38.25	97.15	40.08	35.75	90.80	32.02	17.25	43.81	51.78
38.50	97.79	40.35	36.00	91.44	32.24	17.50	44.45	52.54
38.75	98.42	40.61	36.25	92.07	32.46	17.75	45.08	53.28
39.00	99.06	40.87	36.50	92.71	32.69	18.00	45.72	54.04
39.25	99.69	41.13	36.75	93.34	32.91	18.25	46.35	54.78
39.50	100.33	41.39	37.00	93.98	33.14			
39.75	100.96	41.66	37.25	94.61	33.36			
40.00	101.60	41.92	37.50	95.25	33.58			
40.25	102.23	42.18	37.75	95.88	33.81			
40.50	102.87	42.44	38.00	96.52	34.03			
40.75	103.50	42.70	38.25	97.15	34.26			
41.00	104.14	42.97	38.50	97.79	34.48			
42.25	104.77	43.23	38.75	98.42	34.70			
42.50	105.41	43.49	39.00	99.06	34.93			
41.75	106.04	43.75	39.25	99.69	35.15			
42.00	106.68	44.02	39.50	100.33	35.38			
42.25	107.31	44.28	39.75	100.96	35.59			
42.50	107.95	44.54	40.00	101.60	35.82			
42.75	108.58	44.80	40.25	102.23	36.05			
43.00	109.22	45.06	40.50	102.87	36.27			
43.25	109.85	45.32	40.75	103.50	36.49			
43.50	110.49	45.59	41.00	104.14	36.72			
43.75	111.12	45.85	41.25	104.77	36.94			
44.00	111.76	46.12	41.50	105.41	37.17			
44.25	112.39	46.37	41.75	106.04	37.39			
44.50	113.03	46.64	42.00	106.68	37.62			

Activity

Circuit weight t
  Free weight:
  Hydra-Fitnes
  Nautilus
  Universal

Cycling
  leisure, 5.5 r
  leisure, 9.4 r
  racing, fast

Gardening
  digging
  raking

Ironing clothes

Jumping rope
  70 per min
  80 per min
  125 per min
  145 per min

Paddleball

Running, on flat
  9 min per mil
  6 min per mil

Stock clerking

Swimming
  front crawl, sl

Walking, leisure
  asphalt road

*These examples hav
includes over 250 se
To order a copy of t
Technologies, Inc., 1

CHART 4-2. *continued*

BUTTOCKS			ABDOMEN			FOREARM		
in	cm	Constant A	in	cm	Constant B	in	cm	Constant C
44.75	113.66	46.89	42.25	107.31	37.87			
45.00	114.30	47.16	42.50	107.95	38.06			
42.25	114.93	47.42	42.75	108.58	38.28			
45.50	115.57	47.68	43.00	109.22	38.51			
45.75	116.20	47.94	43.25	109.85	38.73			
46.00	116.84	48.21	43.50	110.49	38.96			
46.25	117.47	48.47	43.75	111.12	39.18			
46.50	118.11	48.73	44.00	111.76	39.41			
46.75	118.74	48.99	44.25	112.39	39.63			
47.00	119.38	49.26	44.50	113.03	39.85			
47.25	120.01	49.52	44.75	113.66	40.08			
47.50	120.65	49.78	45.00	114.30	40.30			
47.75	121.28	50.04						
48.00	121.92	50.30						
48.25	122.55	50.56						
48.50	123.19	50.83						
48.75	123.82	51.09						
49.00	124.46	51.35						

Note: Percent fat = Constant A + Constant B – Constant C – 15.0

CHART 4-3. CONVERSION CONSTANTS TO PREDICT PERCENT BODY FAT FOR YOUNG WOMEN*

ABDOMEN			THIGH			FOREARM		
in	cm	Constant A	in	cm	Constant B	in	cm	Constant C
20.00	50.80	26.74	14.00	35.56	29.13	6.00	15.24	25.86
20.25	51.43	27.07	14.25	36.19	29.65	6.25	15.87	26.94
20.50	52.07	27.41	14.50	36.83	30.17	6.50	16.51	28.02
20.75	52.70	27.74	14.75	37.46	30.69	6.75	17.14	29.10
21.00	53.34	28.07	15.00	38.10	31.21	7.00	17.78	30.17
21.25	53.97	28.41	15.25	38.73	31.73	7.25	18.41	31.25
21.50	54.61	28.74	15.50	39.37	32.25	7.50	19.05	32.33
21.75	55.24	29.08	15.75	40.00	32.77	7.75	19.68	33.41
22.00	55.88	29.41	16.00	40.64	33.29	8.00	20.32	34.48
22.25	56.51	29.74	16.25	41.27	33.81	8.25	20.95	35.56
22.50	57.15	30.08	16.50	41.91	34.33	8.50	21.59	36.64
22.75	57.78	30.41	16.75	42.54	34.85	8.75	22.22	37.72
23.00	58.42	30.75	17.00	43.18	35.37	9.00	22.86	38.79
23.25	59.05	31.08	17.25	43.81	35.89	9.25	23.49	39.87
23.50	59.69	31.42	17.50	44.45	36.41	9.50	24.13	40.95
23.75	60.32	31.75	17.75	45.08	36.93	9.75	24.76	42.03
24.00	60.96	32.08	18.00	45.72	37.45	10.00	25.40	43.10
24.25	61.59	32.42	18.25	46.35	37.97	10.25	26.03	44.18
24.50	62.23	32.75	18.50	46.99	38.49	10.50	26.67	45.26
24.75	62.86	33.09	18.75	47.62	39.01	10.75	27.30	46.34
25.00	63.50	33.42	19.00	48.26	39.53	11.00	27.94	47.41
25.25	64.13	33.76	19.25	48.89	40.05	11.25	28.57	48.49
25.50	64.77	34.09	19.50	49.53	40.57	11.50	29.21	49.57
25.75	65.40	34.42	19.75	50.16	41.09	11.75	29.84	50.65
26.00	66.04	34.76	20.00	50.80	41.61	12.00	30.48	51.73
26.25	66.67	35.09	20.25	51.43	42.13	12.25	31.11	52.80
26.50	67.31	35.43	20.50	52.07	42.65	12.50	31.75	53.88
26.75	67.94	35.76	20.75	52.70	43.17	12.75	32.38	54.96
27.00	68.58	36.10	21.00	53.34	43.69	13.00	33.02	56.04
27.25	69.21	36.43	21.25	53.97	44.21	13.25	33.65	57.11
27.50	69.85	36.76	21.50	54.61	44.73	13.50	34.29	58.19
27.75	70.48	37.10	21.75	55.24	45.25	13.75	34.92	59.27
28.00	71.12	37.43	22.00	55.88	45.77	14.00	35.56	60.35
28.25	71.75	37.77	22.25	56.51	46.29	14.25	36.19	61.42
28.50	72.39	38.10	22.50	57.15	46.81	14.50	36.83	62.50
28.75	73.02	38.43	22.75	57.78	47.33	14.75	37.46	63.58
29.00	73.66	38.77	23.00	58.42	47.85	15.00	38.10	64.66
29.25	74.29	39.10	23.25	59.05	48.37	15.25	38.73	65.73

CHART 4-3. *continued*

ABDOMEN			THIGH			FOREARM		
in	cm	Constant A	in	cm	Constant B	in	cm	Constant C
29.50	74.93	39.44	23.50	59.69	48.89	15.50	39.37	66.81
29.75	75.56	39.77	23.75	60.32	49.41	15.75	40.00	67.89
30.00	76.20	40.11	24.00	60.96	49.93	16.00	40.64	68.97
30.25	76.83	40.44	24.25	61.59	50.45	16.25	41.27	70.04
30.50	77.47	40.77	24.50	62.23	50.97	16.50	41.91	71.12
30.75	78.10	41.11	24.75	62.86	51.49	16.75	42.54	72.20
31.25	78.74	41.44	25.00	63.50	52.01	17.00	43.18	73.28
31.00	79.37	41.78	25.25	64.13	52.53	17.25	43.81	74.36
31.50	80.01	42.11	25.50	64.77	53.05	17.50	44.45	75.43
31.75	80.64	42.45	25.75	65.40	53.57	17.75	45.08	76.51
32.00	81.28	42.78	26.00	66.04	54.09	18.00	45.72	77.59
32.25	81.91	43.11	26.25	66.67	54.61	18.25	46.35	78.67
32.50	82.55	43.45	26.50	67.31	55.13	18.50	46.99	79.74
32.75	83.18	43.78	26.75	67.94	55.65	18.75	47.62	80.82
33.00	83.82	44.12	27.00	68.58	56.17	19.00	48.26	81.90
33.25	84.45	44.45	27.25	69.21	56.69	19.25	48.89	82.98
33.50	85.09	44.78	27.50	69.85	57.21	19.50	49.53	84.05
33.75	85.72	45.12	27.75	70.48	57.73	19.75	50.16	85.13
34.00	86.36	45.45	28.00	71.12	58.26	20.00	50.80	86.21
34.25	86.99	45.79	28.25	71.75	58.78			
34.50	87.63	46.12	28.50	72.39	59.30			
34.75	88.26	46.46	28.75	73.02	59.82			
35.00	88.90	46.79	29.00	73.66	60.34			
35.25	89.53	47.12	29.25	74.29	60.86			
35.50	90.17	47.46	29.50	74.93	61.38			
35.75	90.80	47.79	29.75	75.56	61.90			
36.00	91.44	48.13	30.00	76.20	62.42			
36.25	92.07	48.46	30.25	76.83	62.94			
36.50	92.71	48.80	30.50	77.47	63.46			
36.75	93.34	49.13	30.75	78.10	63.98			
37.00	93.98	49.46	31.00	78.74	64.50			
37.25	94.61	49.80	31.25	79.37	65.02			
37.50	95.25	50.13	31.50	80.01	65.54			
37.75	95.88	50.47	31.75	80.64	66.06			
38.00	96.52	50.80	32.00	81.28	66.58			
38.25	97.15	51.13	32.25	81.91	67.10			
38.50	97.79	51.47	32.50	82.55	67.62			
38.75	98.42	51.80	32.75	83.18	68.14			
39.00	99.06	52.14	33.00	83.82	68.66			
39.25	99.69	52.47	33.25	84.45	69.18			
39.50	100.33	52.81	33.50	85.09	69.70			
39.75	100.96	53.14	33.75	85.72	70.22			
40.00	101.60	53.47	34.00	86.36	70.74			

Note: Percent fat = Constant A + Constant B – Constant C – 19.6

CHART 4-4. CONVERSION CONSTANTS TO PREDICT PERCENT BODY FAT FOR OLDER WOMEN*

ABDOMEN			THIGH			CALF		
in	cm	Constant A	in	cm	Constant B	in	cm	Constant C
25.00	63.50	29.69	14.00	35.56	17.31	10.00	25.40	14.46
25.25	64.13	29.98	14.25	36.19	17.62	10.25	26.03	14.82
25.50	64.77	30.28	14.50	36.83	17.93	10.50	26.67	15.18
25.75	65.40	30.58	14.75	37.46	18.24	10.75	27.30	15.54
26.00	66.04	30.87	15.00	38.10	18.55	11.00	27.94	15.91
26.25	66.67	31.17	15.25	38.73	18.86	11.25	28.57	16.27
26.50	67.31	31.47	15.50	39.37	19.17	11.50	29.21	16.63
26.75	67.94	31.76	15.75	40.00	19.47	11.75	29.84	16.99
27.00	68.58	32.06	16.00	40.64	19.78	12.00	30.48	17.35
27.25	69.21	32.36	16.25	41.27	20.09	12.25	31.11	17.71
27.50	69.85	32.65	16.50	41.91	20.40	12.50	31.75	18.08
27.75	70.48	32.95	16.75	42.54	20.71	12.75	32.38	18.44
28.00	71.12	33.25	17.00	43.18	21.02	13.00	33.02	18.80
28.25	71.75	33.55	17.25	43.81	21.33	13.25	33.65	19.16
28.50	72.39	33.84	17.50	44.45	21.64	13.50	34.29	19.52
28.75	73.02	34.14	17.75	45.08	21.95	13.75	34.92	19.88

CHART 4-4. *continued*

ABDOMEN			THIGH			CALF		
in	cm	Constant A	in	cm	Constant B	in	cm	Constant C
29.00	73.66	34.44	18.00	45.72	22.26	14.00	35.56	20.24
29.25	74.29	34.73	18.25	46.35	22.57	14.25	36.19	20.61
29.50	74.93	35.03	18.50	46.99	22.87	14.50	36.83	20.97
29.75	75.56	35.33	18.75	47.62	23.18	14.75	37.46	21.33
30.00	76.20	35.62	19.00	48.26	23.49	15.00	38.10	21.69
30.25	76.83	35.92	19.25	48.89	23.80	15.25	38.73	22.05
30.50	77.47	36.22	19.50	49.53	24.11	15.50	39.37	22.41
30.75	78.10	36.51	19.75	50.16	24.42	15.75	40.00	22.77
31.00	78.74	36.81	20.00	50.80	24.73	16.00	40.64	23.14
31.25	79.37	37.11	20.25	51.43	25.04	16.25	41.27	23.50
31.50	80.01	37.40	20.50	52.07	25.35	16.50	41.91	23.86
31.75	80.64	37.70	20.75	52.70	25.66	16.75	42.54	24.22
32.00	81.28	38.00	21.00	53.34	25.97	17.00	43.18	24.58
32.25	81.91	38.30	21.25	53.97	26.28	17.25	43.81	24.94
32.50	82.55	38.59	21.50	54.61	26.58	17.50	44.45	25.31
32.75	83.18	38.89	21.75	55.24	26.89	17.75	45.08	25.67
33.00	83.82	39.19	22.00	55.88	27.20	18.00	45.72	26.03
33.25	84.45	39.48	22.25	56.51	27.51	18.25	46.35	26.39
33.50	85.09	39.78	22.50	57.15	27.82	18.50	46.99	26.75
33.75	85.72	40.08	22.75	57.78	28.13	18.75	47.62	27.11
34.00	86.36	40.37	23.00	58.42	28.44	19.00	48.26	27.47
34.25	86.99	40.67	23.25	59.05	28.75	19.25	48.89	27.84
34.50	87.63	40.97	23.50	59.69	29.06	19.50	49.53	28.20
34.75	88.26	41.26	23.75	60.32	29.37	19.75	50.16	28.56
35.00	88.90	41.56	24.00	60.96	29.68	20.00	50.80	28.92
35.25	89.53	41.86	24.25	61.59	29.98	20.25	51.43	29.28
35.50	90.17	42.15	24.50	62.23	30.29	20.50	52.07	29.64
35.75	90.80	42.45	24.75	62.86	30.60	20.75	52.70	30.00
36.00	91.44	42.75	25.00	63.50	30.91	21.00	53.34	30.37
36.25	92.07	43.05	25.25	64.13	31.22	21.25	53.97	30.73
36.50	92.71	43.34	25.50	64.77	31.53	21.50	54.61	31.09
36.75	93.35	43.64	25.75	65.40	31.84	21.75	55.24	31.45
37.00	93.98	43.94	26.00	66.04	32.15	22.00	55.88	31.81
37.25	94.62	44.23	26.25	66.67	32.46	22.25	56.51	32.17
37.50	95.25	44.53	26.50	67.31	32.77	22.50	57.15	32.54
37.75	95.89	44.83	26.75	67.94	33.08	22.75	57.78	32.90
38.00	96.52	45.12	27.00	68.58	33.38	23.00	58.42	33.26
38.25	97.16	45.42	27.25	69.21	33.69	23.25	59.05	33.62
38.50	97.79	45.72	27.50	69.85	34.00	23.50	59.69	33.98
38.75	98.43	46.01	27.75	70.48	34.31	23.75	60.32	34.34
39.00	99.06	46.31	28.00	71.12	34.62	24.00	60.96	34.70
39.25	99.70	46.61	28.25	71.75	34.93	24.25	61.59	35.07
39.50	100.33	46.90	28.50	72.39	35.24	24.50	62.23	35.43
39.75	100.97	47.20	28.75	73.02	35.55	24.75	62.86	35.79
40.00	101.60	47.50	29.00	73.66	35.86	25.00	63.50	36.15
40.25	101.24	47.79	29.25	74.29	36.17			
40.50	102.87	48.09	29.50	74.93	36.48			
40.75	103.51	48.39	29.75	75.56	36.79			
41.00	104.14	48.69	30.00	76.20	37.09			
41.25	104.78	48.98	30.25	76.83	37.40			
41.50	105.41	49.28	30.50	77.47	37.71			
41.75	106.05	49.58	30.75	78.10	38.02			
42.00	106.68	49.87	31.00	78.74	38.33			
42.25	107.32	50.17	31.25	79.37	38.64			
42.50	107.95	50.47	31.50	80.01	38.95			
42.75	108.59	50.76	31.75	80.64	39.26			
43.00	109.22	51.06	32.00	81.28	39.57			
43.25	109.86	51.36	32.25	81.91	39.88			
43.50	110.49	51.65	32.50	82.55	40.19			
43.75	111.13	51.95	32.75	83.18	40.49			
44.00	111.76	52.25	33.00	83.82	40.80			
44.25	112.40	52.54	33.25	84.45	41.11			
44.50	113.03	52.84	33.50	85.09	41.42			
44.75	113.67	53.14	33.75	85.72	41.73			
45.00	114.30	53.44	34.00	86.36	42.04			

Note: Percent fat = Constant A + Constant B − Constant C − 18.4

APPENDIX 5

Frequently Cited Journals in Exercise Physiology

Exercise physiology encompasses numerous scientific areas of inquiry. The following list of journals (with their common abbreviations) has been particularly useful in our own library searches on various topics of interest.

Journal	Abbreviation	Journal	Abbreviation
Acta Medica Scandinavica	Acta Med Scand	International Journal for Vitamin and Nutrition Research	Int J Vitam Nutr Res
Acta Physiologica Scandinavica	Acta Physiol Scand	Journal of Applied Physiology	J Appl Physiol
American Journal of Clinical Nutrition	Am J Clin Nutr	Journal of Applied Sport Science Research	J Appl Sport Sci Res
American Heart Journal	Am Heart J	Journal of Biological Chemistry	J Biol Chem
American Journal of Anatomy	Am J Anat	Journal of Biomechanics	J Biomech
American Journal of Cardiology	Am J Cardiol	Journal of Bone and Joint Surgery	J Bone Joint Surg
American Journal of Epidemiology	Am J Epidemiol	Journal of Clinical Endocrinology and Metabolism	J Clin Endocrinol Metab
American Journal of Human Biology	Am J Hum Biol	Journal of Clinical Investigation	J Clin Invest
American Journal of Obstetrics and Gynecology	Am J Obstet Gynecol	Journal of Gerontology	J Gerontol
American Journal of Physical Anthropology	Am J Phys Anthrop	Journal of Human Movement Studies	J Hum Mov Studies
American Journal of Physics	Am J Physics	Journal of Laboratory and Clinical Medicine	J Lab Clin Med
American Journal of Physiology	Am J Physiol	Journal of Lipid Research	J Lipid Res
American Journal of Public Health	Am J Public Health	Journal of Neurophysiology	J Neurophysiol
American Journal of Sports Medicine	Am J Sports Med	Journal of Nutrition	J Nutr
Annals of Human Biology	Ann Hum Biol	Journal of Parenteral and Environmental Nutrition	JPEN
Annals of Internal Medicine	Ann Intern Med	Journal of Pediatrics	J Pediatr
Appetite	Appetite	Journal of Physical and Medical Rehabilitation	J Phys Med Rehabil
Archives of Environmental Health	Arch Environ Health	Journal of Physiology	J Physiol
Atherosclerosis	Artherosclerosis	Journal of Sports Medicine and Physical Fitness	J Sports Med Phys Fitness
Aviation and Environmental Medicine	Aviat Environ Med	Journal of Sports Psychology	J Sports Psychol
Brain: Journal of Neurology	Brain	Journal of Strength and Conditioning Research	JSCR
British Heart Journal	Br Heart J	Journal of the American Dietetic Association	J Am Diet Assoc
British Journal of Nutrition	Br J Nutr	JAMA (Journal of the American Medical Association)	JAMA
British Journal of Sports Medicine	Br J Sports Med	Journal of Sports Medicine	J Sports Med
British Medical Journal	Br Med J	Lancet	Lancet
Canadian Journal of Applied Sports Sciences	Can J Appl Sport Sci	Medicine and Science in Sports and Exercise	Med Sci Sports Exerc
Canadian Medical Association Journal	Can Med Assoc J	Muscle and Nerve	Muscle/Nerve
Circulation Research	Circ Res	Nature	Nature
Circulation: Journal of the American Heart Association	Circulation	Neuroscience Letters	Neurosci Lett
Clinical Biomechanics	Clin Biomech	New England Journal of Medicine	N Engl J Med
Clinical Chemistry	Clin Chem	Nutrition Abstracts and Reviews	Nutr Abstr Rev
Clinical Neurophysiology plus Electroencephalography	CNEEG	Nutrition and Metabolism	Nutr Abstr Rev
Clinical Science	Clin Sci	Nutrition Reviews	Nutr Rev
Clinical Sports Medicine	Clin Sports Med	Pediatric Exercise Science	Ped Exerc Sci
Diabetes	Diabetes	Pediatrics	Pediatrics
Diabetologia	Diabetologia	Physical Therapy Reviews	Phys Ther Rev
Endocrinology	Endocrinology	Physician and Sportsmedicine	Phys Sportsmed
Ergonomics	Ergonomics	Physiological Reviews	Physiol Rev
European Journal of Applied Physiology	Eur J Appl Physiol	Preventive Medicine	Prev Med
Experientia	Experientia	Proceedings of the Nutrition Society	Proc Nutr Soc
Experimental Brain Research	Exp Brain Res	Psychosomatic Medicine	Psychosom Med
Federation Proceedings	Fed Proc	Public Health Reports	Pub Health Rep
Fertility and Sterility	Fertil Steril	Radiology	Radiology
Geriatrics	Geriatrics	Research Quarterly for Exercise and Sports	Res Q Exerc Sport
Growth	Growth	Scandinavian Journal of Sports Science	Scand J Sports Sci
Human Biology	Hum Biol	Science	Science
Human Movement Science	Hum Mov Sci	Scientific American	Sci Am
International Journal of Obesity	Int J Obes	Sports Medicine	Sports Med
International Journal of Sports Medicine	Int J Sports Med		
International Journal of Sport Nutrition	IJSN		

PHOTO CREDITS

Chapter Openers:

1. Bruno Bade, *Vandystadt/ALLSPORT*
2. Renones Thomas, *Vandystadt/ALLSPORT*
3. Mike Powell, *ALLSPORT*
4. Dan Smith, *ALLSPORT*
5. Michael King, *ALLSPORT*
6. *Vandystadt*
7. Nathan Milow, *ALLSPORT*
8. Mike Powell, *ALLSPORT*
9. Mike Powell, *ALLSPORT*
10. *Vandystadt*
11. Mike Powell, *ALLSPORT*
12. *Vandystadt*
13. Mike Powell, *ALLSPORT*
14. *ALLSPORT*
15. *Vandystadt*
16. Tony Duffy, *ALLSPORT*
17. *Vandystadt/ALLSPORT*
18. *ALLSPORT*

Credit and thanks for photographs supplied by Mark Fox, Mark Fox Photography, Box 113, Silverthorne, Colorado 80498.

Index

Page numbers in italics indicate figures; numbers followed by "t" indicate tables.